Aging and Vulnerability to Environmental Chemicals

Age-related Disorders and their Origins in Environmental Exposures

Issues in Toxicology

Series Editors:
Professor Diana Anderson, *University of Bradford, UK*
Dr Michael D Waters, *Integrated Laboratory Systems, Inc., N Carolina, USA*
Dr Martin F Wilks, *University of Basel, Switzerland*
Dr Timothy C Marrs, *Edentox Associates, Kent, UK*

Titles in the Series:
1: Hair in Toxicology: An Important Bio-Monitor
2: Male-mediated Developmental Toxicity
3: Cytochrome P450: Role in the Metabolism and Toxicity of Drugs and other Xenobiotics
4: Bile Acids: Toxicology and Bioactivity
5: The Comet Assay in Toxicology
6: Silver in Healthcare
7: *In Silico* Toxicology: Principles and Applications
8: Environmental Cardiology
9: Biomarkers and Human Biomonitoring, Volume 1: Ongoing Programs and Exposures
10: Biomarkers and Human Biomonitoring, Volume 2: Selected Biomarkers of Current Interest
11: Hormone-Disruptive Chemical Contaminants in Food
12: Mammalian Toxicology of Insecticides
13: The Cellular Response to the Genotoxic Insult: The Question of Threshold for Genotoxic Carcinogens
14: Toxicological Effects of Veterinary Medicinal Products in Humans: Volume 1
15: Toxicological Effects of Veterinary Medicinal Products in Humans: Volume 2
16: Aging and Vulnerability to Environmental Chemicals: Age-related Disorders and their Origins in Environmental Exposures

How to obtain future titles on publication:
A standing order plan is available for this series. A standing order will bring delivery of each new volume immediately on publication.

For further information please contact:
Book Sales Department, Royal Society of Chemistry, Thomas Graham House, Science Park, Milton Road, Cambridge, CB4 0WF, UK
Telephone: +44 (0)1223 420066, Fax: +44 (0)1223 420247
Email: booksales@rsc.org
Visit our website at www.rsc.org/books

Aging and Vulnerability to Environmental Chemicals
Age-related Disorders and their Origins in Environmental Exposures

Edited by

Bernard Weiss
Department of Environmental Medicine, University of Rochester, NY, USA
Email: bernard_weiss@urmc.rochester.edu

RSC Publishing

Issues in Toxicology No. 16

ISBN: 978-1-84973-418-9
ISSN: 1757-7179

A catalogue record for this book is available from the British Library

Published by The Royal Society of Chemistry,
Thomas Graham House, Science Park, Milton Road,
Cambridge CB4 0WF, UK

Registered Charity Number 207890

For further information see our website at www.rsc.org

Printed in the United Kingdom by Henry Ling Limited, Dorchester, DT1 1HD, UK

Preface

Aging. We all do it from the moment we are born and it could be likened to the finest wine reaching its prime. It sure looked like aging was on our side in the beginning. We liked it. Think back to all the things you looked forward to as a child or a teenager, like reaching "driving age" and then "drinking age". We could not wait until we got "old enough". But while all that took place aging kept plodding on in its phantom-like manner. For some, acknowledging aging has not been easy as they sought surgical options to cover it on the surface. But even with or without wrinkles and sags, reality soon sets in when we realize that aging is no longer an asset. And near the end when more and more of our diverse body systems let us down, un-relentlessly limiting our bounds, that is when we really understand what aging is all about.

But that's normal aging. In this book Dr. Bernard Weiss tackles a serious health problem that has long been ignored, rapid aging, by bridging numerous disciplines and leaning on the most eminent scientists in the field of public health for their perspective. In so doing he opens the door for discussion on how could this have happened? And, why, since the 1950s, accelerated aging has become more prevalent and over the same time period many chronic endocrine related disorders have reached pandemic level, at a tremendous cost to society?

This book could not be more timely. Globally, over the past several decades, hundreds of professional society and government meetings have been devoted to rapid aging and endocrine disruption to the point where it appears that it may be impossible to reverse the trend unless something is done immediately. The technology that has provided this information is based on entirely new laboratory protocols that test genes, molecules, cells, and tissue at realistic concentrations encountered each day in the environment. You might call it a bottom up approach. It is rich in its discoveries and the use of new words

Issues in Toxicology No. 16
Aging and Vulnerability to Environmental Chemicals: Age-related Disorders and their Origins in Environmental Exposures
Edited by Bernard Weiss

Published by the Royal Society of Chemistry, www.rsc.org

creating a whole new vocabulary and a whole new generation of multi-disciplinary researchers. Despite this wealth of knowledge governments have not changed how they test chemicals for their safety. Currently we are at an impasse because the use of toxicological standards based on risk analysis is deeply embedded in the language of federal regulations. While millions have been increasingly succumbing to early onset of chronic disorders, and early mortality, this new language has not been translated into policy for regulatory purposes. For those doing the research who understand the overarching principles of endocrinology it is as though no one has been listening.

Looking back might help understand how this could have happened. Rachel Carson quoted in her 1962 book, *Silent Spring* "A change at one point, in one molecule even, may reverberate throughout the entire system to initiate changes in seemingly unrelated organs and tissues. This concept, familiar in physics, is gaining validity in all fields of biology and medicine." Then she went on to write how difficult it is to demonstrate cause and effect where the ultimate effect may not be expressed for a long time after the initial change in a molecule, or cell, or tissue. Amazingly, she was describing endocrine disruption.

Carson's citations in *Silent Spring* reveal that she had been reading about the changes that were taking place in medical research in the 1950s. I expect that she was looking for clues about cancer, specifically because of her own condition and trying to determine its etiology. She read about the work that was being done in 50s with the adrenal hormones, cortisol and aldosterone, and the anterior pituitary and ACTH. And it was about that time that hormone replacement therapy was being explored and estrogen had caught the interest of the pharmaceutical industry.

I am certain that if Rachel Carson had lived only a few more years she would have discovered the phenomenon called endocrine disruption and I'll just bet that she would have found a better name for it. And perhaps many of the endocrine disorders such as diabetes, obesity, autism, ADHD, fertility problems, Parkinsons, Alzheimers, and the cancers of the sex organs would never have reached current epidemic proportions. There was a big push in the 50s for fundamental research to understand the living organism in order to provide better diagnosis and treatment — and the need to expand on the concept of medicine as a life science and to include biology (Carson's love). Although some advances along these lines have taken place they were not enough to slow down rapid aging.

But there is another reason why it has taken endocrine disruption with its proclivity for rapid aging so long to become accepted as a major threat to humankind. The same trade associations, other industry funded institutions, and corporations that attacked Rachel Carson are still out there 50 years later protecting their products and padding their bottom lines using some of the largest public relations firms in the world to marginalize the science and vilify those doing this 21st century research. And when one takes into consideration that practically every endocrine disrupting chemical in use today was derived from the toxic by-products from coal, oil, and natural gas it becomes even more evident why today, federal health regulations are still based on the odds of getting cancer at one in million or a thousand, not on the most unthinkable odds like diabetes where today one out of every third child born — and if you are among a minority group — every other child born will suffer the disease.

Humankind is in the midst of a dire health crisis that requires immediate intensive care to survive. The paradigm upon which current government policies and regulations have evolved has failed to protect us. A new level of discourse is needed immediately between science and decision makers creating a toxic chemicals platform or framework using a disease-driven approach that employs the principles of endocrinology. This entity should over-see the creation of an entirely new set of 21st century public health rules that would enable governments to reverse the current crisis. This could happen by making possible the merging of the dialogue between the most brilliant statespersons with a record of independence and integrity and the brilliant spokes persons within the community of scientists who understand the endocrine system. I see this book providing the first major break through in that dialogue and contributing to an urgently needed paradigm shift in how governments protect public health.

Theo Colborn
The Endocrine Disruption Exchange,
Paonia, Colorado

Contents

Issues in Toxicology No. 16
Aging and Vulnerability to Environmental Chemicals: Age-related Disorders and their Origins in Environmental Exposures
Edited by Bernard Weiss

Published by the Royal Society of Chemistry, www.rsc.org

Introduction

BERNARD WEISS

Email: bernard_weiss@urmc.rochester.edu

Progressively aging populations introduce a situation never before encountered in human history. Of all the problems this demographic surge creates, the foremost is declining health. As populations age, they impose rising demands on medical care systems and facilities; at the same time, they no longer produce the wealth required to sustain such facilities.

Aging is not a disease. We possess no therapies for it, only for its manifestations. But the stresses it inflicts on society would be more manageable could its burden of disease and disability be diminished or slowed. We have learned during the past four decades that, in fact, it can be. The Framingham Heart study is testimony to that possibility. It identified risk factors that led to new strategies for the prevention and subsequent reduction of coronary heart disease. We have also learned that diet, exercise, and intellectual activity also delay or attenuate the burdens of aging and, in fact, help sustain productive lives. These and other strategies for reducing the health risks of aging now receive profuse publicity.

In this volume, we address another set of risks, one to which we have given hardly more than a glance. These risks arise from the chemical revolution that began about seventy years ago. It flooded the world with chemicals that penetrated every aspect of our lives. Although they have brought us significant benefits, they have also exacted a heavy price. In our ignorance and greed we have so contaminated our environment that we are now exposed to thousands of chemical agents that remain largely untested, despite their residence in our

Issues in Toxicology No. 16
Aging and Vulnerability to Environmental Chemicals: Age-related Disorders and their Origins in Environmental Exposures
Edited by Bernard Weiss

Published by the Royal Society of Chemistry, www.rsc.org

bodies and surroundings. Even those that are permanent residents of our environment, such as metals, have appeared in new guises, such as fuel additives, that spawn new questions.

Now we propose to ask how these chemical agents may alter the health status of aging populations. It is a question currently accorded a relatively low priority by investigators and funding agencies. Early development is the period of the lifespan that has dominated research during the past few decades, with occasional attempts to determine how exposures early in life play out during late adulthood and senescence.

Early development, however, is not the only life stage during which we see heightened responses to the adverse effects of chemicals. Vulnerability to toxic processes climbs again late in life and in many ways recapitulates the imperfect defenses deployed by the immature organism. Traced across the life cycle, this progression takes the form of a U-shaped function, with the greatest potential for damage early and late in life. One feature common to both early and late phases is a reduced capacity to activate defenses against toxic effects. Immature organisms do not yet possess robust defense mechanisms. In aging organisms, they have passed into what might be called a post-mature decline. Older bodies are already high-maintenance properties, so exposure to substances with toxic properties may accelerate the process of decline, or exploit their dwindling capacities to resist such effects. "Aging" is not a mechanistic explanation for the diminished functions we suffer later in life. Sometimes, the roots of such declines merely unfold late in life, having lain dormant for decades, much like the herpes zoster virus. Sometimes, the waning compensatory capacities that accompany aging magnify vulnerability to exposure, a problem with pharmaceuticals and one which is discussed at length in the medical literature.

This volume has assembled a group of scientists who have thought about and investigated the environmental exposures that may imperil what might be called the natural or optimal course of aging. As editor, what I find most striking is how closely and unexpectedly the different chapters fit together and how they intersect.

Six of the chapters touch on metals: lead (two chapters), mercury, cadmium, manganese, and aluminum. Of these, only cadmium doesn't feature brain function directly. There, it is the kidney that receives the most attention, but lead and mercury also affect kidney function. Kidney function, however, exerts potent effects on brain function. For example, chronic kidney disease may induce neurological disorders, such as ischemic brain injury, as well as cognitive impairment. And patients with chronic kidney disease have a higher prevalence of cardiovascular disease, another chapter topic. The liver, too, cannot be overlooked as a source of neurotoxicity. Hepatic encephalopathy is a classic example. The liver can also be the source of the Aβ-amyloid in the brain that is associated with Alzheimer's disease.

Other chapters also examine brain function, and the chapter on Parkinson's disease discusses manganese in detail, but also examines lead. The chapter on polychlorinated biphenyls (PCBs) is focused on the brain, while the chapter on cardiovascular function features related chemicals, the Persistent Organic

Pollutants (POPs) and plastics, as well as PCBs. The chapter on obesity and diabetes also takes account of brain function because food intake is governed by hormonal processes in brain. It is centered on endocrine-disrupting chemicals (EDCs) and what we have learned about their contribution to the current surge in obesity and allied disorders. But we also know that POPs and similar chemicals are also risk factors for diabetes, as well as for cardiovascular disease. And it has now been established, and discussed in the chapter on air pollution, that adverse cardiovascular effects are a major source of the association between air pollution and mortality.

Hormonal function and EDCs are addressed in other chapters as well. One is an extensive review of the compound bisphenol A and exemplifies the range of questions and issues surrounding EDCs. The chapters on prostate and breast cancer also address EDCs, as does the chapter on cardiovascular disease, and all three point to their association with POPs such as dioxins. Like other chapters, these also emphasize the association between exposures early in life and the emergence of adverse effects decades later, a phenomenon termed "silent damage". One reason for the long latency may be the diminution of compensatory mechanisms late in life. But another may stem from earlier, silent damage that renders the target tissues more vulnerable to a second exposure or "hit". Many of the findings that first pointed us to the possibility of environmental chemicals causing endocrine disruption arose from questions about male reproductive function, the subject of one chapter. Many chemicals, we now know, besides those directly associated with the endocrine system, also exert endocrine-disrupting effects. Cadmium, for example, interacts with the estrogen receptor to induce such actions.

Two organ systems in particular play a large role in how we process and defend against environmental exposures. The liver and the immune system carry out these functions, but both suffer diminished efficiency as we age. Chemicals are processed by the liver to detoxify them, but the products (*i.e.* their metabolites) are sometimes the entities carrying the toxic message. The immune system is also a defense system that may respond in such a fashion that the protective response itself inflicts harm on the individual.

Although lead is the focus of the chapter on osteoporosis, cadmium is also stored in bone, and both have a half-life measured in decades. Cadmium, too, is toxic to bone. And both may contribute to osteotoxicity, not only through their effects on calcium but *via* endocrine-disrupting properties acting on estrogenic receptors. Osteoporosis, in effect, also releases lead stored in bone, raising blood lead levels, and in this way contributes to the neurotoxic effects observed in older populations and described in one chapter.

Figure 1 is a schematic depiction of how the course of aging might be influenced by environmental chemical exposures and other factors. The baseline age is taken as 20 years, a time that health statistics indicate is followed by progressively increasing rates of disabilities such as heart disease, for example. With "normal" aging, functional capacity—the ability of the model organ or system to perform its function—has declined to about 50% of its baseline value (shown by the horizontal line) by age 80 years. Exposed individuals are shown

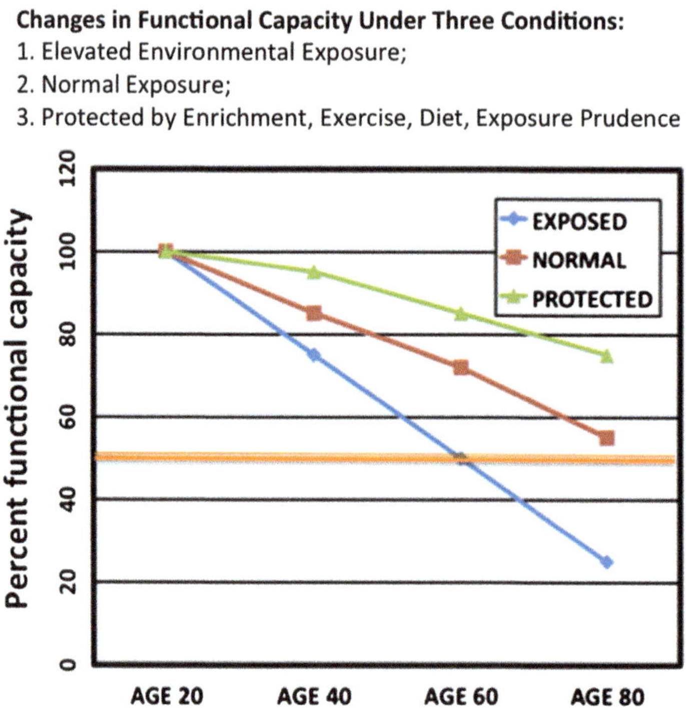

Figure 1 A model depicting changes in functional capacity during the course of aging. Age 20 years is taken as the 100% baseline. Three different progressions are shown: a "normal" rate of decline; a rate accelerated by chemical exposure; and a rate slowed by lower exposures and lifestyle modifications.

to have reached that value by age 60 years, while those who have been able to avoid exposure and undertaken other positive behaviors have suffered a decline of around only 25%. Although only a schematic, the graph emphasizes how different rates of decline can cause the gaps between the different courses of aging to widen with time.

I expect this volume to receive wide recognition and to serve as a foundation for policy decisions. We are all aware of how the combination of aging populations, their health challenges, and rising medical care costs is a priority issue for governments throughout the world. As we gain more knowledge of how our contaminated environment contributes to these disorders and disabilities, I am hopeful that we will act to avert further strains on our beleaguered societies.

The great baseball pitcher Satchel Paige, whose race confined him to the "Negro" baseball leagues until late in his career, was also a philosopher of aging. Taking a somewhat fatalistic view, he observed, "Don't look back. Something may be gaining on you." But he was also sanguine about it, pointing out that, "Aging is a question of mind over matter. If you don't mind, it doesn't matter." This volume aligns itself with those optimists who believe that knowledge gives us the power to make aging matter less.

CHAPTER 1
Exposure to Lead and Cognitive Dysfunction

JENNIFER WEUVE[a,b] AND MARC G. WEISSKOPF*[b,c]

[a] Rush Institute for Healthy Aging, Rush University Medical Center, Chicago, IL, USA; [b] Department of Environmental Health, Harvard School of Public Health, Boston, MA, USA; [c] Department of Epidemiology, Harvard School of Public Health, Boston, MA, USA
*E-mail: mweissko@hsph.harvard.edu

1.1 Lead Exposure: Long at Hand and in Mind

Humans' use of lead dates back at least to 7000 BC.[1] And knowledge of lead's neurotoxicity has been with us since the observations of Nicander, Vitruvius, and the ancient Greek physician, Dioscorides, who wrote that "[l]ead makes the mind give way". Nonetheless, between 1925 and 1980, human exposure to lead in the US environment reached historically high levels owing to the dominance of leaded gasoline for automobile fuel and the widespread use of lead-based paint. In the present US environment, as a result of long-sought regulations that removed lead from gasoline and minimized the use of lead-based paint, exposure to lead happens sporadically, and most individuals' exposures occur at low doses. Nonetheless, exposure to lead remains relevant to the cognitive function of aging adults, because exposures in the past were substantial. These exposures may influence adult cognition either through their effects on the developing nervous system or, because lead is stored in the skeleton for periods of years

Issues in Toxicology No. 16
Aging and Vulnerability to Environmental Chemicals: Age-related Disorders and their Origins in Environmental Exposures
Edited by Bernard Weiss

Published by the Royal Society of Chemistry, www.rsc.org

and decades, through re-exposure to lead in adulthood with age-related bone turnover.

In this chapter, we describe historical and contemporary sources of lead exposure and scientific findings on its effects on cognitive function in adults. We give particular consideration to the history of lead's use in gasoline and the incremental acknowledgement of its neurotoxicity by industrial and regulatory stakeholders. It is this history that underlies an epidemic of elevated lead exposure that spanned several generations and may be responsible for cognitive decrements in many adults. This history is also instructive for how future additives to gasoline and other widely used consumer products should be scrutinized.

1.2 How Humans were and Continue to be Exposed to Lead

1.2.1 Historical Exposures

1.2.1.1 Early Uses: the Emergence of Lead into the Environment

Unlike metals such as iron, copper, and manganese, lead is not essential to physiological function. Yet humans have been introducing lead into their environments—and often directly into their bodies—for millennia.[1–4] In ancient Chinese, Mediterranean, and Middle Eastern societies, lead was a key ingredient in glassware, pots and vessels, solder, paints, cosmetics, eye medicines, and contraceptive methods. It was also used in food and wine as a sweetener and preservative. The Romans, taking advantage of its malleability and availability, made lead the centerpiece of their infrastructure with their extensive web of lead pipes, promoting lead to a quotidian status unprecedented in human civilizations. These uses were joined by new ones—*e.g.*, as an ingredient in inks, ammunitions, and even poisons—and continued throughout the early twentieth century. Then, in the 1920s, humans in the burgeoning US automotive industry, aided and abetted by others in the US government, developed a use for lead that would expose much more of the population, at much higher doses than ever before.

1.2.1.2 How Leaded Gasoline Became the Major Source of Exposure to Lead

The market for automobiles in the US had grown increasingly competitive by the early 1920s, and General Motors (GM) sought to distinguish its automobiles from Ford's reliable but sedate Model T by unveiling new models every year and, critically, improving engine power and efficiency.[5,6] A challenge central to this latter goal was eliminating the pinging "knock" that arose when the fuel ignited prematurely in high-performance, high-compression engines. In

1921, Thomas Midgley, Jr., an engineer at GM, discovered that adding tetraethyl lead (TEL) to gasoline decreased this knock. Curiously, several years earlier, GM's engineers had established that ethyl alcohol (grain alcohol) was also an effective anti-knock agent. However, the competitive advantage of having a proprietary fuel and GM's entwinement with the production of TEL fuel meant that the lead-based agent prevailed while the alcohol-based agent was maligned. This occurred even though, since TEL's first synthesis by a German chemist in 1854, it had a "known deadliness."[7]

In response to protests from industrial hygienists, physiologists, and chemists, the Surgeon General inquired with GM and the DuPont company, a manufacturer of TEL, who responded with evidence-free reassurances. Nonetheless, seeking a governmental "stamp of approval" for their product, GM and DuPont entered into an agreement to study TEL's safety with oversight from the Bureau of Mines.[8] This oversight was merely symbolic, because GM and DuPont negotiated contractual control over all TEL data and any communications regarding it.[5] The first gallon of leaded gasoline was sold in 1923.[5,6]

The momentum behind the ambition of GM and its affiliates was nearly staunched when, in October 1924, five employees at Standard Oil's TEL facility died violent, psychotic deaths, and 35 other workers were smitten with serious neurologic symptoms such as hallucinations, tremors, and palsies. Even though Standard Oil dismissed suspicions with such claims as the victims "had probably worked too hard",[9] officials in New Jersey, Philadelphia, New York state, and New York City were unconvinced and officially banned the sale of leaded gasoline for varying periods – in New York City, the ban lasted for 3 years.[5]

By this time, the Bureau of Mines had formally exonerated leaded gasoline, and yet at the TEL plants, poisonings and deaths continued, many of them closely guarded by industry. Still, the neurotoxicity of lead in these occupational settings was difficult to miss. Among workers at the Standard Oil plant, the TEL building was known as "The Looney Gas Building," and at the DuPont plant, the TEL building was known as "The House of Butterflies," in tribute to its occupants' tendency to have hallucinations involving insects.[6] Yielding to the perception that a governmental body (the Bureau of Mines) was in the pocket of industry, and thus any ill effects of TEL were being ignored, in 1925, the Surgeon General assembled a conference of public health and industry scientists. The argument that prevailed was that TEL would contribute so substantially to the progress of the US as to advance civilization itself, thus making TEL a "gift from God."[5] And although public health advocates argued that it was incumbent on industry to demonstrate TEL's *safety*, ultimately, the Surgeon General commissioned a "Blue Ribbon Panel" to investigate lead's *harm*, giving this panel only seven months to do so.[2] It is not surprising then that the committee concluded that "...at present, there are no good grounds for prohibiting the use of ethyl gasoline...."[5] However, the committee recognized that seven months was insufficient for the job. Presciently, it predicted that, given the insidious and cumulative toxicity of lead poisoning, "[l]onger experience may show that even such slight storage of lead [in the body] as was observed in these studies may lead eventually in susceptible individuals to recognizable or to chronic degenerative diseases. . . ."[5,6] This was the last time for several decades that the US government would come close to considering major regulatory action on leaded gasoline.[8]

1.2.1.3 Lead-Based Paints Added to the Burden of Lead Exposure

Running in parallel to the emergence of leaded gasoline was the emergence of lead-based paint. Humans have been adding lead to paint for centuries, and the neurologic hazards to children of exposure to lead-based paint have been known since at least the early 1900s.[10] The players in the saga of lead-based paint were the archetypes seen in the saga of leaded gasoline. The paint saga differed in its focus on children, both as potential victims of exposure and as subjects in advertising for lead-based paint manufacturers.[11,12] In a perverse twist, the medical director for the Ethyl Gasoline Corporation advocated reducing children's exposures to lead by eliminating lead from paint, but clearly saw no problem with lead in gas.[11]

1.2.1.4 Leaded Gasoline and Lead-Based Paint Were Phased out, but Many Were Exposed

The US Environmental Protection Agency, born in 1970, instituted regulations that initiated the gradual phase-down of lead content in gasoline for on-road vehicles, beginning in 1976 and concluding with a complete ban in 1995.[2,13,14] (Excluded from this phase-down were fuels used for off-road vehicles and marine vessels, and in farming and aviation. In addition, it was only in 2008 that the National Association for Stock Car Racing completely switched its racing fuels to unleaded varieties.[15,16])

In 1978, the Consumer Products Safety Commission banned the sale and use of lead-based paint.[11] By then, human exposures to lead, primarily from leaded gasoline and paint, had reached common and chronic proportions. As of 1980, the estimated *per capita* consumption of lead-based products in the US was 5.2 kilograms per American per year, around 10 times the estimated exposures of ancient Romans.[2] Over the 20th century, the US had burned an estimated 7 million tons of lead in its gasoline,[7] the source of about 90% of the lead emitted into the environment.[17]

While leaded gasoline and paint were being removed from public consumption, interventions were occurring on other sources of exposure. For example, in the 1970s, many US-based food can manufacturers voluntarily ceased using leaded solder in their cans,[18] which resulted in a substantial reduction in human exposure from this source between 1979 and 1989.[17] In 1995, the US Food and Drug Administration formally banned the use of lead-based solder in all canned food sold in the US, including imported food.[18]

The removal of lead from gasoline, paint, and other sources markedly reduced Americans' lead exposures. For example, in early 1976, at the start of the phase-down of lead in gasoline, the *average* blood lead level in the civilian, non-institutionalized US population was 15 μg dL^{-1},[19] well above what is defined today as an elevated level for children (around 5 μg dL^{-1}).[†] (In some areas in the early 1970s, including rural areas, the average blood lead levels among children exceeded 20 μg dL^{-1}.[23–25]) By 1980, the average blood lead level had sunk to 10 μg dL^{-1},[19] and it had plummeted to 2.8 μg dL^{-1} about a decade after that.[‡,26] Nonetheless, millions of children and adults had been exposed to biologically relevant doses of lead, often for many years, and emerging evidence was suggesting that while removing the exposures had established health benefits, the legacies of those exposures could go on to influence myriad health risks, including risks for impaired cognition in adulthood.

1.2.2 Contemporary Sources of Exposure

Lead exposure results from inhalation of air contaminated with lead, or ingestion of food, water, or dust that contains lead. The highest exposures to lead have always been occupational, where workers can experience extremely high levels of exposure. The action level for medical removal from the workplace in the Occupational Safety and Health Administration's (OSHA) standard for blood lead is 50 μg dL^{-1} or above for construction and 60 μg dL^{-1} or above for all other occupation settings;[27–29] that is, when workers are found to have blood lead levels above these levels, they are required to be removed from that work environment until two consecutive blood lead measurements are below 40 μg dL^{-1}. This level is still over 10 times greater than the current average blood lead concentration of adults in the US population (see also Section 1.2.1.4).

In the US, while occupational lead exposure has generally been decreasing, it remains a problem in construction,[30] and this sector has become the dominant source of lead exposure for adults (to a large extent the result of lead in paint). Lead paint can contain up to 50% lead by weight, and workers who remove

---

†In May 2012, the US Centers for Disease Control and Prevention altered and, in effect, lowered its recommended pediatric threshold of concern from 10 μg/dL, the level set in 1991, to any level exceeding the current 97.5th percentile of blood lead levels for children ages 1–5. As of 2012, this was about 5 μg/dL. Sources: [1] Centers for Disease Control. 1991. Preventing lead poisoning in young children 1991. Centers for Disease Control and Prevention. [2] CDC Response to Advisory Committee on Childhood Lead Poisoning Prevention Recommendations in "Low Level Lead Exposure Harms Children: a Renewed Call of Primary Prevention." 2012. Atlanta, GA.

‡Overall, as documented by data from the National Health and Nutrition Examination Survey, blood lead levels in the civilian, non-institutionalized U.S. population dropped from about 15 μg/dL in 1976 to 10 μg/dL in 1980 and then to 2.3, 1.7, 1.5, 1.4 and 1.3 μg/dL, respectively, in the 1991–1994, 1999–2000, 2001–2002, 2003–2004 and 2005–2006 monitoring periods. It remained at 1.3 μg/dL for 2007–2008. Sources: [1] J. L. Annest, J. L. Pirkle, D. Makuc, J. W. Neese, D. D. Bayse, M. G. Kovar. Chronological trend in blood lead levels between 1976 and 1980. *N. Engl. J. Med.*, 1983; **308**(23):1373–1377. [2] Update: blood lead levels–United States, 1991–1994. MMWR Morb Mortal Wkly Rep. 1997; **46**(7):141–146. [3] Centers for Disease Control and Prevention. Fourth National Report on Human Exposure to Environmental Chemicals, Updated Tables, February 2012, Atlanta, Georgia.

paint are at extremely high risk of lead exposure.[31] The majority of houses built before 1978 (estimated at 42–47 million houses in the US) have lead-based paint inside and outside,[32] and lead paint was also used in commercial buildings and other structures such as bridges. Scraping and, in particular, sanding lead paint creates a fine lead dust that can be easily inhaled. Absorption of lead is highly efficient following inhalation, particularly if the particles are small. Hand-to-mouth behavior of construction workers, for example eating and smoking cigarettes without prior hand washing, can also lead to significant absorption of lead. Lead dust on the hands can be ingested and absorbed through the gastrointestinal tract as can lead dust on cigarettes, which can be heated during smoking, generating lead fumes that are especially well absorbed by the lungs. Much more commonly in countries outside the US, Canada, and Europe, workers in many other industries, such as battery manufacturing plants, are also at high risk of extremely high lead exposure.

Aside from occupationally exposed individuals, people who present with blood lead levels that exceed the Centers for Disease Control and Prevention (CDC) current pediatric action limit of $5\,\mu g\,dL^{-1}$ were often exposed from sources such as contaminated traditional medications and cosmetics, accidental exposures to lead from commercial uses (*e.g.*, leaded batteries), or use of lead-containing materials in several common hobbies. For example, persons who create pottery and stained glass often use materials that contain lead, which can result in exposure, as can chewing on or making lead bullets or lead fishing line sinkers. Current exposures can also occur as a result of past activities, unfortunately sometimes unwittingly. Recent reports revealed elevated blood lead levels among children in areas where houses were built on the site of former lead manufacturing plants, of which the residents were unaware.[33,34] In other communities, tap water has been inadvertently contaminated due to partial replacement of service lines,[35] or to water treatment processes that render the chemistry of the water more amenable to dissolving corroded lead in water pipes.[36] Outside of the US, many more examples of very high lead exposures of non-workers are found. A very recent and devastating example of this was the death of an estimated 400 children, and severe lead poisoning of many more, in Nigeria as a result of artisanal gold ore processing in their family compounds.[37,38]

Common current sources of environmental lead exposure in the United States and around the world include lead in plumbing (which can contaminate drinking water), lead paint in older housing, contaminated house dust, contaminated soil, lead crystal, and lead-glazed pottery. However, past exposures to lead are still an important consideration. By far the predominant past general environmental exposure to lead was through exposure to lead in air, which was very largely a result of lead in gasoline. Although a few countries, including Canada and Japan, led the US in banning leaded gasoline, bans in other parts of the world have occurred more recently or not at all, and in these countries, past cumulative exposures are likely to have been much higher.[39–42]

There are many reasons why—even in the US—we may still be seeing the effects of those past high levels of environmental exposures. First, for those who were alive during the times of leaded gasoline, toxic effects of lead exposure at that time may manifest as health impairments later in life. For example, the cumulative exposure to lead in the past could have caused neurotoxicity at the time, which in turn may result in more rapid cognitive decline in later years. Second, while lead initially enters the bloodstream after being inhaled or ingested—from where it is delivered to different tissues and causes different toxicities—the major repository for lead in the body is the skeletal system. Lead deposited in bone stays there a long time—the half life of lead in bone is of the order of years or decades, depending on the bone type[43]—but it is slowly resorbed into blood as bone turnover occurs. Thus bone turnover leads to a remobilization of lead, from exposure potentially many years earlier, back into the bloodstream, where it can again exert toxic effects on other tissues.[44] In fact, in the present environment, in the US and many other countries, of low levels of lead, the current major exposure to lead for many older people may be from lead in their own bones.

1.3 Mechanisms of Neurotoxicity

Several mechanisms by which lead can cause central nervous system dysfunction exist. These have been reviewed elsewhere in greater detail,[45–47] but we will touch on some key aspects of particular relevance to the nervous system here. Many of the neurotoxic actions of lead relate to lead's ability to substitute for calcium, and to a lesser extent zinc. At a very broad view level, nerve cells generally communicate by releasing compounds (neurotransmitters) from one cell (the pre-synaptic neuron) to act on a neighboring cell (the post-synaptic neuron) in some way. The release of these neurotransmitters is finely tuned to the activity of the pre-synaptic neuron in ways that are critically dependent on calcium-dependent mechanisms. The released neurotransmitter acts on the post-synaptic neuron by setting off signalling systems within the neuron; these can have a myriad effects on the intracellular state of the neuron, including altering cytoplasmic molecules as well as intranuclear molecules. Many of these intracellular signalling processes are *also* calcium-dependent. These processes underlie basic neural communication and functioning and underlie the ability of the nervous system to change. This includes changes that drive the establishment and refining of neural architecture during development and the changes that occur in the adult as a result of experience, changes that are thought to underlie learning and memory. Lead is recognized by many of these molecules in much the same way calcium is recognized, but because lead then either blocks or disrupts the function of the protein it interacts with, lead disrupts communication in the nervous system, with the ultimate concern that it thereby disrupts behaviors that are dependent on those neural processes, behaviors such as adult cognitive function.

Many other effects of lead are relevant to adult cognitive function. Gene expression is critical to the normal function of any cell, including neurons, and is also thought to be critical for encoding learning in the brain. Lead can disrupt gene expression in different ways. Many gene transcription factors require calcium or zinc as co-factors, therefore lead's ability to substitute for calcium and zinc can lead to disruption of resultant gene expression.

An exciting new direction of research related to gene expression actions of exposure to lead and other environmental chemicals is epigenetics. Epigenetics refers to several different ways that the read out of the underlying DNA sequence (gene expression) can be modified without an alteration in the DNA sequence itself. An example of this is methylation of the DNA at particular sites. More methylation tends to be associated with less gene expression and *vice versa*. Critical to the importance of epigenetics is that the epigenetic pattern can be altered by the environment and, at the same time, epigenetic changes can persist after the environmental modifier is gone. And in fact these changes can be heritable, *i.e.* passed on to daughter cells. Lead exposure has been found to be associated with increased concentrations of homocysteine.[48] Increased homocysteine reduces the demethylation of *S*-adenosylmethionine (SAM)—which provides methyl groups for DNA methylation—thus possibly reducing DNA methylation levels. In fact, lead exposure has been shown to induce global hypomethylation of hepatic DNA in rats, which was associated with an increase in cell proliferation.[49] Two recent studies in humans found that higher bone lead levels were associated with patterns of lower DNA methylation in adults and the cord blood of newborns.[50,51] Of particular note, epigenetic effects have been proposed to potentially underlie intriguing findings from recent animal studies that link *in utero* and neonatal exposure to lead to Alzheimer's disease neuropathology in later life.[52–54] These findings are related to amyloid beta (Aβ) plaques, which are the pathological hallmark of Alzheimer's disease.[55–57] Aβ is the amyloidogenic product derived from the amyloid precursor protein (APP), with the help of the β-site APP-cleaving enzyme, BACE1. Early life lead exposure—but not later life exposure—in rats has been found to be associated with increased expression of the *APP* gene, increased activity of the Sp1 transcription factor that regulates the *APP* gene, and increased levels of APP and Aβ.[58] Similar changes are seen in early life lead-exposed monkeys, as is increased BACE1 mRNA and amyloid plaques.[59] Moreover, it has been suggested that age-related demethylation—perhaps with a contribution from lead exposure—is related to Aβ production in the brain.[60]

Lead also adversely affects the central nervous system (CNS) through the many ways in which it causes cell damage and death. Lead causes oxidative stress through several pathways, including: the inhibition of enzymes in the heme synthesis pathway (δ-ALA synthetase, δ-ALAD, and ferrochelatase); stimulation of ferrous ion initiated membrane lipid peroxidation;[61,62] changes in the fatty acid composition of membranes;[63] and increased activation of NAD(P)H oxidase.[64,65] Lead also disrupts enzymes involved in antioxidant defense systems. Lead has been shown to alter the function of superoxide dismutase, catalase, glucose-6-phosphate dehydrogenase and enzymes involved in glutathione metabolism, glutathione peroxidase, glutathione-*S*-transferase, and glutathione reductase.[66] Lead also accumulates in and damages the mitochondria, causing release of calcium and apoptotic cell death.[67–70]

In addition to the actions of lead within the nervous system, lead may also affect neural function indirectly: for example, *via* effects on the cardiovascular system. There is abundant evidence of effects of lead on the cardiovascular system, including increasing homocysteine levels, atherosclerosis, blood pressure, and risk of hypertension.[48,71] Homocysteine is toxic to the CNS by influencing neurotransmitter synthesis, and causing excitotoxicity and cell death.[72,73] Atherosclerosis, increased blood pressure, and hypertension can all contribute to silent (or not) cerebrovascular damage, leading to neuronal death. These types of cardiovascular factors are suspected to result in neurobehavioral disturbances and may play a role in other brain disorders as well.

1.4 Assessment of Lead Exposure

The primary biological assessment of exposure to lead is to measure lead in whole blood. The half-life of lead in blood is approximately 30 days, thus a single blood lead concentration measurement only provides a metric of recent exposures, although if external exposures are constant over time, a single blood lead measurement can provide an estimate of exposure to lead over longer periods. In occupational settings where exposures are expected to be high, serial blood lead measurements are often taken at regular intervals for surveillance. These are measured to identify incidents of possible high level exposures (see Sections 2.2 and 2.6), but serial measurements can also be used to construct an index of cumulative exposure over longer work periods, which can be useful for studies of exposures of longer or varying durations. Some epidemiological studies evaluate the effect of lead exposure on the health of workers without access to blood lead measurements. Instead, these studies use job exposure matrices (JEMs), which link specific jobs and tasks to different levels of likely exposure to lead. These exposure levels are inferred from studies in other settings where more direct measures of exposure—*e.g.* workers' blood lead measurements or air lead measurements—are available. In these settings, the relation of specific jobs and tasks to lead exposure levels can be determined to construct a JEM that can then be applied in settings where actual measurements are not available.

Determining exposure levels among those exposed non-occupationally is much more difficult without biomarkers because exposure levels are typically much lower and sources of exposure are more widespread and varied. Although blood lead concentration is by far the most commonly used biomarker of lead exposure, this measure is less useful when one wants to consider the effects of cumulative exposure to lead over a longer time period. While serial blood lead measurements have been used to quantify lead exposure over longer durations in occupational settings, this practice is less commonly used in non-occupational settings as it is time-consuming and labor intensive to implement if not required for surveillance. This conundrum created problems for the study of the effects of lead on cognitive function, and the literature related to blood lead measurements was quite inconsistent.[74] Great advances in these research endeavors came with the development of technology to non-invasively measure lead in bone: x-ray fluorescence (XRF).[44]

Bone is the primary reservoir for lead in the human body, and measures of the concentration of lead in bone provide an integrated estimate of long-term, cumulative exposure to lead. The half-life of lead in the patella—which comprises mainly trabecular bone—is of the order of years, while the half-life of lead in the tibia—which comprises mainly cortical bone—is of the order of decades.[43] It is important to keep in mind however, that bone lead measurements cannot provide information on the temporal pattern of exposures during the years over which it integrates exposure. For example, two people may have the same bone lead concentration, but one may have had uniformly low exposures to lead except for one or more short periods of high exposure, while the other may have experienced a constant level of moderate lead exposure over the same time frame. We may not know whether those differences in exposure patterns matter for the health outcome of interest, but we need to keep in mind that if they do, these are distinctions we cannot make based on bone lead. Distinguishing different effects of those two patterns of exposure would be possible however with serial blood lead measurements.

1.5 Cognitive Effects of Lead Exposures in Adults

Prior to the mid-20th century, the prevailing view of lead poisoning was one of an acute clinical event—involving tremors, vomiting, encephalopathy, and anemia, among other signs—that, if treated prior to encephalopathy, would have no enduring neurologic effects.[75,76] Work in 1943 by Randolph Byers and Elizabeth Lord contradicted both these assumptions.[75] They documented 20 cases of lead exposure among children, most of whom did not exhibit the most severe effects of lead exposure and none of whom exhibited the severe extreme neurologic symptoms believed to be indicative of lead poisoning. However, all of the children exhibited demonstrable neurologic problems, including attention deficits, behavioral problems, and impaired motor function. Over the years that they were followed by their physicians, some of the children's problems resolved, but most had impaired intellectual development and many developed new behavioral problems. In most cases, these enduring effects occurred even after the exposures, mainly from eating chips of lead-based paints, and were removed and treatment given. Indeed, a clinical trial conducted nearly 60 years later indicated that chelation therapy was ineffective at reducing the neurologic effects of lead exposure.[77]

In this section, we describe research on the relation of lead exposure to cognitive function in adulthood. The studies discussed document effects on cognition and subserving brain structures resulting from lead exposure at levels far lower than the doses associated with acute lead poisoning. This body of evidence also extends the pioneering work of Byers and Lord by showing that the cognitive effects of lead exposure may continue well past the point at which the exposure has ended.

1.5.1 Effects of High-Dose, Occupational Exposure

1.5.1.1 Evidence from Studies of Cognition and Cognitive Decline

With the accrual of several decades of research, it is clear that exposure to lead exerts adverse cognitive effects on cognitive functioning in adulthood. The TEL-related events of the 1920s and beyond were sentinels that eventually led to studies focused on adults who experiences high-doses and/or frequent exposures as part of their occupations. The most rigorous early meta-analysis of these study findings included 12 studies, published between 1977 and 1997, that reported quantitative information about the exposed participants' levels of exposure and the cognitive scores, in addition to accounting for age and "premorbid intelligence." Participants' blood lead levels were relatively high by today's standards; among the occupationally exposed participants, study cohort *averages* exceeded $30\,\mu g\,dL^{-1}$, and in over half of the "unexposed" participant groups, the averages exceeded $10\,\mu g\,dL^{-1}$. Overall, higher blood lead levels corresponded to worse performance on tests of visuospatial ability, memory, and motor function.[78] Although these conclusions were contested,[79] the findings were consonant with a subsequent review,[80] as well as several studies that have confirmed and extended these findings by distinguishing the acute effects of exposure from the effects that remain after exposure has ceased and by exploring the realms of cognitive decline over time, cerebral vascular ischemia, and brain volumes.

Since 1997, 16 new studies emerged that, in addition to measuring exposures using blood lead, also measured cumulative exposures.[80] All of these studies were adjusted for several potential sources of confounding, including age (and, unless otherwise specified, this is true of all the other studies that we will discuss in the remainder of this section). In some of the 16 studies, the cumulative exposure estimates came from integrating serial blood lead concentrations. Other studies measured lead concentrations at specific bone sites, taking advantage of *in vivo* K-x-ray fluorescent (KXRF) spectroscopic methods that had been refined for use in research settings (see Section 1.4). As described in a review of these studies,[80] higher blood lead concentration—a measure of recent exposure—predicted worse performance on tests of cognition among workers currently exposed in their occupations. Measures of cumulative exposure were not as strongly associated, a finding that the reviewers attributed to acute effects masking the effects of chronic or past exposures. By contrast, among workers whose occupational exposures had ended, measures of cumulative exposure were more strongly associated with poor performance on cognitive tests than were measures of current exposure (*e.g.* blood lead level). Lead exposure appeared to adversely affect a wide range of cognitive functions, most notably visuospatial ability, executive function, and verbal memory. Higher exposures were also associated with worse performance on tests of motor ability, including dexterity.

Among these studies were two investigations of change in cognition over time. This outcome is of interest because it distinguishes effects of lead that persist over time—*i.e.* cognitive function remains diminished but does not continue to worsen after the exposure ends—from effects that worsen over time.[81] Moreover, decline in cognitive function is more directly related than poor cognition to the pathogenesis and progression of dementia. In these studies, higher cumulative exposure, indicated by tibia bone lead concentration, corresponded to greater decline in several cognitive functions, even after the occupational exposure had ended.[80] These findings were consistent with a subsequent study of 83 previously exposed workers in lead battery plants and 51 unexposed workers.[82] In spite of this study's small size—and even after accounting for factors such as current blood lead level, years of employment with lead, age, education, income, alcohol intake, smoking history, and blood pressure—exposed workers with higher peak tibia lead levels (current tibia bone lead concentration corrected for time since last occupational exposure) experienced significantly faster declines over 22 years on measures of visuospatial ability, general intelligence, and memory ability, as well as overall cognition. Higher peak tibia lead level was also associated with more rapid cognitive decline among the "unexposed" workers, but these findings were not statistically significant.

1.5.1.2 Evidence from Brain Imaging Studies

To further explore the mechanisms by which lead exposure may influence cognitive function and decline in occupationally exposed adults, several researchers have examined findings on brain imaging. A study of 536 men who previously had worked in organolead (*e.g.* tetraethyl lead) manufacturing plants found that higher cumulative exposure to lead, indicated by peak tibia lead level, was associated with significantly elevated cerebral ischemic burden, as assessed by white matter lesion score on magnetic resonance images.[83] This observation provides support for a vascular mechanism underlying at least some of lead's cognitive effects.

In this same study, higher cumulative exposure also appeared to be linked to structural differences in the brain, including reduced total brain volume and total grey matter volume. In addition, frontal, cingulate gyrus and insula volumes were smaller with higher cumulative lead exposure, but cerebellar and occipital volumes were not, consistent with the observed associations of lead exposure with decline in cognitive functions, such as learning and executive abilities, that are subserved by these affected regions.[83] Indeed, a subsequent study found evidence that reduced volumes in brain regions specified *a priori* seemed to explain the association between lead exposure and impaired visuoconstruction ability. Similar but weaker evidence was found for eye-hand coordination and executive function.[84] By contrast, when the investigators examined *changes* in these imaging indices over a five year interval among 362 of the original 536 participants, they found little association with cumulative lead exposure.[85] It is possible that lead exposure has progressive effects on cerebral ischemia and brain structure but that these effects are too modest to be observed in a study of this size that is reliant on these measures of exposure and outcomes. It is also possible that lead's effects on these outcomes are merely persistent rather than progressive and that the progressive effects seen on cognitive function are attributable to other mechanisms, such as effects on microstructure and neural function.

Magnetic resonance spectroscopy (MRS) is another brain imaging technique that integrates data on brain metabolites and structural features of an imaged brain. Because MRS can assess brain metabolites, it can potentially detect changes in brain metabolism that occur before changes in the volume of brain structures can be seen. Using this technique in a study of 71 year old identical twin brothers, Weisskopf and colleagues found additional evidence for the neurotoxic effects of lead.[86] Both twins were retired painters but differed in the extent to which they were involved in paint removal, a task that involves high levels of exposure to lead *via* inhaled leaded paint dust. Despite the twins' many similarities, the MRS results showed lower levels of *N*-acetylaspartate (NAA)—a brain metabolite indicative of neuronal density—in frontal and hippocampal regions in the more highly lead-exposed twin, as well as greater dysfunction on learning, memory, and executive function tasks, which are dependent on frontal and hippocampal regions. A subsequent study of 22 workers at a lead paint factory in Taiwan, along with 18 controls, found similar results, with higher levels of blood and patella lead concentrations exhibiting associations with decreased NAA, particularly in the frontal lobe.[87]

1.5.2 Effects of Low-Dose, Non-Occupational Exposure

Against the backdrop of evidence suggesting that the cognitive effects of earlier occupational exposures linger well into middle and old age, the hypothesis that protracted non-occupational ("community-level"), and therefore lower-level, exposure might also influence cognitive function and cognitive decline in adulthood emerged. This hypothesis is particularly important in light of two demographic phenomena. The first is that an enormous number of individuals experienced relatively high levels of these types of exposures between the 1920s and 1980s, merely by virtue of being exposed to emissions from leaded fuel, lead-based paint, or both. The second demographic feature is the impending surge, fuelled by the aging of the post-war "baby boom" population, in the number of adults expected to develop dementia over the coming decades.[88,89] Impaired cognition and, to a greater extent, cognitive decline in adulthood both signal future dementia risk.[90–93] Thus understanding the relation of community-level lead exposure to impaired cognition and cognitive decline may offer direction toward ameliorating lead's effects among those already exposed and impetus toward continuing to minimize exposures among future generations.

Evidence that the effects of long-term, "low-level" exposure to lead early in life may reverberate to impaired cognition later in life has begun to emerge in studies of animals[52–54] and humans.[94] Additionally, in a recent follow-up study of adults who had participated in a study of prenatal lead exposure, blood plasma indices of Aβ production and deposition were higher among those who had elevated early life blood levels.[95] One mechanism underlying these observations is irreversible change to neural structures and function caused by early exposure. This mechanism may be especially relevant in situations in which exposures have ceased. A second mechanism may involve the cumulative burden of long-term exposure. Such exposure may be exogenous, as for an individual who endured decades of exposure to ambient lead from leaded gasoline. Exposure may also be endogenous, because about 95% of lead in the body is stored in the skeleton (see Section 1.4). The duration of its storage there is a function of the bone characteristics and other metabolic factors that influence the rate of bone turnover. However, when lead-containing bone is resorbed, that lead re-enters the circulation, from where it may access the brain and other susceptible organs and tissues (see Section 1.2.2).

1.5.2.1 Evidence from Studies of Cognition and Cognitive Decline

In comparison with studies of occupational lead exposure, studies of community-level lead exposure and cognitive outcomes in adults are relatively few. However, aided by KXRF technology, their numbers have been increasing. Blood lead levels of most participants in these studies were less than $10\,\mu g\,dL^{-1}$, much lower than those in the occupational studies. A review of 6 such studies, published between 1998 and 2007, in which researchers assessed participants' recent and cumulative exposures to lead, found that higher levels of cumulative exposure—as assessed by KXRF-based bone lead measurements—were associated with worse performance on tests of a variety of cognitive functions, including visuospatial abilities, verbal learning and memory, executive functioning, eye-hand coordination, and overall cognitive ability.[80] Blood lead levels were associated with significantly worse performance on some cognitive tests in some studies, but, overall, these findings were less consistent than those for bone lead.

Since this review, several other studies of community-level exposure to lead and adult cognition have been conducted. In a study of 1812 adults, aged 65 and over and living in rural China, concentration of lead in blood plasma was associated with worse combined performance on 6 cognitive tests, but this result was not statistically significant.[96] Similarly, a study of older adults, aged 60 and over, participating in the US-based National Health and Nutrition Examination Survey (NHANES) found that blood lead levels were associated with increased likelihood of self-reported confusion and problems with memory (N=7277) and worse performance on a test of working memory and attention (N=2299), but neither of these findings was statistically significant.[97] In spite of the large study populations, the findings from these studies are not necessarily surprising. The study in China relied on plasma lead concentrations. Although it is thought that the fraction of lead in plasma represents the most bioavailable lead in blood,[98] levels are typically very low, and this concentration is notoriously difficult to measure.[98,99] Indeed, a large proportion of participants had plasma lead levels that were effectively zero. In the NHANES study, concentrations of lead in whole blood ranged between 0.18 and 54 $\mu g\,dL^{-1}$, but average (2.45 $\mu g\,dL^{-1}$) and median (2.00 $\mu g\,dL^{-1}$) concentrations indicate low levels of recent exposure in most of the study population. More importantly, neither of these studies employed indices of cumulative exposure to lead. These measures would likely have revealed past exposures to leaded gasoline, a major source of community-based exposure in both study's countries, and which had been officially banned by the time these studies were conducted.

Measures of cumulative exposure were available in 3 other studies of community-exposed adults. In a pilot study of 47 adults, aged 55 to 67 years, investigators gauged participants' cumulative exposure to lead by using KXRF-based measurements of lead concentrations in sites representative of both cortical (tibia) and trabecular (calcaneus) bone.[100] They administered a battery of cognitive tests assessing visual memory, as well as the Montreal Cognitive Assessment (MoCA), a separate battery assessing cognitive functions such as visuospatial ability, attention, executive function, and language. Participants with higher calcaneus lead concentrations performed worse on all of the visual memory tests, two of which were borderline significant ($P<0.10$). Findings for the tibia were somewhat similar but less consistent and not statistically significant. In unadjusted analyses, neither bone lead concentration was significantly associated with MoCA score.

A larger study of 587 women, aged 47 to 74, participating in the Nurses' Health Study measured lead concentrations in tibia and patella (representative of trabecular) bone as well as in whole blood.[101] In general, higher levels of all three exposure biomarkers were associated with worse performance on the 6 individual cognitive metrics assessed, which included tests of verbal memory, attention, and executive function. Curiously, the only result that was statistically significant was the single association indicating better performance (on a test of phonemic fluency) with higher exposure (as measured by patellar lead). The investigators also evaluated associations between the lead biomarkers and global cognition, accounting for scores on all cognitive tests completed. They repeated these analyses without the aforementioned fluency test, which was supported by a significant formal test of heterogeneity. Higher levels of all three exposure biomarkers was associated with worse global cognition. In particular, although the women's current exposures to lead were quite low (as indicated by an average blood lead level of 2.9 $\mu g\,dL^{-1}$) higher tibia lead level corresponded to significantly worse global cognition when the fluency test was excluded. (Preliminary data from a subsequent cycle of cognitive testing have failed to confirm the patella lead-fluency association.)

The third study—the Baltimore Memory Study, a population-based cohort of men and women living in a racially diverse collection of neighbourhoods in Baltimore, Maryland—involved 1140 participants, aged from 50 to 70.[102] Investigators measured participants' tibia bone lead concentrations and assessed their cognitive functioning at three study cycles approximately 14 months apart, allowing them to evaluate cumulative exposure to lead in relation to cognitive decline. Decline in all six cognitive domains tested was generally worse with higher levels of tibia lead, although only the association with decline in eye-hand coordination was statistically significant. However, higher tibia lead levels were significantly associated with persistently worse performance on the tests over time (*i.e.*, worse performance but not greater declines in performance). With further adjustment for socioeconomic status, the associations corresponding to executive function, verbal memory, and visual memory remained significant. Nonetheless, in analyses stratified by race, the deleterious association between tibia lead and cognitive function was present only among white participants (and statistically significant only for eye-hand coordination and executive function) and not among African-American participants.

1.5.2.2 Evidence from Brain Imaging Studies

In contrast to the brain imaging research conducted among occupationally exposed individuals, brain imaging research has been scarce among community-exposed individuals. To date, the only such study conducted examined the associations of both patella and tibia bone lead concentration to brain metabolites measured with MRS in 31 older men, none of whom had dementia, participating in the Normative Aging Study.[103] Higher concentrations of lead in both bone sites corresponded to higher levels of hippocampal myoinositol, a metabolite believed to be related to glia (non-neuronal cells in the brain that fill roles including immune function and structural and biochemical support). By contrast, bone lead levels were not associated with neuronal density, as indicated by levels of NAA. While one might expect a reduction in NAA with increasing lead exposure if lead exposure ultimately results in neuronal loss, it is intriguing that others have suggested that one of the earliest spectroscopic signs of Alzheimer's disease is an increase in myoinositol without a change in NAA.[104]

1.5.3 Modification by Psychosocial Factors

An emerging body of animal data suggests that early life exposure to psychological stress may further exacerbate lead exposure's effects on cognitive outcomes.[105–107] This interaction is potentially important because psychological stress and lead exposure frequently occur together in community settings. The mechanism underlying this enhanced susceptibility may involve actions by both factors on the hypothalamic–pituitary–adrenal (HPA) axis, which, via the alteration in cortisol homeostasis[108] and other pathways, is linked to cognitive functioning.[109] Exposure to lead and psychological stress may amplify each other's effects on the HPA axis: lead exposure may alter reactivity to psychological stressors,[110–112] and psychological stress may promote the mobilization of lead from bone into the blood,[113] thus making more lead available to act on the HPA axis and other systems. Both lead and psychological stress also act on the dopaminergic and glutamatergic systems in the brain's mesocorticolimbic regions, which encompass key structures and functions involved in cognition.[105,106]

Because lead exposure and psychological stress may both occur repeatedly over different stages of the lifespan, evaluating their joint effect on cognitive outcomes in adulthood is enormously challenging. Nonetheless, two studies in community-exposed populations offer a start—importantly, using measures of cumulative lead exposure. Their results provide evidence to suggest that adverse effects of lead on cognitive function are worse among persons exposed to greater psychological stress. In a study of 1001 participants, ages 50 to 70 years, of the Baltimore Memory Study, the associations of tibia lead level with poor performance on tests of language, processing speed, and executive function were significantly stronger among those living in neighbourhoods characterized by greater psychosocial hazards (*e.g.* 9-1-1 emergency calls, violent crime).[114] A study of 811 men (mean age, 68 years) participating in the Normative Aging Study found associations between lead exposure biomarkers and performance on a test of global cognition that were more deleterious among men who had experienced greater levels of perceived stress than among men with lower levels of perceived stress.[115] These differences in association were significant or, borderline significant, for both patella bone lead level and blood lead level.

1.5.4 Modification by Genes

Identifying genetic variants that modify the health effects of lead can, in theory, define sub-populations with elevated susceptibility to lead's effects. For example, in the previously discussed cohort of former organolead workers, the adverse association between tibia lead concentration and several cognitive abilities was heightened among men carrying at least one ε4 variant— a variant whose association with increased risk of late-onset alzheimer disease has been well-documented—of the apolipoprotein E gene.[116,117]

Genetic studies may also provide insights into the molecular mechanisms by which cumulative exposure to lead may affect adult cognition. A particularly clear example of this type of inquiry was in a study of variants of the hemochromatosis (*HFE*) gene.[118] Two *HFE* variants are associated with hemochromatosis, a disease of iron overload and consequently excess oxidative stress. Among a group of 358 men in the Normative Aging Study, those who carried at least one of these alleles experienced significantly faster rates of decline in global cognition, compared with non-carriers, for a given increase in bone lead (tibia or patella). These findings provide support for the role of oxidative stress and, potentially, iron–lead interactions in lead's relation to cognition.

These two sets of findings have not, however, been replicated in other settings thus far. And, on the whole, reports on lead–gene interactions have either been isolated, as for the aforementioned interactions, or shown inconsistent results. A well-characterized variant in the gene encoding δ-aminolevulinic acid (ALAD) has received the most attention. This variant, known as *ALAD-2*, produces an enzyme sub-unit that is more electronegative than that produced by the wild type *ALAD-1* variant.[119] Thus lead may have greater affinity for the isozyme composed of a greater number of ALAD-2 sub-units.[120] Whether *ALAD-2* carriers are more susceptible to lead's cognitive effects is unclear. The more electronegative ALAD-2 isozyme could more effectively distribute lead throughout the body or, conversely, bind lead so tightly as to reduce its bioavailability.[121] In addition, lead inhibits ALAD, resulting in an increase in the neurotoxic substrate, 5-aminolevulic acid (ALA). The lead-induced increase in plasma ALA is more pronounced in *ALAD-1* homozygotes,[122–124] implying decreased cognitive susceptibility in *ALAD-2* in carriers. For a given increment in lead exposure biomarker, one study of older adult men found more deleterious associations with cognitive function among *ALAD-2* carriers, although none of these lead exposure-*ALAD* genotype interactions was statistically significant.[125] Findings in two other studies were mixed.[126,127] A fourth study of occupationally exposed and unexposed middle-aged adults found greater susceptibility to lead's effects on motor function among *ALAD*-1 homozygotes.[128]

An emerging area of inquiry, that may produce more promising findings, is how lead exposure affects cognitive function through its effects on the epigenome. Specifically, lead may influence when and how much a particular gene is expressed,[50,51] providing a potentially powerful way, above and beyond lead's interaction with traits of the static genome, for understanding lead's effects on neurodevelopment and cognitive function over the lifespan. (For further discussion on the epigenetic effects of lead, see Section 1.3.)

1.5.5 Does Exposure to Lead Contribute to Dementia Risk?

Taken as a whole, in combination with new findings on childhood lead exposure and adult cognitive functioning, the findings on cumulative exposure to lead among both occupationally and non-occupationally exposed individuals suggest that lead exposure earlier in life has residual neurocognitive ramifications many years later. A mechanistically logical extension of lead exposure's associations with impaired cognition and accelerated cognitive decline is that lead may be associated with increased risk of dementia. Because studies with high-quality assessments of lead exposure rarely also entail high-quality assessments of dementia, and *vice versa*, the data required to answer this important public health question is essentially absent. A few studies have attempted to evaluate this association, but the exposure assessments in these studies were poor, and the studies were underpowered to detect subtle effects, which are common in the study of environmental toxicants on health. With increased interest in the late life effects of early and mid life exposures, more opportunities should arise for addressing the effect of lead exposure on dementia risk.

1.6 Closing Remarks: Shifting Exposures, Continuing Risks

The removal of lead from gasoline and the prohibition of lead-based paint use resulted in substantially reduced exposures for millions of children and adults.

While this achievement has been hailed as a public health victory, the excruciatingly slow pace at which it came about has incurred great costs to the intellectual capacity and economic productivity of the United States,[129] and likely other countries as well, prompting one observer to bemoan the victory as a pyrrhic one.[130]

A surprising dimension of this success is that as average exposure levels have fallen over time, researchers have continued to identify adverse cognitive effects on children at progressively lower levels of exposure.[76] In a recent pooled analysis, adverse effects on children were detectable at levels below 30 $\mu g\,dL^{-1}$ (the screening threshold from 1975–1985), and in fact, the steepest interval of the dose-response curve appeared at the lowest levels of exposure, below 10 μg dL.[131] With these discoveries of cognitive effects at lower blood lead levels, the CDC has lowered its pediatric screening threshold repeatedly over time.[20–22,76] Following advocacy for lowering the threshold even further,[132] the CDC recently changed its recommendations to intervene on children whose levels fall in the 97.5th percentile, effectively reducing the threshold in 2012 to around 5 $\mu g\,dL^{-1}$.[20–22]

In contrast, in occupational settings in the US, the blood lead level thresholds that trigger various actions (*e.g.* removal from the workplace) were last promulgated in an era in which addressing acute toxicity was the primary goal as far as adult health was concerned. The Occupational Health and Safety Administration (OSHA) last set these standards in 1978 and 1993 respectively for construction and general industry. But, as argued by Schwartz and Hu, as well as the American College of Occupational and Environmental Medicine, these current standards may still permit too much risk, especially in light of data that has emerged in the past 15 years.[133,134] For example, a worker with a single blood lead level exceeding 60 $\mu g\,dL^{-1}$ must be removed from further exposure; this level is far in excess of the level at which lead exposure exerts its cognitive effects. In 1978, the average blood lead level in the population exceeded 10 $\mu g\,dL^{-1}$,[19] and even though it had dropped substantially by 1993,[135] most workers who were covered by these standards had started working when average blood lead levels were what are now considered elevated.[133,134]

All told, while lead exposures in the US have been decreasing, they remain relevant to the cognitive well-being of several generations of adults who have sustained substantial exposures during at least parts of their lives. Nearly 90% of US children in 1976 had blood lead levels exceeding 10 $\mu g\,dL^{-1}$.[136] And by the time the most recent OSHA standards for lead exposure came into effect, in 1978 and 1993, most adults had already accrued substantial exposures. Moreover, progress in preventing exposures and their cognitive aftermath will likely not occur at the same pace in all population sectors. Within the US, historic exposures to lead followed marked racial and socioeconomic gradients, with higher exposures more common among individuals of minority race or ethnicity and/or who were economically disadvantaged.[136–138] These gradients have lessened over time, but to a modest degree still remain.[139–141] Progress outside of the US is likely to be uneven as well (see Section 1.2.2). Clearly, the cognitive legacy of lead exposure will likely be a protracted one, as sources of exposure persist or new sources emerge over time.

References

1. M. A. Lessler, *Ohio J. Sci.*, 1988, **88**, 78–84.
2. J. Lewis, *EPA Journal*, 1985. Available online, http://www.epa.gov/aboutepa/history/topics/epa/15c.html.
3. E. H. Schafer, *T'oung Pao*, 1956, **44**, 413–438.
4. S. Hernberg, *Am. J. Ind. Med.*, 2000, **38**, 244–354.
5. D. Rosner and G. Markowitz, *Am. J. Public Health*, 1985, **75**, 344–352.
6. H. L. Needleman, *Environ. Res.*, 1997, **74**, 95–103.
7. J. L. Kitman, in *The Nation*, 2000. Available online, http://www.thenation.com/article/secret-history-lead.
8. D. Ozonoff, *Am. J. Public Health*, 1985, **75**, 338–340.
9. "Odd gas kills one, makes four insane," *New York Times*, October 27, 1924, p. 1.
10. J. L. Gibson, *Public Health Rep.*, 2005, **120**, 301–304.
11. G. Markowitz and D. Rosner, *Am. J. Public Health*, 2000, **90**, 36–46.
12. C. Warren, *Public Health Rep.*, 2005, **120**, 322–329.
13. United States Environmental Protection Agency (1997). Clean Air Act, Section 112(c)(6), Specific Pollutants, Docket N. A097-05; FRL-5843-6, Federal Register. **62**: 33625–33639.
14. United States Environmental Protection Agency, "Press release: EPA takes final step in phaseout of leaded gasoline," January 29,1996.
15. D. Caldwell, "Racing to make the pit stops a little bit greener," *New York Times*, February 25, 2007.
16. V. Bernstein, "Nascar plans to switch to unleaded fuel in '08," *New York Times*, January 20, 2006.
17. Agency for Toxic Substances and Disease Registry, "Toxicological profile for lead" (Public Health Service, US Department of Health and Human Services, Altanta, GA, 2007).
18. Food and Drug Administration, in *21 CFR Part 189* Department of Health and Human Services, ed. (1995), vol. Docket Nos. 82P–0371 and 91N–0165.
19. J. L. Annest, J. L. Pirkle, D. Makuc, J. W. Neese, D. D. Bayse and M. G. Kovar, *N. Engl. J. Med.*, 1983, **308**, 1373–1377.
20. Centers for Disease Control and Prevention, CDC Response to Advisory Committee on Childhood Lead Poisoning Prevention Recommendations in *Low Level Lead Exposure Harms Children: a Renewed Call of Primary Prevention* (Atlanta, GA, 2012).
21. Centers for Disease Control and Prevention (2012). Fourth National Report on Human Exposure to Environmental Chemicals, Updated Tables, February 2012. Atlanta, Georgia.
22. *Morbity and Mortality Weekly Report*, 2012, **61**, 383.
23. I. H. Billick, A. S. Curran and D. R. Shier, *Environ. Health Perspect.*, 1980, **34**, 213–217.
24. P. R. Fine, C. W. Thomas, R. H. Suhs, R. E. Cohnberg and B. A. Flashner, *JAMA*, 1972, **221**, 1475–1479.

25. C. J. Cohen, G. N. Bowers and M. L. Lepow, *JAMA*, 1973, **226**, 1430–1433.
26. J. L. Pirkle, D. J. Brody, E. W. Gunter, R. A. Kramer, D. C. Paschal, K. M. Flegal and T. D. Matte, *JAMA*, 1994, **272**, 284–291.
27. Occupational Safety and Health Administration, in *Subpart D - Occupational Health and Environmental Controls*, 2011, vol. 1926.26(k) - Lead - Medical removal protection.
28. Occupational Safety and Health Administration, in *Subpart Z - Toxic and Hazardous Substances*, 2011, vol. 1926.1025(k) - Lead - Medical removal protection.
29. R. Rabin, D. R. Brooks and L. K. Davis, *Am. J. Public Health*, 1994, **84**, 1483–1485.
30. A. Okun, G. Cooper, A. J. Bailer, J. Bena and L. Stayner, *Am. J. Ind. Med.*, 2004, **45**, 558–572.
31. S. M. Levin and M. Goldberg, *Am. J. Ind. Med.*, 2000, **37**, 23–43.
32. Agency for Toxic Substances and Disease Registry, "Toxicological profile for lead" (Public Health Service, US Department of Health and Human Services, Altanta, GA, 1999).
33. A. Young, "Long gone lead factories leave poisons in nearby yards," *USA Today*, April 19, 2012.
34. A. Young and P. Eisler, "Some neighborhoods dangerously contaminated by lead fallout," *USA Today*, April 19, 2012.
35. R. Renner, *Environ. Health Perspect.*, 2010, **118**, A202–A208.
36. R. Renner, *Environ. Health Perspect.*, 2009, **117**, A542–A547.
37. C. A. Dooyema, A. Neri, Y. C. Lo, J. Durant, P. I. Dargan, T. Swarthout, O. Biya, S. O. Gidado, S. Haladu, N. Sani-Gwarzo, P. M. Nguku, H. Akpan, S. Idris, A. M. Bashir and M. J. Brown, *Environ. Health Perspect.*, 2012, **120**, 601–607.
38. Human Rights Watch. (February 7, 2012). "Nigeria: child lead poisoning crisis." Retrieved April 30, 2012, from http://www.hrw.org/news/2012/02/07/nigeria-child-lead-poisoning-crisis.
39. P. J. Landrigan, "The worldwide problem of lead in petrol." *Bull World Health Organ*, 2002, **80**(10), 768.
40. A. Prüss-Üstün, L. Fewtrell, P. J. Landrigan and J. L. Ayuso-Mateos, in *Comparative Quantification of Health Risks: Global and Regional Burden of Disease Attributable to Selected Major Risk Factors*, eds. M. Ezzati, A. D. Lopex, A. Rodgers and C. J. L. Murray, World Health Organization, Geneva, 2004, vol. 2, pp. 1495–1542.
41. D. Todd and H. Todd, *Outcome and Influence Evaluation of the UNEP Based Partnership for Clean Fuels and Vehicles (PCFV), United Nations Environment Programme*, Nairobi, Kenya, 2010.
42. G. Lean, "UN hails green triumph as leaded petrol banned throughout Africa," *The Independent*, January 1, 2006.
43. E. Wilker, S. Korrick, L. H. Nie, D. Sparrow, P. Vokonas, B. Coull, R. O. Wright, J. Schwartz and H. Hu, *J. Occup. Environ. Med.*, 2011, **53**, 850–855.

44. H. Hu, M. Rabinowitz and D. Smith, *Environ. Health Perspect.*, 1998, **106**, 1–8.
45. J. Bressler, K. A. Kim, T. Chakraborti and G. Goldstein, *Neurochem. Res.*, 1999, **24**, 595–600.
46. A. Garza, R. Vega and E. Soto, *Med. Sci. Monit.*, 2006, **12**, RA57–RA65.
47. T. I. Lidsky and J. S. Schneider, *Brain*, 2003, **126**, 5–19.
48. J. H. Schafer, T. A. Glass, J. Bressler, A. C. Todd and B. S. Schwartz, *Environ. Health Perspect.*, 2005, **113**, 31–35.
49. D. Kanduc, M. R. Rossiello, A. Aresta, C. Cavazza, E. Quagliariello and E. Farber, *Arch. Biochem. Biophys.*, 1991, **286**, 212–216.
50. J. R. Pilsner, H. Hu, A. Ettinger, B. N. Sanchez, R. O. Wright, D. Cantonwine, A. Lazarus, H. Lamadrid-Figueroa, A. Mercado-Garcia, M. M. Tellez-Rojo and M. Hernandez-Avila, *Environ. Health Perspect.*, 2009, **117**, 1466–1471.
51. R. O. Wright, J. Schwartz, R. J. Wright, V. Bollati, L. Tarantini, S. K. Park, H. Hu, D. Sparrow, P. Vokonas and A. Baccarelli, *Environ. Health Perspect.*, 2010, **118**, 790–795.
52. J. Wu, M. R. Basha and N. H. Zawia, *J. Mol. Neurosci.*, 2008, **34**, 1–7.
53. N. H. Zawia and M. R. Basha, *Rev. Neurosci.*, 2005, **16**, 325–337.
54. N. H. Zawia, D. K. Lahiri and F. Cardozo-Pelaez, *Free Radical Biol. Med.*, 2009, **46**, 1241–1249.
55. G. G. Glenner and C. W. Wong, *Biochem. Biophys. Res. Commun.*, 1984, **122**, 1131–1135.
56. D. J. Selkoe, C. R. Abraham, M. B. Podlisny and L. K. Duffy, *J. Neurochem.*, 1986, **46**, 1820–1834.
57. R. E. Tanzi, J. F. Gusella, P. C. Watkins, G. A. Bruns, P. St George-Hyslop, M. L. Van Keuren, D. Patterson, S. Pagan, D. M. Kurnit and R. L. Neve, *Science*, 1987, **235**, 880–884.
58. M. R. Basha, W. Wei, S. A. Bakheet, N. Benitez, H. K. Siddiqi, Y. W. Ge, D. K. Lahiri and N. H. Zawia, *J. Neurosci.*, 2005, **25**, 823–829.
59. J. Wu, M. R. Basha, B. Brock, D. P. Cox, F. Cardozo-Pelaez, C. A. McPherson, J. Harry, D. C. Rice, B. Maloney, D. Chen, D. K. Lahiri and N. H. Zawia, *J. Neurosci.*, 2008, **28**, 3–9.
60. H. Tohgi, K. Utsugisawa, Y. Nagane, M. Yoshimura, Y. Genda and M. Ukitsu, *Brain Research. Molecular Brain Research*, 1999, **70**, 288–292.
61. V. N. Adonaylo and P. I. Oteiza, *Toxicology*, 1999, **132**, 19–32.
62. G. J. Quinlan, B. Halliwell, C. P. Moorhouse and J. M. Gutteridge, *Biochim. Biophys. Acta.*, 1988, **962**, 196–200.
63. L. J. Lawton and W. E. Donaldson, *Biol. Trace Elem. Res.*, 1991, **28**, 83–97.
64. Z. Ni, S. Hou, C. H. Barton and N. D. Vaziri, *Kidney Int.*, 2004, **66**, 2329–2236.
65. N. D. Vaziri, C. Y. Lin, F. Farmand and R. K. Sindhu, *Kidney Int.*, 2003, **63**, 186–194.
66. M. Ahamed and M. K. Siddiqui, *Clin. Chim. Acta*, 2007, **383**, 57–64.

67. A. C. Anderson, S. M. Pueschel and J. G. Linakis, in *Lead Poisoning in Children,* eds. S. M. Pueschel, J. G. Linakis, A. C. Anderson and P.H. Brookes, Baltimore, 1996, pp. 75–96.
68. D. A. Fox, M. L. Campbell and Y. S. Blocker, *Neurotoxicology*, 1997, **18**, 645–664.
69. L. He, A. T. Poblenz, C. J. Medrano and D. A. Fox, *J. Biol. Chem.*, 2000, **275**, 12175–12184.
70. E. K. Silbergeld, *FASEB J.*, 1992, **6**, 3201–3206.
71. A. Navas-Acien, E. Guallar, E. K. Silbergeld and S. J. Rothenberg, *Environ. Health Perspect.*, 2007, **115**, 472–482.
72. A. McCaddon and C. L. Kelly, *Med. Hypotheses*, 1992, **37**, 161–165.
73. L. Parnetti, T. Bottiglieri and D. Lowenthal, *Aging (Milano, Italy)*, 1997, **9**, 241–257.
74. J. M. Balbus-Kornfeld, W. Stewart, K. I. Bolla and B. S. Schwartz, *Occup. Environ. Med.*, 1995, **52**, 2–12.
75. R. K. Byers and E. E. Lord, *Am. J. Dis. Child.*, 1943, **66**, 471–494.
76. D. C. Bellinger and A. M. Bellinger, *J. Clin. Invest.*, 2006, **116**, 853–857.
77. W. J. Rogan, K. N. Dietrich, J. H. Ware, D. W. Dockery, M. Salganik, J. Radcliffc, R. L. Jones, N. B. Ragan, J. J. Chisolm, Jr. and G. G. Rhoads, *N. Engl. J. Med.*, 2001, **344**, 1421–1426.
78. M. Meyer-Baron and A. Seeber, *Arch. Toxicol.*, 2001, **75**, 441–442.
79. M. Goodman, N. LaVerda and J. Mandel, *Arch. Toxicol.*, 2001, **75**, 439–442.
80. R. A. Shih, H. Hu, M. G. Weisskopf and B. S. Schwartz, *Environ. Health Perspect.*, 2007, **115**, 483–942.
81. W. F. Stewart and B. S. Schwartz, *Am. J. Ind. Med.*, 2007, **50**, 729–739.
82. N. Khalil, L. A. Morrow, H. Needleman, E. O. Talbott, J. W. Wilson and J. A. Cauley, *Neuropsychology*, 2009, **23**, 10–109.
83. W. F. Stewart, B. S. Schwartz, C. Davatzikos, D. Shen, D. Liu, X. Wu, A. C. Todd, W. Shi, S. Bassett and D. Youssem, *Neurology*, 2006, **66**, 1476–1484.
84. B. Caffo, S. Chen, W. Stewart, K. Bolla, D. Yousem, C. Davatzikos and B. S. Schwartz, *Am. J. Epidemiol.*, 2008, **167**, 429–437.
85. B. S. Schwartz, B. Caffo, W. F. Stewart, H. Hedlin, B. D. James, D. Yousem and C. Davatzikos, *J. Occup. Environ. Med.*, 2010, **52**, 407–414.
86. M. G. Weisskopf, H. Hu, R. V. Mulkern, R. White, A. Aro, S. Oliveira and R. O. Wright, *Environ. Health Perspect.*, 2004, **112**, 620–625.
87. T. J. Hsieh, Y. C. Chen, C. W. Li, G. C. Liu, Y. W. Chiu and H. Y. Chuang, *Environ. Health Perspect.*, 2009, **117**, 941–945.
88. R. Brookmeyer, S. Gray and C. Kawas, *Am. J. Public Health*, 1998, **88**, 1337–1342.
89. L. E. Hebert, P. A. Scherr, J. L. Bienias, D. A. Bennett and D. A. Evans, *Arch. Neurol.*, 2003, **60**, 1119–1122.
90. R. T. Linn, P. A. Wolf, D. L. Bachman, J. E. Knoefel, J. L. Cobb, A. J. Belanger, E. F. Kaplan and R. B. D'Agostino, *Arch. Neurol.*, 1995, **52**, 485–490.
91. B. J. Small, L. Fratiglioni, M. Viitanen, B. Winblad and L. Backman, *Arch. Neurol.*, 2000, **57**, 839–844.

92. D. A. Bennett, R. S. Wilson, J. A. Schneider, D. A. Evans, L. A. Beckett, N. T. Aggarwal, L. L. Barnes, J. H. Fox and J. Bach, *Neurology*, 2002, **59**, 198–205.
93. C. H. Kawas, M. M. Corrada, R. Brookmeyer, A. Morrison, S. M. Resnick, A. B. Zonderman and D. Arenberg, *Neurology*, 2003, **60**, 1089–1093.
94. M. Mazumdar, D. C. Bellinger, M. Gregas, K. Abanilla, J. Bacic and H. L. Needleman, *Environ. Health*, 2011, **10**, 24.
95. M. Mazumdar, W. Xia, O. Hofmann, M. Gregas, S. Ho Sui, W. Hide, T. Yang, H. L. Needleman and D. C. Bellinger, *Environ. Health Perspect.*, 2012, **120**(5), 702–707.
96. S. Gao, Y. Jin, F. W. Unverzagt, F. Ma, K. S. Hall, J. R. Murrell, Y. Cheng, J. Shen, B. Ying, R. Ji, J. Matesan, C. Liang and H. C. Hendrie, *J. Gerontol., Ser. A*, 2008, **63**, 635–641.
97. E. van Wijngaarden, P. C. Winters and D. A. Cory-Slechta, *Neurotoxicology*, 2011, **32**, 110–115.
98. F. Barbosa, Jr. and J. E. Tanus-Santos, *et al.*, A critical review of biomarkers used for monitoring human exposure to lead: advantages, limitations, and future needs. *Environ. Health Perspect.*, 2005, **113**(12), 1669–1674.
99. D. Smith, M. Hernandez-Avila, M. M. Tellez-Rojo, A. Mercado and H. Hu, *Environ. Health Perspect.*, 2002, **110**, 263–268.
100. E. van Wijngaarden, J. R. Campbell and D. A. Cory-Slechta, *Neurotoxicology*, 2009, **30**, 572–580.
101. J. Weuve, S. A. Korrick, M. A. Weisskopf, L. M. Ryan, J. Schwartz, H. Nie, F. Grodstein and H. Hu, *Environ. Health Perspect.*, 2009, **117**, 574–580.
102. K. Bandeen-Roche, T. A. Glass, K. I. Bolla, A. C. Todd and B. S. Schwartz, *Epidemiology*, 2009, **20**, 831–839.
103. M. G. Weisskopf, H. Hu, D. Sparrow, R. E. Lenkinski and R. O. Wright, *Environ. Health Perspect.*, 2007, **115**, 519–523.
104. K. Kantarci, C. R. Jack, Jr., Y. C. Xu, N. G. Campeau, P. C. O'Brien, G. E. Smith, R. J. Ivnik, B. F. Boeve, E. Kokmen, E. G. Tangalos and R. C. Petersen, *Neurology*, 2000, **55**, 210–217.
105. D. A. Cory-Slechta, S. Stern, D. Weston and J. L. Allen, S. Liu, *Toxicol. Sci.*, 2010, **117**, 427–438.
106. D. A. Cory-Slechta, M. B. Virgolini, A. Rossi-George, M. Thiruchelvam, R. Lisek and D. Weston, *Basic Clin. Pharmacol. Toxicol.*, 2008, **102**, 218–227.
107. M. B. Virgolini, A. Rossi-George, R. Lisek, D. D. Weston, M. Thiruchelvam and D. A. Cory-Slechta, *Neurotoxicology*, 2008, **29**, 812–827.
108. S. J. Lupien, M. de Leon, S. de Santi, A. Convit, C. Tarshish, N. P. Nair, M. Thakur, B. S. McEwen, R. L. Hauger and M. J. Meaney, *Nat. Neurosci.*, 1998, **1**, 69–73.
109. B. S. McEwen and P. J. Gianaros, *Annu. Rev. Med.*, 2011, **62**, 431–445.
110. M. B. Virgolini, M. R. Bauter, D. D. Weston and D. A. Cory-Slechta, *Neurotoxicology*, 2006, **27**, 11–21.

111. B. B. Gump, P. Stewart, J. Reihman, E. Lonky, T. Darvill, P. J. Parsons and D. A. Granger, *Environ. Health Perspect.*, 2008, **116**, 249–255.
112. M. B. Virgolini, A. Rossi-George, D. Weston and D. A. Cory-Slechta, *Neurotoxicology*, 2008, **29**, 928–939.
113. P. J. Bushnell, S. E. Shelton and R. E. Bowman, *Bull. Environ. Contam. Toxicol.*, 1979, **22**, 819–826.
114. T. A. Glass, K. Bandeen-Roche, M. McAtee, K. Bolla, A. C. Todd and B. S. Schwartz, *Am. J. Epidemiol.*, 2009, **169**, 683–692.
115. J. L. Peters, M. G. Weisskopf, A. Spiro, 3rd, J. Schwartz, D. Sparrow, H. Nie, H. Hu, R. O. Wright and R. J. Wright, *Environ. Health Perspect.*, 2010, **118**, 505–510.
116. W. F. Stewart, B. S. Schwartz, D. Simon, K. Kelsey and A. C. Todd, *Environ. Health Perspect.*, 2002, **110**, 501–505.
117. L. Bertram, M. B. McQueen, K. Mullin, D. Blacker and R. E. Tanzi, *Nat. Genet.*, 2007, **39**, 17–23.
118. F. T. Wang, H. Hu, J. Schwartz, J. Weuve, A. S. Spiro, D. Sparrow, H. Nie, E. K. Silverman, S. T. Weiss and R. O. Wright, *Environ. Health Perspect.*, 2007, **115**, 1210–1215.
119. J. G. Wetmur, A. H. Kaya, M. Plewinska and R. J. Desnick, *Am. J. Hum. Genet.*, 1991, **49**, 757–763.
120. J. G. Wetmur, *Environ. Health Perspect.*, 1994, **102**(Suppl 3), 215–219.
121. A. O. Onalaja and L. Claudio, *Environ. Health Perspect.*, 2000, **108**(Suppl 1), 23–28.
122. S. E. Chia, E. Yap and K. S. Chia, *Neurotoxicology*, 2004, **25**, 1041–1047.
123. T. Sakai, Y. Morita, T. Araki, M. Kano and T. Yoshida, *Am. J. Ind. Med.*, 2000, **38**, 355–360.
124. P. Sithisarankul, B. S. Schwartz, B. K. Lee, K. T. Kelsey and P. T. Strickland, *Am. J. Ind. Med.*, 1997, **32**, 15–20.
125. J. Weuve, K. T. Kelsey, J. Schwartz, D. Bellinger, R. O. Wright, P. Rajan, A. Spiro, 3rd, D. Sparrow, A. Aro and H. Hu, *Occup. Environ. Med.*, 2006, **63**, 746–753.
126. P. Rajan, K. T. Kelsey, J. D. Schwartz, D. C. Bellinger, J. Weuve, A. Spiro, 3rd, D. Sparrow, T. J. Smith, H. Nie, M. G. Weisskopf, H. Hu and R. O. Wright, *J. Occup. Environ. Med.*, 2008, **50**, 1053–1061.
127. E. F. Krieg, Jr., M. A. Butler, M. H. Chang, T. Liu, A. Yesupriya, M. L. Lindegren and N. Dowling, *Neurotoxicol. Teratol.*, 2009, **31**, 364–371.
128. G. Zheng, L. Tian, Y. Liang, K. Broberg, L. Lei, W. Guo, J. Nilsson, I. A. Bergdahl, S. Skerfving and T. Jin, *Neurotoxicology*, 2011, **32**, 374–382.
129. S. D. Grosse, T. D. Matte, J. Schwartz and R. J. Jackson, *Environ. Health Perspect.*, 2002, **110**, 563–569.
130. B. P. Lanphear, *Environ. Health Perspect.*, 2007, **115**, A484–A485.
131. B. P. Lanphear, R. Hornung, J. Khoury, K. Yolton, P. Baghurst, D. C. Bellinger, R. L. Canfield, K. N. Dietrich, R. Bornschein, T. Greene, S. J. Rothenberg, H. L. Needleman, L. Schnaas, G. Wasserman, J. Graziano and R. Roberts, *Environ. Health Perspect.*, 2005, **113**, 894–899.

132. Advisory Committee on Childhood Lead Poisoning Prevention, "Low Level Lead Exposure Harms Children: a Renewed Call for Primary Prevention" (Centers for Disease Control and Prevention, 2012).
133. B. S. Schwartz and H. Hu, *Environ. Health Perspect.*, 2007, **115**, 451–454.
134. American College of Occupational and Environmental Medicine Task Force on Blood Lead, "Recommendation to OSHA Regarding Blood Lead Levels" (American College of Occupational and Environmental Medicine, 2010).
135. P. Muntner, A. Menke, K. B. DeSalvo, F. A. Rabito and V. Batuman, *Arch. Intern. Med.*, 2005, **165**, 2155–2161.
136. K. R. Mahaffey, J. L. Annest, J. Roberts and R. S. Murphy, *N. Engl. J. Med.*, 1982, **307**, 573–579.
137. R. A. Shih, T. A. Glass, K. Bandeen-Roche, M. C. Carlson, K. I. Bolla, A. C. Todd and B. S. Schwartz, *Neurology*, 2006, **67**, 1556–1562.
138. J. L. Peters, L. D. Kubzansky, A. Ikeda, A. Spiro, 3rd, R. O. Wright, M. G. Weisskopf, D. Kim, D. Sparrow, L. H. Nie, H. Hu and J. Schwartz, *Am. J. Epidemiol.*, 2011, **174**, 1345–1353.
139. *MMWR Morb Mortal Wkly Rep.*, 2005, **54**, 513–516.
140. Centers for Disease Control and Prevention, "Fourth National Report on Human Exposure to Environmental Chemicals, Updated Tables, February 2012" (Atlanta, Georgia, 2012).
141. M. Bouchard, F. Laforest, L. Vandelac, D. Bellinger and D. Mergler, *Environ. Health Perspect.*, 2007, **115**, 122–127.

CHAPTER 2

Cognitive Deterioration and Related Neuropathology in Older People with Alzheimer's Disease could Result from Life-Long Exposure to Aluminium Compounds

J. R. WALTON

University of New South Wales, St George Hospital Campus, Sydney, NSW 2217, Australia
E-mail: j.walton@unsw.edu.au

2.1 Introduction

Some records are available that reliably describe the health of older humans in the early industrial era. A monograph entitled *Old Age*, published in Cambridge in 1889, and papers published in the *British Medical Journal* between 1886 and 1889 describe results of a health survey carried out by the British Medical Council,[1] where British general practitioners systematically assessed the health of their oldest patients during the mid-1880s. The study group consisted of almost 900 subjects, aged 80 years and older, including 74 centenarians.

Issues in Toxicology No. 16
Aging and Vulnerability to Environmental Chemicals: Age-related Disorders and their Origins in Environmental Exposures
Edited by Bernard Weiss

Published by the Royal Society of Chemistry, www.rsc.org

The author states: "[Dementia, the] saddest state of all, was witnessed only in two of our centenarians... Indeed, the brain in many held out as well or better than other organs – which may be regarded one of the bright rays, if not the brightest, in the centenarian landscape". In contrast, a study conducted at the beginning of the 21st century found that 88%, of all centenarians, or 15 out of the 17, living in three Dutch towns with populations of at least 250 000 had dementia and the other two could not be examined.[2] This dementia increase could relate to living conditions that changed during the 20th century.

Before the industrial era, most humans lived in villages, towns and developing cities, where they consumed food produced from their own gardens or market gardens, and from local or traded farm crops. They drank water from naturally-occurring sources (rivers, springs and ground water from wells) and without chemical treatment. Urban life today has changed again with the increasing consolidation of industrialized products and practices, including drinking water treatment, industrialized food production and marketing, pharmaceutical treatments (as opposed to herbal treatments), and greater reliance on vaccinations and topical applications to treat or prevent medical problems.

Such change in human behaviors can significantly alter the prevalence of a disease in a relatively short time span, such as one to three decades. Between 1997 and 2010, health behaviors, such as dietary choices and rates of physical exercise, increased the number of overweight or obese adults from 42% to 54% in the Australian state of New South Wales. The number of overweight or obese adults correlates with a greater prevalence of self-reported diabetes, which rose from 4.7% to 7.4% over the same 13 year time period in this largely urban population.[3]

In 1907, Alzheimer described a 51–year old woman as the first known case of the disease that now bears his name as a new phenomenon, stating, "The case presented even in the clinic such a different picture, that it could not be categorised under known disease headings, and also anatomically it provided a result which departed from all previously known disease pathology."[4] Several years later, Alzheimer realized that Alzheimer's Disease (AD) also affects older patients, writing, "Similar cases of disease appear in advanced age".[5] Over the 20th century, the prevalence of AD markedly increased in industrialized countries with little if any prevalence in rural regions of some developing countries.[6,7] Estimates indicate that 35.6 million people throughout the world are currently living with dementia.[8] Around 75% of this population,[9] or 27 million people, are currently affected by AD.

Epidemiological studies based on identical and fraternal twin pairs have consistently shown that AD causality has both environmental and genetic components.[10–12] The vast majority of AD patients have late-onset "sporadic AD", lacking the mutations found in familial AD, a minority subgroup with autosomal dominant inheritance and early-onset AD. The observation that old age is a main risk factor for AD has prompted the suggestion that AD involves accrual of a toxic substance that produces biological insult on brain tissue over time.[13] Aluminium (Al) is a candidate for that role.

2.2 The Context for Aluminium in AD Causality

Aluminium, an element that is non-essential to cell metabolism, is classified as definitely neurotoxic to humans.[14] Al salts have been linked to AD causality since 1973,[15] and they remain the most likely candidate for AD's environmental component. The genetic component may represent how well the individual's body is able to absorb, exclude or chelate Al and limit its effects therein. Al salts are now available for many applications in everyday life.

In 1906, the US Congress passed the Food and Drugs Act, which prohibits the use of poisonous agents in confectionery and for coloring food. Responsibility for enforcing this act was given to the United States Food and Drug Administration (FDA), established in 1927.[16]

There were warnings against Al usage both well before and around that time.[17,18] For example, a Columbia University biochemist wrote: "During a period of about seven years I have occasionally conducted experiments on the effects of aluminium salts. These studies have convinced me that the use in food of alum or any other aluminium compound is a dangerous practice. That the aluminium ion is very toxic is well known. That 'aluminized' food yields soluble aluminium compounds to gastric juice (and stomach contents) has been demonstrated. That such soluble aluminium is in part absorbed and carried to all parts of the body by the blood can no longer be doubted. That the organism can 'tolerate' such treatment without suffering harmful consequences has not been shown. It is believed that the facts in this paper will give emphasis to my conviction that aluminium should be excluded from food".[19] The US FDA rates Al as "GRAS" (Generally Recognized As Safe), despite the early warnings about Al and subsequent publications on Al neurotoxicity.

Government regulatory agencies currently allow various Al compounds to be included in store-bought and take-away foods, bottled waters and urban drinking water supplies. Al compounds have versatile properties and serve many useful functions in these applications: as anti-caking agents in salt, coffee whitener, pancake mix and other powdered foods, emulsifiers and melting agents in cheeses, clarifying agents in water, puddings and other processed foods where precipitates may form, pickling agents, meat binders for sausages and luncheon meats, hardening agents for candied fruits, gravy and sauce thickeners, rising agents in baking powder, self-raising flour and baked goods, as buffering and neutralizing agents and as an agent that binds food dyes to confectionaries to make them colorful.

Americans, representative of humans living in a contemporary westernized society, consume 1–10 mg Al each day from natural sources such as fresh fruits, vegetables and meat.[20] In addition, 50% of Americans are now estimated to consume up to 25 mg per day, 45% between 25 and 95 mg per day, and 5% more than 95 mg per day in the form of additives.[20,21] For an average-sized (70 kg) human, these amounts involve up to 0.4 mg kg^{-1} bodyweight (bw) per day, between 0.4 and 1.5 mg kg^{-1} bw per day, and more than 1.5 mg kg^{-1} bw per day or more, respectively. Higher and lower estimates of total dietary Al ingestion have been reported. The described figures are more accurate since these estimates consider survey data from food manufacturers listing Al quantity added.[22]

Other significant sources of Al exposure are Al-based pharmaceuticals, topical applications, Al-adjuvanted vaccines and certain other medical treatments, including some that have caused fatal encephalopathies.[23,24]

2.2.1 Some Ingested Al is Absorbed into Blood and Taken up by the Brain

2.2.1.1 Al Absorption into Plasma

The body's first and main line of defence against dietary Al is the mucus layer that lines the gastrointestinal tract (GIT). GIT mucus traps most ingested Al, including precipitates of larger Al complexes[25] that are excreted together with enterocyes that have sloughed from the GIT lining and undigested food.[26]

Soluble Al salts (*e.g.* Al sulfate, or "alum", and Al chloride) more readily traverse the mucus layer and are more easily absorbed than poorly soluble salts (*e.g.* Al phosphate). Salts of Al with food acids, in particular Al citrate, Al lactate and Al maltolate, remain soluble over a relatively wide pH range, including neutrality. Some Al-food acid salts, previously available only in minute amounts, are now synthesized for use as food additives. Even poorly soluble forms can raise plasma Al levels in normal humans.[27] As we shall see, routine Al exposure, particularly at the high end of the human dietary Al range, can overwhelm the protective barrier of the GIT mucus layer.

Normally, 0.1% to 0.3% of ingested Al passes through the mucus layer and enterocyte lining of the GIT to reach the circulation.[28,29] Some plasma Al is available for uptake into the brain and other tissues. Al values in the plasma or serum of typical humans are usually 6 $\mu g\,L^{-1}$ or less.[30] Around 80–85% of absorbed Al binds to transferrin (Al-transferrin), an iron transport protein, about 10% to albumin and 5% to low molecular weight species, mainly citrate, that are excretable by the kidneys.[31,32]

Many experiments have shown that some asymptomatic humans and laboratory animals have plasma or serum Al levels that are 2- to 3-fold higher than others after ingesting a standardized amount of Al (for an example, see Figure 2.1[33]). Efficient Al absorption may increase an individual's susceptibility to chronic Al neurotoxicity and/or AD.

2.2.1.2 Al Uptake into the Brain

Approximately 0.01% of plasma Al passes through the blood-brain barrier into the brain.[34] Al uptake into the human brain from drinking a single glass of alum-treated water was simulated by gavaging rats with nanomolar quantities of aqueous ^{26}Al, a synthetic radioactive tracer.[35] Measurable ^{26}Al levels were detected in the rat brains two weeks later.The presence of ^{26}Al in brain tissue can only be explained by ^{26}Al exposure, since it is virtually absent in nature. Other laboratories have confirmed brain ^{26}Al uptake following oral ^{26}Al consumption.[36,37]

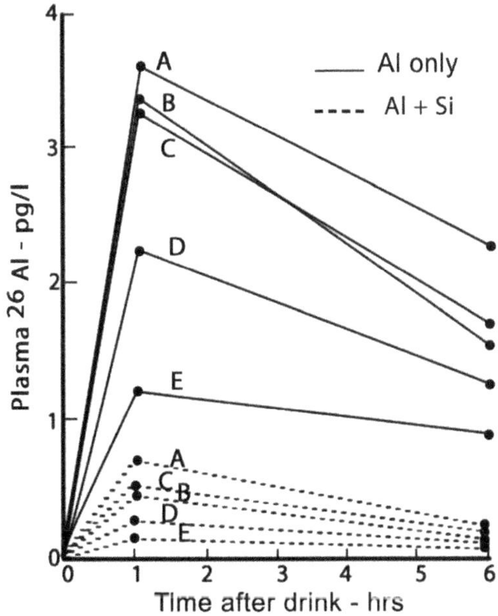

Figure 2.1 Plasma ^{26}Al levels in humans who drank ^{26}alum-treated water and then ^{26}alum-treated water supplemented by silica. Silica lowers the amount of Al absorbed. Note the spread of values from A to E. Notice that the ranking of subjects' absorption values is almost in the same order under both conditions.
Reproduced from reference 33 with permission from Elsevier.

Al exposure occurs continuously throughout life. Many newborn humans, with their immature blood-brain barriers, are exposed to Al. Sucklings take up Al from their mothers' milk[38] and from soy-based infant formulae that have Al levels of up to 700 μg L^{1}.[39] Infants are injected with a course of Al-adjuvanted diphtheria-pertussis-tetanus (DPT) vaccines.[40] Injections bypass the mucus and enterocyte barriers of the intestine, increasing the exposure level to a given dose of bioavailable Al up to 1000 fold. Intraperitoneal injection of a simulated Al hydroxide-adjuvanted DPT vaccine into mice produces a surge in their brain Al level that peaks at 2–3 days post-injection.[41]

Each individual exposure, from one vaccine with an Al adjuvant, or one meal containing Al-rich foods, might produce an insignificant effect with respect to the risk of developing dementia; but above all, cumulative exposure from multiple sources,—such as decades of exposure to alum-treated drinking water—leads to slow but progressive Al increase in the brain. Brain Al measurements confirm that more Al enters the brain than exits, resulting in a gradual net Al accumulation in the hippocampus and cortex with advancing age, even in the brains of non-demented controls.[15,42–44] Brain concentrations of the essential metals remain stable or decrease with age.[45] The significant age-related increase in brain Al that occurs reflects accumulation from the environment.

Al is already the recognized cause of another dementia, dialysis encephalopathy, or dialysis dementia.[46] It is also a contributing factor to other dementias, including amyotrophic lateral sclerosis/parkinsonism-dementia (ALS/PD) of Guam[47–49] and Balint's syndrome, which results from occupational Al exposure.[50]

2.2.1.3 Al accumulates in Aged Pyramidal Neurons either Without or With Neurofibrillary Tangles (NFTs)

Al can be visualized in most large pyramidal cells, particularly in the cortex and hippocampus of aged humans and laboratory animals, processed either with the Walton histological stain for Al or a monoclonal antibody stain for Al.[51–54] Al is first recognizable in the nucleolus and later in the condensed chromatin of post-mortem human pyramidal cells. As Al continues to accumulate, it distributes throughout the nucleoplasm of cells without NFTs.[52–54] Eighty-nine percent of ^{26}Al in rat neurons was observed to be chromatin-bound following subcutaneous injection of ^{26}Al.[55] Rat and human hippocampal and cortical pyramidal neurons without NFTs show the same stages of nuclear Al accumulation (Figure 2.2).[54]

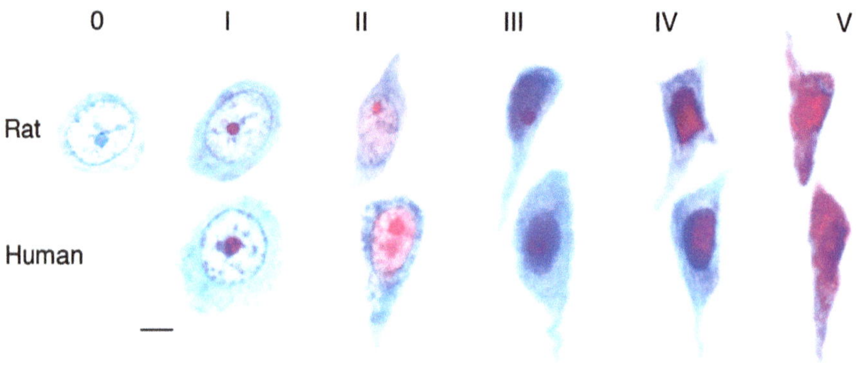

Figure 2.2 Stages of Al accumulation in rat and human hippocampal neurons. Stage I: All sections of hippocampal pyramidal neurons from older human brain, that contained a visible nucleolus, exhibited at least stage I Al accumulation (staining only the nucleolus). Neuronal shape appears normal in stage I cells. Stages II and III: The nucleoplasm progressively deepens in hue, appearing pink at stage II and purple at stage III. The nucleus and overall cell shape show subtle shrinkage and dendritic changes at these stages. Stages IV and V: By stage IV, the nuclear Al appears bright magenta. The cell is obviously shrunken and its neurites appear tortuous and retracted. At stage V, Al is distributed throughout the nucleus plus cytoplasm. These deformed cells are still viable (exhibiting neither necrosis nor apoptosis) but are apparently dysfunctional as they no longer immunostain for neuron-specific proteins. Magnification bar = 5 μM. Reproduced from reference 54 with permission from Elsevier.

Al also appears in the cytoplasm of cells able to form NFTs, specifically staining these fibrillar structures.[56] NFT formation affects only a portion of the pyramidal cells in the AD hippocampal CA1 field and cortex. Pyramidal cells that either exhibit Al in the form of NFTs or throughout the nucleus (stages IV and V) first appear sporadically, then in clusters and eventually as large bands of cells.[54,57–59] Al-affected cell bands are referred to here as "lesions". Before exploring potential consequences of these lesions it is useful to review the nature of Al toxicity.

2.3 Al Neurotoxicity

Ionic Al (Al^{3+}) is regarded as the most toxic form of Al. Al^{3+} has unique physical properties. Neurotoxicity of Al^{3+} usually requires chronic exposure as most Al activity depends on its accumulation in brain cells, unlike many other toxicants and toxins that produce acute systemic effects.[60]

2.3.1 Al Disrupts Cell Metabolism by Substituting for Essential Metal Ions in Key Regulatory Proteins

Al^{3+} is a small ion with a high (3+) fixed charge.[61] Picomolar quantities of Al can successfully compete with the mM quantities of Mg^{2+} that occur in cells.[62] The small size of Al allows it to substitute for essential metal ions such as Mg^{2+} in active sites of proteins and protein co-factors such as ATP and GTP.[63,64]

Mg^{2+} regulates over 300 proteins, giving Al^{3+} many opportunities to disrupt cellular metabolism. The larger electrochemical charge of Al^{3+} results in a much higher association constant than that of Mg^{2+} for Mg^{2+} binding sites. The association constant of Al for GTP and transducin is approximately 10^7 times higher than that for Mg^{2+}, the physiological regulator of microtubules within neurons. This allows Al^{3+} to substitute for Mg^{2+} in the Mg^{2+}/GTP/tubulin complex,[64] with damaging consequences for microtubule function.

Al^{3+} dissociates from biological ligands 10^5 times more slowly than Mg^{2+} and 10^8 times more slowly than Ca^{2+}.[61] Rapid dissociation is required for biological reactions, and the slow dissociation of Al^{3+} from its biological ligands precludes Al^{3+} from being useful in cellular metabolism.

2.3.2 Al Produces Oxidative Damage in Cells

Al^{3+} is a highly reactive ion. The nearly maximal charge density of ionic Al promotes its binding to almost any oxygen or nitrogen atom.[60] Al generates reactive oxygen species (ROS) despite its non-redox status.[65] Al^{3+} acts as a strong Lewis acid, attracting pairs of electrons from oxygen in phosphates and other small ligand groups. Al is thus a pro-oxidant, both on its own and synergistically with iron.[65–67] In view of its Lewis acidity, $AlO_2^{\bullet 2+}$ is expected to be a stronger oxidant than either $HO_2^{-\bullet}$ or $O_2^{-\bullet}$.[67] Al facilitates the production of the superoxide ion ($O_2^{-\bullet}$) in biological oxidations that can be photochemical, enzymatic, chemical or biomolecular.[67–69] Al oxidative reactions are countered by superoxide dismutase and vitamin E.[67,70,71]

Al^{3+} cross-links proteins with proteins, proteins with nucleic acids, and nucleic acids with each other.[72] Al has polymerizing properties, *e.g.* as a Ziegler-Natta catalyst. Al has a particularly high affinity for myelin membranes[73] and Al incorporation in membranes changes their fluidity. Al^{3+} can thus a substitute for essential metals in important regulatory reactions in cells and cause oxidative damage.

2.3.3 All Epidemiological Studies Evaluating the Al Exposure-AD Link have been Based on Crude Estimates of Single Sources of Al Exposure and are Rife with Confounders

The highest standard of proof is generally considered to be a prospective, well-designed, randomly-controlled study, based on a large number of participants. We need to consider whether this standard is reasonable and necessary for assessing the toxicity of neurotoxicants, particularly those with a long prodromal phase.

Many epidemiological studies have already investigated the putative relationship between Al ingestion and an increased risk for AD (reviewed by Flaten).[74] Most of these studies have shown an increased risk of AD in people who have routinely consumed water containing more than $0.1\,mg\,L^{-1}$Al.

To date, the most rigorous of these studies was conducted by Rondeau and her colleagues[75] and consisted of a prospective trial carried out on a sample of 1925 normal subjects at baseline, with 15 years of follow-up. The study showed that the risk for cognitive decline was significantly greater in subjects that lived in districts supplied by water with an Al content greater than $0.1\ mg\,L^{-1}$ and/or drank bottled waters clarified by alum, compared to those living in a region supplied by water with a lower Al content ($p=0.005$).[75] Food Al was not taken into account.

A single study has investigated AD risk in subjects who routinely consumed processed foods with high levels of Al additives. In this case, water Al levels were not taken into account. The crude odds ratio of this small case-control study was equal to 8.6 when adjusted for covariates.[76]

Most routine exposure to Al is from the diet: from food, water and Al additives. Each of the epidemiological studies performed to date has investigated a single source of Al exposure, usually Al levels in drinking water. While their almost-consistent results suggest a relationship between chronic Al exposure and AD, all are plagued by confounding factors that make the relationship appear considerably weaker than it probably is.

Epidemiological studies that take into account human exposure to total dietary Al^{3+} from both food and drinking water have yet to be carried out. Such studies are necessary to control for confounding. Otherwise, studies based on people who live in a region with low Al content in their municipal drinking water supply (the low Al group) may consume a fast food diet with Al-rich foods and drink alum-treated bottled water; this would elevate their plasma Al levels and cancel out the potentially beneficial effect of low Al content in the public drinking water supply. Thus, unless total Al ingestion from all dietary Al sources is taken into consideration, the results are severely confounded.

2.3.4 A Randomly Controlled Human Study of Total Chronic Al Exposure would be Impractical to Perform and Most Likely be Unethical

Information as to whether or not the total dietary amounts of Al that contemporary humans routinely ingest can be safely tolerated over the life span could theoretically be obtained in a human study that requires the participants to measure and record the total amount of Al they consume each day from their food and beverages, including water and Al additives. An accurate study would take five to eight decades to complete. This should be sufficient to learn whether, and how, people are affected in old age from continuous Al exposure over the life span.

Such studies would be made more difficult by dietary products that are constantly entering and leaving the marketplace. Humans have very different lifestyles and are exposed to Al in many different forms, some without their knowledge. Current labeling laws do not require the Al content of packaged foods to be revealed in milligram quantities. Al additives on food packaging are only identified by code numbers in some countries. Thus, the task of determining how much Al one routinely consumes from their foods and beverages would be close to insurmountable.

The second approach would require groups of blinded human subjects to adhere to one of several prescribed diets that provide specific amounts of low, medium and high levels of Al additives, contained in measured amounts of food and drinking water, throughout their youth, middle age and old age. If true that AD is a form of human aluminum neurotoxicity, a dose-dependent effect should occur with more subjects in the high Al group developing AD. This approach would obviously be impractical to administer and unethical to perform. Nevertheless, that is what would be needed for a human study to convincingly prove that aluminum causes AD.

Participants of the study would have to restrict their caloric intake to the prescribed dietary regimen over the five or more decades of the study and would also have to measure and record the amounts of food and water they consume.

Ganrot[60] notes the difficulty in performing such a study, of a disease with insidious onset that requires decades of exposure to an etiological agent (to which most humans are abundantly exposed) and to then link the disease to that agent.

It is therefore necessary, and much more convenient, to rely on long-term studies involving surrogate animals given known amounts of Al at equivalent levels and duration to those experienced by humans, thus mimicking human Al exposure conditions.

2.3.5 Surrogate Animals are Required to Investigate the Effects of Chronic Exposure to the Al Neurotoxicant

Towards this end we carried out two animal studies: a pilot study[77] with two rat groups, and a main study[78] with three rat groups. Both were designed as randomly-controlled longitudinal studies to learn whether outbred Wistar rats could age successfully while ingesting known quantities of Al—at equivalent levels to those routinely ingested by humans from their foods and beverages, including alum-treated drinking water—throughout much of their lives. Al treatment was postponed until early middle age in order to ensure normal brain development. Inclusion criteria included: (1) survival till at least age 28 months and (2) ability to complete the 11–choice rewarded continuous alternation T-maze task within five minutes. The experimental design and timeline for treatment of rats in the main study are shown in Figure 2.3.

At age 6 months, the rats were trained to perform the continuous alternation T-maze task,[78] which is commonly used to assess memory performance.[79] They were fed twice weekly from this age onwards, with their diet consisting of measured amounts of a feed formulated for mature animals, in quantities just sufficient to maintain their bodies at a healthy weight of 500 ± 50 g. The Al content of their feed was 9 ppm. With this protocol the rats drank some water on an empty stomach[77,78] to simulate its consumption by humans, who often drink water on a fasted stomach. The low pH of the empty stomach increases the ionic Al^{3+} level of ingested alum-treated drinking water and facilitates Al^{3+} absorption.[36,61] Some rats on this protocol developed cognitive deterioration in old age after chronic Al exposure; this is described in more detail in the next section.

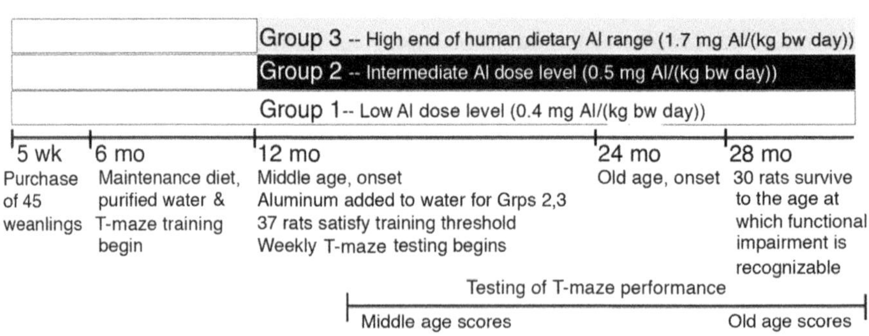

Figure 2.3 Experimental design and timeline for treatment of the three rat groups. Reproduced from reference 78 with permission from Elsevier.

2.4 Evidence that Supports Al Causality of AD

2.4.1 Cognitive Deterioration in Animals with Chronic Al Neurotoxicity and Humans with AD is Associated with More Efficient Al Absorption and Higher Serum/Plasma Al Levels

2.4.1.1 Al Absorption in Humans with AD

^{26}Al absorption measurements showed that AD-affected humans absorbed 1.4 times as much ^{26}Al from a standardized ^{26}Al dose contained in an orange drink than age-matched non-demented controls.[80] Plasma and serum Al levels of AD-affected humans were also reported to be higher than in those without AD.[30,81–84] Moreover, serum Al levels were higher in patients with AD than in controls with vascular dementia.[85] Only one small study was unable to find such difference. This study has very low statistical power so it is susceptible to a type II error, *i.e.* a false negative error.[86]

Subjects with Down's syndrome (DS) absorbed 6 times more ^{26}Al than age-matched controls from a dietary Al dose (140 ng) added to a citric drink. The DS group also absorbed four times more Al than age-matched controls from a pharmacological (antacid-sized) dose equating to 280 mg of Al with citrate.[87] DS is commonly regarded as a human model for AD in that DS is associated with an unusually high rate of dementia.[88] DS brains exhibit AD neuropathology prematurely, by 50 years of age.[89]

2.4.1.2 Al Absorption in Rats that Develop Cognitive Deterioration

The serum Al values of the three rat groups[78] in the main study were measured and found to be proportional to the rats' Al dose levels. The high Al group had serum levels that were significantly higher than those of the low Al group ($p < 0.05$). The latter remained cognitively intact. The range of serum Al values for rats in the high Al group was much larger than those of the two lower dose groups. Rats that developed cognitive deterioration also had significantly higher serum Al levels than the low Al rats ($p < 0.01$). Moreover, the rats that developed cognitive deterioration in the intermediate and high Al groups were those with the highest serum Al levels in their treatment group, implying more efficient Al absorption than the others.[78]

2.4.2 Certain Brain Regions Show More Damage than Others in AD and Chronic Al Neurotoxicity

2.4.2.1 Damaged Cell Types and Brain Regions in AD

Pyramidal cells that project over great distances—especially those located in the transentorhinal and entorhinal cortex, hippocampus, subiculum, temporal, parietal and frontal cortices, amygdala, olfactory bulb, nucleus basalis, locus coeruleus and the dorsal raphe nucleus—are particularly damaged in AD.[90,91] These are the regions in humans that show NFT damage.[90,92,93] These brain regions are connected by cortico-cortical projections, implying that pathology in AD brains may spread across synaptic connections.[58]

2.4.2.2 Pyramidal Cells and Stellate Cells in Brain Regions Preferentially Damaged in Humans and Rats with Chronic Al Neurotoxicity and Humans with Renal Failure Associated with High Serum Al Levels are the Same or Equivalent to those Preferentially Damaged in AD

Al is most prone to concentrate in large pyramidal cells, that project over great distances, in the entorhinal cortex, hippocampus, subiculum, temporal, parietal and frontal cortices, amygdala, nucleus basalis, olfactory lobe and other AD-vulnerable brain regions of experimental animals subjected to chronic Al exposure.[78,94] Al also deposits in these brain regions of humans with renal failure, and who have had high serum Al levels arising from their use of Al-based phosphate binders and/or dialysis with Al-contaminated water, despite their limited renal capacity for efficient Al removal.[95,96]

Fe-transferrin and Al-transferrin complexes circulating in the plasma attach to transferrin receptors located on the surface of blood-brain barrier capillaries.[97] The transferrin complexes transcytose the endothelium and enter the neuropil, where they can attach to, and become internalized by, transferrin receptors on large pyramidal cells.[98]

Elevated Al levels in AD cortex and hippocampus have been demonstrated by instrumental Al measurements,[15,44,99] as well as staining techniques.[52–54]

2.4.2.3 Al Levels are Higher in AD-Vulnerable Regions of AD-Affected Brains than in Age-Matched Controls

At least seven laboratories have reported that AD neocortex has higher Al levels than the neocortex of non-demented age-matched controls.[99–105] AD-vulnerable brain regions in AD cases contain mean Al values of approximately $4\,\mu g\,g^{-1}$ brain tissue (dry weight), whereas the same regions in age-matched non-demented cases average $\leq 2\,\mu g\,g^{-1}$ brain tissue.[15,99,100] Approximately 1/4 of the AD samples contain Al levels up to $11\,\mu g\,g^{-1}$ brain tissue.[15]

Thus AD hippocampus and cortex generally contain 1.4 to 4 times more Al than the same regions of controls.[99,100] By comparison, brain Al levels in subjects with dialysis encephalopathy, a condition that develops in renal failure patients over months or 1–2 years, are 10–15 times higher than in controls.[46] The cytotoxic concentration for Al in human neurons is unknown, but in cat cerebral neurons this concentration lies between 4 and $6\,\mu g\,Al\,g^{-1}$ brain (dry weight).[102]

Two studies have reported that AD brains show no more Al than controls.[42,43] Ganrot[60] has described methodological flaws in both studies.

2.4.3 Cognitive Deterioration in AD and Chronic Al Neurotoxicity

2.4.3.1 Cognitive Deterioration in AD

AD is the most common dementia. Neuropathological change in the cerebral cortex and limbic system leads to deficits in learning, memory processing, visuospatial and language skills. The first sign of AD cognitive deterioration is often recognized as short-term memory impairment involving, for example, forgetfulness of recent events. The patient may exhibit confusion, perseverative behaviors and incontinence. At a later stage of the disease, a person with AD may no longer recognize their own image in a mirror. The progression of AD symptoms varies from person to person.

2.4.3.2 Rats that Mimic the Long-Term Total Dietary Al Levels Ingested by Americans can Develop Cognitive Deterioration in Old Age

By the time the rats in our longitudinal study were 12 months of age, they were skillful in their T-maze task performance. At this age they were randomly assigned to three Al treatment groups (low, intermediate and high).[78] The only treatment difference between the animals concerned the quantities of Al they ingested in the form of drinking water. The quantities of water consumed were also measured.

Rat middle age is, by convention, between their 12th and 24th months. Wistar rats age approximately 35 times faster than humans,[106] so middle age for rats is considered to extend from 35 years to 70 years in human age-equivalence. The mean T-maze performance score for all rats was 78% during middle age, indicating that they made almost 8 out of 10 correct choices on each weekly test. During old age, the low Al dose rats exceeded this standard, obtaining a mean score of 82%. None of the rats in the low Al dose group, two (20%) in the intermediate Al dose group and seven (70%) in the group that consumed Al at the high end of the human range for total dietary Al exhibited significantly lower mean scores on their T-maze task in old age than in middle age, as well as showing dementia-like behaviors such as confusion, inability to focus attention on the task, perseverative activities and incontinence while in the T-maze.[†] These are the rats described as having cognitive deterioration.[54,77,78]

T-maze performance scores of the rats that developed cognitive deterioration in old age decreased to 45.5%, indicating that the choice accuracy of these aged

[†]Videos attached to the electronic version of reference 77 show a rat from the high Al group in the T-maze in middle age, then old age, with firstly normal, and subsequently abnormal behaviors.

rats was no better than random. Results from the main study[78] were consistent with, and validated, those of the pilot study.[77] The rats were euthanized when they showed indications of a terminal condition and their brains were examined for evidence of neuropathology.[54,107,108]

These studies concluded that most rats that consumed Al at the high end of the human total dietary Al range developed cognitive deterioration in old age, accompanied by AD-relevant neuropathology. Interestingly, the rats developed cognitive deterioration without developing fully-formed plaques and tangles. Nevertheless, stages that lead to plaque and tangle formation in humans were observed in their brains. The rats with Al-induced cognitive deterioration exhibited additional neuropathological changes known to occur in AD that have received less attention than amyloid. These additional neuropathological changes explain cognitive deterioration more readily than the amyloid hypothesis.

2.4.4 Cognitive Deterioration in AD and Chronic Al Neurotoxicity Occur from the Same Mechanism of Damage

The entorhinal cortex (Brodmann's area 28) occupies the anterior part of the parahippocampal gyrus in humans.[109] Large stellate and pyramidal cells in superficial layers of the entorhinal cortex receive projections from many neocortical regions, including the olfactory, auditory, visual and somatosensory cortices, as well as multimodal areas and the amygdala.[110] The stellate and pyramidal cells are the cells of origin for the perforant path of the entorhinal cortex. Their axons collect in an angular bundle (Figure 2.4) and then project massively to the hippocampal formation in the form of distinct fascicles that perforate grey matter of the subicular cortex on their way to the hippocampal formation.[110]

Most fascicles project to the dentate gyrus, where they terminate on distal dendrites of granule cells in the outer two thirds of the molecular layer. Others terminate on distal dendrites of pyramidal cells in the CA1/subiculum zone. The perforant path thereby activates a sequence of intrinsic connections within the hippocampal formation, allowing the hippocampus to remain informed of ongoing cortical sensory activity.[110,111]

Stimulation of this circuitry culminates in hippocampal and subicular output, and reciprocates the perforant path, by projecting back to the deeper part of the entorhinal cortex.[112,113] The entorhinal cortex thus serves as a pivotal two-way station with the dual roles of: (1) funneling input from the neocortex and amygdala *via* the perforant path into the hippocampal formation, and (2) funneling reciprocal output from the CA1 and subiculum of the hippocampal formation back to the neocortex *via* layer IV.[110] This activity of the entorhinal cortex is crucial for acquisition into long-term memory.[113]

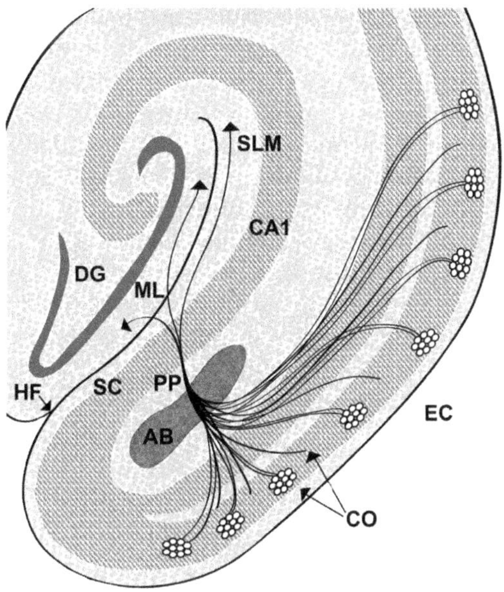

Figure 2.4 Schematic representation of the perforant path. The perforant path is similar for humans and rats, except for minor variations. (1) The cells of origin (CO) for the perforant path (PP) reside in layer II (shown as cell islands) and in the superficial part of layer III of the entorhinal cortex (EC). The cells of origin receive information from many cortical regions. (2) Axons of the cells of origin converge in the angular bundle (AB) from which the perforant path emerges. (3) Upon leaving the angular bundle, the axons (4) diverge into fascicles known as the perforant path (PP), perforating the subicular cortex (SC) on their way to the hippocampal formation. (5) A contingent of fascicles enters the stratum lacunosum moleculare (SLM) of the CA1/subicular zone (CA1). (6) More fascicles cross the hippocampal fissure (HF) (7) to enter the molecular layer (ML) of the dentate gyrus (DG).
Reproduced from reference 117 with permission from the Hindawi Publishing Corporation.

2.4.4.1 Disruption of the Perforant Path in Humans with AD Isolates the Hippocampal Formation from the Neocortex

The entorhinal cortex is the most affected region of the AD brain. It has by far more NFTs than any other of Brodmann's areas.[114] By the time AD is evident, many NFTs in the cells of origin for the perforant path have become extracellular "ghost" NFTs that have outlived their host cells.[110] Such damage destroys the perforant path. AD hippocampal sections also reveal discrete lesions of NFT-containing cells in the hippocampal subiculum/CA1 zone.[54] Intraneuronal Al is involved in the formation and growth of human NFTs that capture and sequester Al in the cell cytoplasm, thereby slowing its accumulation in the nucleus.[56] Instrumental techniques have also shown high Al content in NFTs.[115,116] For these reasons, NFTs can be regarded as a marker for human pyramidal cells that contain considerable amounts of accumulated Al.

These pathological changes effectively disconnect the hippocampal formation from the limbic and association cortices.[113] Cortical regions depend upon the hippocampal formation for memory consolidation. The structural changes that occur with AD in these brain regions preclude the normal acquisition of episodic or contextual knowledge.[113]

Severe damage to the perforant path thus provides a structural basis for the learning and memory changes that occur in AD. Confusion and inability to recall new episodes occurs relatively early in the course of AD and directly affects cognition.[110] As perforant path terminals deteriorate, a layer of neuritic plaques forms in the center of the dentate gyrus molecular layer, precisely where the glutamatergic terminals of the perforant path were previously located.[113]

2.4.4.2 Disruption of the Perforant Path in Rats with Al-Induced Cognitive Deterioration Isolates the Hippocampal Formation from the Neocortex

Two conditions have been recognized as necessary for cognitive deterioration in the Al-inducible rat model that mimicked consumption of human dietary Al levels over most of the life span. The first condition is that large numbers of pyramidal cells in the rats' entorhinal cortex showed high-stage (IV) Al accumulation. Pyramidal cells with stage IV Al accumulation exhibit microtubule depletion, dendritic dieback and loss of synapse density.[54]

The cells of origin for the perforant path in the entorhinal cortex stain for Al to a greater extent than for cells in any other brain region. Computer-assisted cell counts showed that, on average, $60 \pm 7\%$ of the cells of origin for the perforant path of the entorhinal cortex exhibited stage VI Al accumulation in the brains of rats with cognitive deterioration compared to $23 \pm 7\%$ in the low Al controls ($p < 0.001$)[54] (Figure 2.5, A&B).

Association area 3 of the temporal cortex is another AD-vulnerable brain region. In the rats with cognitive deterioration, $40 \pm 7\%$ of pyramidal cells exhibited stage IV Al accumulation compared to $13 \pm 3\%$ in the low Al controls ($p < 0.01$). The percentages of entorhinal cortical cells with stage IV Al accumulation correlated with the extent of change in the animals' T-maze performance scores between middle age and old age ($r = 0.76$; $p < 0.0005$).[54]

The second condition for cognitive deterioration in this rat model is the presence of at least one substantial lesion consisting of cells with high stage (IV) Al accumulation in the subiculum/CA1 zone of the hippocampal formation (Figure 2.5, C). Equivalent damage in the hippocampal formation of humans results in hippocampal failure to reciprocate output back to deeper layers of the entorhinal cortex, and from there to the neocortex.[110]

The presence of the two conditions in the brains of rats results in cognitive deterioration. The two conditions are analogous to those that result in disconnection of the hippocampal formation from the neocortex in humans,

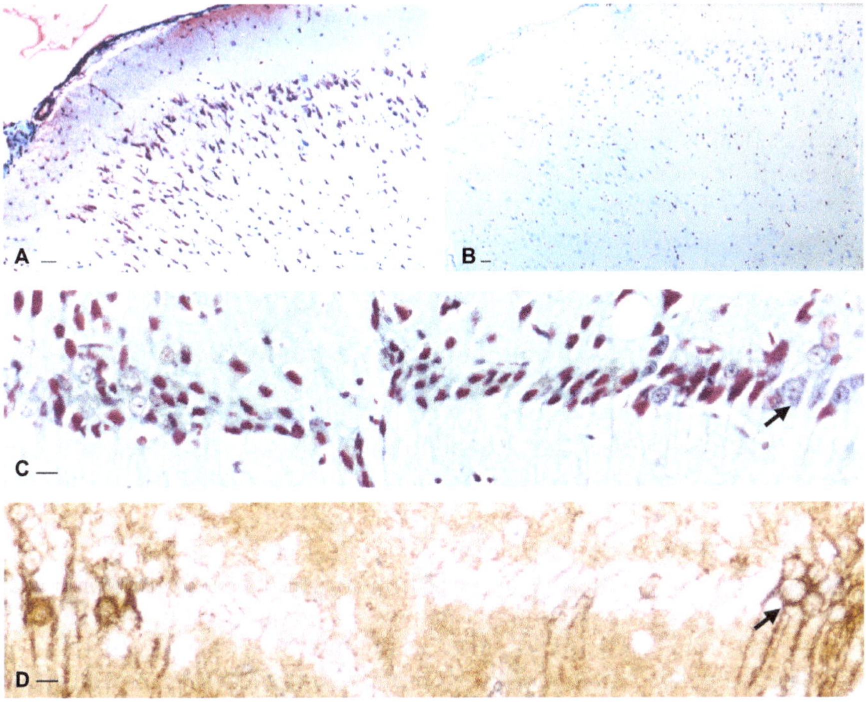

Figure 2.5 Al staining of cells of origin for the perforant pathway in the entorhinal cortex and in a lesion consisting of hippocampal CA1 cells that coincides with microtubule depletion in the brain of an aged rat with cognitive deterioration. A – Al stains large pyramidal and stellate cells of the entorhinal cortex magenta to purple in a rat with cognitive deterioration; B – Al staining is primarily localized in glial cells in superficial layers of the entorhinal cortex of a low Al rat control. Cells with low Al stain blue; C – Stage IV pyramidal cells stain magenta for nuclear Al within a hippocampal CA1 lesion of an aged rat with cognitive deterioration. The lesion is situated in the center of this micrograph. Pyramidal cells with a more normal appearance (*e.g.*, arrow) occur along the edges of the lesion; and D – An adjacent immunostained section shows that cells within the same lesion fail to immunostain for microtubules, whereas microtubules can be clearly seen in the more normal cells along the edges of the lesion (*e.g.*, arrow). Magnification bar = 50 μM for A and B, and 10 μM for C and D.
Reproduced from reference 54 with permission from Elsevier.

thereby isolating the hippocampus, as occurs in AD.[113] Thus the Al-inducible model is a translational animal model that replicates the process by which cognitive deterioration develops in AD.[117] Conversely, all low Al rats retained normal cognition. Low Al rats (1) had smaller percentages of stage IV Al accumulation in their cells of origin for the perforant path and (2) lacked any sign of a lesion in the CA1 field or subiculum.[54]

Previously, the selective vulnerability of entorhinal, hippocampal and cortical cells in AD was described as a mystery.[110] This Al-inducible rat model for chronic Al neurotoxicity and AD demonstrates that Al derived from dietary exposure at human-relevant levels preferentially accumulates in these and other AD-vulnerable brain regions and can accumulate to the point of interference with cognition.[54,111]

More widespread changes take place in the human brain as AD continues to progress. This is consistent with Al levels increasing over time to neurotoxic thresholds in additional AD-vulnerable brain regions—as evidenced by the spread of NFT damage—as a result of continuing human exposure to Al in foods, water and other sources. Chronic Al neurotoxicity also involves changes in calcium and iron metabolism and in neurotransmission.

2.4.5 Calcium (Ca^{2+}) Metabolism is Disrupted in AD and Chronic Al Neurotoxicity

2.4.5.1 Disruption of Ca^{2+} Metabolism in AD

Many reports describe significantly higher Ca^{2+} levels in fresh hippocampal and cortical brain cell samples obtained from aged rats, rabbits and monkeys compared to those of younger animals.[118] Actual intraneuronal Ca^{2+} levels, and Ca^{2+} movement into and out of neurons, of aged non-demented humans and humans with AD are resistant to analysis, owing to post-mortem change.[119] However, it is known that Ca^{2+} metabolism is disturbed on several levels in AD. The amount of ^{45}Ca that is absorbed across the GIT of humans with AD is significantly lower than that of age-matched controls in the presence of normal plasma concentrations of vitamin D metabolites, parathyroid hormone and serum Ca^{2+}.[120] Also, Ca^{2+} extrusion by plasma membrane Ca^{2+}-ATPase is impaired in AD neurons relative to that of non-demented controls.[121]

Ca^{2+}/phosphoinositide signalling pathways are also impaired in AD pyramidal cells. These pathways depend on G-proteins. G-proteins and their activation by GDP/GTP exchange exhibit general dysfunction in AD brain cells.[122–124] Protein kinase C (PKC) is normally activated by Ca^{2+}/phosphoinositide signaling pathways, the impairment of which may in part explain why PKC shows reduced activation in AD-affected cortical regions.[125,126]

Calmodulin (CaM) activity, essential for Ca^{2+} signaling, is also impaired in AD.[52] Immunostaining techniques show that monoclonal antibodies raised against CaM have a poor ability to recognize CaM protein in AD brain tissue. Ca^{2+} influx through activated NMDA receptors and heightened activities of CaM and PKC are all essential for long-term potentiation (LTP), a Ca^{2+}-dependent process involving sustained synaptic activity that underlies certain types of memory formation.[127] Changes in the levels of any of these proteins and/or their activities could contribute to the LTP deficit observed in AD.[127–130]

2.4.5.2 Disruption of Ca^{2+} Metabolism in Chronic Al Neurotoxicity is Comparable with that which Occurs in AD

Al inhibits calbindin and thereby impairs transcellular absorption of Ca^{2+} in the intestine.[131,132] Al also competes with Ca^{2+} for Ca^{2+}-binding sites on proteins, membranes and in Ca^{2+} channels, disrupting Ca^{2+} metabolism in the same ways that are altered with aging and AD.[118]

Al blocks voltage-gated Ca^{2+} channels, N-methyl-D-aspartate (NMDA), α-amino-3-hydroxy-5-methyl-4-isoxazolepropionic acid (AMPA) and glutamate-mediated currents in isolated hippocampal and dorsal ganglion neurons[133,134] and irreversibly blocks Ca^{2+} channels formed in bilayer membrane by high levels of β-amyloid.[135]

Al elevates Ca^{2+} levels in resting neurons.[136–138] Al interference occurs at several stages of the Ca^{2+}/phosphoinositide signaling pathways, inhibiting: (1) G protein activation[62,63]; (2) hydrolysis of PIP_2 by PI-PLC[139]; (3) phosphoinositide accumulation[140]; and, consequently, (4) PKC activation by diacylglycerol, a product of PIP_2 hydrolysis. Exposure to nanomolar quantities of Al also inhibits 90% of PKC activity in rat brain extracts.[141]

Al binds to CaM, forming an Al-CaM complex that has reduced ability to interact with CaM-dependent proteins needed for translating Ca^{2+} signals into cellular activities.[142,143] Monoclonal antibodies raised against normal CaM have poor recognition of the Al-CaM complex.[143,144] Thus efficacy of CaM for activating CaM kinase in the brains of Al-treated rats and phosphodiesterase in the brains of Al-treated rabbits declines progressively to approximately 50% and 30%, respectively, of their control values.[136,145] *In vitro* exposure of synaptosomes to 100 μM Al reduces their CaM activity to 40% of control value.[146]

Al^{3+} substitutes for Mg^{2+} in the ATP co-factor of Mg^{2+}-ATPase.[63] Chronic Al exposure also alters plasma membrane Ca^{2+}-ATPase activity in a way that depresses Ca^{2+} extrusion from neurons.[136] These results are completely reversible by desferrioxamine, an Al (and iron) chelator. Al accumulation in AD neurons and its ability to inhibit Ca^{2+}-ATPase activity, which normally plays a large role in extruding excess Ca^{2+} from cells, may explain why Ca^{2+} levels are generally elevated in neurons isolated from Al-exposed and older animal brains.

Al inhibits, in a dose-dependent manner, the activity of several enzymes important to Ca^{2+} metabolism: PKC, G proteins, CaM, and plasma membrane Ca^{2+}-ATPase.[62–64,136,141,145,146] Interference with either Ca^{2+} uptake through NMDA receptors, PKC or CaM activities on their own would disrupt LTP. LTP and long-term depression (LTD), an activity-dependent reduction in the synapse efficacy, were strongly disrupted in the brains of rats subjected to daily intracerebral Al injection over a 5–day period, which elevated the brain Al content to a local concentration estimated at 2.7 $\mu g\, mL^{-1}$.[147] Oral Al exposure since weaning has also produced LTP and LTD deficits in the brains of young rats.[148,149]

2.4.6 Iron Metabolism is Disrupted in AD and in Chronic Al Neurotoxicity

Iron is essential for energy production and cell health. Intracellular iron must be rigorously regulated to limit the amount of iron that would otherwise be freely available in cells. Free iron is a major source of oxidative damage.

The highest concentrations of (non-heme) iron in the adult human brain are normally found in ferritin deposits of oligodendrocytes and microglial cells in the globus pallidus and substantia nigra, followed by the red nucleus, putamen, caudate nucleus, dentate nucleus and subthalamic body. The cerebral and cerebellar cortex, anterior nucleus of the thalamus, mammillary body, tectum of the midbrain and the central grey matter of the third ventricle have considerably less iron. The medulla oblongata, spinal cord grey matter, spinal and sympathetic ganglia and white matter of the brain and spinal cord fail to stain for iron altogether.[150] Neurons of most brain regions contain granular iron deposits that increase with age.

The main usage of iron in neurons is for the synthesis of heme-containing enzymes, namely cytochrome oxidase and succinate dehydrogenase in mitochondrial respiratory chains, and iron-sulfur proteins such as iron regulatory protein 1 (IRP1).[151] Brain regions that contain neurons with high energy needs have large demands for heme iron and they also have a high density of transferrin receptors on their surface. High levels of transferrin receptors are found in the cortex, hippocampus, amygdala, dorsal raphe nucleus and cerebellar Purkinje cells.[151] High transferrin receptor levels show an almost identical distribution to that of cytochrome oxidase, which is an indicator of high energy needs.[151]

IRP1 and IRP2 are iron sensor proteins that normally govern intracellular iron homeostasis by controlling iron-transferrin uptake *via* transferrin receptors and storage of free iron in cytoplasmic ferritin deposits.[152] When intracellular iron is deficient, IRP2 avidly binds to iron responsive elements (IREs) in the 3'-untranslated region (UTR) of transferrin receptor mRNA, stimulating the formation of transferrin receptors. Transferrin receptors promote cellular iron uptake and restore the deficient intracellular iron levels. When iron levels are adequate, IRP2 normally dissociates from IREs and is rapidly degraded. IRP1 binds to IREs in the UTR of ferritin receptor mRNA and stimulates ferritin formation as IRP2 degrades.[152]

2.4.6.1 Disruption of Iron Metabolism in AD

In AD, iron levels increase in all AD-vulnerable brain regions, particularly in the hippocampus and amygdale, and to a lesser extent in temporal and parietal cortical regions.[153] IRP2 is stabilized in AD hippocampal neurons.[154] AD pyramidal cells with IRP2 stabilization behave as if they are in a permanent state of iron deficiency. These pyramidal cells continue to synthesize transferrin receptors, leading to abnormally high levels of intracellular free iron ions and oxidative damage, while ferritin synthesis is inhibited. Intraneuronal iron causes oxidative stress by its redox reactions, particularly those that involve the highly reactive Fenton reaction.[155] IRP1 is apparently unchanged in AD hippocampal pyramidal cells.[154]

2.4.6.2 Disruption of Iron Metabolism in Chronic Al Neurotoxicity is Comparable to that which Occurs in AD

Al-loading of laboratory rats concurrently induces significant increases in iron, proportional to Al increase, in pyramidal cells of the cortex, amygdala and hippocampus.[71] Al stimulates the uptake of both transferrin-bound iron and non-transferrin-bound iron in human cells.[156] Intraneuronal Al disrupts iron metabolism in neurons by interacting with IRP2.[157]

Al pre-treatment of cultured neural cells also increases their free iron uptake,[158,159] disrupts their iron homeostasis by inducing IRE binding activity of IRP2, and stabilises IRP2 by interfering with iron-catalysed oxidation in a way that prevents IRP2 breakdown.[157] IRP1 shows no change in Al-exposed neural cells,[157] just as IRP1 is unchanged in AD.[154] Immunostaining shows that IRP2 is abnormally localised in AD-affected hippocampal cells, with strong IRP2 immunoreactivity appearing on NFTs[152] where Al is particularly concentrated.[53,56,115,116]

Al and iron both generate oxidative stress in the brain.[65–67] Oxidative stress is one of the earliest changes observed in AD.[160] Al enhances iron-initiated lipid peroxidation several-fold.[67,161] Al also stabilises iron in its ferrous form (Fe^{2+}),[162] thereby increasing lipid peroxidation. The ferrous iron ion drives the Fenton reaction in cells. Individual contributions to oxidative stress from Al and iron in AD cells are probably indissociable, owing to the multiple synergistic interactions that occur between Al and iron ions.

2.4.7 Neurotransmitter Levels are Diminished in AD and Al Neurotoxicity

2.4.7.1 Neurotransmitter Levels are Diminished in AD

In AD, acetylcholine, glutamate, dopamine, norepinephrine and serotonin levels are diminished in cortical, hippocampal and striatal regions of the brain.[163–165] The main neurotransmitter-related change in AD brains is a 40–90% decrease in choline acetyltransferase (ChAT) in the hippocampus and cerebral cortex.[166] The ChAT decrease is already noticeable in the first year that symptoms appear[167] and is accompanied by a large (*e.g.*, 45%) loss of cholinergic activation of phosphoinositide signaling.[168]

The ChAT enzyme catalyses the synthesis of acetylcholine from its choline and acetyl coenzyme A precursors.[169] Normally, ChAT is functionally regulated by PKC phosphorylation on serine-440.[170,171] However, PKC levels are abnormally low in AD.[125] The reduced ChAT levels can explain the lowered acetylcholine availability for attaching to acetylcholine receptors and stimulating Ca^{2+}/phosphoinositide signaling pathways in AD.[123]

Noradrenergic and serotonergic neurotransmitters also show reductions in AD but are less than those of the cholinergic system.[166] Tetrahydrobiopterin (BH_4) is a co-factor required for the hydroxylation of phenylalanine and tyrosine in the synthesis of the monoaminergic neurotransmitters dopamine and noradrenaline, and for the hydroxylation of tryptophan in the case of serotonin.[172] BH_4 synthesis is significantly reduced in the temporal lobe of post-mortem AD brain samples[173] and BH_4 deficiency is regarded as a characteristic of late-stage AD.[174]

2.4.7.2 *Neurotransmitter Levels are Diminished in Chronic Al Neurotoxicity as in AD*

Acetylcholine, glutamate, dopamine, noradrenaline and serotonin levels are significantly diminished in cortical, hippocampal and striatal brain regions of Al-exposed animals as in AD.[175–177] Al accumulates in cholinergic neurons[78,94] and interferes with several aspects of acetylcholine metabolism.[178] Brains of Al-exposed rabbits show significant reductions in ChAT activity in the entorhinal cortex (27%), hippocampus (36%-40%), and striatum (53%) after CNS Al injection.[175]

A possible explanation for ChAT inhibition by Al and low acetylcholine levels in AD is that nanomolar amounts of Al inhibit 90% of PKC activity[141] and PKC activity is needed for ChAT phosphorylation.[171] Al also inhibits acetylcholine synthesis by interfering with choline uptake, lowering the content of acetyl-coenzyme A[178] and inhibiting acetylcholine release.[179,180] Al produces a biphasic effect on acetylcholinesterase levels in experimental animals, initially stimulating, and then depressing its rate of synthesis.[181] Al inhibition of ChAT activity and acetylcholine synthesis has flow-on effects, reducing acetylcholine receptor-stimulated Ca^{2+}/phosphoinositide signaling pathways in Al-affected neurons.[139,146]

Al also reduces the levels of glutamatergic and monoaminergic neurotransmitters but to a lesser extent than ChAT.[175,177] Rats that drank water containing Al acetate had reduced total brain biopterins and less BH_4 synthesis than controls,[182] and low BH_4 levels could help to explain the monoaminergic neurotransmitter deficit. It is currently unknown whether Al directly inhibits BH_4 synthesis or indirectly inhibits its synthesis by interfering with BH_4 phosphorylation. The terminal enzyme in the biosynthetic pathway for BH_4 is normally phosphorylated by PKC and/or CaM kinase II.[183] Both enzymes are inhibited by Al at low concentrations.[141,145]

2.4.8 AD and Chronic Al Neurotoxicity are Inflammatory Conditions

2.4.8.1 *Inflammatory Effects are Observed in AD*

AD is a mildly inflammatory condition.[184] Gene microarray experiments[185] analyzed for 12 633 gene, and expressed sequence, expression levels and indicated a generalized down-regulation of normal gene expression in the AD hippocampus. Specifically, AD hippocampal tissue exhibited statistically-significant decreases in reporter signal intensity mainly for genes that encode transcription and neurotrophic factors, signal transduction elements and metal ion-sensitive factors. AD hippocampal tissue showed increased expression levels of 24 genes. In both cases (increase and decrease), the differences were altered by a factor equal to or greater than three-fold compared to controls ($p<0.04$).[13,185] Greater increases in gene expression were found for inflammatory transcription factors and their subunits (NFκBp52/p100, HIF-1, hypoxia-inducible factor-1) and inflammatory proteins [β-amyloid precursor protein (β-APP), NF-IL6, IL precursor, cytochrome oxidase-2 (COX-2), interleukin 1L-1β (IL-1β), tumor necrosis factor (TNFα) and death-associated protein 6 (DAXX), a regulatory protein that represses transcription and induces apoptosis].[185] Reactive astrocytes and activated microglial cells are abundant in AD brain tissue and T-cells marginate along post-capillary venules of inflamed areas.[184]

2.4.8.2 Inflammatory Effects are Observed in Chronic Al Neurotoxicity

Al-generated ROS initiate an inflammatory cascade in brain tissue.[186–188] Chronic Al exposure up-regulates the expression of the NFκB transduction factor as well as IL-β and TNFα cytokines in brains of laboratory mice.[177,188] High density gene microarrays have revealed that cultured human neural cells exposed to 100 nM Al emulate many stress response gene expression changes previously reported in late-stage AD brain tissue at, or more than three times, the gene expression of control cultures. Specifically, 7 out of 8 genes (87.5%) significantly up-regulated in AD are up-regulated by Al exposure. Similarly, 17 out of the 24 (71%) genes that are significantly down-regulated in AD are down-regulated by Al.[13] Pro-inflammatory and pro-apoptotic genes are over expressed in these Al-exposed human neural cells, including subunits for nuclear factor kappa B (NFκB) and HIF-1 transduction factors, IL-1β precursor, β-APP, COX-2 and DAXX.[13] Co-exposure of human neural cells to Al and iron produces a synergistic effect on the expression of the same up-regulated and down-regulated genes.[189] Hence Al accumulation in the AD brain could account for observations that AD involves inflammation.

Al activates astrocytes and microglial cells in studies performed *in vivo* and *in vitro*.[190–194] Cultured rat astrocytes exposed to Al for up to 41 days have interrupted gap junctions that interfere with their intercellular communication and ability to buffer ions and transmitters in the extracellular environment of neurons.[192]

2.5 Al and Neuropathological Hallmarks of AD

Neuropathological features of AD include microtubule depletion, dendritic dieback, loss of synapse density, cortical atrophy, hyperphosphorylated tau and NFTs, hippocampal granulovacuolar degeneration, and changes in the metabolism of amyloid protein precursor and presenilins that lead to the formation of amyloid plaques.

2.5.1 Microtubules

Neurons require microtubules, to maintain the structure and shape of the cell body and its dendritic/axonal processes. Microtubules provide the infrastructure for fast axonal flow and transport of nutrients, neurotransmitters, and organelles between the cell body and its distant synaptic terminals.[195]

2.5.1.1 Microtubule Depletion and its Consequences in AD

Microtubule depletion is a neuropathological hallmark of AD that results in dendritic dieback, loss of synapse density and cortical atrophy. Microtubule depletion is much less conspicuous than the formation of plaques and tangles, yet is potentially more important to AD-type dementia than any other AD hallmark. Microtubule depletion has long been known to occur in NFT-containing pyramidal cells of the AD cortex and hippocampus,[196,197] but its significance has been under-estimated. Microtubule depletion also occurs in certain pyramidal cells of AD-vulnerable brain regions without NFTs.[54] Direct morphological consequences of microtubule depletion are dendritic dieback and loss of synapse density.[54] Dendritic dieback is revealed by Golgi staining in pyramidal cells of the AD hippocampus (Figure 2.6) and entorhinal cortex.[198]

Dendritic branches are the main target for synaptic input to neurons, accounting for 95% of a neuron's surface area.[199] Pyramidal neurons from the parahippocampal gyrus of non-demented older humans (mean age, 79.6 years) have more extensive dendritic trees than those of normal middle-aged humans (mean age, 51.2 years). The greatest increase is in the number of terminal segments of the dendritic tree and their average length.[199]

The hippocampal CA1 field shows dendritic stability in normal old age,[200] whereas the dentate gyrus shows regressive dendritic change, particularly in the oldest-old.[201] Neocortical synapse loss is normally confined to certain regions, these being the regions where compensatory re-innervation occurs in response to cellular injury.[202,203]

A final surge in compensatory neuroplasticity occurs in intermediate stage AD in response to the increasing cell damage.[204] After this surge, many more pyramidal cells are incapable of forming new dendritic branches, spines and synapses. By way of example, pyramidal neurons in the anterior part of the parahippocampal gyrus (*i.e.*, the entorhinal cortex) of humans with AD are no longer able to mount a compensatory response.[203] This inability results in

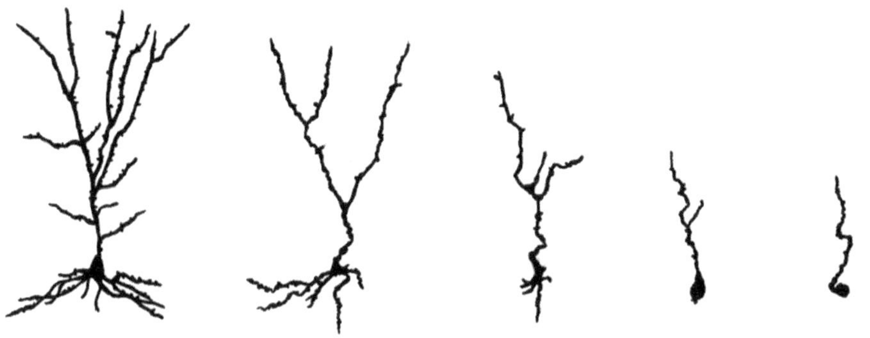

Figure 2.6 Camera lucida drawings of AD Golgi-stained pyramidal cells, illustrating the process of dendritic dieback (left to right). The deteriorated cell on the right resembles the Al-rich cells in the lesion of Figure 8.5. Redrawn from reference 198 with permission from Elsevier.

progressive, marked atrophy of dendrites with loss of spines and synapses. The apical dendrites are shorter and less branched than in controls. All brains with dementia contain cells with shrunken dendritic trees.[205] Progressive reduction in the dendritic tree involves sequential loss in distoproximal synapses.[206] AD-altered pyramidal cells occur in groups, forming expanding lesions surrounded by other pyramidal cells with a more normal appearance.[54] Loss of synapse density is regarded as a better diagnostic feature of AD than either plaques or tangles.[207]

2.5.1.2 Microtubule Depletion and its Consequences in Chronic Al Neurotoxicity

Al produces a biphasic toxic effect on microtubules. *In vitro* Al exposure at picomolar concentrations results in Al binding to the site on tubulin-GTP (normally occupied by Mg^{2+}, the physiological mediator of microtubule assembly) and stimulates tubulin polymerization. Al-induced microtubules appear identical to normal microtubules, even at the ultrastructural level.[64] However, Al-induced microtubules are physiologically abnormal. They fail to disassemble under normal conditions, being resistant to PP2B-induced depolymerization.[64]

Al is a microtubule disruptor at the μM concentrations that typically occur in aged pyramidal cells. Microtubule density is reduced as NFTs form in pyramidal cells of the entorhinal cortex, hippocampus and neocortex of cats in response to intraventricular Al injection.[208] Microtubule counts in TEM micrographs of NFT-containing cat pyramidal cells showed they contained 0–3 microtubules per μm^2 compared to pyramidal cells of sham-operated cats, which contained a mean count of 71 ± 26 microtubules per μm^2. Microtubule depletion in the hippocampus of the Al-exposed cats correlates with impairments in learning and retention.[208] Other animal species given intracerebral, intracisternal or intraperitoneal Al injections also experience performance difficulties on behavioral tests for memory and learning.[206,208–210]

Intracerebral Al injection into rabbit brains results in a sharp and progressive reduction in the length and number of apical and basal dendritic branches, beginning with those furthest from the cell body, and progressing towards the cell body.[206] This dendritic change is indicative of the dieback process and resembles that which occurs in AD.[198] Al-induced dendritic dieback also resembles dendritic dieback induced by colchicine, another microtubule disruptor.[211] Dendritic dieback is a slow process that continues for 200–300 days after animals have experienced acute Al exposure.[212] Dendritic changes are accompanied by significant loss of synapse density over the same time frame.[213] Dendritic change induced in brains of rabbits injected intracerebrally with Al also coincides with impairment in memory and learning activities.[206]

Microtubule depletion and dendritic dieback also occur with high stage Al accumulation in hippocampal pyramidal cells of rats that developed cognitive deterioration after chronically consuming Al at human-relevant levels. Aged pyramidal cells that stain for stage IV Al accumulation (Figure 2.5, C) fail to immunostain for microtubules (Figure 2.5, D).[54] In contrast, microtubules are clearly demonstrable in aged pyramidal cells where Al staining is at lower stages of Al accumulation.[54]

Examination of brain sections in the hippocampal stratum radiatum of rats with Al-induced cognitive deterioration showed glial cells in the course of pruning dendritic processes.[54] High stage Al accumulation causes the cell structure to collapse so the cell bodies appear shrunken with a serpentine-shaped apical dendrite, as described by Simchowicz[214] for AD pyramidal cells. Neurites shrivel, synapses break down and neuronal connectivity is lost. Cells with high stage Al accumulation are sufficiently structurally compromised that they hardly resemble neurons.[54]

Substantial lesions consisting of Al-rich microtubule-depleted cells are observed in brains of humans with AD and in rats with cognitive deterioration. The lesion illustrated in Figure 2.5 was from a serially-sectioned rat cerebrum that showed this lesion extended along the entire anteroposterior axis of the rat hippocampus. Extensive Al damage to the cells of origin for the perforant path and one substantial hippocampal lesion consisting of cells with high stage Al accumulation are sufficient to distinguish the brains of rats with cognitive deterioration from those of rats that remain cognitively-intact. Loss of synapse density is another consequence of the high stage Al accumulation and dendritic dieback that feature in the brains of rats with cognitive deterioration.[54,215]

2.5.2 Cortical Atrophy in AD

Localized cell loss occurs in AD, particularly affecting the hippocampal CA1 field, where cell counts indicated an average loss of 68%.[216] Several earlier reports[217] indicated more widespread neuronal loss, relative to age-matched controls, in cortical regions of AD-affected brains and was suggested as a cause for the cortical atrophy that accompanies AD. Other reports indicated that neuronal densities in AD brains and brains of age-matched controls were similar.[218] Stereological counting techniques that allow more precise estimates of neuron numbers have since developed. These techniques provide evidence that any observed difference between cortical neuron density in AD and age-matched controls is insufficient to account for cortical atrophy. Instead, degenerative reduction occurs in the axon/dendritic/synapse compartment of these neurons, resulting in dieback that diminishes the cortical volume and increases ventricular size.[219] Change in the axon/dendritic/synapse compartment can significantly increase or decrease cortical thickness.[220]

2.5.3 Hyperphosphorylated Tau and NFTs

NFTs, originally described by Alzheimer,[4] represent an AD hallmark that parallels the duration and severity of AD.[221] NFTs primarily develop in large pyramidal cells. They are resistant to degradation and can outlast the cells in which they form.[222]

2.5.3.1 *Hyperphosphorylated Tau and NFTs in AD*

Protein phosphatase 2A (PP2A), the main phosphatase that dephosphorylates tau, is inhibited by approximately 30% in AD brain tissue.[223,224] This inhibition of phosphatase activity upsets the normal balance between tau phosphorylation by kinases and tau dephosphorylation by protein phosphatases. Such imbalance leads to the hyperphosphorylation of tau.[224] Consequently, a massive increase occurs in the hyperphosphorylated tau: normal tau ratio of the brain as AD develops.[225]

Human hyperphosphorylated tau is truncated by caspase.[226] The truncated hyperphosphorylated tau aggregates and initially precipitates in the cytoplasm of pyramidal cells in the form of granules.[227] Eventually, in some cells, the granules give rise to polymerized filaments[228] that are now recognized to have the form of twisted ribbons[229] rather than paired helical filaments as originally described.[230] Some NFT filaments are straight, and others are half-straight and half-twisted. Masses of these filaments constitute NFTs. Cortical NFTs appear as tangles, whereas hippocampal NFTs appear flame-shaped.

NFT-containing cells are recognized as having down-regulated oxidative phosphorylation and low respiration.[231,232] They can survive in certain brain regions for decades without contributing to neural function.[233] Extracellular tangles known as "ghost tangles" result when NFTs become sufficiently large to enucleate the pyramidal cells that contain them.[53] Cell death follows enucleation.

Alzheimer observed, "As these fibrils stain with dyes differently from normal neurofibrils, a chemical change to the fibril substance must have taken place. This may well be the reason why the fibrils outlive the destruction of the cell."[4]

2.5.3.2 *Hyperphosphorylated Tau and NFTs in Brains of Al-Exposed Experimental Animals and Humans with AD*

Al inhibits the activity of protein phosphatases (PP1, PP2A and PP2B) that normally remove phosphate from tau in brain tissue.[234,235] The massive increase in the hyperphosphorylated tau: normal tau ratio that occurs in AD also occurs in the brains of dialysis patients that have had high Al exposure.[236]

Al exposure causes tau hyperphosphorylation in: (1) solutions of isolated tau;[237] (2) cultured human neuroblastoma cells;[238] and (3) brains of rats chronically-exposed to dietary Al at human-relevant levels.[108] Al aggregates hyperphosphorylated tau *in vitro*, while sparing normal tau.[222] The fact that hyperphosphorylated tau can be aggregated by Al *in vitro* suggests that intracytoplasmic Al can also aggregate hyperphosphorylated tau in human cells where NFTs form.

An observed sequence of events can provide a reasonable explanation for the development of NFTs in human brain.[56] The Al/hyperphosphorylated tau granules fuse and grow (Figure 2.7, A&B) in human pyramidal cells of the CA1 hippocampal field and cortex of AD brains. Granule fusion results in a homogeneous-textured Al/hyperphosphorylated tau complex in the form of

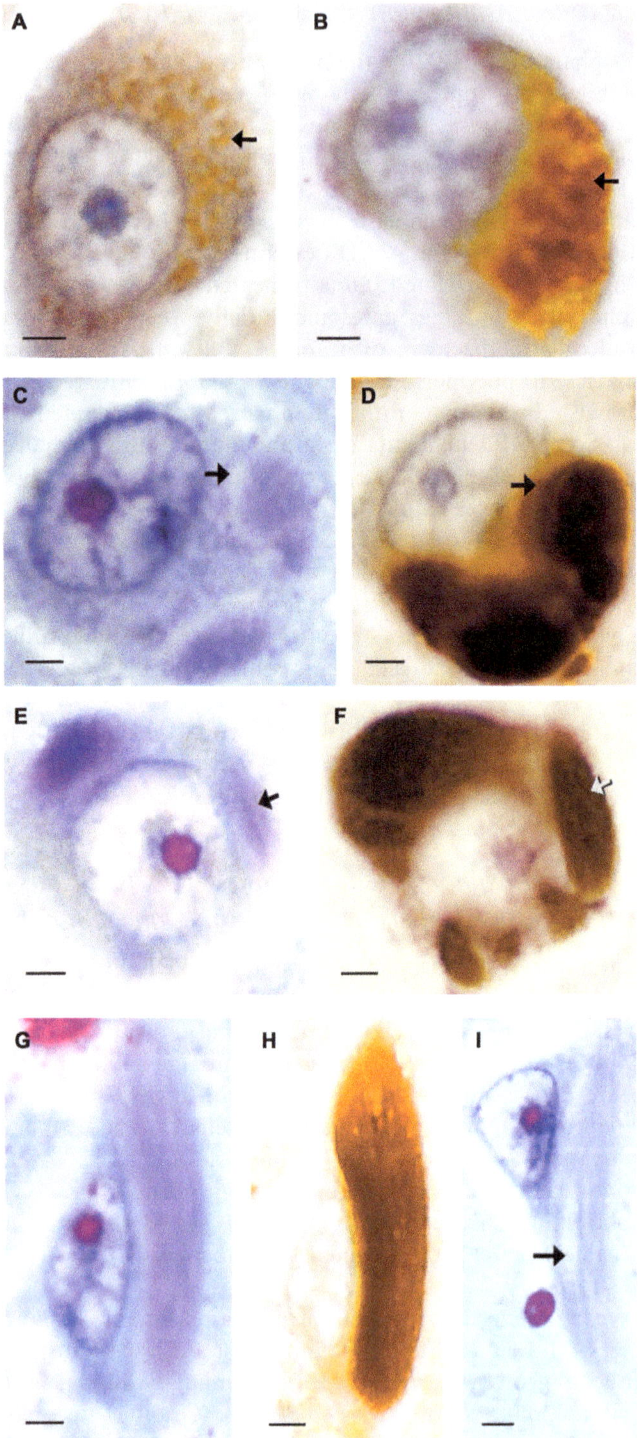
A
B
C
D
E
F
G
H
I

pools that occupy much of the cytoplasm. These pools stain for both Al and hyperphosphorylated tau (Figure 2.7, C&D). Nascent NFT filaments polymerize within the Al-hyperphosphorylated tau complex of the cytoplasmic pools (Figure 2.7, E&F). The NFTs grow and mature, consuming the surrounding Al-hyperphosphorylated tau complex (Figure 2.7, G-I). The implication is that NFTs are a protective neuronal response that sequesters Al in the cytoplasm, thereby slowing Al uptake into the nucleus.[56]

The Al in AD NFTs was originally described by scanning electron microscopy with X-ray spectroscopy.[115] NFTs also form in the brains of patients with Down's syndrome.[89] The NFTs of ALS/PD contain both Al and Ca^{2+}.[239] Al content in human NFTs has been measured at 250 ppm.[240]

NFT formation is species-specific and rat neurons are unable to form NFTs.[241] Brains of rats that develop cognitive deterioration from chronic Al ingestion have abundant amounts of hyperphosphorylated tau yet they lack NFTs.[108] Intracerebral Al injection can induce NFT formation in rabbit and cat brain within 96 hours.[242] NFTs form much more slowly in monkey brain.[243] Al-induced NFTs form in rabbits in brain regions equivalent to those where NFTs form in humans with AD.[94,243] Al-induced NFTs in animals are neurofilament-based rather than tau-based. The neurofilament/tau difference could represent species difference and/or temporal difference. It is possible that neurofilament-based NFTs serve as a scaffold for the formation of tau-based NFTs. For example, rabbit NFTs are reported to change within days of their formation as they acquire tau and other proteins that increase their similarity to human NFTs.[244,245]

2.5.4 Hippocampal Granulovacuolar Degeneration (GVD)

Granulovacuolar degeneration (GVD) has been recognized as an AD hallmark since 1914, when first described by one of Alzheimer's students.[246]

2.5.4.1 Hippocampal GVD in AD

GVD affects many hippocampal pyramidal neurons, appearing in the cytoplasm either as several large vacuoles or, more commonly, as numerous

Figure 2.7 Development of NFTs in AD hippocampal neurons. A&B – Pre-tangle pyramidal cells stained for hyperphosphorylated tau show small and larger (fused) granules (arrows); C&D – Cytoplasmic pools form *via* granule fusion and stain for (C) Al and (D) hyperphosphorylated tau. Arrows denote the thinner margins of the pools consisting of an Al/hyperphosphorylated tau complex; E&F – Thin filamentous structures, just visible in the cytoplasmic pools, stained for (E) Al and (F) hyperphosphorylated tau, represent nascent filaments that develop into NFTs; G&H – Mature NFTs continue to stain for (G) Al and (H) hyperphosphorylated tau; and I – A large NFT stained to show Al (pale purple filaments) has consumed the cytoplasmic pool so individual filaments are more clearly seen (arrow). Magnification bars = 2.5 µM for A-F, 2 µM for G and H, 1 µM for I.
Reproduced from reference 56 with permission from IOS Press.

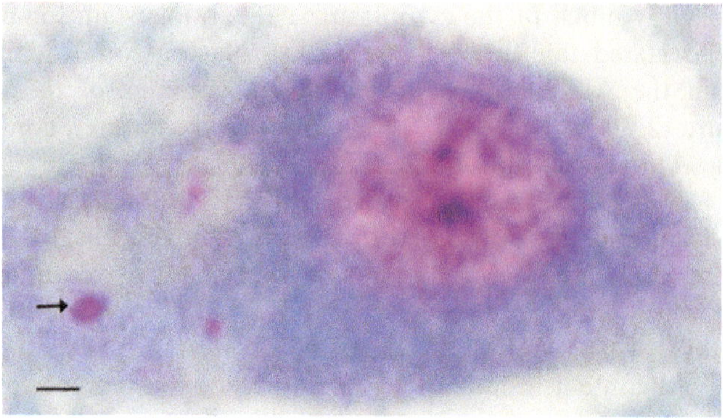

Figure 2.8 Granules stain for Al in vacuoles of a GVD-affected AD hippocampal neuron. Magnification Bar = 2.5 μM.
Reproduced from reference 53 with permission from Elsevier.

small vacuoles. Each of the vacuoles contains a single dense granule (Figure 2.8). The granules stain for Al and for abnormal forms of tau, caspase-cleaved APP, activated caspase-3 and amyloid.[53,247,248] Figure 2.8 shows the appearance of large GVD vacuoles, stained for Al, in a hippocampal pyramidal cell from an AD brain.

2.5.4.2 Hippocampal GVD in Chronic Al Neurotoxicity

GVD develops in the brains of rats chronically exposed to dietary Al at human-relevant dietary levels.[108] GVD formation can also be induced in the rat hippocampus by repeated intraperitoneal injections.[210,249] Al is the only agent that has, to date, been reported to induce hippocampal GVD in experimental animals. Hippocampal GVD also occurs in the brains of humans affected by Down's syndrome,[89] and in those with ALS/PD[250] which, as previously noted, is an Al-associated dementia.

2.5.5 β-Amyloid and Presenilins in AD and Al Neurotoxicity

Amyloid is a congo red-staining waxy material that occurs in blood vessels and in plaques located in the extracellular matrix of aged brains, particularly those with AD. The main sequence of events that lead to amyloid plaque formation is reasonably well-understood.

2.5.5.1 APP, β-Amyloid and Presenilins in Neurons

The inflammatory transduction factors NFκB and HIF-1 up-regulate the synthesis of amyloid precursor protein (APP) in the human brain.[251] APP is normally cleaved by α-secretase to form secreted APP (sAPPα). sAPPα is a non-amyloidogenic product that regulates APP participation in neurite budding and branching for neurodevelopment and repair.[252] sAPPα formation from APP requires phosphorylation by PKC.[253,254] Low PKC phosphorylation in AD[125] results in APP cleavage at alternate sites, mediated by β- and γ-secretases and giving rise to β-amyloid and cytoplasmic fragments.[255]

Monomeric β-amyloid peptide is soluble. However, amino acid oxidation and protein cross-linking reactions convert this soluble peptide into oligomers and fibrils that aggregate[256] and give rise to amyloid plaques in the extracellular matrix, particularly in the hippocampus and cortex. AD patients generally have significantly larger amounts of β-amyloid plaque in AD-vulnerable brain regions than non-demented controls, although some mentally-alert humans have a considerable volume of β-amyloid in their brains.[257]

The wild-type rat/mouse sequence for β-amyloid differs from the human β-amyloid sequence by three amino acid residues.[258] This species-specific difference is sufficient to block β-amyloid fibrillization and amyloid plaque formation in aged wild-type rats and mice.[256,258] Rodent brains can form human-like amyloid plaques only if they have been genetically altered to over-express human mutant APP genes. Some animal models have been engineered to express human mutant genes for both APP and presenilin. Such gene change enables mouse brains to produce large amounts of human β-amyloid, which can fibrillize and form amyloid plaques similar to those that occur in brains of aged humans.[259,260]

Presenilins normally control APP maturation, and mutant forms of presenilin can block this maturational process. A variant form of the presenilin-2 gene is diagnostic for sporadic AD, being found in 100% (10/10) of brains tested from sporadic AD cases and only in 1/10 of those from elderly, non-demented controls.[261] This aberrantly-spliced variant of the presenilin-2 gene gives rise to mRNA lacking the exon 5 sequence which produces a presenilin-2 variant-encoding protein (PS2V), truncated at its N-terminus. PS2V resembles normal presenilin proteins in that PS2V localizes in membranes of the endoplasmic reticulum and Golgi complex of pyramidal neurons, particularly in the temporal cortex and the CA1 hippocampal field.[262] However, PS2V prevents the correct folding and maturation of APP and causes significant increases in both β-amyloid$_{1-40}$ and β-amyloid$_{1-42}$.[262] CA1 pyramidal neurons that are highly immunoreactive for PS2V exhibit shrinkage and dendritic dieback. PS2V expression can be blocked by antioxidants, suggesting that PS2V formation is induced by a metal that produces oxidative damage.[261]

2.5.5.2 Al Induces the Formation of the Presenilin-2 Variant of Sporadic AD and β-Amyloid in Laboratory Animals and Other Experimental Systems

Several ROS-producing metals were tested to determine whether they might be involved in PS2V formation.[263] Neuroblastoma cells were exposed to $CuCl_2$, $CuSO_4$, $ZnCl_2$, $FeCl_2$, $FeCl_3$, $AlCl_3$ and Al-maltol. Al (both $AlCl_3$ and Al-maltol) was the only metal that consistently induced the PS2V isoform and did so at a low concentration (25 μM Al).[263] The shrinkage of hippocampal

CA1 neurons and dieback described in human neural cells highly immunoreactive for PS2V are consistent with indications of chronic Al neurotoxicity.[54]

Al plays significant roles in amyloidogenesis, contributing to the formation of β-amyloid peptides, amyloid oligomers and amyloid plaques. *In vitro* and *in vivo* experiments have shown that Al affects every major stage of human amyloidogenesis,[107,264–267] giving rise to the likelihood that β-amyloid is a by-product of Al activity in the brain. Al is also associated with another type of amyloid that deposits in the joints of long-term renal dialysis patients.[268]

Al accumulation in cells generates ROS that stimulate the activity of the transduction factors, NFκB and HIF-1. Al-induced up-regulation of these transduction factors in turn up-regulates gene expression for APP and other inflammatory response proteins in gene microarrays of Al-exposed cultured human neural cells.[13,189] APP mRNA and protein are elevated in the brains of rats that develop cognitive deterioration after chronic exposure to Al under conditions that mimic human Al exposure.[107] Hippocampal and cortical sections immunostained for APP, from brains of these Al-exposed rats, exhibit neurites of irregular caliber that stain strongly for APP, indicating impaired axoplasmic flow. The neurites appear tortuous, with constrictions in some places and varicosities in others. A similar neuritic phenomenon has been observed in APP-immunostained brain sections of rats four days after they received an intrastriatal Al injection.[269] Al also suppresses transport of newly synthesized RNA in dendrites of cultured hippocampal neurons.[270] Swollen neurites and suppression of RNA transport were not observed in controls for these experiments.[107,270]

Al inhibits the phosphorylation by PKC[141] necessary for normal APP cleavage by α-secretase.[253,254] Consequently, APP metabolism is redirected from its non-amyloidogenic soluble APP (s-APPα) form to its amyloidogenic form in the presence of Al, becoming cleaved by β and γ secretases to produce β-amyloid. Al stabilises β-amyloid oligomers.[271] Al or iron addition to human β-amyloid$_{1-42}$ both convert β-amyloid$_{1-42}$ from a soluble peptide with random structure to a fibrillar beta-pleated precipitate that forms β-amyloid sheets.[264–266] The fact that this reaction can be reversed by Al/iron chelators confirms that amyloid fibrillization is Al- and iron-induced.[265] Zinc inhibits the formation of β-amyloid$_{1-42}$ sheets, whereas copper prevents their formation. Al also aggregates human β-amyloid$_{1-42}$ fibrils, causing them to form deposits that stain for thioflavin S as do amyloid plaques in AD brain tissue.[267]

Exposure of APP-transgenic mice to a diet supplemented by Al for 12 months significantly augments oxidative reactions and increases the volume of β-amyloid that forms in their brains, compared to oxidative reactions and β-amyloid volume in brains from a transgenic control group without Al supplementation.[70] The plaques that form in response to Al exposure are both more numerous and larger in size. A third transgenic mouse cohort, supplemented with both vitamin E and Al, showed less oxidative stress with smaller and fewer amyloid plaques comparable to the amyloid plaques that form in brains of APP-transgenic mice without any Al supplementation.[70] This indicates that Al-generated ROS, and the oxidative stress that up-regulates

APP and increases amyloidogenesis were ameliorated by the vitamin E anti-oxidant.

In experimental animals, Al exposure also induces an amyloid condition that is homologous to congophilic β-amyloid angiopathy in humans,[272] being a specialized type of sporadic AD shown to coincide with very high brain Al levels.[273] Al forms a complex with plasma β-amyloid$_{1-42}$, increasing amyloid transport across the blood-brain barrier and causing the formation of β-amyloid deposits in brain tissue.[274]

2.5.6 APOE-Dependent Neuroplasticity

Neuroplasticity is the brain's potential to reorganize itself by creating new neural pathways to compensate for cell dysfunction, cell death and denervation, such as that which occurs in the AD brain. Astrocytes enable neuroplasticity by synthesizing and secreting APOE,[275] the main lipid carrier in the mammalian brain.[276] Astrocyte-secreted APOE stimulates compensatory neuroplasticity by recycling cholesterol and cholesterol esters from neurons with deteriorating synapses and delivering them to other neurons that can use this cholesterol to sprout buds, grow new axonal branches, undergo synaptogenesis and re-inervate deafferented neurons.[276]

Humans express three forms of this protein: APOE2, APOE3 and APOE4.[277] APOE2 and APOE3 are capable of stimulating neuroplasticity in response to injury-induced denervation. The molecular structure of APOE4 impairs its ability to transport cholesterol. This impairs APOE4's ability to promote sprouting and re-innervation.[278]

AD progresses with severe loss of entorhinal cortical cells and cells in the subiculum/CA1 zone. Perforant path fibers, emanating from damaged cells of origin, shrivel and withdraw from the cells to which they were formerly connected. Consequently, other afferent fibers to the dentate gyrus vigourously sprout to form new synapses with deafferented target cells in the dentate gyrus. Commissural and associational fibres from less affected perforant path neurons can re-innervate and temporarily restore original connections between the neocortex and dentate gyrus.[279]

2.5.6.1 Failure of APOE-Dependent Neuroplasticity in AD

As AD continues to progress, damage to the entorhinal cortex and its cells of origin for the perforant pathway becomes too extensive to be effectively countered by compensatory neuroplasticity. APOE-dependent neuroplasticity continues for some time, but with diminishing returns. For example, AD patients with intact septal cholinergic input to the hippocampus show intensified acetylcholinesterase activity in an expanded region of the dentate gyrus molecular layer previously occupied by perforant path glutamateric terminals.[204] This inappropriate reinnervation is incapable of restoring connections between the hippocampal formation and neocortex because neurons from the septum connect the hippocampus to brain structures other than the entorhinal cortex. The sprouting/re-innervation response to dendritic dieback and cell death eventually exhausts,[199,203] resulting in re-innervation failure.

The effectiveness of APOE-dependent neuroplasticity, when operating correctly, is to postpone overt AD. This is indicated by the mean (± SEM) age of AD onset in humans with APOE2 and/or APOE3 alleles; *i.e.*, without any APOE4 allele (84.3 ± 1.3 years), in those with one APOE2 or APOE3 allele and one APOE4 allele (75.5 ± 1.0 years) and in those with two APOE4 alleles (68.4 ± 1.2 years).[277] The earlier age at which AD occurs in individuals with APOE4 alleles most likely results from APOE4's inability to hold and transport the cholesterol and cholesterol esters needed for neuroplasticity and re-innervation.

2.5.6.2 ApoE-dependent Neuroplasticity in Animal Models for AD with Perforant Path Lesions or Chronic Al Neurotoxicity

Rats with unilateral lesions of the entorhinal cortex temporarily lose their ability to perform continuous alternation in the T-maze immediately after surgery.[79] Compensatory sprouting from the contralateral entorhinal cortex offsets perforant path damage by re-innervating the deafferented hippocampal formation. If tested three days after lesioning the rat cannot perform, but if allowed to recover for ten days, their T-maze performance is restored to the pre-lesion level.[79] Acetylcholinesterase staining, indicative of re-innervation by cholinergic fibers, is also faintly detectable in the brains of rats with unilateral lesions of the perforant path at 15 days post-lesioning.[280] At 30 days, the molecular layer of the dentate gyrus shows a strong acetylcholinesterase staining pattern. Cholinergic re-innervation is completely inhibited if a secondary lesion is made in the medial septal nucleus 30 days after the original lesioning of the entorhinal cortex.[280]

However, rats that receive bilateral lesions of the entorhinal cortex, thereby destroying the perforant path on both sides of the brain, develop neuropathology and behaviors similar to those observed in humans with AD.[281] Re-innervation is restricted to septal and other afferents that have no obvious relationship with the glutamatergic perforant path innervation destroyed by the lesions. This attempt at compensatory neuroplasticity is unable to restore the rat brains' original connections and hence their T-maze performance. Instead, the rats are left with severe memory deficits as in AD.[281]

In our longitudinal study, the rats that developed cognitive deterioration from chronic Al neurotoxicity showed remarkable similarities in neuropathology and T-maze performance to rats with bilateral lesions. They also shared striking similarities to humans with AD in relation to their neuropathology and some abnormal behaviours. Chronic Al exposure produces damage to the entorhinal cortex over a much longer prodromal period than in lesioned animals that develop equivalent damage. Thus chronic Al

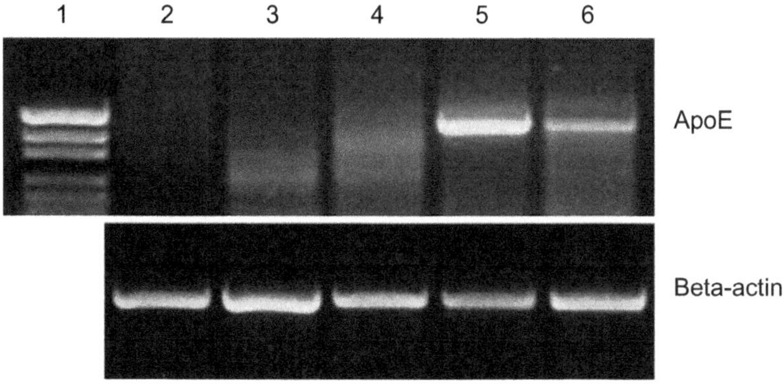

Figure 2.9 RT-PCR analysis for ApoE mRNA in rat brain. Lane 1, pUC19; lane 2, negative control (macrophage cell line RAW 264); lanes 3 and 4, brain tissue from cognitively-intact rats; lanes 5 and 6, brain tissue from rats that exhibited cognitive deterioration. Beta-actin bands are shown as controls.

neurotoxicity shows closer resemblance to the slowly developing process of cognitive deterioration than occurs in AD.

Most rats that develop chronic Al neurotoxicity from Al supplementation in their diet began to show evidence of cognitive deterioration around age 27 months, equivalent to about 79 years in humans.[78] ApoE mRNA was significantly higher in their cortical/hippocampal tissue than for the same brain regions of low-Al controls, suggesting that ApoE-dependent neuroplasticity was stimulated in the brains of rats with cognitive deterioration (Figure 2.9). However, sprouting, re-innervation and synaptogenesis were eventually unable to compensate for the continuous Al insult that causes microtubule depletion and dieback in pyramidal cells of the entorhinal cortex, neocortex, hippocampal formation and other AD-vulnerable brain regions.[54]

2.6 Aging Increases Human Vulnerability to AD and Chronic Al Neurotoxicity

During aging, certain physical changes occur that could contribute to the risk of developing AD in humans and chronic Al neurotoxicity in experimental animals. The passage of time allows more Al accumulation in the brain. However, additional changes also occur in aging that probably contribute to the relentless process of high stage Al accumulation in increasing numbers of neurons throughout the brain.

2.6.1 Kidney Aging and Functional Loss

Humans are estimated to lose approximately 50% of their kidney function between the ages of 45 and 80 years as nephrons are progressively lost.[282] In general, the rate of decline in kidney function increases as subjects age.[282]

This was shown in 254 normal volunteers who prospectively participated in the Baltimore Longitudinal Study of Aging with 23 years of follow-up (1958–1981).[283] However, a significant proportion of the subjects showed no absolute decrease in kidney function in old age.

Age-related decline in kidney function may impact on Al removal from blood, elevating the plasma Al level, with more Al bioavailable for uptake into brain. Al nephrotoxicity research should determine whether age-related decline in kidney function results in less efficient Al removal from plasma. The continuing need for kidney tubule cells to remove plasma Al from the blood may inflict damage on those same cells and contribute to the age-related decline in kidney function seen in most older humans and to kidney dysfunction in renal failure patients.[284] At least one large prospective study has shown that poor kidney function correlates with cognitive decline in elderly humans.[285]

2.6.2 Bone Aging and Osteoporosis

The periosteum consists primarily of osteogenic cells and osteoblasts, which normally cover the bone surface. This cellular layer controls Ca^{2+} and PO_{4-} fluxes into and out of bone.[286] As age advances, the periosteum thins and the osteogenic layer has fewer cells, giving less coverage of the bone surface. Eventually, osteoblasts are almost absent and there is poor control of ion flux both into and out of bone.[286]

Bone serves as a repository for excess plasma Al in humans. Al that deposits in the skeleton has a long half-life in human bone, possibly lasting for decades.[287] Histological stains show that most bone Al deposits at the interface between the osteoid (unmineralized matrix) and the mineralized zone. Al is the recognized cause of several types of bone disease in renal failure patients, including vitamin D-resistant osteomalacia and aplastic bone disease, where little if any osteoblast activity is evident.

Idiopathic osteoporosis is an age-related disease of unknown origin that occurs when the rate of bone breakdown by osteoclasts outpaces the rate of bone building by osteoblasts. This involves dissolution of the mineralized bone matrix with loss of bone density and increased risk for fracture.

Experimental Al exposure produces a biphasic effect on osteoblasts. Very low Al concentrations (10^{-8} M to 1.5×10^{-6} M) are mitogenic. Al concentrations above 1.5×10^{-6} M inhibit the replication of osteoblasts and their specialized activities.[288] Bone Al delays the formation of amorphous calcium phosphate by osteoblasts, its transformation into calcium hydroxyapatite crystals and subsequent crystal growth.[289]

Al also affects osteoclast activity. Al adsorbs to the surface of hydroxyapatite crystals in the osteoid/mineralized bone interface and slows their rate of dissolution by osteoclast-generated acid.[290] Some acid diffuses below the Al-protected crystals into calcified bone, leading to crystal dissolution relatively deep in calcified bone and to a weakening of bone strength. In effect, Al disrupts the balance between osteoblast and osteoclast activities, causing osteoporosis-like bone change. Only a small portion of bone crystals have to be protected by Al before giving rise to a pathological state.[290]

Some reports have noted an association between osteoporosis and Alzheimer's disease.[291–293] AD often co-occurs with osteoporosis in clinical practices.[293] Trabecular bone biopsies from AD patients with hip fracture generally reveal high bone Al content.[294] However, not all humans who have high Al content in their bone biopsy samples have AD, suggesting that Al uptake rates, into different tissues that tend to store Al, vary from one individual to another.

The past 50 years has seen an epidemic of hip fractures in the older population.[294] The association between Al and fractures has received little research attention. Al content in trabecular bone biopsies from osteoporosis patients is intermediate between those with renal failure and healthy controls.[295] Osteoporosis can, in principle, accelerate the release of stores of Al, Ca^{2+} and phosphate from bone into the blood of aged, osteoporotic humans. This would result in higher levels of Al available for uptake into the brain.

2.6.3 Brain Aging and Loss of Neuroplasticity

As mentioned previously, Al measurements using spectroscopic techniques have shown a net Al increase in brain tissue as humans age.[15,42–44] Cumulative damage to CNS neurons is to some extent offset by (1) neuron redundancy; (2) compensatory neuroplasticity involving axonal and dendritic sprouting; and (3) synaptogenesis. Here, we examine some possible reasons that, in view of these resources, older brains are more vulnerable to Al neurotoxicity and AD than younger brains.

Firstly, some age-related attrition of pyramidal cells occurs, reducing neuronal redundancy.[296] On average, cortical neurons show a 9.5% decrease in their numbers between ages 20 and 90 years.[297] Around 85 000 neurons are lost each day of the life span, equivalent to approximately one per second.[296] Also, 40–50% of the length of the myelinated nerve fiber is lost in advanced old age. Some brain regions, such as the entorhinal cortex and the subiculum/CA1 zone, have precise requirements for their connections and relatively low redundancy. Modest cell losses in these brain regions may produce dramatic deficits.[296] Exhaustion of compensatory neuroplasticity leads to continuing damage in these brain regions and loss of cognition.[198–200,202]

Secondly, the vast majority of neurons are established during fetal growth[298] and survive into old age. Neurons are very long-lived cells that show structural and functional differences as they age. Older neurons have lower rates of RNA and protein synthesis than younger neurons.[299,300] Older cells have less capacity for RNA and DNA repair.[301]

Thirdly, neural plasticity has reduced efficacy with increasing age. Older neurons have less ability than young neurons for sprouting and re-innervation of damaged brain areas. For example, sprouting in the rat olfactory bulb increases during the growth phase and up to the onset of old age (*i.e.*, between 3 and 24 months). Sprouting decreases slightly between 24 and 27 months and then decreases sharply after 27 months.[302] This age-related decrease in neural sprouting and re-innervation may explain why most rats that developed cognitive deterioration after chronic Al exposure showed decline in their T-maze performance scores from 27 months of age onwards, and why AD incidence increases exponentially after age 65.

2.6.4 Al-Containing Dietary Supplements Specifically Marketed for Older Individuals

Most very old people who are still alive at time of writing (2012) were born and raised in an era before the currently available array of Al-containing supplements gained popularity, and have had relatively low Al exposure for at least part of their lives. However, certain of these supplements have high Al content and are currently being marketed specifically for the older consumer.

Digestive disorders are common in elderly people, and many routinely consume Al hydroxide- or Al phosphate-based antacids, even though magnesium-based antacids are also effective and potentially less toxic. Some people consume between 840 and 5000 mg Al per day from antacids.[303] These Al salts are poorly soluble and are largely trapped by intestinal mucus, so the ingested amount is disproportional to the amount absorbed. Nevertheless, a study involving healthy human volunteers has shown some Al absorption occurs from antacid ingestion.[27]

Supplemental calcium is often recommended for older people, especially for post-menopausal women. Calcium supplements are typically contaminated with Al; for example, supplements derived from oyster shells provide a source of Ca^{2+}, but they also provide about 12 mg Al per day.[304] Influenza vaccines, recommended annually for older people, are Al-adjuvanted in the UK and some other British Commonwealth countries. As mentioned, Al adjuvant in vaccines delivers at least 100 times more Al than a comparable oral Al dose because injections bypass the gastrointestinal mucosal barrier.

2.7 Conclusions

Alzheimer's disease is a relatively new form of dementia. The history of AD is associated with increasing urbanization, changes in diet and other health practices such as immunization rates. The author has reviewed evidence that routine and chronic exposure to relatively low Al doses from the diet produces a slow but progressive increase in Al content throughout life in the brains of laboratory rats and humans. Susceptible individuals that develop chronic Al neurotoxicity show neuropathological characteristics essentially the same as those observed in AD, apart from species-specific differences, and share some behavioral characteristics. Dietary Al doses, delivered to animals over a prolonged time period, faithfully replicate the progression of AD and reveal its potential consequences in human brains.

Modern evidence reveals that the most salient pathological features in the AD brain are high stage Al accumulation in pyramidal cells, accompanied by microtubule depletion. A cascade of effects follows. Al-induced microtubule depletion results in dieback of the axon and dendrites, and loss of synapse density, accounting for the loss of connectivity between affected neurons and the cortical atrophy that eventually occurs. These characteristics affect sporadic pyramid cells as well as groups of adjacent cells with high-stage aluminum accumulation that constitute expanding lesions in AD-vulnerable brain regions.

All brains of rats with cognitive deterioration were distinguished by extensive damage to the cells of origin for the perforant path in the entorhinal cortex and the presence of at least one substantial lesion in the subiculum/CA1 zone, consisting of pyramidal cells with high stage nuclear Al staining, microtubule depletion and dendritic dieback. Taken together, these lesions cause cognitive deterioration by effectively isolating the hippocampal formation from the neocortex.

NFTs in AD-affected human brains have been shown to involve Al accumulation in their formation and growth. NFTs apparently form as a protective mechanism, binding neurotoxic Al in the cytoplasm and slowing Al accumulation in the nucleus. Granulovacuolar degeneration is another characteristic shared between Al neurotoxicity and AD.

Al-exposed animal brains reproduce all major stages of amyloid formation, from up-regulation of APP to the laying down of neuritic plaques in the neuropil. On a biochemical level, Al competes with essential metal ions, disrupting calcium and iron metabolism. Al also produces ROS that oxidize cell proteins and membranes and provoke an inflammatory response in the brain. These pathological features are all characteristic of AD.

Age-related changes in the kidneys, bone and brain increase the amount of bioavailable Al in circulation and contribute to the development of AD. The slow but relentless net accumulation of Al in neurons over decades produces a continuous insult on large pyramidal neurons in certain AD-vulnerable brain regions. Eventually, APOE-dependent neuroplasticity is up-regulated, requiring other neurons to compensate for Al damage by re-innervation. Cells have finite repair capacities which eventually exhaust, thereby leading to re-innervation failure. The number of decades required to reach this stage explains why old age has been recognized as the main risk factor for AD.

Chronic Al neurotoxicity is virtually the same as AD when species-specific differences are taken into account. Chronic Al neurotoxicity is the only proposed cause of AD that shows so many consistent characteristics. Apparent inconsistencies between chronic Al neurotoxicity and AD have now been explained.

Some people, including scientists, may challenge the link between Al and AD, despite the extensive data that support the link. Consensus on industry-sensitive subjects may be hard to reach, just as some continue to question the evidence for smoking as a cause of lung cancer.

However, regulatory agencies such as the US FDA should now consider whether Al deserves to retain its GRAS rating, and whether to place strict limitations on its inclusion in products that can contribute to the Al burden of the brain in AD-vulnerable regions.

Declaration

The author has no conflict of interest to declare.

Acknowledgments

The author is most grateful to Don Bryson-Taylor for his generous offer to review this chapter and for his helpful editorial suggestions. The author also appreciates the skillful help of Dirce Everett with the illustrations.

References

1. G. M. Humphry, *Old Age: The Results of Information Received Respecting Nearly Nine Hundred Persons who had Attained the Age of Eighty Years, Including Seventy-four Centenarians*, MacMillan and Bowes, Cambridge, 1889, p. 48.
2. B. A. Blansjaar, R. Thomassen and H. W. Van Schaick, *Int. J. Geriatr. Psychiatry*, 2000, **15**, 219–225.
3. Centre for Epidemiology and Research, *2010 Report on Adult Health from the New South Wales Population Health Survey,* NSW Department of Health, Sydney, 2011, pp. 87–89 and 102–104. http://www.health.nsw.gov.au/resources/publichealth/surveys/pdf/hsa_10pub.pdf (last accessed November 2011).
4. A. Alzheimer, *Zentralbl. Nevenheilkunde Psychiatrie*, 1907, **30**, 177–179.
5. A. Alzheimer, *Z. Gesamte Neurol. Psychiatrie*, 1911, **4**, 356–385.
6. B. O. Osuntokun, A. Ogunniyi, E. E. U. Akang, P. U. Aghadiuno, A. Ilori, E. A. Bamgboye, K. Beyreuther and C. Masters, *Lancet*, 1994, **343**, 56.
7. V. Chandra, R. Pandav, H. H. Dodge, J. M. Johnston, S. H. Belle, S. T. DeKosky and M. Ganguli, *Neurology*, 2001, **57**, 985–989.
8. World Health Organization and Alzheimer's Disease International, *Dementia: A Public Health Priority*, WHO Press, Geneva, 2012.
9. J. C. Morris, *Clin. Geriatr. Med.*, 1994, **10**, 257–276.
10. L. E. Nee, R. Eldridge, T. Sunderland, C. B. Thomas, D. Katz, B. S. Thompson, H. Weingartner, H. Weiss, C. Julian and R. Cohen, *Neurology*, 1987, **37**, 359–363.
11. H. Creasey, A. Jorm, W. Longley, G. A. Broe and A. S. Henderson, *Neurology*, 1989, **39**, 1474–1476.
12. I. Räihä, J. Kaprio, M. Koskenvuo, T. Rajala and L. Sourander, *Lancet*, 1996, **347**, 573–578.
13. W. J. Lukiw, M. E. Percy and T. P. Kruck, *J. Inorg. Biochem.*, 2005, **99**, 1895–1898.
14. L. Simonsen, H. Johnsen, S. P. Lund, E. Matikainen, U. Midtgard and A. Wennberg, *Scand. J. Work Environ. Health*, 1994, **20**, 1–12.
15. D. R. Crapper, S. S. Krishnan and A. J. Dalton, *Science*, 1973, **180**, 511–513.

16. US FDA. http://www.fda.gov/ForIndustry/ColorAdditives/Regulatory Process HistoricalPerspectives/default.htm (last accessed November, 2011).
17. J. Snow, *Lancet*, 1857, (ii), 4-5; reprinted in *Int. J. Epidemiol.* 2003, 32, 336–337.
18. F. P. Underhill, F. I. Peterman and S. L. Steel, *J. Physiol. (London)*, 1929, **90**, 52–61.
19. W. J. Gies, *JAMA*, 1911, **57**, 816–821.
20. J. S. Greger, *Annu. Rev. Nutr.*, 1993, **13**, 42–63.
21. J. S. Greger and J. E. Sutherland, *Crit. Rev. Clin. Lab. Sci.*, 1997, **34**, 439–474.
22. Committee on the GRAS List Survey, Phase III, Estimates of daily intake in *The 1977 Survey of Industry on the Use of Food Additives*, National Academy of Science, Washington, DC, 1979, Vol. 3.
23. L. R. Kavoussi, L. D. Gelstein and G. L. Andriole, *J. Urol.*, 1986, **136**, 665–667.
24. P. Hantson, P. Mahieu, M. Gersdorff, C. Sindic and R. Lauwerys, *Clin. Toxicol.*, 1995, **33**, 645–648.
25. M. W. Whitehead, G. Farrar, G. L. Christie, J. A. Blair, R. P. H. Thompson and J. J. Powell, *Am. J. Clin. Nutr.*, 1997, **65**, 1446–1452.
26. J. J. Powell, C. C. Ainley, R. Evans and R. P. H. Thompson, *Gut*, 1994, **35**, 1053–1057.
27. R. R. Recker, A. J. Blotcky, J. A. Leffler and E. P. Rack, *J. Lab. Clin. Med.*, 1977, **90**, 810–815.
28. R. A. Yokel, S. S. Rhineheimer, P. Sharma, D. Elmore, D and P. J. McNamara, *Toxicol. Sci.*, 2001, **64**, 77–82.
29. T. B. Drüeke, *Nephrol., Dial., Transplant.*, 2002, **17**, 13–16.
30. G. J. Naylor, A. H. W. Smith, A. McHarg, P. Walker, B. Shepherd, N. I. Ward and M. Harper, *Trace Elem. Psychiatry*, 1989, **6**, 93–95.
31. J. P. Day, J. Barker, L. J. A. Evans, J. Perks, P. J. Seabright, P. Ackrill, J. S. Lilley, P. V. Drumm and G. W. A. Newton, *Lancet*, 1991, **337**, 1345.
32. G. A. Trapp, *Life Sci.*, 1983, **33**, 311–316.
33. J. A. Edwardson, P. B. Moore, I. N. Ferrier, J. S. Lilley, G. W. A. Newton, J. Barker, J. Templar and J. P. Day, *Lancet*, 1993, **342**, 211–212.
34. S. Yumoto, H. Nagai, M. Imamura, H. Matsuzaki, K. Hayashi, A. Masuda, H. Kumazawa, H. Ohashi and K. Kobayashi, *Nucl. Inst. Method. Physics. Res. B*, 1997, **123**, 279–282.
35. J. Walton, C. Tuniz, D. Fink, G. Jacobsen and D. Wilcox, *Neurotoxicology*, 1995, **16**, 187–190.
36. T. B. Drüeke, P. Jouhanneau, H. Banide and B. Lacour, *Clin. Sci.*, 1997, **92**, 63–67.
37. T. A. Zafar, C. M. Weaver, B. R. Martin, R. Flarend and D. Elmore, *Proc. Soc. Exp. Biol. Med.*, 1997, **216**, 81–85.
38. S. Yumoto, H. Nagai, K. Kobayashi, A. Tamate, S. Kakimi and H. Matsuzaki, *J. Inorg. Biochem.*, 2003, **97**, 155–160.

39. S. A. Burrell and C. Exley, *BMC Pediatr.*, 2010, **10**, 63.
40. N. W. Baylor, W. Egan and P. Richman, *Vaccine*, 2002, **20**(Suppl. 3), S18–S23.
41. K. Redhead, G. J. Quinlan, R. G. Das and J. M. C. Gutteridge, *Pharmacol. Toxicol.*, 1992, **70**, 278–280.
42. W. R. Markesbery, W. D. Ehmann, T. I. Hossain, M. Alauddin and D. T. Goodin, *Ann. Neurol.*, 1981, **10**, 511–516.
43. J. R. McDermott, A. I. Smith, K. Iqbal and H. M. Wisniewski, *Neurology*, 1979, **29**, 809–814.
44. H. Shimizu, T. Mori, M. Koama, M. Sekiya and H. Ooami, *Nihon Ronen Igakkai Zasshi - Jpn. J. Geriatr.* (Tokyo), 1994, **31**, 950–960.
45. W. R. Markesbery, W. D. Ehmann, M. Alauddin and T. I. M. Hossain, *Neurobiol., Aging*, 1984, **5**, 19–28.
46. A. C. Alfrey, G. R. LeGendre and W. D. Kaehny, *N. Engl. J. Med.*, 1976, **294**, 184–188.
47. M. Yasui, Y. Yase, K. Ota and R.M. Garruto, *Neurotoxicology*, 1991, **12**, 603–614.
48. M. Yasui, Y. Yase, K. Ota and R. M. Garruto, *Neurotoxicology*, 1991, **12**, 615–620.
49. R. M. Garruto, *Curr. Alzheimer Res.*, 2006, **3**, 397–401.
50. S. Kobayashi, N. Hirota and K. Saito, *Acta Neuropathol.*, 1987, **74**, 47–52.
51. J. R. Walton, *Biotech. Histochem.*, 2004, **79**, 169–176.
52. B. Solomon, R. Koppel and J. Jossiphov, *Brain Res. Bull.*, 2001, **55**, 253–256.
53. J. R. Walton, *Neurotoxicology*, 2006, **27**, 385–394.
54. J. R. Walton, *Neurotoxicology*, 2009, **30**, 1059–1069.
55. S. Yumoto, H. Nagai, M. Imamura, H. Matsuzaki, K. Hayashi, A. Masuda, H. Kumazawa, H. Ohashi and K. Kobayashi, *Nucl. Instr. Meth. Physics Res. B*, 1997, **123**, 279–282.
56. J. R. Walton, *J. Alzheimer's Dis.*, 2010, **22**, 65–72.
57. R. C. A. Pearson, M. M. Esiri, R. W. Hiorns, G. K. Wilcock and T. P. Powell, *Proc. Natl. Acad. Sci. U.S.A.*, 1985, **82**, 4531–4534.
58. R. A. Armstrong, *Neurosci. Lett.*, 1993, **160**, 57–60.
59. M. M. Esiri and S. A. Chance, *J. Alzheimer's Dis.*, 2006, **9**, 79–89.
60. P. O. Ganrot, *Environ. Health Persp.*, 1986, **65**, 363–441.
61. R. B. Martin, *Clin. Chem.*, 1986, **32**, 1797–1806.
62. J. L. Miller, C. M. Hubbard, B. J. Litman and T. L. Macdonald, *J. Biol. Chem.*, 1989, **264**, 243–250.
63. G. A. Trapp, *Kidney Int.*, 1986, **29**, S12–S16.
64. T. L. Macdonald, W. G. Humphreys and R. B. Martin, *Science*, 1987, **236**, 183–186.
65. S. C. Bondy, S. F. Ali and S. Guo-Ross, *Mol. Chem. Neuropathol.*, 1998A, **34**, 219–232.
66. S. C. Bondy, S. X. Guo-Ross and J. Pien, *Neurotoxicology*, 1998B, **19**, 65–71.
67. C. Exley, *Free Radic. Biol. Med.*, 2004, **36**, 380–387.

68. S. Kong, S. Liochev and I. Fridovich, *Free Radic. Biol. Med.*, 1992, **13**, 79–81.
69. L. Meglio and P. I. Oteiza, *Neurochem. Res.*, 1999, **24**, 1001–1008.
70. D. Pratico, K. Uryu, S. Sung, S. Tang, J. W. Trojanowski and V.M.-Y. Lee, *FASEB J.*, 2002, **16**, 1138–1141.
71. R. M. Ward, Y. Zhang and R. R. Crichton, *J. Inorg. Biochem.*, 2001, **87**, 9–14.
72. S. J. Karlik, G. L. Eichhorn, P. N. Lewis and D. R. Crapper, *Biochemistry*, 1980, **19**, 5991–5998.
73. S. V. Verstraeten, M. S. Golub, C. L. Keen and P. I. Oteiza, *Arch. Biochem. Biophys.*, 1997, **344**, 289–294.
74. T. P. Flaten, *Brain Res. Bull.*, 2001, **55**, 187–196.
75. V. Rondeau, H. Jacmin-Gadda, D. Commenges, C. Helmer and J.-F. Dartigues, *Am. J. Epidemiol.*, 2009, **169**, 489–496.
76. M. A. Rogers and D. G. Simon, *Age Ageing*, 1999, **28**, 205–209.
77. J. R. Walton, *Neurosci. Lett.*, 2007, **412**, 29–33.
78. J. R. Walton, *Neurotoxicology*, 2009, **30**, 182–193.
79. J. Loesche and O. Steward, *Brain Res. Bull.*, 1977, **2**, 31–39.
80. P. B. Moore, J. P. Day, G. A. Taylor, I. N. Ferrier, L. K. Fifield and J. A. Edwardson, *Dement. Geriatr. Cogn. Disord.*, 2000, **11**, 66–69.
81. J. M. Kellet, A. Taylor and J. J. Oram, *Lancet*, 1986, **i**, 682.
82. A. Van Rhijn, F. M. Corrigan and N. I. Ward, *Trace Elem. Med*, 1989, **6**, 24–26.
83. F. M. Corrigan, J. S. Crichton, A. G. Van Rhijn, E. R. Skinner and N. I. Ward, *Clin. Chim. Acta*, 1992, **211**, 121–123.
84. N. B. Roberts, A. Clough, J. P. Bellia and J. Y. Kim, *J. Inorg. Biochem.*, 1998, **69**, 171–176.
85. C. Smorgon, E. Mari, A. R. Atti, E. Dalla Nora, P. F. Zamboni, F. Calzoni, A. Passaro and R. Fellin, *Arch. Gerontol. Geriatr., Suppl.*, 2004, **9**, 393–402.
86. D. Shore, M. Millson, J. L. Holtz, S. W. King, T. P. Bridge and R. J. Wyatt, *Biol. Psychiatry*, 1980, **15**, 971–977.
87. P. B. Moore, J. A. Edwardson, I. N. Ferrier, G. A. Taylor, D. Lett, S. P. Tyrer, J. P. Day, S. J. King and J. S. Lilley, *Biol. Psychiatry*, 1997, **41**, 488–492.
88. A. H. Ropper and K. R. S. Williams, *Neurology*, 1980, **30**, 639–644.
89. D. M. A. Mann in *Down Syndrome and Alzheimer's Disease*, ed. V.P. Prasher, Radcliffe Publishing Ltd, Milton Keynes, 2006, pp. 15–36.
90. H. Braak and E. Braak, *Acta Neuropathol.*, 1991, **82**, 239–259.
91. T. Kovács, N. J. Cairns and P. L. Lantos, *NeuroReport*, 2001, **12**, 285–288.
92. D. Holland, J. B. Brewer, D. L. Hagler, C. Fennema-Notestine and A. M. Dale, *Proc. Natl. Acad. Sci. U.S.A.*, 2009, **106**, 20954–20959.
93. S. E. Arnold, B. T. Hyman, J. Flory, A. R. Damasio and G. W. Van Hoesen, *Cerebral Cortex*, 1991, **1**, 103–116.
94. N. W. Kowall, W. W. Pendlebury, J. B. Kessler, D. P. Perl and M. F. Beal, *Neuroscience*, 1989, **29**, 329–337.

95. J. A. Edwardson, I. N. Ferrier, F. K. McArthur, I. G. McKeith, I. McLaughlin, C. M. Morris, A. E. Oakley, S. A. Mountfort, A. E. Oakley, G. A. Taylor, M. K. Ward and J. M. Candy in *Aluminum in Chemistry Biology and Medicine, A Series of Advances*, eds. M. Nicolini, P.F. Zatta and B. Corain, Raven Press, New York, 1991, vol. 1, pp. 85–96.
96. C. M. Morris, J. M. Candy, A. E. Oakley, G. A. Taylor, S. Mountfort, H. Bishop, M. K. Ward, C. A. Bloxham and J. A. Edwardson, *J Neurol. Sci.*, 1989, **94**, 295–306.
97. W. A. Jefferies, M. R. Brandon, S. V. Hunt, A. F. Williams, K. C. Gatter and D. Y. Mason, *Nature*, 1984, **312**, 162–163.
98. A. J. Roskams and J. R. Connor, *Proc. Natl. Acad. Sci. U.S.A.*, 1990, **87**, 9024–9027.
99. E. Andrasi, N. Pali, Z. Molnar and S. Kosel, *J. Alzheimer's Dis.*, 2005, **7**, 273–284.
100. R. Rusina, R. Matěj, L. Kašparová, J. Kukal and P. Urban, *Neurotox. Res.*, 2011, **20**, 329–330.
101. G. A. Trapp, *Biol. Psychiatry*, 1978, **13**, 709–718.
102. D. R. Crapper, S. S. Krishnan and S. Quittkat, *Brain*, 1976, **99**, 67–80.
103. R. D. Traub, T. C. Rains, R. M. Garruto, D. C. Gajdusek and C. J. Gibbs, *Neurology*, 1981, **31**, 986–990.
104. N. Xu, V. Majidi, W. R. Markesbery and W. D. Ehmann, *Neurotoxicology*, 1992, **13**, 735–743.
105. F. M. Corrigan, G. P. Reynolds and N. I. Ward, *BioMetals*, 1993, **6**, 149–154.
106. A. V. Everitt, *Proc. Aust. Assoc. Gerontol.*, 1991, **26**, 79–82.
107. J. R. Walton and M. X. Wang, *J. Inorg. Biochem.*, 2009, **103**, 1548–1554.
108. J. R. Walton, *J. Inorg. Biochem.*, 2007, **101**, 1275–1284.
109. G. W. Van Hoesen and D. N. Pandya, *Brain Res.*, 1975, **95**, 39–59.
110. G. W. Van Hoesen, B. T. Hyman and A. R. Damasio, *Hippocampus*, 1991, **1**, 1–8.
111. S. A. Bayer in The Rat Central Nervous System: *Forebrain and Midbrain*, ed. G. Paxinos, 1st edn, Academic Press, San Diego, 1985, pp. 335–352.
112. R. M. Beckstead, *Brain Res.*, 1978, **152**, 249–264.
113. B. T. Hyman, G. W. Van Hoesen, L. J. Kromer and A. R. Damasio, *Ann. Neurol.*, 1986, **20**, 472–481.
114. S. E. Arnold, B. T. Hyman, J. Florey, A. R. Damasio and D. W. Van Hoesen, *Cerebral Cortex*, 1991, **1**, 103–116.
115. D. P. Perl and A. R. Brody, *Science*, 1980, **208**, 297–299.
116. P. F. Good, D. P. Perl, L. M. Bierer and J. Schmeidler, *Ann. Neurol.*, 1992, **31**, 286–292.
117. J. R. Walton, *Int. J. Alzheimer's Dis.*, 2012, p. 17, doi:10.1155/2012/914947.
118. J. R. Walton, *J. Alzheimer's Dis.*, 2012, **29**, 255–273.
119. K. N. Green and F. M. LaFerla, *Neuron*, 2008, **59**, 190–194.

120. I. N. Ferrier, A. Leake, G. A. Taylor, I. G. McKeith, A. F. Fairbairn, C. J. Robinson, R. M. Francis and J. A. Edwardson, *Age Ageing*, 1990, **19**, 368–375.
121. M. Berrocal, D. Marcos, M. R. Sepulveda, M. Perez, J. Avila and A. M. Mata, *FASEB J.*, 2009, **23**, 1826–1834.
122. R. S. Jope, L. Song, X. Li and R. Powers, *Neurobiol. Aging*, 1994, **15**, 221–226.
123. R. S. Jope, *J. Alzheimer's Dis.*, 1999, **1**, 231–247.
124. A. F. Greenwood, R. E. Powers and R. S. Jope, *Neuroscience*, 1995, **69**, 125–138.
125. G. Cole, K. R. Dobkins, L. A. Hansen, R. D. Terry and T. Saitoh, *Brain Res.*, 1988, **452**, 165–174.
126. H. Matsushima, S. Shimohama, M. Chachin, T. Taniguchi and J. Kimura, *J. Neurochem.*, 1996, **67**, 317–323.
127. M. F. Bear and A. Kirkwood, *Curr. Opin. Neurobiol.*, 1993, **3**, 197–202.
128. W. R. Holmes, *J. Comput. Neurosci.*, 2000, **8**, 65–85.
129. M. E. Gnegy, *Crit. Rev. Neurobiol.*, 2000, **14**, 91–129.
130. F. Battaglia, H.-Y. Wang, M. F. Ghilardi, E. Gashi, A. Quartarone, E. Friedman and R. A. Nixon, *Biol. Psychiatry*, 2007, **62**, 1405–1412.
131. D. Orihuela, V. Meichtry and M. Pizarro, *J. Inorg. Biochem.*, 2005, **99**, 1879–1886.
132. K. A. Cox and M. A. Dunn, *J. Nutr.*, 2001, **131**, 2007–2013.
133. B. Platt and D. Busselberg, *Cell. Mol. Neurobiol.*, 1994, **14**, 819–829.
134. B. Platt, H. Haas and D. Büsselberg, *NeuroReport*, 1994, **5**, 2329–2332.
135. N. Arispe, E. Rojas and H. B. Pollas, *Proc. Natl. Acad. Sci. U.S.A.*, 1993, **90**, 567–571.
136. D. Julka and K. D. Gill, *Biochim. Biophys. Acta*, 1996, **1315**, 47–54.
137. S. Sarin, D. Julka D and K. D. Gill, *Mol. Cell. Biochem.*, 1997, **168**, 95–100.
138. S. Kirischuk, N. Pronchur and A. Verkhratsky, *Neuroscience*, 1992, **50**, 947–951.
139. A. C. Nostrandt, T. J. Shafer, W. R. Mundy and S. Padilla, *Toxicol. Appl. Pharmacol.*, 1996, **136**, 118–125.
140. L. J. McDonald and M. D. Mamrack, *Biochem. Biophys. Res. Commun.*, 1988, **155**, 203–208.
141. M. Cochran, D. C. Elliott, P. Brennan and V. Chawtur, *Clin. Chim. Acta*, 1990, **194**, 167–172.
142. H. Kurita, A. Nakatomi, H. Shimahara, M. Yazawa and S.-Y. Ohki, *Biochem. Biophys. Res. Commun.*, 2005, **333**, 1060–1065.
143. T. Wolf, B. Solomon, D. Ivnitski, J. Rishpon and G. Fleminger, *J. Mol. Recogn.*, 1998, **11**, 14–19.
144. R. Levi, T. Wolf, G. Fleminger and B. Solomon, *Mol. Cell. Biochem.*, 1998, **189**, 41–46.
145. B. J. Farnell, D. R. Crapper McLachlan, K. Baimbridge, U. De Boni, L. Wong and P. L. Wood, *Exp. Neurol.*, 1985, **88**, 68–83.
146. B. Shi, K. Chou and A. Haug, *Mol. Cell. Biochem.*, 1993, **121**, 109–118.

147. B. Platt, D. O. Carpenter, D. Busselberg, K. G. Reymann and G. Riedel, *Exp. Neurol.*, 1995, **134**, 73–86.
148. M. Wang, D.-Y. Ruan, J.-T. Chen and Y.-Z. Xu, *Food Chem. Toxicol.*, 2002, **40**, 471–478.
149. J. Chen, M. Wang, D. Ruan and J. She, *Neuroscience*, 2002, **112**, 879–887.
150. B. Hallgren and P. Sourander, *J. Neurochem.*, 1958, **3**, 41–51.
151. C. M. Morris, J. M. Candy, C. A. Bloxham and J. A. Edwardson, *Biochem. Soc. Trans.*, 1989, **18**, 647–648.
152. K. Pantopoulos, *Ann. N.Y. Acad. Sci.*, 2004, **1012**, 1–13.
153. M. A. Deibel, W. D. Ehmann and W. R. Markesbery, *J. Neurol. Sci.*, 1996, **143**, 137–142.
154. M. A. Smith, K. Wehr, P. L. Harris, S. L. Siedlak, J. R. Connor and G. Perry G, *Brain Res.*, 1998, **788**, 232–236.
155. C. C. Winterbourn, *Toxicol. Lett.*, 1995, **82–83**, 969–974.
156. Y. Kim, L. Olivi, J. H. Cheong, A. Maertens and J. P. Bressler, *Toxicol. Appl. Pharmacol.*, 2007, **230**, 349–356.
157. K. Yamanaka, N. Minato and K. Iwai, *FEBS Lett.*, 1999, **462**, 216–220.
158. K. Abreo, F. Abreo, M. L. Sella and S. Jain, *J. Neurochem.*, 1999, **72**, 2059–2064.
159. S. Oshiro, M. Kawahara, S. Mika, K. Muramoto, K. Kobayashi, R. Ishige, K. Nozawa, M. Hori, C. Yung, S. Kitajima and Y. Kuroda, *J. Biochem.*, 1998, **123**, 42–46.
160. A. Nunomura, G. Perry, A. Gjumrakch, K. Hirai, A. Takeda, E. K. Balraj, P. K. Jones, H. Ghanbari, T. Wataya, S. Shimohama, S. Chiba, C. S. Atwood, R. B. Petersen and M. A. Smith, *J. Neuropathol. Exp. Neurol.*, 2001, **60**, 759–767.
161. O. I. Aruoma, B. Halliwell, M. J. Laughton, G. J. Quinlan and J. M. C. Gutteridge, *Biochem. J.*, 1989, **258**, 617–620.
162. E. Y. Yang, S. X. Guo-Ross and S. C. Bondy, *Brain Res.*, 1999, **839**, 221–226.
163. H. Arai, K. Kosaka and R. Iizuka, *J. Neurochem.*, 1984, **43**, 388–393.
164. P. T. Francis, A. M. Palmer, N. R. Sims, D. M. Bowen, A. N. Davidson, M. M. Esiri, D. Neary, J. S. Snowden and G. K. Wilcock, *New Engl. J. Med.*, 1985, **313**, 7–11.
165. C. M. Yates, J. Simpson and A. Gordon, *Neurosci. Lett.*, 1986, **65**, 189–192.
166. R. Katzman, Alzheimer's disease, *New Engl. J. Med.*, 1986, **314**, 964–973.
167. D. M. Bowen, J. S. Benton, J. A. Spillane, C. C. T. Smith and S. J. Allen, *J. Neurol. Sci.*, 1982, **57**, 191–202.
168. R. S. Jope, L. Song and R. E. Powers, *Neurobiol Aging*, 1997, **18**, 111–120.
169. J. K. Blusztajn, M. Liscovitch and U. I. Richardson, *Proc. Natl. Acad. Sci. U.S.A.*, 1987, **84**, 5474–5477.
170. P.W. Schenk and B. E. Snaar-Jagalska, *Biochim. Biophys. Acta*, **1449**, 1–24.
171. T. Dobransky, W. L. Davis and R. J. Rylett, *J. Biol. Chem.*, 2001, **276**, 22244–22250.

172. C. Sumi-Ichinose, F. Urano, R. Kuroda, T. Ohye, M. Kojima, M. Tazawa, H. Shiraishi, Y. Hagino, T. Nagatsu, T. Nomura and H. Ichinose, *J. Biol. Chem.*, 2001, **276**, 41150–41160.
173. J. M. Anderson, C. G. B. Hamon, R. A. Armstrong and J. A. Blair in *Chemistry and Biology of Pteridines,* eds. B. A. Cooper and V. M. Whitehead, Walter de Gruyter & Co., Berlin, 1986, pp. 327–330.
174. A. D. Kay, S. Milstien, S. Kaufman, H. Creasey, J. V. Haxby, N. R. Cutler and S. I. Rapoport, *Arch. Neurol.*, 1986, **43**, 996–999.
175. J. R. Hofstetter, I. Vincent, O. Bugiani, B. Ghetti and J. A. Richter, *Neurochem. Pathol.*, 1987, **6**, 177–193.
176. M. F. Beal, M. F. Mazurek, D. W. Ellison, N. W. Kowall, P. R. Solomon and W. W. Pendlebury, *Neuroscience*, 1989, **29**, 339–346.
177. M. Tsunoda and R. P. Sharma, *J. Trace Elements Med. Biol.*, 1996, **13**, 224–231.
178. P. P. Gonçalves and V. S. Silva, *J. Inorg. Biochem.*, 2007, **101**, 1291–1338.
179. A. Szutowicz, M. Tomaszewicz, A. Jankowska, B. Madziar and H. Bielarczyk, *Metabol. Brain Dis.*, 2000, **15**, 29–44.
180. V. S. Silva, M. A. Nunes, J. M. Cordeiro, A. I. Calejo, S. Santos, P. Neves, A. Sykes, F. Morgado, Y. Dunant and P. P. Gonçalves, *Toxicology*, 2007, **236**, 158–177.
181. S. Kumar, *Med. Hypothesis*, 1999, **52**, 557–559.
182. R. A. Armstrong, J. Anderson, J. D. Cowburn, J. Cox and J. A. Blair, *Biol. Chem. Hoppe-Seyler*, 1992, **373**, 1075–1078.
183. S. Katoh, T. Sueoka, Y. Yamamoto and S. Y. Takahashi, *FEBS Lett.*, 1994, **341**, 227–232.
184. E. G. McGeer and P. I. McGeer, *Neuropsychopharmacol. Biol. Psychiatry*, 2003, **27**, 741–749.
185. V. Colangelo, J. Schurr, M. J. Ball, R. P. Pelaez, N. G. Bazan and W. J. Lukiw, *J. Neurosci. Res.*, 2002, **70**, 462–473.
186. A. Campbell and S. C. Bondy, *Cell Mol. Biol.*, 2000, **46**, 721–730.
187. A. Campbell, E. Y. Yang, M. Tsai-Turton and S. C. Bondy, *Brain Res.*, 2002, **933**, 60–65.
188. A. Campbell, A. Becaria, D. K. Lahiri, K. Sharman and S. C. Bondy, *J. Neurosci. Res.*, 2004, **75**, 565–572.
189. P. N. Alexandrov, Y. Zhao, A. I. Pogue, M. A. Tarr, T. P. Kruck, M. E. Percy, J. G. Cui and W. J. Lukiw, *J. Alzheimer's Dis.*, 2005, **8**, 117–127.
190. R. A. Yokel and J. P. O'Callaghan, *Neurotoxicol. Teratol.*, 1998, **20**, 55–60.
191. B. Platt, G. Fiddler, G. Riedel and Z. Henderson, *Brain Res. Bull.*, 2001, **55**, 257–267.
192. C. Theiss and K. Meller, *Cell Tissue Res.*, 2002, **310**, 143–154.
193. D. A. Aremu and S. Meshitsuka, *Brain Res. Rev.*, 2006, **52**, 193–200.
194. X. B. Li, H. Zheng, Z. R. Zhang, M. Li, Z. Y. Huang, H. J. Schluesener, Y. Y. Li and S. Q. Xu, *Nanomedicine*, 2009, **5**, 473–479.
195. P. W. Baas, *Int. Rev. Cytol.*, 2002, **212**, 41–62.

196. E. G. Gray, M. Paula-Barbosa and A. Roher, *Neuropathol. Appl. Neurobiol.*, 1987, **13**, 91–110.
197. B. Hempen and J.-P. Brion, *J. Neuropathol. Exp. Neurol.*, 1996, **55**, 964–972.
198. M. E. Scheibel, R. D. Lindsay, U. Tomiyasu and A. B. Scheibel, *Exp. Neurol.*, 1976, **53**, 420–430.
199. S. J. Buell and P. D. Coleman, *Brain Res*, 1981, **214**, 33–41.
200. S. D. Hanks and D. G. Flood, *Brain Res.*, 1991, **540**, 63–82.
201. D. G. Flood, S. J. Buell, C. H. Defiore, G. J. Horwitz and P. D. Coleman, *Brain Res.*, 1985, **345**, 366–368.
202. I. Adams, *Brain Res.*, 1987, **424**, 343–351.
203. D. G. Flood and P. D. Coleman, *Can. J. Neurol. Sci.*, 1986, **13**, 475–479.
204. J. W. Geddes, D. T. Monaghan, C. W. Cotman, I. T. Lott, R. C. Kim and H.C., *Science*, 1985, **230**, 1179–1181.
205. S. J. Buell and P. D. Coleman, *Brain Res.*, 1981, **214**, 23–41.
206. T. L. Petit, G. B. Biederman and P. A. McMullen, *Exp. Neurol.*, 1980, **67**, 152–162.
207. R. D. Terry, E. Masliah, D. P. Salmon, N. Butters, R. DeTeresa, R. Hill, L. A. Hansen and R. Katzman, *Ann. Neurol.*, 1991, **30**, 572–580.
208. D. R. Crapper and A. J. Dalton, *Physiol. Behav.*, 1973, **10**, 935–945.
209. D. R. Crapper and A. J. Dalton, *Physiol. Behav.*, 1973, **10**, 925–933.
210. A. C. Miu, A. I. Olteanu and M. Miclea, *J. Alzheimer's Dis.*, 2004, **6**, 315–328.
211. T. L. Petit, *Soc. Neurosci. Abstr.*, 1977, **3**, 351.
212. E. Uemura and W. P. Ireland, *Exp. Neurol.*, 1985, **89**, 530–542.
213. E. Uemura and W. P. Ireland, *Exp. Neurol.*, 1984, **85**, 1–9.
214. T. Simchowicz, in *Histologische und histopathologische Arbeiten über die Grosshirnrinde mit besonderer Berücksichtigung der pathologischen Anatomie der Geisteskranken,* ed. F. Nissl and A. Alzheimer, Gustav Fischer Verlag, Jena, 1911, pp. 267–443.
215. Y. Jing, Z. Wang and Y. Song, *Synapse*, 2004, **52**, 292–298.
216. M. J. West, P. D. Coleman, D. G. Flood and J. C. Troncosa, *Lancet*, 1994, **344**, 769–772.
217. R. D. Terry, A. Peck, R. DeTeresa, R. Schechter and D. S. Horoupian, *Ann. Neurol.*, 1981, **10**, 184–192.
218. C. Q. Mountjoy, M. Roth, N. J. R. Evans and H. M. Evans, *Neurobiol. Aging*, 1983, **4**, 1–11.
219. L. Regeur, G. Badsberg Jensen, H. Pakkenberg, S. M. Evans and B. Pakkenberg, *Neurobiol. Aging*, 1994, **15**, 347–352.
220. M. C. Diamond, *An. Acad. Bras. Cienc.*, 2001, **73**, 211–220.
221. P. V. Arriagada, J. H. Growdon, E. T. Hedley-Whyte and B. T. Hyman, *Neurology*, 1992, **42**, 631–639.
222. R. W. Shin, V. M. Lee and J. Q. Trojanowski, *J. Neurosci.*, 1994, **14**, 7221–7233.
223. C. X. Gong, T. J. Singh, I. Grundke-Iqbal and K. Iqbal, *J. Neurochem.*, 1993, **61**, 921–927.

224. C. X. Gong, S. Shaikh, J. Z. Wang, T. Zaidi, I. Grundke-Iqbal and K. Iqbal, *J. Neurochem.*, 1995, **65**, 732–738.
225. R.-W. Shin, T. Iwaki, T. Kitamoto, Y. Sato and J. Tateishi, *Am. J. Pathol.*, 1992, **140**, 937–945.
226. A. de Calignon, L. M. Fox, R. Pitstick, G. A. Carlson, B. J. Bacskai, T. L. Spires and B. T. Hyman, *Nature*, 2010, **464**, 1201–1203.
227. C. Bancher, C. Brunner, H. Lassmann, H. Budka, K. Jellinger, G. Wiche, F. Seitelberger, I. Grundke-Iqbal, K. Iqbal and H. M. Wisniewski, *Brain Res.*, 1989, **477**, 90–99.
228. C. M. Wischik, M. Novak, H. C. Thøgersen, P. C. Edwards, M. J. Runswick, R. Jakes, J. E. Walker, C. Milstein, M. Roth and A. Klug, *Proc. Natl. Acad. Sci. U.S.A.*, 1988, **85**, 4506–4510.
229. G. C. Ruben, J. Z. Wang, K. Iqbal and I. Grundke-Iqbal, *Microsc. Res. Tech.*, 2005, **67**, 175–195.
230. M. Kidd, *Nature*, 1963, **197**, 192–193.
231. K. Hatanpää, D. R. Brady, J. Stoll, S. I. Rapoport and K. Chandrasekaran, *Ann. Neurol.*, 1996, **40**, 411–420.
232. S. I. Rapoport, K. Hatanpaa, D. R. Brady and K. Chandrasekaran, *Neurodegeneration*, 1996, **5**, 473–476.
233. R. Morsch, W. Simon and P. D. Coleman, *J. Neuropathol. Exp. Neurol.*, 1999, **58**, 188–197.
234. F. C. Amador, A. G. Henriques, O. A. B. da Cruz e Silva and E. F. da Cruz e Silva, *Neurotox. Teratol.*, 2004, **26**, 387–395.
235. J. M. Cordeiro, V. S. Silva, C. R. Oliveira and P. P. Gonçalves, *J. Inorg. Biochem.*, 2003, **97**, 132–142.
236. C. R. Harrington, C. M. Wischik, F. K. McArthur, G. A. Taylor, J. A. Edwardson and J. M. Candy, *Lancet*, 1994, **343**, 993–997.
237. H. Yamamoto, Y. Saitoh, S. Yasugawa and E. Miyamoto, *J. Neurochem*, 1990, **55**, 683–690.
238. S. P. Guy, D. Jones, D. M. A. Mann and R. Itzaki, *Neurosci. Lett.*, 1991, **121**, 166–168.
239. P. Piccardo, R. Yanagihara, R. M. Garruto, C. J. Gibbs, Jr and D. C. Gajdusek, *Acta Neuropathol.*, 1988, **77**, 1–4.
240. D. P. Perl, D. Munoz-Garcia, P. F. Good and W. W. Pendlebury, *J. Neuropath. Exp. Neurol.*, 1986, **45**, 379.
241. G. A. King, U. DeBoni and D. R. Crapper, *Pharmacol. Biochem. Behav.*, 1975, **3**, 1003–1009.
242. D. R. Crapper in *Neurobiology of Aging*, eds. R.D. Terry and S. Gershon, Raven Press, New York, 1976, pp. 405–432.
243. U. D. Boni, A. Otvos, J. W. Scott and D. R. Crapper, *Acta Neuropathol.*, 1976, **35**, 285–294.
244. J. Savory, Y. Huang, M. M. Herman, M. R. Reyes and M. R. Wills, *Brain Res.*, 1995, **669**, 325–329.
245. Y. Huang, M. M. Herman, J. Liu, C. D. Katsetos, M. R. Wills and J. Savory, *Brain Res.*, 1997, **771**, 213–220.
246. T. Simchowicz, *L'Encéphale*, 1914, 218–231.

247. D. W. Dickson, W.-K. Liu, Y. Kress, J. Ku, O. DeJesus and S.-H.C. Yen, *Acta Neuropathol.*, 1993, **85**, 463–470.
248. J. S. Su, J. P. Kesslak, E. Head and C. W. Cotman, *Acta Neuropathol.*, 2002, **104**, 1–6.
249. X. Sun, Z. Liu, X. Zhang and Z. Zhang, *J. Hygiene Res. Wei Sheng Yen Chiu*, 1999, **28**, 164–166.
250. A. Hirano, L. T. Kurland, R. S. Krooth and S. Lessell, *Brain*, 1961, **84**, 642–661.
251. W. J. Lukiw, *Neurochem. Res.*, 2004, **29**, 1287–1297.
252. T. L. Young-Pearse, A. C. Chen, R. Chang, C. Marquez and D. J. Selkoe, *Neural Develop.*, 2008, **3**, 15–28.
253. G. L. Caporaso, S. E. Gandy, J. D. Buxbaum, T. V. Ramabhadran and P. Greengard, *Proc. Natl. Acad. Sci. U.S.A.*, 1992, **89**, 3055–3059.
254. A. Y. Hung and D. J. Selkoe, *EMBO J.*, 1994, **13**, 534–542.
255. Y.-H. Suh and F. Checler, *Pharmacol. Rev.*, 2002, **54**, 469–525.
256. T. Dyrks, E. Dyrks and C. L. Masters, *FEBS Lett.*, 1993, **324**, 231–236.
257. H. Crystal, D. Dickson, P. Fuld, D. Masur, R. Scott, M. Mehler, J. Masdeu, C. Kawas, M. Aronson and L. Wolfson, *Neurology*, 1988, **38**, 1682–1687.
258. B. D. Shivers, C. Hilbich, G Multhaup, M. Salbaum, K. Beyreuther and P. H. Seeburg, *EMBO J.*, 1988, **7**, 1365–1370.
259. D. Games, D. Adams, R. Alessandrini, R. Barbour, P. Berthelette, C. Blackwell, T. Carr, J. Clemens, T. Donaldson, F. Gillespie, S. Guido Hagoplan, K. Johnson-Wood, K. Khan, M. Lee, P. Leibowitz, I. Lieberburg, S. Little, E. Masliah, L. McConlogue, M. Montoya-Zavala, L. Mucke, L. Paganinin, E. Penniman, M. Power, D. Schenk, P. Seubert, B. Snyder, F. Soriano, H. Tan, J. Vitale, S. Wadsworth, B. Wolozin and J. Zhao, *Nature*, 1995, **373**, 523–527.
260. K. Hsiao, P. Chapman, S. Nilsen, C. Eckman, Y. Harigaya, S. Younkin, F. Yang and G. Cole, *Science*, 1996, **274**, 99–102.
261. N. Sato, K. Imaizumi, T. Manabe, M. Taniguchi, J. Hitomi, T. Katayama, T. Yoneda, T. Morihara, Y. Yasuda, T. Takagi, T. Kudo, T. Tsuda, Y. Itoyama, T. Makifuchi, P. E. Fraser, P. George-Hyslop and M. Tohyama, *J. Biol. Chem.*, 2001, **276**, 2108–2114.
262. N. Sato, O. Hori, A. Yamaguchi, J.-C. Lambert, M.-C. Chartier-Harlin, P. A. Robinson, A. Delacourte, A. M. Schmidt, T. Furuyama, K. Imaizumi, M. Tohyama and T. Takagi, *J. Neurochem.*, 1999, **72**, 2498–2505.
263. S. Matsuzaki, T. Manabe, T. Katayama, A. Nishikawa, T. Yanagita, H. Okuda, Y. S. Yasuda, S. Miyata, S. Meshitsuka and M. Tohyama, *J. Neurochem.*, 2004, **88**, 1345–1351.
264. C. Exley, N. C. Price, S. M. Kelly and J. D. Birchall, *FEBS Lett.*, 1993, **324**, 293–295.
265. E. House, J. Collingwood, A. Khan, O. Korchazkina, G. Berthon and C. Exley, *J. Alzheimer's Dis.*, 2004, **6**, 291–301.

266. F. Ricchelli, D. Drago, B. Filippi, G. Tognon and P. Zatta P, *Cell. Mol. Life Sci.*, 2005, **62**, 1724–1733.
267. M. Kawahara, K. Muramoto, K. Kobayashi, H. Mori and Y. Kuroda, *Biophys. Res. Commun.*, 1994, **198**, 531–535.
268. P. Netter, M. Kessler, A. Gaucher and B. Bannworth, *Ann. Rheum. Dis.*, 1990, **49**, 573–575.
269. K. Shigematsu and P. L. McGeer, *Brain Res.*, 1992, **593**, 117–123.
270. I. Wakayama, K. J. Song, V.R. Nerurkar, S. Yoshida and R. Garruto, *Brain Res.*, 1997, **748**, 237–240.
271. D. Drago, S. Bolognin and P. Zatta, *Curr. Alzheimer Res.*, 2008, **5**, 500–507.
272. L. F. Rodella, F. Ricci, E. Borsani, A. Stacchiotti, E. Foglio, G. Favero, R. Rezzani, C. Mariani and R. Bianchi, *Histol. Histopathol.*, 2008, **23**, 433–439.
273. C. Exley and M. M. Esiri, *J. Neurol. Neurosurg. Psychiatry*, 2006, **77**, 877–879.
274. W. A. Banks, M. I. Niehoff, D. Drago and P. Zatta, *Brain Res.*, 2006, **1116**, 215–221.
275. B. A. Barres and S. J. Smith, *Science*, 2001, **294**, 1296–1297.
276. J. Poirier, A. Baccichet, D. Dea and S. Gauthier, *Neuroscience*, 1993, **55**, 81–90.
277. E. H. Corder, A. M. Saunders, W. J. Strittmatter, D. E. Schmechel, P. C. Gaskell, Jr., J. B. Rimmler, P. A. Locke, P. M. Conneally, K. E. Schmader, R. E. Tanzi, J. F. Gusella, G. W. Small, A. D. Roses, M. A. Pericak Vance and J. L. Haines, *Neurology*, 1995, **45**, 1323–1328.
278. B. Teter, *J. Mol. Neurosci.*, 2004, **23**, 167–179.
279. G. Raisman, *Brain Res.*, 1969, **14**, 25–48.
280. G. Lynch, D. A. Matthews, S. Mosko, T. Parks and C. Cotman, *Brain Res.*, 1972, **42**, 311–318.
281. O. Steward, J. Loesche and W. C. Horton, *Brain Res. Bull.*, 1977, **2**, 41–48.
282. P. S. Ebersole, P. A. Hess and A. S. Luggen in *Toward Healthy Aging: Human Needs and Nursing Response,* ed. M.S. Ledbetter and L.K. Gower, Mosby Inc., St Louis, MO, 2004, pp. 79–108.
283. R. D. Lindeman, J. Tobin and N. W. Shock, *J. Am. Geriatr. Soc.*, 1985, **33**, 278–285.
284. E. H. Jeffery, K. Abreo, E. Burgess, J. Cannata and J. L. Greger, *J. Toxicol. Environ. Health*, 1996, **48**, 649–665.
285. A. S. Buchman, D. Tanne, P. A. Boyle, R. C. Shah, S. E. Leurgans and D. A. Bennett, *Neurology*, 2009, **73**, 920–927.
286. E. A. Tonna, *J. Gerontol.*, 1978, **33**, 163–177.
287. N.D. Priest, D. Newton and R.J. Talbot, *UKAEA Report AEA-EE-0206*, 1991, Harwell, UKAEA.
288. M. Lieberherr, B. Gross, G. Cournot-Witmer, M. P. M. Hermann-Erlee and S. Balsan, *Kidney Int.*, 1987, **31**, 736–743.
289. N. C. Blumenthal and A. S. Posner, *Calcif. Tissue Int.*, 1984, **36**, 439–441.

290. M. R. Christoffersen and J. Christoffersen, *Calcif. Tiss. Int.*, 1983, **37**, 673–676.
291. T. Sato, J. Iwamoto, T. Kanoko and K. Satoh, *J Bone Min. Res.*, 2005, **20**, 1327–1333.
292. C. Luckhaus, B. Mahabadi, B. Grass-Kapanke, M. Janner, H. Willenberg, M. Jager, T. Supprian and K. Fehsel, *J. Neural Transm.*, 2009, **117**, 905–911.
293. M. Tysiewicz-Dudek, F. Pietraszkiewicz and B. Drozdzowska, *Ortop. Traumatol. Rehabil.*, 2008, **10**, 315–323.
294. B. Mjoberg, *Calcif. Tissue Int.*, 1990, **47**, 2959–2960.
295. J. R. Walton, T. H. Diamond, S. Kumar and G. A. C. Murrell, *J. Inorg. Biochem.*, 2007, **101**, 1285–1290.
296. D. A. Drachman, *Neurology*, 2005, **64**, 2004–2005.
297. B. Pakkenberg, D. Pelvig, L. Marner, M. J. Bundgaard, H. J. Gundersen, J. R. Nyengaard and L. Regeur, *Exp. Gerontol.*, 2003, **38**, 95–99.
298. J. Dobbing and J. Sands, *Nature*, 1970, **226**, 639–640.
299. A. Richardson and M. C. Birchenall-Sparks, *Rev. Biol. Res. Aging*, 1983, **1**, 255–273.
300. D. M. Lindholm, *J. Neurochem.*, 1986, **47**, 1503–1506.
301. K. S. Rao, V. V. Annapurna and N. S. Raji, *Ann. N.Y. Acad. Sci.*, 2001, **928**, 113–120.
302. J. W. Hinds and N. A. McNelly, *J. Comp. Neurol.*, 1977, **72**, 345–367.
303. A. Lione, *Pharmacol. Ther.*, 1985, **29**, 255–285.
304. B. P. Bourgoin, *Bull. Environ. Contam. Toxicol.*, 1992, **48**, 803–808.

CHAPTER 3

Do Polychlorinated Biphenyls and Associated Chemicals Exacerbate Aging-Related Declines in Brain Function?

R. F. SEEGAL[a,b]

[a] Wadsworth Center, New York State Department of Health, Empire State Plaza, P.O. Box 509, Albany, NY, 12201, USA; [b] Departments of Environmental Health Sciences and Biomedical Sciences, School of Public Health, University at Albany, Albany, NY, 12222, USA
E-mail: seegal@wadsworth.org

3.1 Introduction

Age-related declines in health, including increased incidence of neurodegenerative disorders (*e.g.*, Parkinson's disease, Alzheimer's disease), reductions in cognitive function, cardiac disease, diabetes and an increased incidence of cancer are inevitable.[1,2] Exacerbation of these changes (*i.e.*, observation of deleterious changes in younger populations or increased incidence and severity in aging populations) following exposure to environmental contaminants, including polychlorinated biphenyls (PCBs), however, should not be.

This review differs from previous ones I have written, because the primary focus will be on the neurological (neurocognitive and neurodegenerative) health consequences to aged individuals of *adult* human exposure to PCBs,

Issues in Toxicology No. 16
Aging and Vulnerability to Environmental Chemicals: Age-related Disorders and their Origins in Environmental Exposures
Edited by Bernard Weiss

Published by the Royal Society of Chemistry, www.rsc.org

rather than the much larger literature describing the developmental consequences of exposure of infants, children or experimental animals to PCBs or contaminated foods containing PCBs. Reference will be made to laboratory studies only when deemed necessary to clarify findings from studies of adult and aging human populations.

This review also differs in that I will discuss not only the 'direct' effects of PCBs on the adult human nervous system, but also epidemiological and, to a lesser extent, laboratory studies that describe the consequences of adult human exposure to PCBs on non-nervous system disorders, particularly the relationship between PCBs, diabetes and obesity that can negatively impact the quality of life and lead to disabilities or death occurring at an age earlier than might otherwise occur. This approach is justified not only because the concept of the brain as a 'privileged' organ, insensitive to contaminant-induced or age-related changes in other organ systems, is no longer valid, but also because of accumulating evidence that adult human exposure to PCBs is associated with increased obesity,[3] diabetes and insulin resistance,[4–6] cancer[7,8] and cardiac disease.[9] These contaminant-associated diseases not only decrease quality of life in their own right, but also play important roles in reducing cognitive function and increasing the incidence of neurodegenerative disorders.[10–13]

As I questioned in a previous review,[14] 'Have we not devoted sufficient resources and time to the study of the developmental consequences of these toxicants (*i.e.*, PCBs)? Aging 'baby-boomers' constitute a large and rapidly growing portion of the adult population of the United States and many European countries. The consequences of either current or prior exposure to PCBs, and their putative interactions with aging processes, demand further investigation'. I also wish to emphasize that the 'obesity epidemic' and associated increases in Type 2 diabetes is a risk factor for central nervous system (CNS) function/dysfunction that has only recently been recognized as a risk factor for CNS dysfunction, particularly in adults and in the aged (Figure 3.1).

3.2 What are PCBs?

PCBs are members of a large class of organic compounds known collectively as halogenated aromatic hydrocarbons (HAHs).[15] This class includes not only PCBs, but also structurally related compounds, including 2,3,7,8-tetrachlorodibenzo-*p*-dioxin (TCDD) and 2,3,7,8-tetrachlorodibenzofuran (TCDF). PCBs were used as non-flammable dielectric fluids in power capacitors and transformers, in die and machine cutting oils, as heat exchange fluids in preparation of edible oils, in paints and plastics, in fluorescent ballasts, in carbon-free copy paper and as weather proof sealants in many buildings.[16]

The molecular structures of PCBs are illustrated in Figure 3.2. PCBs can theoretically be chlorinated in any of ten positions on the biphenyl structure, resulting in isomers or congeners ranging from mono- to decachlorinated biphenyls. Thus there are a possible 209 congeners;[17] commercial synthesis,

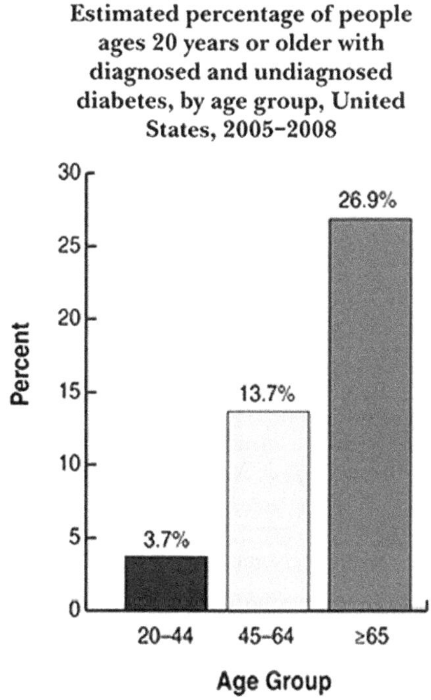

Figure 3.1 Age and diabetes.
(Source: National Institutes of Health).

however, yields approximately 135 congeners.[18] In addition to the number of chlorines, the location of the chlorines on the biphenyl moiety plays an important role in influencing their potential toxicity. Based on the location of chlorines on the biphenyl moiety, there are two major classes of PCB congeners. One class, known as coplanar, has only laterally substituted chlorines and shares many of its mechanisms of action (and toxicity)—including the ability to bind to the aryl hydrocarbon (Ah) receptor—with TCDDs and TCDFs.[19] In turn, binding to the Ah receptor is associated with alterations in endocrine function[20] and an increased risk of developing cancer.[7,8] Coplanar PCB congeners, also bind to the Ah receptor, albeit at significantly lower affinities than either TCDDs or TCDFs.[19,21] Because all coplanar halogenated aromatic hydrocarbons bind to this receptor, it was possible to develop a means of summing the activities of mixtures of coplanar contaminants known as toxic equivalent factors, or TEFs, as first described by Safe.[19,22]

In contrast, the second major class of PCB congeners, *ortho*-substituted or non-coplanar, have chlorine substitutions adjacent to the biphenyl bond, thus inhibiting the planar confirmation required for binding to or activation of the Ah receptor.[15] Indeed, until the early 1990's, it was thought that *ortho*-substituted PCB congeners were not a significant health concern. Initial studies conducted by Seegal and colleagues at the Wadsworth Center of the New York

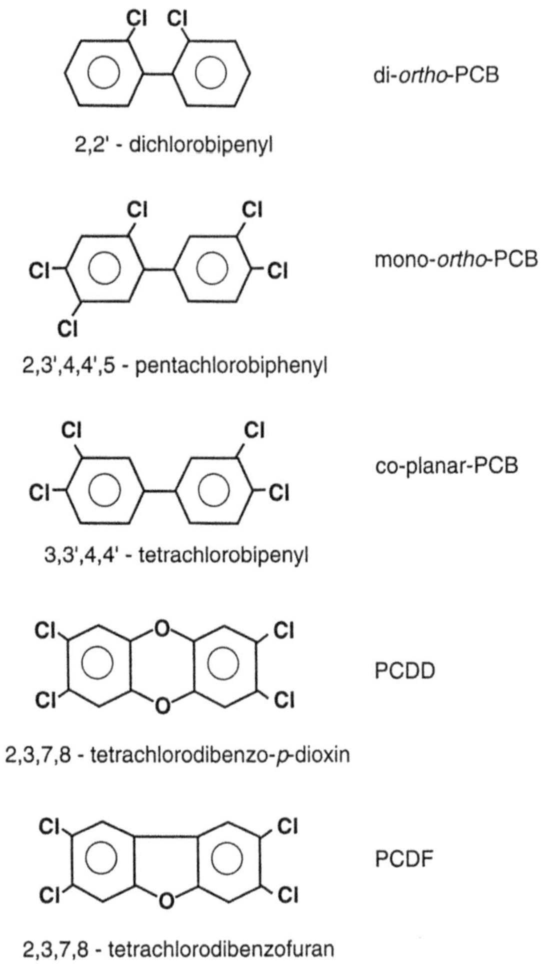

Figure 3.2 Chemical structures of representative compounds from different classes of halogenated aromatic hydrocarbons.
(Reproduced with permission from ref. 15).

State Department of Health, however, demonstrated that *ortho*-substituted congeners were particularly active in reducing neurotransmitter [dopamine (DA)] concentration in cells in culture[23] and in experimental animals[24,25] while, in contrast, coplanar congeners and TCDD were inactive. An abbreviated table (Table 3.1) describing this structure–activity relationship is presented below. Nevertheless, despite what, at the time, were considered 'revolutionary' findings, I would, after presenting these findings at national and international meetings, often listen to other speakers discussing the role(s) of the 'toxic PCBs' *i.e.*, coplanar PCBs. Indeed it took many years, and confirmation by other investigators of the nervous system activity of *ortho*-substituted congeners, for the PCB community to accept the notion that *ortho*-substituted PCBs may pose

Table 3.1 PCB Structure Activity Relationships: Three Approaches. EC50 values for PCB congeners determined by PC12 cellular dopamine content[a], cerebellar granule cell [^{3}H]phorbol ester binding[b] and brain or muscle sarcoplasmic/endoplasmic reticulum RyR/Ca^{2+}-Release Channel [^{3}H]ryanodine binding.[c]

PCB Congener		*EC50 (μM)*			
		PC12	*Cerebellar*	*RyR/Ca^{2+}-Release Channel*	
BZ #	*Structure*	*Cells*	*Granule Cells*	*Brain*	*Skeletal*
4	2,2′	64	43	34.3	
11	3,3′	195	60		
14	3,5	>201	74		
15	4,4	NEO[d]	NEO[e]		
28	2,4,4′	196	>100		
47	2,4,2′,4′	115	89		
50	2,4,6,2′	71	41		
52	2,5,2′,5′	86	28	52.1	
54	2,6,2′,6′	NEO[d]	NEO[e]		
66	2,4,3′,4′	>201		Inactive[f]	
70	2,5,3′,4′			166	
77	3,4,3′,4′	NEO[d]	NEO[e]		
82	2,3,4,2′,3′				1.2
88	2,3,4,6,2′			89.3	
95	2,3,6,2′,5′			17.1	0.33
103	2,4,6,2′,5′	157		50.8	
104	2,4,6,2′,6′	93	38	157	0.57
105	2,3,4,3′,4′		95		0.3
126	3,4,5,3′,4′	NEO[d]	NEO[e]	Inactive[f]	Inactive[g]
153	2,4,5,2′,4′,5′		>100	178	

[a]Adapted from ref. 23.
[b]Adapted from ref. 26.
[c]Adapted from refs. 28 and 29.
[d]No effect observed up to 200 μM.
[e]No effect observed up to 100 μM.
[f]Inactive up to 200 μM.
[g]Inactive up to 10 μM.

a health risk. Important additional studies were conducted at the United States Environmental Protection Agency by Kodavanti and colleagues, who demonstrated that non-dioxin-like PCB congeners increased phorbol ester binding to protein kinase C (PKC)[26] and elevated cytosolic calcium concentration in rat cerebellar granule cells.[27] This SAR fully recapitulated the SAR for non-dioxin-like reductions in neuronal DA concentrations, as seen by Seegal and colleagues. Additional important work by Pessah and colleagues provided an explanation for the observed elevations in cytosolic calcium by determining the mechanism by which *ortho*-substituted PCBs elevated intra-cellular calcium concentrations, *i.e.*, ryanodine receptor activation and a resulting increase in the open probability of its channel.[28,29] Given the disparity in the measures examined, it is surprising (and somewhat satisfying) that the SARs demonstrating the activity of *ortho*-substituted PCB congeners are so remarkably similar.

Although information on the toxicity of the two major classes of congeners has increased our understanding of the potential mechanisms by which PCBs alter brain, immune and endocrine function, the composition of PCB congeners in the environment—and consequently both the body burdens of congeners and their potential toxicity—are influenced by a number of factors that complicate the ability, particularly in epidemiological studies, to determine which congeners, or mixture of congeners and/or their metabolites, contribute to these untoward changes.

Firstly, commercial mixtures of PCBs, known in the US as Aroclors, differ in their congener composition,[18] and differences in the physical properties of these congeners (*e.g.*, their partition coefficients and rates of degradation, including photodegradation) make it unlikely that contaminated foodstuffs (the major route of exposure of humans to PCBs) contain the same congener patterns found in the original Aroclor mixtures. Hence laboratory studies (including those of the author) using either Aroclor mixtures or individual PCB congeners only partially recapitulate human non-occupational exposure due to consumption of PCB-contaminated food products.

Secondly, PCB body burdens, most often measured in serum, contain a large number of congeners, making it difficult to statistically determine which individual congeners are causally associated with changes in nervous and endocrine function.

Thirdly, because of genetic differences in ability to metabolize PCBs, as well as coexposure to other halogenated aromatic hydrocarbons that may enhance metabolism, PCB body burdens vary dramatically between exposed individuals. Finally, despite the fact that serum PCB levels are often measured, PCB-contaminated foods often contain additional contaminants, including methyl mercury and pesticides,[10,30] that we and others have shown[31–33] enhance the toxicity associated with exposure to complex mixtures of contaminants.

3.3 Why are PCBs Still of Concern in the 21st Century?

PCBs have, on occasion, been described as a toxicant most relevant to the 20th Century (Wolff, personal communication), since manufacture and use of PCBs ceased in the mid to late 1970's.[16] Hence it is necessary to explain why a review of the health consequences of exposure of adults and aging individuals to PCBs is still important in 2012. There are, however, several reasons for continued interest in the roles of PCBs in altering CNS and endocrine changes in adults and the elderly.

Firstly, there has been widespread use of PCBs. Indeed it has been estimated that, in the period between 1930 and 1970, approximately 30 000 tons were released into the air, 60 000 tons into fresh and coastal waters and more than 300 000 tons into dumps and landfills.[34] Given their persistence and widespread distribution, in both the environment and in foodstuffs including fish and dairy products, exposure to PCBs still remains a valid concern. Indeed levels of PCBs in fish from contaminated sites, including the Hudson River in New York State, still require fish consumption advisories.[35]

Secondly, since this review focuses on aging and vulnerability to environmental chemicals, levels of PCBs in the environment were dramatically higher in the past;[36,37] hence the elderly were more likely than younger individuals of today to have been exposed to higher levels of PCBs. In support of this statement, it is widely recognized that body burdens of PCBs (as well as other environmental contaminants) are positively associated with the age of the individual.[38] Furthermore, Seegal and colleagues recently described the half-lives of individual PCB congeners in a subset of former capacitor workers who had been exposed more than 28 years ago to extraordinarily high levels of PCBs.[39] Despite the passage of almost three decades, serum PCB levels in these former workers were more than twice those seen in individuals of similar age who were living in the same area but had not been occupationally-exposed to PCBs. Half-lives of PCB congeners were dependent on two factors: the degree of chlorination of the congener (more highly chlorinated congeners had longer half-lives than did lightly chlorinated congeners) and the initial levels of PCBs (the greater the initial PCB body burden, the shorter the half-lives of the congeners). Thus, persistent, relatively low body burdens of PCBs may either continue to contribute to dysfunctions of the nervous and endocrine systems in elderly populations or provide a biomarker of prior exposure to much higher PCB levels that may have contributed to the observed reductions in the health of elderly individuals.

This latter point is supported by results from a study in which adult non-human primates (NHPs) were exposed to either Aroclor 1016 (a mixture consisting primarily of lightly chlorinated *ortho*-substituted congeners) or Aroclor 1260 (a mixture of more highly chlorinated congeners) (0.8, 1.6 or 3.2 mg/kg/day) on a daily basis for 20 weeks. This exposure paradigm significantly reduced basal ganglia (nigral and striatal) DA concentrations[25] and resulted in serum PCB concentration near the upper level reported in capacitor workers.[40] In order to determine whether these reductions in central DA concentrations were permanent, an additional cohort of NHP was exposed to the same concentrations of Aroclors 1260 or 1016 for the same duration, but maintained for an additional 20 weeks following PCB exposure prior to sacrifice.[41] Despite significant reductions in serum PCB concentrations during this 'wash-out' period, basal ganglia DA concentrations failed to return to levels seen in control animals. Because the serum (and brain) concentrations of PCBs following the wash-out were similar to those seen in animals exposed to lower levels of PCBs for 20 weeks and then immediately sacrificed, but failed to show significant reductions in basal ganglia DA concentrations, these findings strongly suggest that the high levels of PCBs seen during exposure, rather than residual levels following removal from PCBs, were responsible for the reductions in central DA. Thus, although current PCB body burdens may provide an estimate of prior exposure, it is most likely that any deleterious consequences are the result of prior, higher level exposure, further supporting the hypothesis that any PCB-induced deficits in aged or elderly humans were likely due to prior exposure.

3.4 Neurological Sequelae of High Level Occupational Exposure to PCBs in Adults

I have chosen to first discuss the neurological consequences of occupational exposure to PCBs for two reasons. Firstly, levels of exposure (and resulting body burdens of PCBs) were dramatically higher those than seen in non-occupationally exposed individuals. Secondly, exposures to other putative neurotoxicants were either absent or at lower levels (on a percentage basis) than environmental exposures.

Occupational exposure to PCBs, which occurred primarily in factories that manufactured power capacitors that used PCBs as dielectric fluids, resulted in extraordinarily high serum levels of PCBs measured shortly after the use of PCBs was banned in the late 1970's.[16] Serum levels were approximately 100-fold higher in the serum of these workers (approximate geometric mean of 363 ppb for lower PCBs and 30 ppb for higher PCBs)[40] compared to those seen in non-occupationally-exposed individuals in the same geographical region (3.6 ppb for total PCBs).[13]

Steenland *et al.*,[42] in a retrospective mortality study of male and female former capacitor workers whose average birth date was 1934, found an excess mortality associated with amyotrophic lateral sclerosis and, in the most highly exposed women, an excess mortality associated with Parkinson's disease. Although these findings were based on mortality, rather than incidence, the authors suggest that, particularly for aging women, exposure to PCBs is associated with increased mortality due to neurological disorders.

Seegal and colleagues, because of the previously mentioned studies in NHPs—which demonstrated that exposure to PCBs resulted in long-term if not permanent reductions in basal ganglia DA concentrations—undertook a study, *using a cohort nearly identical to that used by Steenland* et al, to determine if prior occupational exposure to PCBs would also result in a decrease in measures of central DA. To test that hypothesis, we used single positron emission computerized tomography (SPECT) imaging with the DA transporter ligand, [^{123}I] Beta CIT to determine changes in the density of DA terminals in the striatum of male and female former capacitor workers whose median age at the time these measures were collected was 63.5 years. Reductions in striatal DA terminals are seen in PD, and these decreases become greater during disease progression.[43] Women, but not men, showed an inverse relationship between lipid-adjusted total serum PCB concentrations and the density of DA terminals, even though serum PCB concentrations did not differ significantly between them. Most importantly, these findings were still significant after controlling for a number of potential confounders that have been shown to influence the rate and severity of PD progression. These include the age of the individual, their body mass index, their level of education, the number

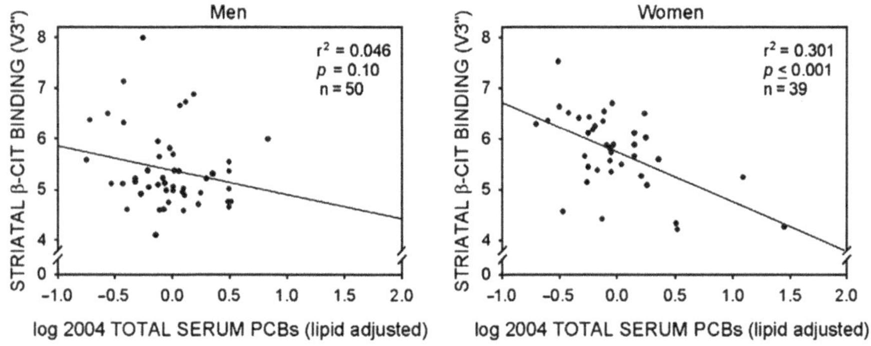

Figure 3.3 Dopamine transporter density, as measured by β-CIT SPECT imaging, as a function of the log of current serum PCB concentrations (expressed on a lipid-adjusted basis, ppm) by sex, prior to adjusting for potential confounders, in former capacitor factory workers. (Reproduced with permission from ref. 53).

of caffeinated beverages consumed and the number of cigarettes smoked (Figure 3.3).

Although the Steenland *et al.* and the Seegal *et al.* studies were conducted at different times—Steenland *et al.* published their findings in 2006 while Seegal *et al.* published their findings in 2010—both studies reached similar conclusions, *i.e.*, only women who were highly exposed to PCBs demonstrated increased PD associated mortality[42] and a decrease in the number of striatal DA terminals indicative of PD.[11] It is tempting to conclude that the sex-specific reductions in DA terminal densities serve as an early biomarker of PD.

3.5 Sequelae of High Level Non-Occupational Exposure to PCBs on Cognitive Function

Unfortunately, high level exposure to PCBs and related HAHs, including dibenzofurans, has not been limited to occupational settings. First in Japan, noted in 1968 (Yusho),[44] and then, approximately ten years later, in Taiwan (YuCheng),[45] adults, children, infants and fetuses were exposed to rice oil that had been contaminated with PCBs and dibenzofurans. Existing literature[46–48] describes the devastating neurological and morphological changes that resulted in children and infants that had been exposed due to maternal consumption of the contaminated rice oil. The effects of exposure to the contaminated rice oil were, however, not limited to those individuals exposed during development. Lin *et al.*[12,49] describe the neurocognitive changes seen in adults who were more than 60 years of age at the time of assessment. These changes included reduced attention during performance of a digit span test, visual memory span and verbal memory recall. Most importantly, these changes were significant *only* in exposed women. In the later study, Lin *et al.* noted deficits in the Mini-Mental Status examination that were negatively associated with the subjects' body burden of PCBs.

Thus in at least three epidemiological studies,[11,12,42] associations were seen between body burdens of PCBs and related HAHs and deficits in neurological and neurocognitive performance in women but not in men, despite the fact that the age of the men and women did not differ significantly. Why are aging women more susceptible to the neurotoxic effects of PCBs than men?

We suggest that a highly relevant factor, common to these studies, is the age of the subjects and their consequent reproductive status. For example, in the Seegal *et al.* study, the median age of the subjects was 65 years, hence both men and women had either segued into, or had begun the process of reproductive senescence associated with, a decrease in gonadal hormones.[50] We further suggest that age-related decline in central gonadal hormones, either of ovarian origin or conversion of testosterone to estrogen in the brain,[51] has different consequences in men and women following exposure to known DA neurotoxicants. This suggestion is supported by data from Murray *et al.*[52] and Tamas *et al.*,[53] who have shown that, following administration of 6-OHDA, a potent DA neurotoxicant, (1) ovariectomy increases the loss of basal ganglia DA, compared to that seen in the intact female; (2) castration reduces the loss of basal ganglia DA, compared to that seen in the intact male; (3) estrogen supplementation in the ovariectomized rat restores DA to levels seen in the intact female and (4) estrogen supplementation in the castrated male reduces the protection following castration to levels seen in the intact male rat. These findings strongly suggest that estrogen is neuroprotective in the female, while estrogen (from aromatization of testosterone) may be a risk factor in the male brain. Thus reductions in ovarian hormones following menopause (all women in the above described epidemiological studies were postmenopausal) are posited to result in the loss of known neuroprotective factor(s), while reductions in circulating testosterone and central aromatase activity in the aging male may result in the loss of a neuro-risk factor (*i.e.*, central estrogen due to enzymatic conversion of testosterone to estrogen).

In order to test that hypothesis in a laboratory setting, we recently conducted studies using intact, gonadectomized and sham-gonadectomized adult male and female mice exposed to PCBs and determined changes in striatal DA concentrations. Although experimental gonadectomy only partially recapitulates the hormonal and neurological changes associated with natural menopause, this approach best models the changes seen in reproductively senescent women and men. As seen in Figure 3.4, PCBs significantly reduced striatal DA concentrations in intact, reproductively competent male mice, but not in intact reproductively competent female mice. These findings closely approximate the observations reported by DiPaolo and colleagues,[54,55] Murray *et al.*[52] and Gillies *et al.*[56] following exposure of in intact male and female mice or rats to either MPTP or 6-OHDA. Furthermore, in our study, ovariectomized mice exposed to PCBs showed significant reductions in striatal DA following exposure to PCBs compared to levels seen in intact PCB-exposed mice, findings similar to those seen by Morissette *et al.*[54] These findings further support the hypothesis that ovarian hormones are neuroprotective and that the loss of ovarian hormones (due to ovariectomy) increases susceptibility to DA

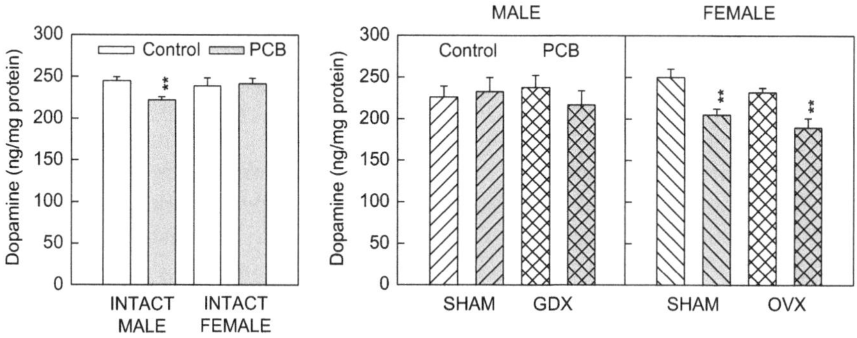

Figure 3.4 Dopamine levels in the striatum of control and PCB exposed (70-day subchronic exposure to food containing 500 ppm of Aroclor 1254) adult intact male and female mice or mice that had undergone gonadectomy or sham gonadectomy surgery.

neurotoxicants. However, unlike other studies that have used ovariectomized rodents to examine the role of estrogen as a neuroprotective factor, we chose to compare the neurochemical consequences of exposure to PCBs in gonadectomized mice against those seen in sham-gonadectomized mice (*i.e.*, mice that were exposed to the same anesthetics and analgesics and who had been surgically manipulated but did not have their gonads removed). Surprisingly, PCB-exposed, sham-ovariectomized mice showed the same reductions in striatal DA as seen in ovariectomized mice, despite no significant changes in circulating ovarian hormones.

Why have I spent so much effort describing these results, particularly since the focus of this review is concerned with aging and increased vulnerability to environmental contaminants? Firstly, these unexpected findings suggest that surgical trauma, and by analogy, significant psychological trauma, may interact with environmental contaminants to induce changes in the CNS, thereby increasing the likelihood of developing PD or associated movement disorders. Thus trauma, including the death of a spouse or a loved one, *in combination* with prior exposure to environmental contaminants, may trigger Parkinson's disease or other neurological or neurocognitive disorders. Obviously, this novel hypothesis requires additional research. Furthermore, there is evidence, both epidemiological[57,58] and laboratory-based[59,60] demonstrating that PCB exposure leads to menopause at an earlier age.

3.6 Effects of Environmental Exposure to PCBs on Motor and Cognitive Function in Adults

A number of studies have examined the behavioral consequences of developmental exposure to PCBs[61–64] and have noted long-lasting deficits in cognition and behavior in infants and children born to mothers who consumed contaminated fish from the Great Lakes. A much smaller series of studies, however, have examined the behavioral consequences of exposure of adults to environmental levels of PCBs.

An early study by Schantz *et al.*[65] examined the effects of exposure to PCBs and DDE on motor function in 50–90 year old Michigan residents who reported that they had eaten more than 24 pounds of contaminated fish per year. Higher fish consumption, and by inference, elevations in PCB body burdens, was associated with significantly poorer performance on tests of motor function, including the Grooved Peg Board and the Static Motor Steadiness Test. However, when statistically correcting for relevant confounders, including age and gender, the associations between exposure to PCBs and/or DDE became only marginally significant.

These largely negative results have been, in part, obviated by findings from the same cohort when measures of neurocognitive were obtained. Schantz *et al.*[10] found significant associations between consumption of contaminated fish and impairments of memory and learning. Furthermore, these authors noted that PCBs, but not DDE, were statistically and negatively associated with lower scores on several measures of memory and learning, including the Weschler Memory Scale and the California Verbal Learning test (CVLT).

A similar study was more recently conducted by Fitzgerald *et al.*,[13] who determined the neuropsychological status among older residents of Upper Hudson River communities. The subjects were of similar age to those examined by Schantz *et al.* (55–74 years of age), although information on consumption of contaminated fish was not included. Furthermore, serum PCB levels (lipid-adjusted) were less than half the levels reported in the studies by Schantz *et al.* (3.2 ppb *versus* 7.9 ppb). Nevertheless, negative associations between serum PCB levels and decrements in the CVLT, as well as increased depression, measured by the Beck Depression Index, were seen in the Fitzgerald study. Thus even at lower PCB body burdens, residents of the upper Hudson River demonstrated deficits in the CVLT, thereby partially recapitulating the earlier findings of Schantz *et al.* The findings of both authors are of particular importance because they suggest that either current or prior exposure to contaminated fish (Schantz) or living adjacent to PCB contaminated sites (Fitzgerald) is associated with decrements in neurocognitive function in adults, even after controlling for age.

Somewhat similar findings were reported by Haase *et al.*,[66] from a study supported by the NIEHS Superfund. They examined the relationship between exposure to PCBs and neuropsychological function in a Native American population of Mohawk people who were residing in upstate New York and who had been environmentally exposed to PCBs and pesticides. Interestingly, the age of the subject significantly affected the relationships between PCBs, but not pesticides, and cognitive function; only individuals who were more than 49 years of age demonstrated deficits on the Trail Making Test, the Stroop test, the Wisconsin Card Sorting Test and Visual memory performance.

Finally, Kilburn *et al.* published a series of manuscripts describing the behavioral consequences of adult exposure to PCBs and related contaminants. In a 1989 publication,[67] the author described neurobehavioral dysfunctions in firemen exposed to PCBs and their by-products in a transformer fire. Behavioral deficits included memory impairments for story recalls, visual images and number recall. Improvement in some of their behaviors following an experimental detoxification program consisting of a medically supervised diet, exercise and sauna, was also reported. There was, however, no relationship between reported deficits in behavior and serum measures of PCBs raising concerns since exposure to combustion products of PCBs, including dioxins, may have contributed to the reported neurocognitive deficits. Furthermore, McCaffrey and Westervelt[68] criticized the purported improvements following detoxification, since many of the tests were subject to practice effects, *i.e.*, performance on these tests would have shown an increase regardless of intervention simply because the tests were repeated. Kilburn[69] also described visual and neurobehavioral impairment in residents living near a natural gas pipeline pumping station (the pumps were lubricated with a compound that consisted of 50–80% PCBs) that resulted in dispersion of PCBs from compressed air used to start the pumps. Exposed subjects were reported to have slower simple and choice reaction times, increased body sway and deficits in performance of the grooved peg board test and the Trail Making Test. Concerns have been raised, however, because many of the exposed subjects were involved in a lawsuit against the gas pipeline company. Hence these subjects would, perhaps, be motivated to show deficits in neurocognitive function. However, in a later publication, Kilburn[70] stated that being involved in a lawsuit against a company that owned an electronic manufacturing plant that resulted in exposure of residents to tricholoroethylene did not affect performance. These issues would have been either partially or fully negated if the author had administered the Test of Memory Malingering, which is designed to help psychologists and psychiatrists distinguish between malingered and true memory deficits.[71]

Nevertheless, the concerns raised about the aforementioned studies illustrate the complexity, and the necessity for extreme care, in conducting epidemiological studies. These concerns include: controlling for potential confounders, determining, using power analyses, whether the cohort is sufficiently large to allow appropriate conclusions to be drawn, whether other known or putative environmental agents may contribute to deficits in central function and if the subjects have or have had a vested interest in the outcome of the neurocognitive or neurological measures.

3.7 Are PCBs the only 'Bad Actors'?

It is appropriate at this time to discuss concerns that I and others have that environmental exposure to PCBs rarely, if ever, occurs in the absence of coexposure to other neurotoxicants. This statement is particularly true in the case of consumption of contaminated fish and other foodstuffs (Figure 3.5).[10,37,72] Indeed, in a 1999 publication entitled 'Are PCBs the Major Neurotoxicant in Great Lakes Salmon?',[30] I demonstrated that, in rats exposed to diets adulterated with lyophilized salmon (from either Lake Huron or Lake Ontario) that resulted in daily exposure of as little as 13.9 μg/kg/day of PCBs,

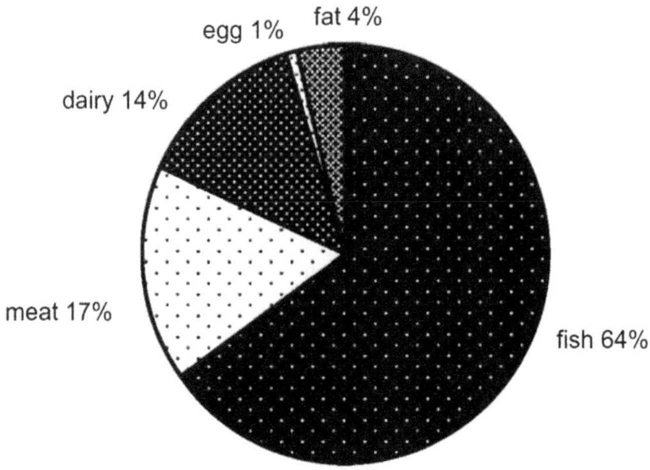

Figure 3.5 Relative contribution of food groups to the intake of total PCBs, determined from a Swedish market basket in 2005.
(Reproduced with permission from ref. 38).

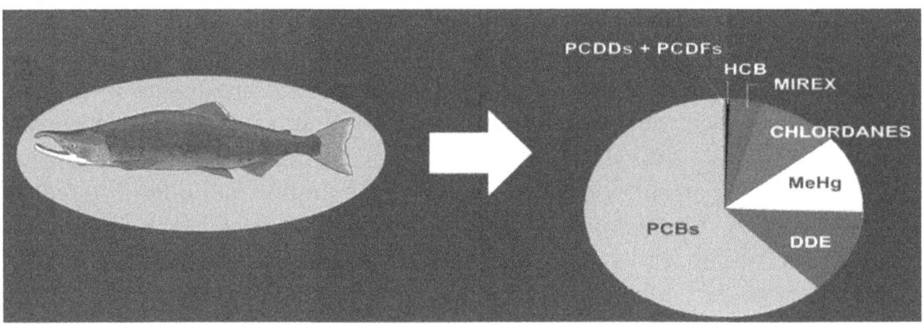

Figure 3.6 Relative proportion of the major organic contaminants found in Lake Ontario salmon fillets.
(Reproduced with permission from ref. 78).

reductions in striatal DA were similar to those seen following exposure to 10 mg/kg/day of an *ortho*-substituted congener (2,4,2′,4′-tetrachlorinated PCB). However, the concentration of this congener required to yield changes in striatal DA similar to those following consumption of diets containing lyophilized Great Lakes salmon were approximately 100-fold higher!

What other contaminants found in salmon from the Great Lakes may contribute to this much greater activity? As shown in Figure 3.6, contaminated salmon from the Great Lakes contains many other known neurotoxicants, including methyl mercury and pesticides.[10,73,74] To reinforce this point, we later examined, using an *in vitro* tissue model and measuring DA content, whether PCBs would interact with methylmercury.[31] This study clearly demonstrated that coexposure to two recognized environmental neurotoxicants resulted in greater decreases in DA than did exposure to either contaminant alone.

These studies also serve as a caveat for epidemiological studies that examine the relationships between consumption of contaminated foods and neurocognitive deficits, since many studies examine only the statistical relationships between serum PCB levels and behavioral deficits. This is because techniques for their quantification are readily available and are used as a biomarker of exposure, leading perhaps to the fallacious conclusion that it is only the PCBs that contribute to the behavioral/cognitive deficits.

3.8 PCBs as Etiologic Factors in Diabetes/Insulin Resistance

Major non-neurological health consequences of both occupational and environmental exposure to PCBs include evidence for increased risk of cancer,[8] as well as diabetes/insulin resistance.[75] Although the mechanisms responsible for the relationship between obesity and cancer are not fully understood, there is compelling evidence that elevations in circulating levels of insulin, and associated increases in cellular insulin-like growth factor, are associated with obesity and increase the availability of glucose to cells within the body.[76] In turn, because cancer cells require large amounts of glucose, the obesity/diabetes-induced elevations in insulin are thought to play an important role in tumorigenesis.

Because the major focus of this review is on the neurological/neurocognitive effects of PCBs in adults and the elderly, I will focus, in this section, on the role that PCB-induced diabetes/insulin resistance plays in altering CNS function, including neurodegenerative disorders. Before that discussion, however, it is necessary to review research that demonstrates that PCBs lead to an increase in either diabetes or insulin resistance.

Persky *et al.*[75] examined the associations between PCB exposure, determined by measuring serum PCB levels, and diabetes in post-menopausal women who had been previously employed at a capacitor manufacturing plant. All PCB-exposed women demonstrated an increase in self-reported diabetes, but not in insulin resistance, after controlling for relevant confounders, *e.g.*, body mass index, triglycerides and alcohol consumption. This relationship was seen only for dioxin-like and not *ortho*-substituted PCB congeners. However, for those women who did not report having diabetes, a measure of insulin resistance (homeostatic model of insulin resistance) was significantly associated with total PCB body burden. Potential mechanisms for the association between dioxin-like PCB congeners and self-reports of diabetes may involve autoimmune effects associated with increased glutamic acid decarboxylase, which is often seen in individuals diagnosed with either Type I or Type II diabetes.[77]

Environmental exposure to PCBs has also been associated with an increase in diabetes. A 2009 study from Persky's group[78] determined that organochlorine exposure in Great Lakes sport fish consumers was associated with increased risk of diabetes. However, in a cohort of individuals originally studied because of widespread polybrominated biphenyl (PBB) exposure due to accidental contamination of feed for dairy cows, Vasiliu *et al.*[3] demonstrated, for women, but not men, that PCBs, *but not PBBs,* were associated with a 2.3-fold increased risk for diabetes. In both the Persky and the Vasiliu *et al.* study, the concept of 'reverse causation' *i.e.*, either increased body mass index or serum lipid levels, that may have confounded the relationship between elevated halogenated aromatic hydrocarbon levels and diabetes, was shown not to influence the observed relationship between exposure and diabetes.

Finally, in a series of studies, Lee *et al.*[4,5,79] demonstrated, using results obtained from the National Health and Nutrition Examination Survey (NHANES), an association between serum concentrations of persistent organic pollutants and diabetes in non-diabetic adults. In the first publication,[4] the authors reported a strong dose–response relationship between serum concentrations of persistent organic pollutants, including an *ortho*-substituted PCB congener (2,4,5,2′,4′,5-hexachlorobiphenyl), as well as hepta- and octa-chlorodibenzo-*p*-dioxin, oxychlordane, *p,p*′-dichlorodiphenyltrichloroethane, trans-nonachlor) and incidence of diabetes. The authors caution, however, that, particularly for cross-sectional studies, it is not possible to determine whether those individuals who had diabetes metabolized the halogenated aromatic hydrocarbons at a lower rate than individuals who did not have diabetes, which could result in a confounding of the causal relationship between these contaminants and diabetes. In a follow-up report, again using data from NHANES, Lee *et al.*[5] found that both *ortho*-substituted PCB congeners and organochlorine pesticides were associated with increased incidence of diabetes. Finally, the same authors[79] concluded that dioxin-like and not *ortho*-substituted PCB congeners were associated with increased risk of diabetes.

The lack of agreement between the aforementioned studies highlights the difficulties in carrying out retrospective epidemiological studies, including sample selection, measurement of body burdens of relevant contaminants and determining the relationships between various classes of halogenated aromatic hydrocarbons, including whether the dose responses for these contaminants are linear. Nevertheless, in total, the studies suggest that halogenated aromatic hydrocarbons, including PCBs, are associated with an increased risk of diabetes and that this risk may initially be independent of the body mass index of the subject.

Why have I spent so much of this chapter describing the relationships between occupational and environmental exposures to PCBs and related contaminants and diabetes/insulin resistance if the goal of this review is to highlight the role of PCBs in the etiology of disorders of the central nervous system in adults? The perhaps less than obvious reason is that diabetes is often associated with elevated circulating levels of insulin resulting in a clinical insulin resistance.[80] Furthermore, these elevations can influence the CNS by reducing the activity of growth factors essential for the maintenance of neuronal viability and synaptic connectivity.[81] These changes are associated with decreased cognitive function,[82] as well as an increased risk for developing Parkinson's and Alzheimer's disease.[83,84] Potential mechanisms by which alterations in circulating (and brain) levels of insulin and increased cognitive dysfunctions are associated with age, as well as Alzheimer' disease, have been reviewed by Bosco *et al.*[84] These authors suggest that hyperglycemia, associated with diabetes, increases peripheral usage of insulin, resulting in decreased insulin transport into the brain. In turn, alterations in central insulin and insulin-like growth factors influence neuronal survival, longevity and learning and memory. Hence reductions in brain insulin, combined with an age-related decrease in central insulin receptor densities, may interact to increase the likelihood of both mild cognitive deficits and Alzheimer's disease, most likely by increasing inflammation, oxidative stress and levels of β-amyloid and tau.

Similar to Alzheimer's disease, clinical studies[85,86] have demonstrated an association between obesity, diabetes/insulin resistance and Parkinson's disease.[83] Potential mechanisms include, as with Alzheimer's disease, reduced central energy balance, increased oxidative stress and—in an animal model of diabetes, induced by placing rats on a high-fat diet—increased nigral iron levels, which has been associated with a significant reduction in nigral dopaminergic neurons[87] due to Fenton reaction-induced increases in oxidative stress.

I began this review by stating that declines in cognitive function, as well as an increased risk for developing neurodegenerative disorders, including Parkinson's disease and Alzheimer's disease, are an inevitable consequence of aging. I have hopefully presented sufficient data to indicate that exposure to *ortho*-substituted PCBs and related coplanar halogenated aromatic hydrocarbons, including dioxin, may exacerbate these deficits in brain function, particularly in adults and the elderly. I do not, however, wish to leave the reader with the impression that prior or current exposure to these and other contaminants represents a 'death sentence', resulting in contaminant-accelerated decline in cognitive function and an increase in aging-related neurodegenerative diseases. Because of the strong associations between obesity, diabetes/insulin resistance and neurocognitive and neurodegenerative disorders, it has been suggested—and seconded by this author—that regulating obesity at both the national and personal level must be made an extremely high priority, since reductions in Type 2 diabetes is likely to decrease diabetes-associated deficits in CNS function in adults and the aged. Furthermore, as is well known, regular exercise reduces body weight and diabetes, as well as increasing a process of cell death known as apoptosis.[88] Although this may appear to be ominous and counter-intuitive, recent studies have suggested that the positive association between exercise and health is likely to include death/removal of cells that have been injured or damaged, for example by contaminants or the aging process itself. Thus, as our mothers were wont to say (or at least mine was!), 'eat healthy and exercise (both your body and your brain)!'.

References

1. G. Wick, P. Jansen-Durr, P. Berger, I. Blasko and B. Grubeck-Loebenstein, *Vaccine*, 2000, **18**, 1567.
2. E. R. Stadtman, *Ann. N. Y. Acad. Sci.*, 2001, **928**, 22.

3. O. Vasiliu, L. Cameron, J. Gardiner, P. Deguire and W. Karmaus, *Epidemiology*, 2006, **17**, 352.
4. D. H. Lee, I. K. Lee, K. Song, M. Steffes, W. Toscano, B. A. Baker and D. R. Jacobs, Jr., *Diabetes Care*, 2006, **29**, 1638.
5. D. H. Lee, I. K. Lee, S. H. Jin, M. Steffes and D. R. Jacobs, Jr., *Diabetes Care*, 2007, **30**, 622.
6. J. Ruzzin, R. Petersen, E. Meugnier, L. Madsen, E. J. Lock, H. Lillefosse, T. Ma, S. Pesenti, S. B. Sonne, T. T. Marstrand, M. K. Malde, Z. Y. Du, C. Chavey, L. Fajas, A. K. Lundebye, C. L. Brand, H. Vidal, K. Kristiansen and L. Froyland, *Environ. Health Perspect.*, 2010, **118**, 465.
7. P. A. Bertazzi, L. Riboldi, A. Pesatori, L. Radice and C. Zocchetti, *Am. J. Ind. Med.*, 1987, **11**, 165.
8. K. Mallin, K. McCann, A. D'Aloisio, S. Freels, J. Piorkowski, J. Dimos and V. Persky, *J. Occup. Environ. Med.*, 2004, **46**, 565.
9. R. A. DeFronzo and E. Ferrannini, *Diabetes Care*, 1991, **14**, 173.
10. S. L. Schantz, D. M. Gasior, E. Polverejan, R. J. McCaffrey, A. M. Sweeney, H. E. B. Humphrey and J. C. Gardiner, *Environ. Health Perspect.*, 2001, **109**, 605.
11. R. F. Seegal, K. L. Marek, J. P. Seibyl, D. L. Jennings, E. S. Molho, D. S. Higgins, S. A. Factor, E. F. Fitzgerald, E. A. Hills, S. A. Korrick, M. S. Wolff, R. F. Haase, A. C. Todd, P. Parsons and R. J. McCaffrey, *Neurobiol. Dis.*, 2010, **38**, 219.
12. K. C. Lin, N.-W. Guo, P.-C. Tsai, C.-Y. Yang and Y. L. Guo, *Environ. Health Perspect.*, 2008, **116**, 184.
13. E. F. Fitzgerald, E. E. Belanger, M. I. Gomez, M. Cayo, R. McCaffrey, R. Seegal, R. L. Jansing, S.-A. Hwang and H. E. Hicks, *Environ. Health Perspect.*, 2008, **116**, 209.
14. R. F. Seegal, *Organohalogen Compd.*, 2004, **66**, 3548.
15. R. F. Seegal, *Crit. Rev. Toxicol.*, 1996, **26**, 709.
16. National Research Council, in *Polychlorinated Biphenyls*, National Academy of Sciences, Washington, DC, 1979, p. 1.
17. M. D. Mullin, C. M. Pochini, S. McCrindle, M. Romkes, S. H. Safe and L. M. Safe, *Environ. Sci. Technol.*, 1984, **18**, 468.
18. M. D. Erickson, in *Analytical Chemistry of PCBs*, CRC Press, Boca Raton, 2 ed., 1997.
19. S. Safe, *CRC Crit. Rev. Toxicol.*, 1990, **21**, 51.
20. S. Safe, B. Astroff, M. Harris, T. Zacharewski, R. Dickerson, M. Romkes and L. Biegel, *Pharmacol. Toxicol.*, 1991, **69**, 400.
21. A. Parkinson and S. Safe, in *Polychlorinated Biphenyls (PCBs): Mammalian and Environmental Toxicology*, eds. S. Safe and O. Hutzinger, Springer-Verlag, New York, 1987, pp. 49–75.
22. S. H. Safe, *CRC Crit. Rev. Toxicol.*, 1994, **24**, 87.
23. W. Shain, B. Bush and R. F. Seegal, *Toxicol. Appl. Pharmacol.*, 1991, **111**, 33.
24. R. F. Seegal, B. Bush and W. Shain, *Toxicol. Appl.Pharmacol.*, 1990, **106**, 136.

25. R. F. Seegal, B. Bush and K. O. Brosch, *Toxicology*, 1991, **66**, 145.
26. P. R. S. Kodavanti, T. R. Ward, J. D. McKinney and H. A. Tilson, *Toxicol. Appl. Pharmacol.*, 1995, **130**, 140.
27. W. R. Mundy, T. J. Shafer, H. A. Tilson and P. R. S. Kodavanti, *Toxicology*, 1999, **136**, 27.
28. P. W. Wong and I. N. Pessah, *Molec. Pharmacol.*, 1996, **49**, 740.
29. P. W. Wong, W. R. Brackney and I. N. Pessah, *J. Biol. Chem.*, 1997, **272**, 15145.
30. R. F. Seegal, *Environ. Res., Sect. A*, 1999, **80**, S38.
31. J. C. Bemis and R. F. Seegal, *Environ. Health Perspect.*, 1999, **107**, 879.
32. J. C. Bemis and R. F. Seegal, *Neurotoxicology*, 2000, **21**, 1123.
33. C. S. Roegge, J. R. Morris, S. Villareal, V. C. Wang, B. E. Powers, A. Y. Klintsova, W. T. Greenough, I. N. Pessah and S. L. Schantz, *Neurotoxicol. Teratol.*, 2006, **28**, 74.
34. M. A. Q. Khan, S. F. Khan, and F. Shattari, in *Ecotoxicology* ed. Erik Jorgensen, Academic Press, Amsterdam, 2010, p. 251.
35. New York State Department of Health. Health Advice on Eating Sportfish and Game. NYSDOH website, 27 February, 2012.
36. S. Y. Huestis, M. R. Servos, D. M. Whittle and D. G. Dixon, *J. Great Lakes Res.*, 1996, **22**, 310.
37. A. Tornkvist, A. Glynn, M. Aune, P. O. Darnerud and E. H. Ankarberg, *Chemosphere*, 2011, **83**, 193.
38. R. B. Jain and R. Y. Wang, *Chemosphere*, 2010, **79**, 243.
39. R. F. Seegal, E. F. Fitzgerald, E. A. Hills, M. S. Wolff, R. F. Haase, A. C. Todd, P. Parsons, E. S. Molho, D. S. Higgins, S. A. Factor, K. L. Marek, J. P. Seibyl, D. L. Jennings and R. J. McCaffrey, *J. Expo. Sci. Environ. Epidemiol.*, 2011, **21**, 234.
40. R. W. Lawton, M. R. Ross, J. Feingold and J. F. Brown, Jr., *Environ. Health Perspect.*, 1985, **60**, 165.
41. R. F. Seegal, B. Bush and K. O. Brosch, *Toxicology*, 1994, **86**, 71.
42. K. Steenland, M. J. Hein, R. T. I. Cassinelli, M. M. Prince, N. B. Nilsen, E. A. Whelan, M. A. Waters, A. M. Ruder and T. M. Schnorr, *Epidemiology*, 2006, **17**, 8.
43. K. Marek, R. Innis, C. Van Dyke, B. Fussell, M. Early, S. Eberly, D. Oakes and J. Seibyl, *Neurology*, 2001, **57**, 2089.
44. M. Kuratsune, T. Youshimara, J. Matsuzaka and A. Yamaguchi, *Environ. Health Perspect.*, 1972, **1**, 119.
45. S.-T. Hsu, C.-I. Ma, S. K. H. Hsu, S.-S. Wu, N. H. M. Hsu, C.-C. Yeh and S.-B. Wu, *Environ. Health Perspect.*, 1985, **59**, 5.
46. W. J. Rogan, B. C. Gladen, K. L. Hung, S. L. Koong, L. Y. Shih, J. S. Taylor, Y. C. Wu, D. Yang, N. B. Rogan and C.-C. Hsu, *Science*, 1988, **241**, 334.
47. Y.-C. J. Chen, Y.-L. Guo, C.-C. Hsu and W. J. Rogan, *JAMA*, 1992, **268**, 3213.
48. Y.-C. J. Chen, M.-L. M. Yu, W. J. Rogan, B. C. Gladen and C.-C. Hsu, *Am. J. Public Health*, 1994, **84**, 415.

49. K. C. Lin, P. C. Huang, P. S. Yeh, J. R. Kuo and D. S. Ke, *Psychogeriatrics*, 2010, **10**, 191.
50. T. R. Chakraborty and A. C. Gore, *Exp. Biol. Med.*, 2004, **229**, 977.
51. S. Veiga, R. C. Melcangi, L. L. DonCarlos, L. M. Garcia-Segura and I. Azcoitia, *Exp. Gerontol.*, 2004, **39**, 1623.
52. H. E. Murray, A. V. Pillai, S. R. McArthur, N. Razvi, K. P. Datla, D. T. Dexter and G. E. Gillies, *Neuroscience*, 2003, **116**, 213.
53. A. Tamás, A. Lubics, I. Lengvári and D. Reglödi, *Endocrine*, 2006, **29**, 275.
54. M. Morissette, S. Jourdain, S. A. Sweidi, F. S. Menniti, A. D. Ramirez and T. Di Paolo, *Neuropharmacology*, 2007, **52**, 1509.
55. S. Jourdain, M. Morissette, N. Morin and T. Di Paolo, *J. Neuroendocrinol.*, 2005, **17**, 509.
56. G. E. Gillies, H. E. Murray, D. Dexter and S. McArthur, *Pharmacol. Biochem. Behav.*, 2004, **78**, 513.
57. A. Axmon, L. Rylander, L. Stromberg and L. Hagmar, *Chemosphere*, 2004, **56**, 813.
58. H. M. Blanck, M. Marcus, P. E. Tolbert, C. Schuch, C. Rubin, A. K. Henderson, R. H. Zhang and H. S. Vicki, *Maturitas*, 2004, **49**, 97.
59. D. B. Sager and D. M. Girard, *Environ. Res.*, 1994, **66**, 52.
60. A. C. Gore, T. J. Wu, T. Oung, J. B. Lee and M. J. Woller, *J. Neuroendocrinol.*, 2002, **14**, 814.
61. J. L. Jacobson, S. W. Jacobson and H. E. B. Humphrey, *J. Pediatr.*, 1990, **116**, 38.
62. J. L. Jacobson, S. W. Jacobson, R. J. Padgett, G. A. Brumitt and R. L. Billings, *Dev. Psychol.*, 1992, **28**, 297.
63. P. Stewart, J. Reihman, E. Lonky, T. Darvill and J. Pagano, *Neurotoxicol. Teratol.*, 2000, **22**, 21.
64. P. Stewart, S. Fitzgerald, J. Reihman, B. Gump, E. Lonky, T. Darvill, J. Pagano and P. Hauser, *Environ. Health Perspect.*, 2003, **111**, 1670.
65. S. L. Schantz, J. Gardiner, D. Gasior, A. Sweeney, D. W. Humphrey and R. McCaffrey, *Environ. Res.*, 1999, **80**, S46.
66. R. F. Haase, R. J. McCaffrey, A. L. Santiago-Rivera, G. S. Morse and A. Tarbell, *Environ. Res.*, 2009, **109**, 73.
67. K. H. Kilburn, R. H. Warsaw and M. G. Shields, *Arch. Environ. Health*, 1989, **44**(6), 345.
68. R. J. McCaffrey and H. J. Westervelt, *Neuropsychol. Rev.*, 1995, **5**, 203.
69. K. H. Kilburn, *Neurotoxicology*, 2000, **21**, 489.
70. K. H. Kilburn, *Arch. Environ. Health*, 2002, **57**, 121.
71. T. N. Tombaugh, in *Test of Memory Malingering*, Multi-Health Systems, Inc., North Tonawanda, NY, 1996.
72. R. Duarte-Davidson and K. C. Jones, *Sci. Total Environ.*, 1994, **151**, 131.
73. R. F. Seegal, in *PCBs: Recent Advances in Environmental Toxicology and Health Effects*, eds. L. W. Robertson and L. G. Hansen, The University Press of Kentucky, Lexington, 2001, pp. 241–255.
74. R. Seegal and W. J. Bowers, *Environ. Toxicol. Pharmacol.*, 2002, **12**, 63.

75. V. Persky, J. Piorkowski, M. Turyk, S. Freels, R. Chatterton, Jr., J. Dimos, H. L. Bradlow, L. K. Chary, V. Burse, T. Unterman, D. Sepkovic and K. McCann, *Environ. Res.*, 2011, **111**, 817.
76. G. Taubes, *Science*, 2012, **335**, 28, 30.
77. P. Langer, M. Tajtakova, H. J. Guretzki, A. Kocan, J. Petrik, J. Chovancova, B. Drobna, S. Jursa, M. Pavuk, T. Trnovec, E. Sebokova and I. Klimes, *Arch. Environ. Health*, 2002, **57**, 412.
78. M. Turyk, H. Anderson, L. Knobeloch, P. Imm and V. Persky, *Environ. Health Perspect.*, 2009, **117**, 1076.
79. D. H. Lee, I. K. Lee, M. Steffes and D. R. Jacobs, Jr., *Diabetes Care*, 2007, **30**, 1596.
80. M. R. Meyer, C. F. Lichti, R. R. Townsend and A. G. Rao, *Biochemistry*, 2011, **50**, 2170.
81. A. M. Stranahan, E. D. Norman, K. Lee, R. G. Cutler, R. S. Telljohann, J. M. Egan and M. P. Mattson, *Hippocampus*, 2008, **18**, 1085.
82. J. A. Luchsinger, *J. Neurol. Sci.*, 2010, **299**, 35.
83. E. Schernhammer, J. Hansen, K. Rugbjerg, L. Wermuth and B. Ritz, *Diabetes Care*, 2011, **34**, 1102.
84. D. Bosco, A. Fava, M. Plastino, T. Montalcini and A. Pujia, *J. Cell Mol. Med.*, 2011, **15**, 1807.
85. R. Sandyk, *Int. J. Neurosci.*, 1993, **69**, 125.
86. K. R. Wilhelm, K. Yanamandra, M. A. Gruden, V. Zamotin, M. Malisauskas, V. Casaite, A. Darinskas, L. Forsgren and L. A. Morozova-Roche, *Eur. J. Neurol.*, 2007, **14**, 327.
87. J. K. Morris, G. L. Bomhoff, B. K. Gorres, V. A. Davis, J. Kim, P. P. Lee, W. M. Brooks, G. A. Gerhardt, P. C. Geiger and J. A. Stanford, *Exp. Neurol.*, 2011, **231**, 171.
88. S. Phaneuf and C. Leeuwenburgh, *Med. Sci. Sports Exerc.*, 2001, **33**, 393.

CHAPTER 4

Parkinson Disease

G. NELSON AND B. A. RACETTE*

University of the Witwatersrand, Division of Biostatistics and Epidemiology, School of Public Health, Faculty of Health Sciences, 7 York Rd, Parktown, 2193 South Africa

4.1 Introduction

Parkinsonism is a clinical syndrome characterized by bradykinesia, postural instability, rest tremor, and rigidity. The most common degenerative parkinsonism is Parkinson disease (PD), a progressive condition that affects approximately 2% of people over the age of 65.[1] PD is associated with degeneration of substantia nigra and intraneuronal deposition of alpha synuclein (either Lewy bodies or Lewy neurites), and clinical improvement of symptoms with the dopamine precursor, levodopa. Parkinsonism is also commonly seen with aging.[2] Age-related parkinsonism is associated with functional disability[3] and may serve as a marker for degenerative brain pathologies.[4]

Patients with PD display resting tremor, bradykinesia, a paucity of spontaneous movement, rigidity, and postural instability. Disease progression is gradual but relentless, and eventually leads to substantial disability for most of those afflicted. Pathologically, there is selective neuronal loss in the substantia nigra with the presence of cytoplasmic inclusions (Lewy bodies) in remaining cells, reduced nigrostriatal neuronal projection, and subsequent striatal dopamine deficiency.[5] Although symptomatic treatment with levodopa focuses on replacing striatal dopamine, the progression of the disease cannot be slowed or halted.[6,7]

Issues in Toxicology No. 16
Aging and Vulnerability to Environmental Chemicals: Age-related Disorders and their Origins in Environmental Exposures
Edited by Bernard Weiss

Published by the Royal Society of Chemistry, www.rsc.org

PD is primarily viewed as a disease of aging. The average age of onset is around 60 years, with only 5–10% of cases occurring before the age of 50.[8] However, it is widely believed that PD develops from multiple risk factors, including aging, genetic predisposition, and environmental exposure. Several gene mutations have been identified as risk factors for PD, but these account for only 5–10% of cases of PD.[9] This suggests that exogenous or environmental factors influence the risk of development of PD, either independently or in conjunction with genetic predisposition.[8]

PD has been linked to exposure to a number of toxins, including metals, such as manganese, lead, and copper; pesticides, often associated with farming and gardening activities; and solvents, such as trichloroethylene. The source of these exposures can be occupational or community/residential, including rural pesticide application or urban industrial emissions. Although there are numerous studies implicating specific occupations in the aetiology of PD, the majority of PD cases do not have clear occupational exposure, suggesting that residential/community exposures may be critical in PD pathogenesis.

Many studies have compared PD incidence and/or prevalence amongst rural and urban populations in attempts to compare the relative roles of residential and industrial exposures in the aetiology of PD. Some have shown a higher risk of PD in individuals living in rural areas of Europe and North America,[10–13] which would potentially link PD to exposure to pesticides and herbicides used in farming, in addition to well water; however, the results are inconsistent.[14] The largest population-based study of the relationship between residence and PD—which used Medicare ICD-9 diagnosed cases and the US Department of Agriculture rural–urban continuum classification (United States Department of Agriculture Economic Research Service, 2008) to classify 'rurality'—found no dose-dependent relationship between PD and rural living but a higher PD prevalence and incidence in the most urban counties as compared to the most rural counties.[1] This study suggests that urban living may be an important risk factor for PD. Most studies investigate only current residence, and not lifetime residence, and risk of PD.

Studies suggesting that industrialization may increase the risk of PD include a comparison between similar populations in the USA and Nigeria;[15] a population-based study in Michigan, USA, which showed higher mortality rates in counties with higher concentrations of industries with potential heavy metal emissions;[16] and comparisons of urban and rural populations in Italy,[17] Bulgaria,[18] and Taiwan[19] (Table 4.1). Although figures were not estimated, a Swedish study suggested that there was an increased prevalence of PD in a county where the economy was predominated by steel and wood manufacturing industries, in comparison to three other less-industrialized counties, based on levodopa prescription records, a common method for identifying cases given the almost universal treatment of patients with levodopa during the course of their disease.[20] A mortality study of World War II veterans found higher PD death rates in the more industrialized Northern states than in the less industrialized Southern states.[21]

Table 4.1 Studies comparing PD in different populations.

			PD prevalence ($\times 10^{-5}$)	
Authors	*Measurement*	*Country(ies)*	*Industrialized region*	*Non/less industrialized region*
Schoenberg *et al.*, 1988[15]	Age-adjusted prevalence ratio	USA and Nigeria (>39 years)	341 (rural USA)	67 (rural Nigeria)
Rybicki *et al.*, 1993[16]	Mortality rate	USA	27	16
Taba and Asser, 2002[22]	Age-adjusted prevalence rate	Estonia	159 (urban)	139 (rural)
Taba and Asser, 2003[23]	Age-adjusted incidence rate	Estonia	19 (urban)	14 (rural)
Totaro *et al.*, 2005[17]	Age- and sex-adjusted prevalence rate	Italy	245 (urban)	215 (rural)
Peters *et al.*, 2006[25]	Prevalence rate (unadjusted)	Australia	130 (urban)	164 (rural)
Chen *et al.*, 2009[19]	Age-standardized prevalence rate	Taiwan (>50 years)	939 (urban)	544 (rural)
Hristova *et al.*, 2010[18]	Age-adjusted incidence rate	Bulgaria	13 (urban)	10 (rural)
Walker *et al.*, 2010[24]	Age-adjusted prevalence rate	England	139 (urban)	142 (rural)
Willis *et al.*, 2010[1]	Age-adjusted prevalence rate	USA	1 706 (pop. >1 m)	1 371 (pop. <2500)

However, differences in rural–urban PD prevalence have not been found consistently worldwide. Similar PD prevalence and incidence rates were found amongst residents in urban and rural areas in Estonia,[22,23] and in England,[24] and an Australian study reported lower prevalence rates of PD in urban areas[25] (Table 4.1). A case-control study in Serbia did not find any difference in the odds ratio (OR) for PD between rural and urban areas,[26] and a case-control study in Quebec, Canada, reported a lower adjusted OR of 0.15 (95% CI 0.04–0.55) for PD associated with living in industrial or mining areas.[14]

Different study designs, case-finding methods, and definitions of PD, as well as the difficulty in classifying rural and urban living, prevent direct comparison of the above studies. In many of the studies, small sample size also affects the validity of the findings. A recent study investigated rural–urban risk for PD using standard, population density-based definitions for rural living.[1] More than 500 000 prevalent PD cases older than 65 years were identified from USA population-based Medicare data. The authors found a significantly higher prevalence of PD in the most urban USA counties compared to the most rural (Table 4.1 and Figure 4.1).

Studies analyzing PD incidence trends potentially test the hypothesis that industrialization is a risk factor for PD. A study investigating the longitudinal risk of PD in a small, relatively rural region in Minnesota, USA, from 1967 to 1979,[27] found no change in the annual incidence of PD during that time period.

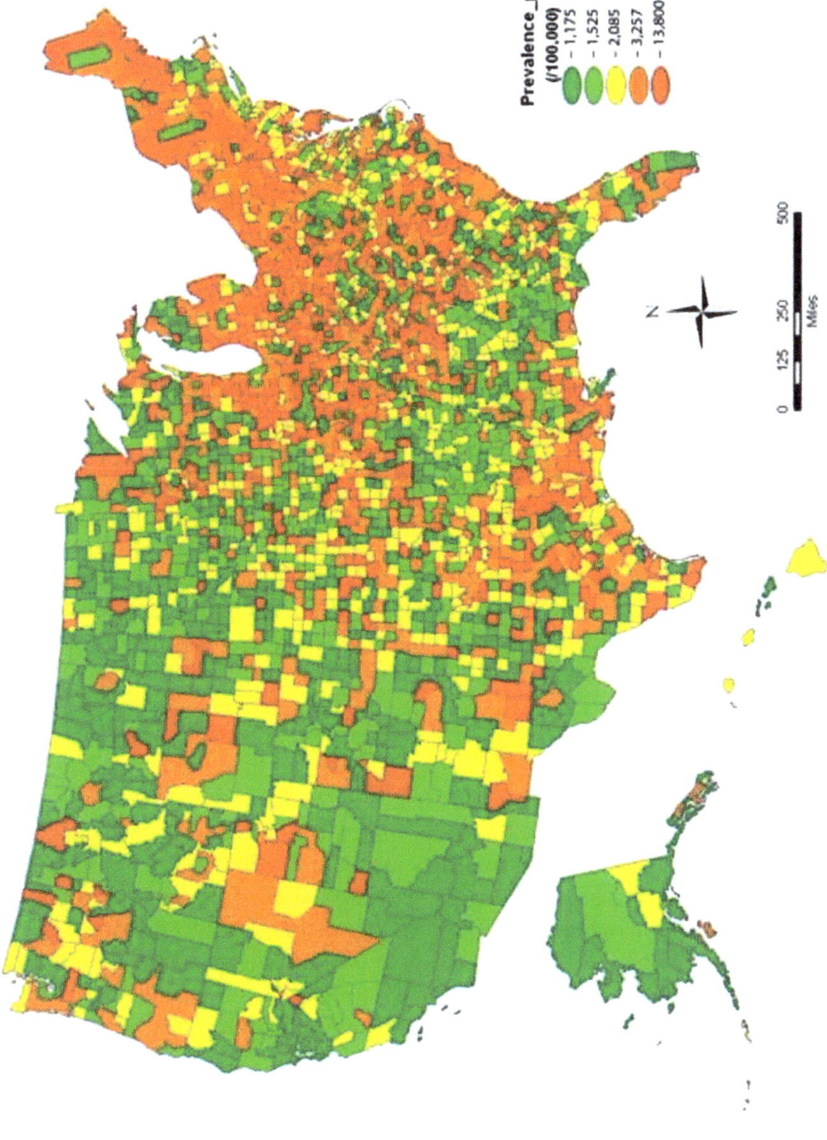

Figure 4.1 County level age- and race-standardized prevalence (per 100 000) of Parkinson disease among Medicare beneficiaries in the USA (year = 2003).[1]

It is also unlikely that there was a substantial change in industrialization in that rural region of the USA over the 12-year period. Similarly, a more recent population-based study of USA Medicare beneficiaries, reporting PD incidence rates for a 4-year period from 2002 to 2005, also showed no change.[1] This same study also found a stable PD prevalence rate from 1995 to 2005. A population prevalence study in the English Midlands did show an increase in PD from 1982 to 1992,[28] but this may have been due to increased medical and public awareness, rather than industrialization.

4.2 Environmental Toxins

Risk factors for PD include modifiable and non-modifiable factors. Non-modifiable factors include increasing age, male gender, and White race.[1,29,30] Modifiable risk factors, such as environment or occupation, have been relatively under-studied, especially in urban areas where the overwhelming majority of PD patients reside. Understanding community level exposures to environmental toxins is critical in determining the causes of most cases of PD and in developing strategies to reduce the burden of the disease in the future.

4.2.1 Metals

There are a number of studies that suggest that heavy metals are associated with PD,[16,31–34] and that exposure may accelerate some of the pathologic findings characteristic of PD. The metal for which the most evidence exists for an association with PD is manganese, but lead, copper, and mercury have also been implicated.[34–36] Most studies have been conducted on occupationally exposed populations; very little research has been conducted on the effects of community exposure.

4.2.1.1 Manganese

Manganese is a known neurotoxin that has been associated with damage to some of the same structures in the brain that are affected in PD.[37–39] Exposure to acute, high levels of manganese is clearly associated with parkinsonism, and lower-level exposure is associated with parkinsonian motor abnormalities. Evidence implicating manganese in the aetiology of PD is contradictory.

There is strong evidence for an association of parkinsonism and occupational exposure to manganese. In 1837, the first case series of parkinsonism in manganese miners was published. The neurological effects of manganese exposure in four ore crushers were described as lower extremity predominant muscular weakness, festination, postural instability, facial masking, hypophonia, and sialorrhea.[40] More than 100 years later, in 1955, Rodier described similar neurological symptoms in a group of 150 Moroccan underground manganese miners,[41] with latency from exposure ranging from one month to more than 10 years. He described a syndrome characterized by typical parkinsonian findings (rigidity, bradykinesia, tremor, flexed posture, shuffling gait, postural instability) and atypical findings (psychosis, personality change, dystonic 'cock' gait, emotional lability). In most cases, the disease progressed to total disability, despite discontinuing exposure.

There are a number of clinical reports of atypical parkinsonism in similar and other manganese-exposed workers. Two case series in the 1960s described manganese poisoning: one in 13 Chilean miners,[42] and the other in seven workers from various industries in Pennsylvania, USA.[43] Another report of six men who developed manganese poisoning in a manganese ore crushing plant where reported levels were as high as 21.9 mg m^{-3} was published in 1974.[44]

Manganese is the primary exposure in the steel industry and there is some evidence that workers with acute exposures to fumes present with an atypical parkinsonian syndrome. In 1966, Whitlock *et al.* reported two cases of manganese poisoning in a manganese steel plant.[45] Both men were exposed to manganese levels of 2.3–4.7 mg m^{-3} during the process of cleaning manganese steel castings. In 1989, Wang *et al.* described parkinsonism in six of eight workers, exposed to even higher concentrations of manganese (>28.8 mg m^{-3}) in a Taiwanese ferromanganese smelter,[46] one of whom later developed a 'cock' gait.[47]

While it is clear that manganese causes an atypical parkinsonian disorder, evidence implicating manganese in the aetiology of PD is contradictory. Although one population-based case-control study showed an OR of 10.6 for PD with occupational exposure to manganese for more than 20 years, the findings were based on three cases and one control.[35,48] A Canadian study found an increased risk of PD in a small case-control study of 42 PD patients exposed to a combination of metals, including manganese, but did not calculate risks for exposure to individual metals.[14] Conversely, two other case-control studies, in Germany and Canada, found no association between exposure to heavy metals, including manganese, and PD.[34,49] Contradictory findings were likely due to differences in study design and study population exposures, and small sample sizes.

There are many clinical reports on the effects of exposure to manganese fumes in welders.[45,50–52] Manganese is commonly found in welding fumes, and many welders are regularly overexposed to the American Conference of Governmental Industrial Hygienists threshold limit value of 0.2 mg m^{-3}, which was primarily set in regard to neurological effects.[53,54] Although the dose–response relationship between welding exposures and motor function remain to be established, one small study suggested that performance on pegboard and timed motor tasks might be slower in 12 manganese-exposed welders when compared to a control group of 39 railway track welders who had welded for less than 25 hours in total.[52] A large study of 1 423 Alabama welders found a substantially higher prevalence of parkinsonism compared with the general population of Copiah County, Mississippi, USA. The estimated prevalence of parkinsonism among active male welders aged 40–69 years was 977–1 336 per 100 000, and was higher among welders when compared to age-standardized data for the general population (prevalence ratio 10.19; 95% CI 4.43–23.43).[55]

Table 4.2 Parkinsonian motor abnormalities in workers exposed to low levels of manganese.

Authors	*Country*	*Study population*	*Mean ambient manganese level ($mg\,m^{-3}$)*	*Clinical signs*
Roels *et al.*, 1987[115]	Belgium	141 manganese oxide and salt producing plant workers	0.94 (0.07–8.61)	Slowed simple reaction times, increased hand tremor
Iregren, 1990[116] Wennberg *et al.*, 1991[117] Wennberg *et al.*, 1992[118]	Sweden	30 steel smelting workers; 60 controls	0.18–1.41	Slower reaction times, reduced finger tapping speeds, reduced tapping endurance, diadochokinesis
Mergler *et al.*, 1994[119]	Canada	115 ferro-manganese and silicomanganese alloy workers; 145 controls	0.89	Slower computerized finger tapping scores, less hand steadiness
Lucchini *et al.*, 1999[120]	Italy	61 ferroalloy plant workers; 87 controls	0.07	Tremor, coordination, bradykinesia

This study specifically addressed parkinsonism, not PD. Several cross-sectional studies have shown that occupational exposure to manganese at low levels, *viz.* below the Occupational Safety and Health Administration's permissible exposure limit of $5\,mg\,m^{-3}$, may be associated with parkinsonian motor abnormalities (Table 4.2), with the most consistent symptom being slowed finger tapping. Such studies have been conducted primarily in workers employed in the metal industry and in welders.

These findings are supported by a number of studies in manganese-exposed communities (Table 4.3). One such study on 273 people in Quebec, Canada, showed an association of raised blood manganese levels with slowing of motor tasks and difficulty with pointing tasks consistent with tremor.[56] Two more recent Italian studies have also suggested that residential exposure to manganese is associated with an increased prevalence of parkinsonian disturbances.[57,58]

Although there is some evidence that welders may have a higher risk of parkinsonism, findings of epidemiologic studies, including large welder cohorts, provide contradictory results regarding the relationship between welding and PD. A survey of three specialty-based practices found only three welders among 2 249 consecutive patients with PD.[59] However, it is possible that welders were underrepresented in these relatively white collar communities. In a death certificate study of neurodegenerative disease and PD, welding-related occupations were not among the highest ranked occupations in PD-related deaths.[60]

Table 4.3 Studies of community manganese exposure and parkinsonism or PD.

Authors	*Country*	*Study design*	*Study population*	*Findings*
Mergler *et al.*, 1999[56]	Canada	Cross-sectional	273 residents exposed to manganese	Slowing of motor tasks; difficulty with pointing tasks consistent with tremor
Lucchini *et al.*, 2007[57]	Italy	Cross-sectional	903 997 residents in 206 municipalities	Prevalence in municipalities in vicinities of ferromanganese plants 492/100 000 *vs* 321/100 000 in others
Lucchini *et al.*, 2012[58]	Italy	Cross-sectional	154 adolescents in vicinity of ferroalloy plants 157 controls	Historical manganese exposure from ferroalloy emission reflected by the concentration in soil and biomarkers as associated with sub-clinical deficits in olfactory and motor function
Dick *et al.*, 2007[66]	Scotland, Italy, Sweden, Romania, Malta	Case-control	767 PD patients 1 989 controls	No association of manganese exposure with PD
Finkelstein and Jerrett, 2007[67]	Canada	Nested case control	509 PD patients 52 477 controls	OR 1.03 (95% CI 1.00–1.07) per 10 ng m^{-3} increase in particulate manganese; exposure to ambient manganese advances the age of diagnosis of PD
Willis *et al.*, 2010[68]	USA	Cross-sectional	34 584 PD patients	RR 1.78 (95% CI 1.54–2.07)
Willis *et al.*, 2012[63]	USA	Cohort	138 000 Medicare beneficiaries with PD	Adjusted HR 1.19 (95% CI 1.10–1.29)

However, death certificates may underestimate the prevalence of parkinsonism or PD, given the long clinical course and rarity of death due to PD-related morbidity. Two studies in Sweden and Denmark, using hospitalization for PD to identify cases, found no increased risk of PD in welders.[61,62] However, a recent survival study in PD patients found that only 1% of patients with PD are ever hospitalized for PD, making this a very insensitive method of case identification.[63] Finally, there is some evidence that welding exposure may accelerate the age of onset of,[64] and death due to, PD.[65]

There is also a growing body of evidence implicating community level exposures to manganese as a risk factor for PD (Table 4.3). Although a European study did not demonstrate an association with manganese exposure, based on occupation, hobbies, and water supply,[66] three subsequent large studies, using GIS (geographic information system) coding, did report increased risks. The first, using markers of exposure to ambient manganese, found no association with markers for traffic-generated air pollution, but reported an increased OR for markers for industrial emissions containing manganese.[67] Using Medicare data for PD case identification and exposure lagging, a second study reported a higher incidence of neurologist-diagnosed PD in urban USA counties with high manganese release compared to those with none[68] (Figure 4.2). This was specific to manganese as there was no increased incidence in counties with high industrial lead or zinc emissions. While these two studies suggest that community manganese exposures may be a risk factor for PD, the third, more recent GIS study suggests that manganese may modulate PD progression. This large retrospective cohort study of Medicare beneficiaries with incident PD demonstrated higher risk of death in patients living in urban areas with high industrial manganese emissions than in those in areas with low emissions.[63] This finding was specific to manganese as PD patients living in regions with high copper emissions had no elevated risk of PD.

The pathophysiology of manganese-associated neurotoxicity has been studied using molecular imaging in manganese-exposed welders. The same technology provides an opportunity to understand the relationship between manganese exposure and PD. [^{18}F]Fluorodopa ([^{18}F]FDOPA) Positron Emission Tomography imaging in two welders with PD demonstrated reduced [^{18}F]FDOPA uptake to be more prominent in the posterior putamen contralateral to the most affected side.[64] A recent study of asymptomatic, active welders found reductions in [^{18}F]FDOPA uptake preferentially involving the caudate, with relative preservation of the posterior putamen.[69] Workers imaged in this study had only mild abnormalities on a quantified motor exam for parkinsonism (Unified Parkinson Disease Rating Scale motor scale). However, further work to investigate the spectrum of dopaminergic dysfunction in manganese-exposed workers is needed in order to understand the toxic effects of manganese on the substantia nigra.

4.2.1.2 Lead

Long-term exposure to lead has been suggested as a possible risk factor for PD. Parkinsonism has been reported in workers exposed to lead-sulfate

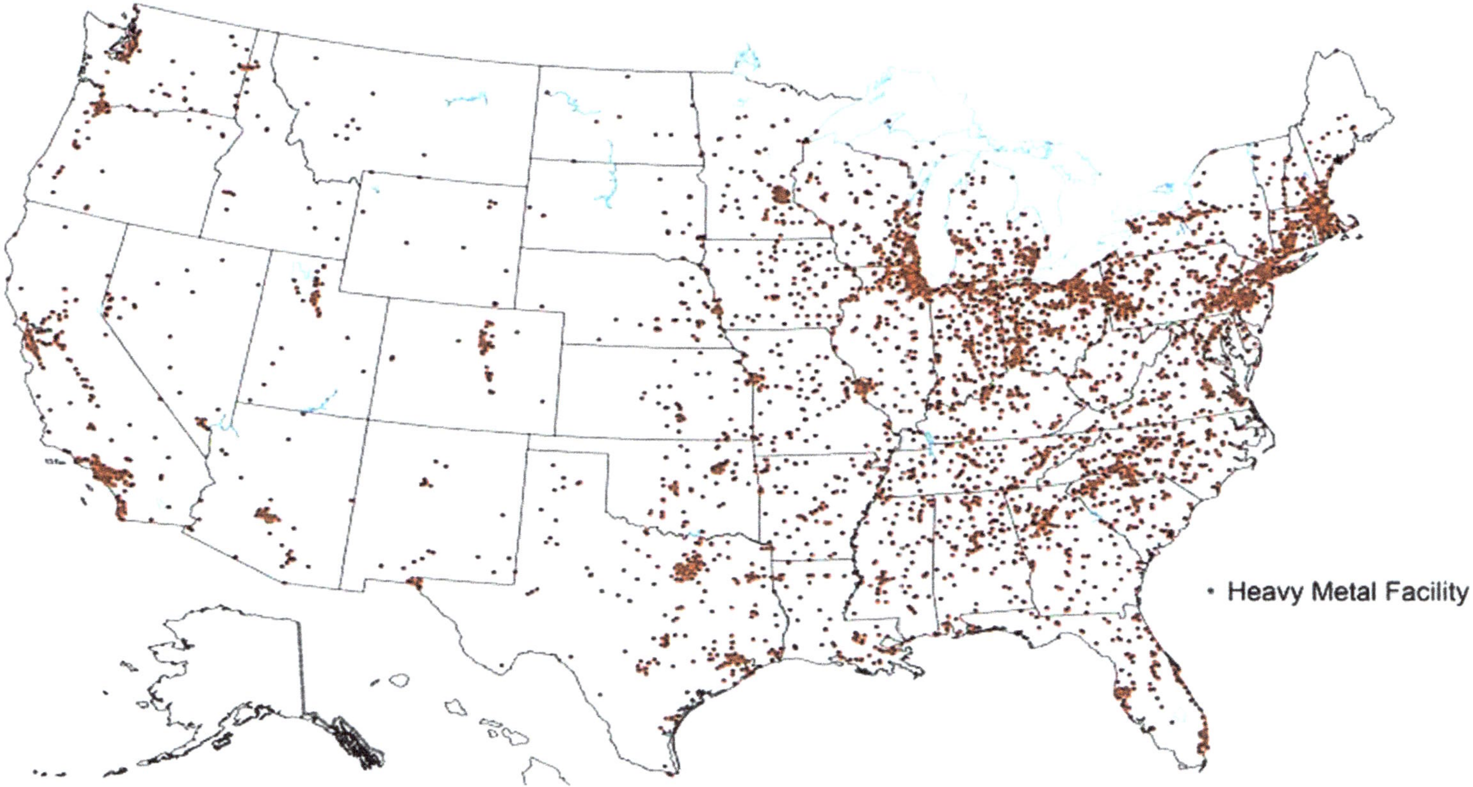

Figure 4.2 Map of USA showing heavy metal emitting facilities (manganese, copper, or lead). Produced by A. Wright Willis, using Environmental Protection Agency Toxic Release Inventory Facility data, 1988–2005, using ESRI ARC MAP, version 9 software.

batteries.[70–72] A USA case-control study, published in 2006, reported a two-fold increase in the risk of PD with occupational lead exposure, measured as cumulative lead in bone tissue.[73] While lead in blood is a good biomarker for recent exposure, cumulative exposure, which can be measured in bone where the half-life for lead is decades, is more relevant when studying PD. A second, much larger case-control study, carried out in the USA and published in 2010, confirmed a role for lead in the development of PD.[74] However, Willis *et al.* found no relationship between industrial lead emissions and the incidence of PD in the USA in a cross-sectional GIS study, using Medicare data.[68] Residential lead exposure differs from manganese in that it has many potential sources. The role of environmental lead exposure in PD thus needs to be investigated more thoroughly.

4.2.1.3 Copper

As for lead, the evidence for an association between residential exposure to copper and PD is tenuous. While occupational exposure to copper was associated with a two-fold increased risk for PD in a population-based case-control study in the USA,[35] no association was found in a case-control study conducted in Germany.[34]

An earlier population-based mortality study showed that USA counties with a higher concentration of paper-, chemical-, iron- or copper-related industries had statistically significantly higher PD death rates than counties without these industries,[16] suggesting a geographic association between PD mortality and the industrial use of heavy metals. Using GIS, Willis *et al.* analyzed Medicare data for the risk of PD in counties with high emissions of copper and found no relationship between industrial copper emissions and the incidence of PD.[68]

4.2.1.4 Combinations of Metals

Studies suggest that exposures to combinations of metals present a higher risk for PD than exposures to single metals. Gorell *et al.* calculated increased risks for PD with occupational exposures to lead and copper (OR 5.24), lead and iron (OR 2.83), and iron and copper (OR 3.69) over more than 20 years.[35] Another study demonstrated an increased risk for PD in those occupationally exposed to a combination of manganese, iron, and aluminium (OR 2.28), which increased when exposure was longer than 30 years (OR 13.64).[14] However, the number of subjects was small in both studies.

4.2.1.5 Other Metals

Other metals that have been studied include iron, zinc, cadmium, aluminium, and nickel. Although more central nervous system symptoms and decreased motor function were reported in 38 aluminium exposed welders compared to 39 controls,[52] a small case-control study of 130 patients with PD, compared to sex- and age-matched community controls selected by random-digit dialing, showed no difference in work-related contact with aluminium.[49] One case-control study of only 54 patients in the 1980s demonstrated an association between blood mercury levels and PD.[36] All subsequent studies on mercury have shown no association.[34,35,75] There is no other evidence of an association of exposure to any of these metals with PD[76] (when not combined with exposure to other metals, as discussed in Section 4.2.1.4).

4.2.2 Pesticides

Numerous studies have investigated the association between exposure to pesticides and the risk of PD. Products most consistently implicated as risk factors for PD are the widely-used broad-spectrum herbicide, paraquat (1,1′-dimethyl-4,4′-bipyridylium dichloride), and the manganese-containing fungicide, maneb (manganese ethylene bisdithiocarbamate), although neurological effects of other pesticides have also been reported.

There are reports of the development of parkinsonism after acute exposure to diquat,[77] paraquat,[78] and glyphosate.[79] In addition, a study comparing 50 maneb-exposed, with 19 non-exposed, agricultural workers found that the exposed group was significantly more likely to have rigidity than the non-exposed group.[80] A case-control study conducted in eight movement disorders centers in North America compared lifelong occupational and job task histories to determine associations with parkinsonism and certain clinical subtypes in 519 cases and 511 controls.[81] Risk of parkinsonism increased with pesticide use (OR 1.90; 95% CI 1.12–3.21), use of any of eight pesticides mechanistically associated with experimental parkinsonism (OR 2.20; 95% CI 1.02–4.75), and use of the herbicide 2,4-dichlorophenoxyacetic acid (OR 2.59; 95% CI 1.03–6.48).

Studies investigating risk of PD associated with pesticides are conflicting. There are several case-control studies demonstrating increased risk of PD associated with occupational exposure to pesticides, herbicides, fungicides, and/or insecticides.[11,82–87] Many of these studies were based on small numbers of PD cases. On the other hand, a large cross-sectional study found a dose–response relationship between self-reported incident, but not prevalent, PD and pesticide use in more than 52 000 pesticide applicators.[88] However, there was no association with specific pesticides. In a cohort study, a relative risk of 1.7 (95% CI 1.2–2.3) was calculated for PD and pesticide use.[89]

A recently published Finnish nested case-control study, using serum biomarkers of organochlorine pesticides collected from 101 cases and 349 matched controls from 1968 to 1972, demonstrated weak evidence for an association between PD and pesticide exposure.[90] A dose-dependent increased risk of PD was found for only one of the five pesticides tested (dieldrin) and only among non-smokers.

Fewer studies have looked at associations of PD with community exposure to pesticides. A case-control study in California, using death certificates to identify PD cases, found that PD mortality was higher in counties using agricultural pesticides than in those where pesticides were not used (ORs ranged from 1.19 to 1.45).[91] However, studies that use GIS methodologies to estimate exposure, rather than relying on subjective self-reported exposure data, provide the most convincing evidence of the link between pesticides and PD. GIS modeling was used in a second case-control study to calculate residential exposure to maneb and paraquat in more than 300 cases and controls over 10 years.[92,93] High residential exposures to these pesticides significantly increased the risk of PD.

Other studies have attempted to estimate the risk of PD from community exposure to pesticides by using well water consumption as a surrogate measure of pesticide or herbicide exposure. Only one study, however, has measured pesticide contamination of well water and attempted to correlate these levels with PD risk. Gatto *et al.* used a case-control GIS model to investigate whether drinking water from wells in areas with documented historical agricultural pesticide use was associated with an increased risk of PD among residents in a farming-intensive area of California.[94] A comparison of 368 PD cases, diagnosed by movement disorder specialists, with 341 non-PD controls, was made. The risk of PD increased for consumption of well water contaminated with methomyl (OR 1.67; 95% CI 1.00–2.78), chlorpyrifos (OR 1.87; 95% CI 1.05–3.31), and propargite (OR 1.92; 95% CI 1.15–3.20) and also increased as the number of pesticides in the water increased. The authors concluded that consuming well water, presumably contaminated with pesticides, may play a role in the aetiology of PD.

4.2.3 Solvents

Parkinsonism has been reported in patients following exposure to solvents, including lacquer thinner,[95] n-hexane,[96] carbon tetrachloride,[97] and mixed solvent exposures from petroleum waste.[98] Parkinsonian features have also been described in painters exposed to various solvents, including toluene, xylene, carbon disulfide, thinner, methanol, and methylethylketone.[99,100] Parkinsonism has been described in a number of case reports as a consequence of a methanol poisoning,[101–106] but no studies have shown an association with PD for this or any other solvent, other than trichloroethylene.

Although a case-control study in Italy identified occupational exposure to organic solvents as the only significant risk factor for PD among several industrial chemicals investigated (OR 2.78; 95% CI 1.23–6.26),[107] the numbers of cases and controls were small (86 of each) and no specific solvents were identified. Epidemiological studies have only been conducted to test associations of parkinsonism and/or PD with trichloroethylene and carbon disulfide. However, all studies have been performed in occupationally exposed individuals, and no data are available for residential exposures.

4.2.3.1 Trichloroethylene

Trichloroethylene (TCE) is a chlorinated hydrocarbon commonly used as a solvent in the industrial degreasing of metals. It is also used in adhesive paint and polyvinyl chloride production, in the textile industry, and in the manufacturing of pesticides and other chemicals. TCE is also the most common organic contaminant of groundwater.[108]

There have been several case reports of PD associated with occupational exposure to TCE. A 47-year old women developed PD after exposure to TCE, first as a house cleaner, and then in the plastics industry.[109] Three cases were also reported by Kochen *et al.* in 2003.[110] In a report published in 2008, Gash *et al.* described three factory workers, using TCE as a degreasing agent, who developed PD.[111] An additional 24 workers demonstrated parkinsonian motor features.

More recently, Goldman *et al.* tested the hypothesis that exposure to specific solvents is associated with PD risk. They interviewed 99 twin pairs discordant for PD and estimated exposures to six different solvents. Only exposure to TCE was associated with a significantly increased risk of PD (OR 6.1; 95% CI 1.2–33).[108] However, the number of subjects was small and exposure assessments were based on jobs that may have involved exposure to multiple agents. Studies with more detailed dose reconstruction and larger numbers are necessary to confirm these findings, as solvents are common environmental toxins.

Hydrocarbon exposure has also been investigated as a risk factor for PD in other epidemiological studies. A nested case-control study of 188 patients with PD found that those occupationally exposed to hydrocarbons were significantly younger at onset of disease ($p = 0.014$), suggesting that hydrocarbons may be an environmental accelerant for PD.[112]

4.2.3.2 Carbon Disulfide

Carbon disulfide is used primarily in the manufacture of regenerated cellulose rayon but is also used in many other industries. Atypical parkinsonism in 21 grain workers (grain inspectors, malt laboratory workers, and grain elevator workers) was attributed to exposure to carbon disulfide in the 1980s.[113] Symptoms included bradykinesia, rest tremor, cerebellar signs, and sensory neuropathy. In a more recent cross-sectional study of 85 viscose rayon plant workers and 66 unexposed controls, exposed workers performed more poorly on finger tapping tests, and displayed postural tremor and peripheral polyneuropathy, even at exposure levels below the threshold limit value.[114] No associations with typical PD have been demonstrated.

4.3 Conclusion

This chapter identifies several common environmental chemicals as risk factors for PD. The metals for which most evidence exists for an association with parkinsonism and/or PD are manganese, lead, and copper. The products in the agricultural industry that are most consistently implicated as risk factors for PD and/or parkinsonism are paraquat and maneb. There is some evidence for an association of parkinsonism with carbon disulfide, but TCE is the only solvent for which there is modest evidence for a risk of PD. Future studies, providing converging evidence for the aetiologic role of these environmental chemicals are needed in order to demonstrate dose–response and to establish critical thresholds of exposure to inform environmental regulation. Despite some contradictory findings, reducing environmental exposures may well result in a substantial reduction in the number of new cases of PD.

Acknowledgements

Dr Racette's research is supported by the National Institute for Environmental Health Sciences (R01 ES013743, K24 ES017765, P42ES04696), the Michael J. Fox Foundation, National Institute of Neurological Disorders and Stroke (NINDS) Grant Number 5T32NS007205-27, National Center for Research Resources (NCRR0) and National Institutes of Health (NIH) Roadmap for Medical Research Grant Number UL1 RR024992, the American Parkinson Disease Association, and the Greater St. Louis Chapter of the American Parkinson Disease Association. Both Dr Racette's and Dr Nelson's research is further supported by Washington University: Grant Numbers ICTS NCRR UL1RR024992 and R21 ES017504.

Permission to reproduce Figure 4.1 was obtained from authors Dr Allison Wright Willis and Dr Brad Racette, and from S. Karger AG, Basel. Permission to use Figure 4.2 was obtained from Dr Allison Wright Willis.

References

1. A. Wright Willis, B. A. Evanoff, M. Lian, S. R. Criswell and B. A. Racette, *Neuroepidemiology*, 2010, **34**, 143–151.
2. E. D. Louis, J. A. Luchsinger, M. X. Tang and R. Mayeux, *Neurology*, 2003, **61**, 24–28.
3. E. D. Louis, M. X. Tang, N. Schupf and R. Mayeux, *Arch. Neurol.*, 2005, **62**, 297–302.
4. E. D. Louis, K. Marder, M. H. Tabert and D. P. Devanand, *Mov. Disord*, 2008, **23**, 524–530.
5. W. R. Gibb and A. J. Lees, *Neuropathol. Appl. Neurobiol.*, 1989, **15**, 27–44.
6. Parkinson Study Group PRECEPT Investigators, *Neurology*, 2007, **69**, 1480–1490.
7. I. Shoulson, *Ann. Neurol.*, 1998, **44**, S160–S166.
8. H. M. Gao and J. S. Hong, *Prog. Neurobiol. (N.Y.)*, 2011, **94**, 1–19.
9. W. M. Caudle, T. S. Guillot, C. R. Lazo and G. W. Miller, *Neurotoxicology*, 2012, **33**, 178–188.
10. E. Granieri, M. Carreras, I. Casetta, V. Govoni, M. R. Tola, E. Paolino, V. C. Monetti and P. De Bastiani, *Arch. Neurol.*, 1991, **48**, 854–857.
11. J. P. Hubble, T. Cao, R. E. Hassanein, J. S. Neuberger and W. C. Koller, *Neurology*, 1993, **43**, 1693–1697.
12. W. Koller, B. Vetere-Overfield, C. Gray, C. Alexander, T. Chin, J. Dolezal, R. Hassanein and C. Tanner, *Neurology*, 1990, **40**, 1218–1221.

13. L. W. Svenson, G. H. Platt and S. E. Woodhead, *Can. J. Neurol. Sci.*, 1993, **20**, 307–311.
14. J. Zayed, S. Ducic, G. Campanella, J. C. Panisset, P. Andre, H. Masson and M. Roy, *Can. J. Neurol. Sci.*, 1990, **17**, 286–291.
15. B. S. Schoenberg, B. O. Osuntokun, A. O. Adeuja, O. Bademosi, V. Nottidge, D. W. Anderson and A. F. Haerer, *Neurology*, 1988, **38**, 645–646.
16. B. A. Rybicki, C. C. Johnson, J. Uman and J. M. Gorell, *Mov. Disord*, 1993, **8**, 87–92.
17. R. Totaro, C. Marini, F. Pistoia, S. Sacco, T. Russo and A. Carolei, *Acta. Neurol. Scand.*, 2005, **112**, 24–28.
18. D. Hristova, Z. Zachariev, N. Mateva and I. Grozdev, *Neuroepidemiology*, 2010, **34**, 76–82.
19. C. C. Chen, T. F. Chen, Y. C. Hwang, Y. R. Wen, Y. H. Chiu, C. Y. Wu, R. C. Chen, J. J. Tai, T. H. Chen and H. H. Liou, *Neuroepidemiology*, 2009, **33**, 350–357.
20. S. M. Aquilonius and P. Hartvig, *Acta. Neurol. Scand.*, 1986, **74**, 379–382.
21. W. E. Lux and J. F. Kurtzke, *Neurology*, 1987, **37**, 467–471.
22. P. Taba and T. Asscr, *Acta. Ncurol. Scand.*, 2002, **106**, 276–281.
23. P. Taba and T. Asser, *Neuroepidemiology*, 2003, **22**, 41–45.
24. R. W. Walker, A. Hand, C. Jones, B. H. Wood and W. K. Gray, *Parkinsonism Relat. Disord.*, 2010, **16**, 572–575.
25. C. M. Peters, C. E. Gartner, P. A. Silburn and G. D. Mellick, *J. Clin. Neurosci.*, 2006, **13**, 343–348.
26. H. D. Vlajinac, S. B. Sipetic, J. M. Maksimovic, J. M. Marinkovic, E. D. Dzoljic, I. S. Ratkov and V. S. Kostic, *Int. J. Neurosci.*, 2010, **120**, 361–367.
27. A. H. Rajput, K. P. Offord, C. M. Beard and L. T. Kurland, *Ann. Neurol.*, 1984, **16**, 278–282.
28. R. L. Sutcliffe and J. R. Meara, *Acta. Neurol. Scand.*, 1995, **92**, 443–350.
29. K. Marder, G. Logroscino, B. Alfaro, H. Mejia, A. Halim, E. Louis, L. Cote and R. Mayeux, *Neurology*, 1998, **50**, 279–281.
30. S. K. Van Den Eeden, C. M. Tanner, A. L. Bernstein, R. D. Fross, A. Leimpeter, D. A. Bloch and L. M. Nelson, *Am. J. Epidemiol.*, 2003, **157**, 1015–1022.
31. T. Fukushima, X. Tan, Y. Luo and H. Kanda, *Neuroepidemiology*, 2010, **34**, 18–24.
32. R. Lucchini, E. Albini, L. Benedetti, S. Zoni, A. Caruso, E. Nan, P. Pasqualetti, P. M. Rossini, G. Binetti, L. Benussi, G. Parrinello, R. Gasparotti, A. Padovani, F. Draicchio and L. Alessio, *G. Ital. Med. Lav. Ergon*, 2007, **29**, 280–281.
33. R. Lucchini, L. Benedetti, S. Borghesi, S. Garattini, G. Parrinello and L. Alessio, *G. Ital. Med. Lav. Ergon*, 2003, **25**(Suppl), 88–89.
34. A. Seidler, W. Hellenbrand, B. P. Robra, P. Vieregge, P. Nischan, J. Joerg, W. H. Oertel, G. Ulm and E. Schneider, *Neurology*, 1996, **46**, 1275–1284.

35. J. M. Gorell, C. C. Johnson, B. A. Rybicki, E. L. Peterson, G. X. Kortsha, G. G. Brown and R. J. Richardson, *Neurology*, 1997, **48**, 650–658.
36. C. H. Ngim and G. Devathasan, *Neuroepidemiology*, 1989, **8**, 128–141.
37. L. Casamajor, *J. Am. Med. Assoc*, 1913, **60**, 646–649.
38. M. Yamada, S. Ohno, I. Okayasu, R. Okeda, S. Hatakeyama, H. Watanabc, K. Ushio and H. Tsukagoshi, *Acta. Neuropathol.*, 1986, **70**, 273–278.
39. M. M. Canavan, W. Cobb and B. Drnovsek, *Arch. Neurol. Psychiatry*, 1934, **32**, 501–512.
40. J. Couper, *Brit. Ann. Med. Pharm.*, 1837, **1**, 41–42.
41. J. Rodier, *Br. J. Ind. Med.*, 1955, **12**, 21–35.
42. I. Mena, O. Marin, S. Fuenzalida and G. C. Cotzias, *Neurology*, 1967, **17**, 128–136.
43. S. Tanaka and J. Lieben, *Arch. Environ. Health*, 1969, **19**, 674–684.
44. D. G. Cook, S. Fahn and K. A. Brait, *Arch. Neurol.*, 1974, **30**, 59–64.
45. C. M. Whitlock, Jr., S. J. Amuso and J. B. Bittenbender, *Am. Ind. Hyg. Assoc. J.*, 1966, **27**, 454–459.
46. J. D. Wang, C. C. Huang, Y. H. Hwang, J. R. Chiang, J. M. Lin and J. S. Chen, *Br. J. Ind. Med.*, 1989, **46**, 856–859.
47. C. C. Huang, C. S. Lu, N. S. Chu, F. Hochberg, D. Lilienfeld, W. Olanowa and D. B. Calne, *Neurology*, 1993, **43**, 1479–1483.
48. J. M. Gorell, C. C. Johnson, B. A. Rybicki, E. L. Peterson, G. X. Kortsha, G. G. Brown and R. J. Richardson, *Neurotoxicology*, 1999, **20**, 239–247.
49. K. M. Semchuk, E. J. Love and R. G. Lee, *Neurology*, 1993, **43**, 1173–1180.
50. S. V. Chandra, G. S. Shukla, R. S. Srivastava, H. Singh and V. P. Gupta, *Clin. Toxicol.*, 1981, **18**, 407–416.
51. K. Nelson, J. Golnick, T. Korn and C. Angle, *Br. J. Ind. Med.*, 1993, **50**, 510–513.
52. B. Sjogren, A. Iregren, W. Frech, M. Hagman, L. Johansson, M. Tesarz and A. Wennberg, *Occup. Environ. Med.*, 1996, **53**, 32–40.
53. R. E. Korczynski, *Appl. Occup. Environ. Hyg*, 2000, **15**, 936–945.
54. P. Susi, M. Goldberg, P. Barnes and E. Stafford, *Appl. Occup. Environ. Hyg*, 2000, **15**, 26–38.
55. B. A. Racette, S. D. Tabbal, D. Jennings, L. Good, J. S. Perlmutter and B. Evanoff, *Neurology*, 2005, **64**, 230–235.
56. D. Mergler, M. Baldwin, S. Belanger, F. Larribe, A. Beuter, R. Bowler, M. Panisset, R. Edwards, A. de Geoffroy, M. P. Sassine and K. Hudnell, *Neurotoxicology*, 1999, **20**, 327–342.
57. R. G. Lucchini, E. Albini, L. Benedetti, S. Borghesi, R. Coccaglio, E. C. Malara, G. Parrinello, S. Garattini, S. Resola and L. Alessio, *Am. J. Ind. Med.*, 2007, **50**, 788–800.
58. R. G. Lucchini, S. Guazzetti, S. Zoni, F. Donna, S. Peter, A. Zacco, M. Salmistraro, E. Bontempi, N. J. Zimmerman and D. R. Smith, *Neurotoxicology*, 2012, **33**, 687–696.

59. S. M. Goldman, C. M. Tanner, C. W. Olanow, R. L. Watts, R. D. Field and J. W. Langston, *Neurology*, 2005, **65**, 1430–1435.
60. P. A. Schulte, C. A. Burnett, M. F. Boeniger and J. Johnson, *Am. J. Public Health*, 1996, **86**, 1281–1288.
61. C. M. Fored, J. P. Fryzek, L. Brandt, G. Nise, B. Sjogren, J. K. McLaughlin, W. J. Blot and A. Ekbom, *Occup. Environ. Med.*, 2006, **63**, 135–140.
62. J. P. Fryzek, J. Hansen, S. Cohen, J. P. Bonde, M. T. Llambias, H. A. Kolstad, A. Skytthe, L. Lipworth, W. J. Blot and J. H. Olsen, *J. Occup. Environ. Med.*, 2005, **47**, 466–472.
63. A. W. Willis, M. Schootman, N. Kung, B. A. Evanoff, J. S. Perlmutter and B. A. Racette, *Arch. Neurol.*, 2012, **69**, 601–607.
64. B. A. Racette, L. McGee-Minnich, S. M. Moerlein, J. W. Mink, T. O. Videen and J. S. Perlmutter, *Neurology*, 2001, **56**, 8–13.
65. R. M. Park, R. M. Bowler, D. E. Eggerth, E. Diamond, K. J. Spencer, D. Smith and R. Gwiazda, *Neurotoxicology*, 2006, **27**, 373–384.
66. F. D. Dick, G. De Palma, A. Ahmadi, N. W. Scott, G. J. Prescott, J. Bennett, S. Semple, S. Dick, C. Counsell, P. Mozzoni, N. Haites, S. B. Wettinger, A. Mutti, M. Otelea, A. Seaton, P. Soderkvist and A. Felice, *Occup. Environ. Med.*, 2007, **64**, 666–672.
67. M. M. Finkelstein and M. Jerrett, *Environ. Res.*, 2007, **104**, 420–432.
68. A. W. Willis, B. A. Evanoff, M. Lian, A. Galarza, A. Wegrzyn, M. Schootman and B. A. Racette, *Am. J. Epidemiol.*, 2010, **172**, 1357–1363.
69. S. R. Criswell, J. S. Perlmutter, T. O. Videen, S. M. Moerlein, H. P. Flores, A. M. Birke and B. A. Racette, *Neurology*, 2011, **76**, 1296–1301.
70. W. Kuhn, R. Winkel, D. Woitalla, S. Meves, H. Przuntek and T. Muller, *Neurology*, 1998, **50**, 1885–1886.
71. P. Sanz, S. Nogue, D. Vilchez, J. Vilchez, A. Casal and G. Logroscino, *J. Int. Med. Res.*, 2007, **35**, 159–163.
72. R. Winkel, W. Kuhn and H. Przuntek, *J. Neural. Transm. Suppl.*, 1995, **46**, 183–187.
73. S. Coon, A. Stark, E. Peterson, A. Gloi, G. Kortsha, J. Pounds, D. Chettle and J. Gorell, *Environ. Health Perspect.*, 2006, **114**, 1872–1876.
74. M. G. Weisskopf, J. Weuve, H. Nie, M. H. Saint-Hilaire, L. Sudarsky, D. K. Simon, B. Hersh, J. Schwartz, R. O. Wright and H. Hu, *Environ. Health Perspect.*, 2010, **118**, 1609–1613.
75. C. G. Ohlson and C. Hogstedt, *Scand. J. Work Environ. Health*, 1981, **7**, 252–256.
76. J. M. Gorell, B. A. Rybicki, C. Cole Johnson and E. L. Peterson, *Neuroepidemiology*, 1999, **18**, 303–308.
77. G. P. Sechi, V. Agnetti, M. Piredda, M. Canu, F. Deserra, H. A. Omar and G. Rosati, *Neurology*, 1992, **42**, 261–263.
78. J. R. Sanchez-Ramos, F. Hefti and W. J. Weiner, *Neurology*, 1987, **37**, 728.

79. E. R. Barbosa, M. D. Leiros da Costa, L. A. Bacheschi, M. Scaff and C. C. Leite, *Mov. Disord*, 2001, **16**, 565–568.
80. H. B. Ferraz, P. H. Bertolucci, J. S. Pereira, J. G. Lima and L. A. Andrade, *Neurology*, 1988, **38**, 550–553.
81. C. M. Tanner, G. W. Ross, S. A. Jewell, R. A. Hauser, J. Jankovic, S. A. Factor, S. Bressman, A. Deligtisch, C. Marras, K. E. Lyons, G. S. Bhudhikanok, D. F. Roucoux, C. Meng, R. D. Abbott and J. W. Langston, *Arch. Neurol.*, 2009, **66**, 1106–1113.
82. F. Duzcan, M. Zencir, F. Ozdemir, G. O. Cetin, H. Bagci, P. Heutink, V. Bonifati and T. Sahiner, *Mov. Disord*, 2003, **18**, 799–804.
83. R. Frigerio, K. R. Sanft, B. R. Grossardt, B. J. Peterson, A. Elbaz, J. H. Bower, J. E. Ahlskog, M. de Andrade, D. M. Maraganore and W. A. Rocca, *Mov. Disord*, 2006, **21**, 1688–1692.
84. J. M. Gorell, C. C. Johnson, B. A. Rybicki, E. L. Peterson and R. J. Richardson, *Neurology*, 1998, **50**, 1346–1350.
85. H. H. Liou, M. C. Tsai, C. J. Chen, J. S. Jeng, Y. C. Chang, S. Y. Chen and R. C. Chen, *Neurology*, 1997, **48**, 1583–1588.
86. C. M. Tanner, F. Kamel, G. W. Ross, J. A. Hoppin, S. M. Goldman, M. Korell, C. Marras, G. S. Bhudhikanok, M. Kasten, A. R. Chade, K. Comyns, M. B. Richards, C. Meng, B. Priestley, H. H. Fernandez, F. Cambi, D. M. Umbach, A. Blair, D. P. Sandler and J. W. Langston, *Environ. Health Perspect.*, 2011, **119**, 866–872.
87. A. Menegon, P. G. Board, A. C. Blackburn, G. D. Mellick and D. G. Le Couteur, *Lancet*, 1998, **352**, 1344–1346.
88. F. Kamel, C. Tanner, D. Umbach, J. Hoppin, M. Alavanja, A. Blair, K. Comyns, S. Goldman, M. Korell, J. Langston, G. Ross and D. Sandler, *Am. J. Epidemiol.*, 2007, **165**, 364–374.
89. A. Ascherio, H. Chen, M. G. Weisskopf, E. O'Reilly, M. L. McCullough, E. E. Calle, M. A. Schwarzschild and M. J. Thun, *Ann. Neurol.*, 2006, **60**, 197–203.
90. M. G. Weisskopf, P. Knekt, E. J. O'Reilly, J. Lyytinen, A. Reunanen, F. Laden, L. Altshul and A. Ascherio, *Neurology*, 2010, **74**, 1055–1061.
91. B. Ritz and F. Yu, *Int. J. Epidemiol.*, 2000, **29**, 323–329.
92. S. Costello, M. Cockburn, J. Bronstein, X. Zhang and B. Ritz, *Am. J. Epidemiol.*, 2009, **169**, 919–926.
93. B. R. Ritz, A. D. Manthripragada, S. Costello, S. J. Lincoln, M. J. Farrer, M. Cockburn and J. Bronstein, *Environ. Health Perspect.*, 2009, **117**, 964–969.
94. N. M. Gatto, M. Cockburn, J. Bronstein, A. D. Manthripragada and B. Ritz, *Environ. Health Perspect.*, 2009, **117**, 1912–1918.
95. R. J. Uitti, B. J. Snow, H. Shinotoh, F. J. Vingerhoets, M. Hayward, S. Hashimoto, J. Richmond, S. P. Markey, C. J. Markey and D. B. Calne, *Ann. Neurol.*, 1994, **35**, 616–619.
96. G. Pezzoli, A. Antonini, S. Barbieri, M. Canesi, L. Perbellini, A. Zecchinelli, C. B. Mariani, A. Bonetti and K. L. Leenders, *Mov. Disord*, 1995, **10**, 279–282.

97. E. Melamed and S. Lavy, *Lancet*, 1977, **309**(8019), 1015.
98. J. W. Tetrud, J. W. Langston, I. Irwin and B. Snow, *Neurology*, 1994, **44**, 1051–1054.
99. G. Hageman, J. van der Hoek, M. van Hout, G. van der Laan, E. J. Steur, W. de Bruin and K. Herholz, *J. Neurol.*, 1999, **246**, 198–206.
100. R. Kuriwaka, T. Mitsui, S. Fujiwara, Y. Nishida and T. Matsumoto, *Eur. Neurol.*, 2002, **47**, 85–87.
101. M. A. Guggenheim, J. R. Couch and W. Weinberg, *Arch. Neurol.*, 1971, **24**, 550–554.
102. D. R. McLean, H. Jacobs and B. W. Mielke, *Ann. Neurol.*, 1980, **8**, 161–167.
103. M. J. Mozaz, M. A. Wyke and B. Indakoetxea, *J. Neurol. Neurosurg. Psychiatry*, 1991, **54**, 843–844.
104. W. Verslegers, M. Van den Kerchove, R. Crols, W. De Potter, B. Appel and A. Lowenthal, *Acta. Neurol. Belg.*, 1988, **88**, 163–171.
105. Y. Finkelstein and J. Vardi, *Neurotoxicology*, 2002, **23**, 521–525.
106. N. J. Reddy, L. D. Lewis, T. B. Gardner, W. Osterling, C. J. Eskey and D. W. Nierenberg, *Clin. Pharmacol. Ther. (N. Y., NY, U. S.)*, 2007, **81**, 114–121.
107. A. Smargiassi, A. Mutti, A. De Rosa, G. De Palma, A. Negrotti and S. Calzetti, *Neurotoxicology*, 1998, **19**, 709–712.
108. S. M. Goldman, P. J. Quinlan, G. W. Ross, C. Marras, C. Meng, G. S. Bhudhikanok, K. Comyns, M. Korell, A. R. Chade, M. Kasten, B. Priestley, K. L. Chou, H. H. Fernandez, F. Cambi, J. W. Langston and C. M. Tanner, *Ann. Neurol.*, 2011, **71**, 776–784.
109. D. Guehl, E. Bezard, S. Dovero, T. Boraud, B. Bioulac and C. Gross, *Eur. J. Neurol.*, 1999, **6**, 609–611.
110. W. Kochen, D. Kohlmuller, P. De Biasi and R. Ramsay, *Adv. Exp. Med. Biol.*, 2003, **527**, 253–263.
111. D. M. Gash, K. Rutland, N. L. Hudson, P. G. Sullivan, G. Bing, W. A. Cass, J. D. Pandya, M. Liu, D. Y. Choi, R. L. Hunter, G. A. Gerhardt, C. D. Smith, J. T. Slevin and T. S. Prince, *Ann. Neurol.*, 2008, **63**, 184–192.
112. G. Pezzoli, M. Canesi, A. Antonini, A. Righini, L. Perbellini, M. Barichella, C. B. Mariani, F. Tenconi, S. Tesei, A. Zecchinelli and K. L. Leenders, *Neurology*, 2000, **55**, 667–673.
113. H. A. Peters, R. L. Levine, C. G. Matthews and L. J. Chapman, *Arch. Neurol.*, 1988, **45**, 537–540.
114. L. Godderis, L. Braeckman, M. Vanhoorne and M. Viaene, *Int. J. Hyg. Environ. Health*, 2006, **209**, 139–150.
115. H. Roels, R. Lauwerys, J. P. Buchet, P. Genet, M. J. Sarhan, I. Hanotiau, M. de Fays, A. Bernard and D. Stanescu, *Am. J. Ind. Med.*, 1987, **11**, 307–327.
116. A. Iregren, *Neurotoxicol. Teratol.*, 1990, **12**, 673–675.
117. A. Wennberg, A. Iregren, G. Struwe, G. Cizinsky, M. Hagman and L. Johansson, *Scand. J. Work Environ. Health*, 1991, **17**, 255–262.

118. A. Wennberg, M. Hagman and L. Johansson, *Neurotoxicology*, 1992, **13**, 271–274.
119. D. Mergler, G. Huel, R. Bowler, A. Iregren, S. Belanger, M. Baldwin, R. Tardif, A. Smargiassi and L. Martin, *Environ. Res.*, 1994, **64**, 151–180.
120. R. Lucchini, P. Apostoli, C. Perrone, D. Placidi, E. Albini, P. Migliorati, D. Mergler, M. P. Sassine, S. Palmi and L. Alessio, *Neurotoxicology*, 1999, **20**, 287–297.

CHAPTER 5

Mercury

HIROSHI SATOH

Professor Emeritus, Tohoku University, Food Safety Commission, Akasaka Park Bld. 22F 5-2-20 Akasaka, Minato-ku, Tokyo 107-6122
E-mail: h.satoh@med.tohoku.ac.jp

5.1 Mercury and its Compounds

5.1.1 Classification of Mercury Compounds

Mercury (Hg) is a metal that exists in liquid form at room temperature. Metallic mercury easily evaporates in air to become mercury vapor (elemental mercury). Mercury creates various compounds which are classified into two general groups: inorganic mercury compounds and organic mercury compounds. Inorganic mercury compounds include mercurous mercury (monovalent) and mercuric mercury (divalent) compounds. Mercurous mercury compounds are easily broken down into mercuric mercury and elemental mercury. Organic mercury compounds are chemicals in which mercury is covalently bound to carbon, for example $R–Hg^+$ or $R–Hg–R'$, where R or R' represent organic moieties. Three major organic mercury compound groups are alkylmercury, arylmercury, and alkoxyalkylmercury.

It is noteworthy that different mercury compounds have different toxicological profiles, including routes of exposure, metabolism in the body, and health effects. For metallic mercury, inhalation of mercury vapor is a significant exposure route, while oral exposure *via* ingestion is not. A typical health effect of mercuric mercury compounds is nephrotoxicity, while that of alkylmercury compounds is neurotoxicity. It is also recognized that exposure at different

Issues in Toxicology No. 16
Aging and Vulnerability to Environmental Chemicals: Age-related Disorders and their Origins in Environmental Exposures
Edited by Bernard Weiss

Published by the Royal Society of Chemistry, www.rsc.org

stages of life causes different health effects. In the disasters of Minamata Disease and Iraqi methyl mercury poisoning, infants born to mothers with minimal signs and symptoms of methylmercury exposure showed severe neurological damage and developmental delays. Therefore, fetuses are considered to be more susceptible than their mothers.

5.2 Mercury Vapor (Elemental Mercury)

5.2.1 Physical and Chemical Properties

The physical and chemical properties of metallic mercury are as follows:[1] atomic weight, 200.6; atomic number, 80; density, 13.6; melting point, −38.90 °C; boiling point, 356.60 °C. Since the melting point of metallic mercury is −38.90 °C, it exists in liquid form at room temperature. Metallic mercury is highly volatile. A saturated atmosphere of mercury vapor contains approximately 18 mg Hg/m^3 at 24.0 °C.

5.2.2 Exposure and Metabolism

5.2.2.1 Route of Exposure and Absorption

Substantial exposure to mercury vapor occurs *via* inhalation. Mercury vapor is readily absorbed through the alveolar membrane.[2] Approximately 80% of mercury will be absorbed through the alveolar membrane.

Metallic mercury (in liquid form) is poorly absorbed from the gastrointestinal tract. Therefore, metallic mercury ingested is of no toxicological importance. Dermal absorption is low; uptake of mercury vapor by the forearm skin of volunteers was calculated to be approximately 1% of the uptake from inhalation.[3]

5.2.2.2 Metabolism in the Body

Absorbed mercury vapor is dissolved in the blood stream where it is oxidized mainly in red blood cells.[4,5] While being circulated, remaining elemental mercury is able to penetrate into brain tissue through the blood–brain barrier[6] and into fetal tissues through the placental barrier.[7] The distribution of mercury in neonatal guinea pigs after *in utero* exposure to mercury vapor was found to be highest in the liver,[8] while in adult animals the kidney has the highest distribution. The distribution in the kidney, and other organs accumulating mercury, after exposure to mercury vapor is similar to that seen after exposure to mercuric compounds (see section 5.3.2.).

Following exposure to mercury vapor, mercuric mercury is the main chemical form of eliminated mercury, although exhalation of small quantities of mercury vapor has been demonstrated.[9,10] The biological half-life of mercury in the human body is considered to be approximately 60 days,[10] though the data is limited. The biological half-life of mercury accumulated in the brain is slow and may exceed several years.[11,12]

5.2.3 Health Effects of Mercury Vapor

5.2.3.1 *Acute Poisoning*

Acute accidental exposure to high concentrations of mercury vapor causes erosive bronchitis and bronchiolitis with interstitial pneumonitis. The patient may develop severe respiratory insufficiency. Sometimes signs caused by effects on the central nervous system (CNS), such as tremor or increased excitability, are observed.[13]

5.2.3.2 *Chronic Poisoning*

Repeated and long-term exposure to toxic levels of mercury vapor causes signs and symptoms of the CNS. Relatively low dose exposure produces asthenic-vegetative syndrome, involving weakness, fatigue, anorexia, loss of weight, and disturbance of gastrointestinal functions. This syndrome has been called micromercurialism.[14]

At higher dose exposure, the characteristic tremor appears as fine trembling of the muscles interrupted by coarse shaking movements. This tremor is observed in fingers, eyelids and lips. Mercurial erethism also develops; this is characterized by behavioral and personality changes and increased excitability. Loss of memory and insomnia are also observed. In addition to the effects on the CNS, inflammatory changes of the gums with ptyalism (excessive salivation) may develop.

The toxic effects of mercury vapor exposure on organs other than the CNS, such as the kidneys, the immune system[15] and the endocrine glands, have been reported. It is, however, difficult to differentiate these from the effects of inorganic mercury, because after inhalation, mercury vapor is oxidized in the body.

5.3 Inorganic Mercury Compounds

5.3.1 Mercuric and Mercurous Mercury Compounds

Inorganic mercury compounds consist of two classes; mercuric mercury (divalent) compounds and mercurous (monovalent) mercury compounds. Mercuric compounds include mercury(II) chloride, mercury(II) nitrate, mercury(II) oxide and mercury(II) sulfide. Mercurous compounds include mercury(I) chloride, mercury(I) iodide and mercury(I) sulfate. Mercurous mercury compounds are unstable, especially in the presence of biological molecules; they decompose into elemental mercury and the ion of mercuric mercury. Therefore, mercuric mercury is of toxicological significance.

5.3.2 Exposure and Metabolism

5.3.2.1 *Route of Exposure and Absorption*

Since mercuric mercury compounds are generally stable, inhalation exposure is not important; ingestion (exposure *via* the gastrointestinal tract) is the most significant.

Acute poisoning after accidental or intentional ingestion of mercuric compounds has been observed, indicating absorption of such compounds by ingestion. From experimental studies,[16] approximately 2% of ingested mercuric chloride is absorbed. It is considered that the corrosive action of mercuric chloride may alter the permeability of the gastrointestinal tract, enhancing absorption. In newborn rats, increased absorption of mercury has been reported.[17]

As for the skin (dermal absorption), it has been demonstrated that if mercuric mercury applied to the human skin, penetration of mercury occurs. In animal studies,[18] up to 8% of the mercuric chloride applied to the skin was absorbed within 5 hours.

5.3.2.2 Metabolism in the Body

After exposure to mercuric mercury, the kidneys accumulate the largest amount of mercury, followed by the liver. Mercuric mercury does not readily cross the blood–brain barrier or the placental barrier. However, mercuric mercury does accumulate in the placenta.[19] In placental tissue, mercury coexists with metallothionein (MT), suggesting a defense mechanism by MT.[20]

Twenty-four hours after injection of mercuric chloride (1.5 or 15.0 mmol kg^{-1} BW) to pregnant mice on day 16 of gestation, only 0.03% of the dose was detected in an individual fetus.[19] Whereas when methylmercury chloride was injected, 1.3% of the dose was detected.[21]

Mercuric mercury is excreted by the kidney and the fecal route, with small amounts being excreted from sweat glands, lacrimal glands, mammary glands, and salivary glands.[1] Small amounts of mercuric mercury is exhaled after reduction to mercury vapor.[22] Alcohol enhances exhalation by changing redox status, which involves the inhibition of catalase activity.[23]

5.3.3 Health Effects of Mercuric Mercury Compounds

5.3.3.1 Acute Poisoning

Accidental or suicidal ingestion of mercuric chloride or other mercuric salts induces dysfunction of the kidneys and the intestinal tract.[1] A solution of concentrated mercuric salt produces corrosion on the mucous membranes of the gastrointestinal tract; gastric pain and vomiting may follow. Abdominal pain and bloody diarrhea with necrosis of the intestinal mucosa will occur when the solution of mercuric salts reaches the intestine. Circulatory collapse (shock) and even death are possible. Survivors develop renal failure caused by necrosis of proximal tubular epithelium, and accompanying anuria and uremia.

5.3.3.2 Chronic Poisoning

Chronic poisoning caused by mercuric mercury salts is not considered to exist. Chronic exposure to a mixture of mercury vapor and mercuric mercury actually occurs in an occupational setting. In this case, the kidneys and CNS are target organs. Intake of mercurous chloride (calomel) as a purgative was reported to produce symptoms similar to those of poisoning by exposure to a mixture of mercury vapor and mercuric mercury.[24]

5.4 Organic Mercury Compounds (Methylmercury)

5.4.1 Organic Mercury Described in this Section

Among the organic mercury compounds, including alkylmercury, arylmercury, and alkoxyalkylmercury, methylmercury compounds have toxicological significance. Arylmercury and alkoxyalkylmercury compounds are generally unstable in the environment and in the body of organisms. They easily break down into mercuric mercury. Short-chain alkyl mercury compounds, such as methyl- and ethylmercury compounds, are stable. Ethylmercury compounds have toxicological properties similar to those of the methylmercury compounds but are more rapidly degraded in the body.

Since methylmercury occurs naturally in the environment and is bioconcentrated through the food web, the carnivore fish and sea mammals located at the center of the food web contain methylmercury concentration, therefore there may be health concerns associated with consuming these fish. Methylmercury compounds are the subject of section 5.4.

5.4.2 Exposure and Metabolism

5.4.2.1 Route of Exposure and Absorption

In the occupational setting, the vapor of methylmercury can be absorbed by inhalation. It is also possible that methylmercury salts in the form of fine particles are inhalable. In olden times, methylmercury-related poisoning of workers was reported.[25] Dimethylmercury is liquid at room temperature and easily evaporates. Substantial amounts of vaporized dimethylmercury can be inhaled resulting in poisoning.[26]

Although exposure through inhalation has occurred as described, ingestion of methylmercury in food is an important route of exposure among the general population.

Ingested methylmercury is almost completely (more than 95%) absorbed through the intestinal tract. Absorption of alkylmercury compounds through the skin is also likely to occur, and cases of poisoning caused by local application of ointment containing methylmercury to the skin have been described.[27]

5.4.2.2 Metabolism

Methylmercury absorbed into the body is distributed to tissues and organs *via* the blood stream. In the blood, a large proprotion (>90%) of methylmercury exists in red blood cells. Methylmercury crosses the blood–brain barrier and placental barrier. This was thought to be due to lipid solubility of methylmercury, but was later attributed to formation of a methylmercury–cystine complex that structurally resembles methionine, an essential amino acid. The methylmercury–cystine complex is transported through the barriers.[28,29]

After administration of tracer doses of radioactive methylmercury in man, 10% of the body burden of radioactive mercury was found in the head.[30] A substantial amount of methylmercury is found in the liver and the kidneys. Methylmercury is rather evenly distributed in the rest of the body.

Methylmercury transported through the placenta to the fetus accumulates and concentrates, especially in the brain. Higher mercury concentrations in fetal blood than in maternal blood are probably due to the different chemical structures of fetal and adult hemoglobin.

Methylmercury is decomposed to inorganic mercury by demethylation in the body. In the organs of sea mammals, extremely high concentrations of mercury have been detected in the form of inorganic mercury.[31] The demethylation process and formation of mercury selenide is considered a defense mechanism against methylmercury toxicity, though apparent accumulation is extremely large.

Methylmercury is excreted mainly (approximately 90%) through the liver into the bile, and partly through the kidney into urine. Thus fecal excretion is the main route, though methylmercury excreted in the bile is reabsorbed in the intestine (an enterohepatic circulation). Methylmercury can be decomposed to inorganic mercury by the microflora in the intestine.[32] Since inorganic mercury is far less absorbed than methylmercury, the decomposition contributes to increase fecal excretion. Methylmercury is also excreted into breast milk, the concentration being approximately 5% of the concentration in the maternal blood.[33] A recent study analyzed, using Electron Capture Detector Gas Chromatography, methylmercury in the breast milk of Japanese mothers living in the ordinary environment.[34] An average of 54% (with the range of 17–83%) of total mercury in the milk was identified as methylmercury. Since without specific exposure most mercury in the human blood exists as methylmercury, it is considered that methylmercury is excreted into breast milk less than inorganic mercury is.

Hair has been known as a good indicator of methylmercury exposure, because the tissue of a hair strand takes in methylmercury during hair formation. Thus hair is a route of excretion of methylmercury. The amount taken up is proportional to the blood concentration of mercury at the time of incorporation. The ratio of mercury concentration between blood and hair in man is considered to be 1/250 under steady-state conditions, although the quotient may vary with age[35] and pregnancy. In fact, 1/340 on average was reported among Japanese adults.[36]

The biological half-life of methylmercury is approximately 70 days on average. However, analyses of consecutive hair segments from the populations in Iraq who ingested wheat contaminated with methylmercury[37] suggest that a part of the population has longer biological half-lives, 110–190 days. An intervention study where subjects ingested fish with high methylmercury concentrations revealed biological half-lives of approximately 90 days, from analyses of both hair and blood mercury.[36]

5.4.3 Health Effects of Methyl Mercury Compounds

5.4.3.1 Acute and Chronic Poisoning

In the case of methylmercury poisoning, there is no sharp difference between acute and chronic poisoning. Once a toxic dose has been absorbed in the body, it is retained for a long time, causing functional disturbances and damage. A single toxic dose does not produce signs or symptoms until after a latency period.

The CNS is the critical organ and there are two types of poisoning depending upon timing of exposure: fetal (pre- or perinatal) exposure and adult exposure.

5.4.3.2 Poisoning by Fetal Exposure

As was shown in the Minamata Disease disaster and Iraqi methylmercury poisoning cases, the newborns from the mothers who ingested methylmercury developed signs or symptoms. Severe cases showed an unspecific infantile cerebral palsy accompanied by ataxic motor disturbances and mental retardation. In mild cases, psychomotor retardation has been observed; in Iraqi cases, delayed walking and talking and an increased incidence of seizures[38] were reported. In fish-consuming populations with increased mercury exposure, such as 10 ppm in hair-mercury levels during pregnancy, impaired psychomotor test performance of the child at 7 years of age[39] was reported. Poor performances associated with prenatal methylmercury exposure have been reported among infants whose mothers were living in ordinary environment.[40,41] These reports indicate vulnerability of the fetus to methylmercury. Since methylmercury is excreted through breast milk, postnatal infants can be exposed to methylmercury. It is, however, difficult to differentiate the effects of postnatal exposure from the effects of prenatal exposure. Because mothers exposed to methylmercury during pregnancy had elevated mercury concentrations in breast milk, fetal exposure occurred. A mouse experiment employing a cross-fostering procedure revealed effects of prenatal exposure were larger than those of postnatal exposure.[42]

5.4.3.3 Poisoning by Adult Exposure

In severe and typical poisoning cases, ataxia, concentric constriction of the visual field, impairment of hearing, and extrapyramidal tract symptoms appear. Clonic seizures may be observed and some patients develop encephalitis and can die. Less severe cases show sensitivity disturbances with paresthesia in the distal extremities, in the tongue, and around the lips. These are early signs of Minamata Disease.

5.5 Developmental Toxicity of Mercury

5.5.1 Fetal Minamata Disease Patients

5.5.1.1 Discovery of Fetal Minamata Disease

Fetal Minamata Disease is caused by intrauterine exposure to methylmercury through the ingestion of contaminated seafood by pregnant mothers. It was first detected in 1958 in the Minamata Bay area.[43] Nine infants manifested a severe disease resembling cerebral palsy during the epidemiologic investigation by Kumamoto university. The incidence of the cerebral palsy-like disease was extremely high among infants who were born in or after 1955. By 1974, 40 cases were confirmed as fetal Minamata Disease.

Examination of these children revealed a high incidence of signs and symptoms such as mental retardation, cerebellar ataxia, primitive reflex, dysarthria, seizure, and pyramidal signs. Sensory disturbance, constriction of the visual fields, and hearing impairment could not be examined because of the serious conditions of the patients. It is noteworthy that the mothers of these children manifested minimal signs and symptoms of Minamata Disease, such as paresthesia of the lip and extremities. Therefore, fetuses are much more vulnerable than mothers.

5.5.1.2 Activities of Daily Living (ADL) Scores of Fetal Minamata Disease Patients at Middle Age

Doi[44] suggested an urgent follow-up study for the victims of fetal Minamata Disease, because of his impression of rapid exacerbation of the several fetal Minamata Disease patients of his acquaintance. In 2001, the 6th International Conference on Mercury as a Global Pollutant was held in Minamata, Japan. At the conference, Doi saw a fetal Minamata Disease patient in a wheelchair. Five years previously, at the occasion of the opening of the Minamata exhibition in Tokyo, the patient gave remarks on the stage without any help, though motion did not appear completely smooth. Since he was still 46 years old, Doi noted the rapid exacerbation. People who had cared for the patients told Doi that rapid exacerbation of fetal Minamata Disease patients was observed among several patients, but not all.

In 2002, a survey of 31 fetal Minamata Disease patients was conducted; the survey concerned family structure, present status of care, their demand for care, communication status, and ADL scores.[45] Changes in ADL scores during the past 15 years were also studied among the 22 patients. Their mean ages were 45.5 ± 3.5 ($n = 20$) for males, and 46.1 ± 1.9 ($n = 11$) for females.

Eighteen patients lived in their home and 13 patients lived in a welfare institute. Analysis of ADL showed that around 50% of the patients could not walk or take a bath, and 30 to 40% of the patients could not eat, excrete, change their clothes, or wash their face unaided. Approximately 80% of the patients could understand daily conversation to some degree. Their ability to express their demands and thoughts, put an idea into action, remember events, and live like ordinary people were significantly worse than their ability to understand daily conversation.

The changes in the ADL scores of the 22 patients over the 15 year period were not significant, although two patients showed a rapid decrease for ADL of movement and two other patients died after an interview, before they reached 50 years of age.

This investigation did not involve neurological examination. But these results indicate that the disturbances among the fetal Minamata Disease patients are long lasting, with rapidly deteriorating ADL in some cases. Increased risk of early death is also suggested, although the number of patients who experience this is small.

5.5.1.3 Cardiovascular Autonomic Nervous Functions in Fetal Minamata Disease Patients and Other Populations

Cardiovascular autonomic nervous functions in nine fetal Minamata Disease patients (aged 44.3 ± 1.0 years) were compared with age matched healthy subjects.[46] Electrocardiographic data were collected for 3 min. In the time domain analyses, average R-R interval was significantly shorter for Minamata Disease patients than healthy subjects, while standard deviation of R-R intervals or coefficient of variation were not. Frequency domain analysis by fast Fourier transformation revealed the high frequency component of Minamata Disease patients was significantly lower than that of the healthy subjects.

In contrast, a birth cohort study on 1000 children from the Faroe Islands revealed that prenatal exposure to methylmercury decreased heart rate variability only in boys at age 7 years. Both diastolic and systolic blood pressure elevated with increase of cord blood mercury level. At age 14 years, it was found that prenatal methylmercury exposure was associated with a decrease in low frequency and high frequency powers and the coefficient of variation of the electrocardiographic R-R interval.

Although the study subjects were healthy adults, an intervention study was recently conducted to examine effects of methylmercury on heart rate variability;[47] in the study, healthy adults ate meat of tuna and marline with a high concentration of methylmercury at a dose of the tolerable weekly intake recommended by the government of Japan. After 14 weeks of ingestion, heart rate variability was evaluated. Compared with the baseline data, increases in "low frequency"/"high frequency" ratio and %"low frequency" were observed after fast Fourier transformation of collected electrocardiograms. This change was not detected 15 weeks after stopping the ingestion.

Although details are varying among the reports above described, all the results are involved with cardiovascular autonomic nervous functions. In the case of fetal exposure, the changes in frequency have been long-lasting, while adult exposure, the changes were temporary. Affected parameters were also different.

5.6 Behavioral Teratology Studies of Methylmercury

5.6.1 Behavioral Teratology

Behavioral teratology is a field of science that examines postnatal effects of prenatal exposure to any foreign agent, such as chemical substances and physical stimulants. The concept of behavioral teratology was established by Werboff in the 1960s.[48] Behavioral effects on the offspring of maternal rats given tranquillizer during pregnancy were observed. "The behavior, functional adaptation of offspring to its environment, is susceptible to teratogenic effects of drugs" was described.

The concept of behavioral teratology was expanded so that effects of prenatal exposure to environmental pollutants have been included. Spyker and her colleagues conducted the pioneering study on the postnatal effects of prenatal methylmercury exposure. They revealed impaired swimming ability in offspring mice exposed to methylmercury *in utero*.[49] The offspring mice showed behavioral changes in the open field test. It is important to note that the offspring mice developed apparently normally until being examined under a stressful environment, such as being immersed in a cold water or released in a open space with bright light.

Spyker and colleagues defined "behavioral teratology" as the overlapping area between behavioral toxicology and teratology. The cause of this abnormality occurs during pregnancy, and the effects become overt after birth and persist over the lifetime of an individual.[50]

5.6.2 Postnatal Effects of Prenatal Exposure to Methylmercury in Experimental Animals

A number of investigations on the postnatal effects of prenatal exposure to methylmercury in experimental animals have been conducted (See reviews by Shimai and Satoh, 1985,[51] Watanabe and Satoh, 1996.[52] and Satoh, 2003.)[48] As the framework of behavioral teratology has been developing, postnatal effects have been grouped into "eight Ds". Spyker originally showed that postnatal effects could be categorized into: "birth Defects, abnormal Development, behavioral Deviation, neurological Disorder, immunological Deficiency, generalized Debilitation, and premature Death." These were known as the "seven Ds" in behavioral teratology. Later, Tanimura added reproductive Debility and emphasized birth Defects.[48] Currently, eight Ds are accepted in behavioral teratology.It was emphasized that each D appears in sequence as the individual ages from neonate to senescence.

Findings reported from investigations include: reflexive behavior (such as righting reflex and walking ability) in the neonatal period, ultrasonic vocalization during the lactational period, swimming ability, maze avoidance, and operant learning at in adulthood.[48] The doses administered are varying; in some experiments, the dose corresponded to LD_{50}, but in the other experiments much smaller doses were administered.[51,52] The lowest dose to cause postnatal effects on operant learning was 0.008 mg Hg kg^{-1} body weight (of maternal rats), repeatedly administered during gestational days 6–9.

5.6.3 Effects of Fetal Methylmercury Exposure among Humans Under General Environment

5.6.3.1 Risk Assessment by WHO

As mentioned previously, in the Iraqi outbreak, fetal cases were examined closely.[53–55] A group of mother and infant pairs were examined for the delay in developmental milestones such as walking and talking, and the mothers' exposure to mercury. The mercury content of a hair strand of each mother was longitudinally analyzed to determine the peak mercury concentration during pregnancy. A dose–response relationship was established between the peak mercury concentration during pregnancy and whether first walking or talking was delayed.[56] Based on this dose–response relationship, the World Health Organization (WHO)[57] claimed that "A prudent interpretation of the Iraqi data implies that a 5% risk may be associated with the peak mercury level of 10–20 μg g^{-1} of maternal hair".

5.6.3.2 Fish (or Seafood) Eating Population

Since exposure levels among the fish eating population reach the above mentioned level, effects of fetal methylmercury exposure among this population is of great concern. Thus epidemiological prospective studies with more sophisticated examination methods than simple observation of developmental milestones have been carried out since the mid 1980s.

5.6.3.3 New Zealand

In New Zealand, the development of children prenatally exposed to methylmercury *via* their mothers' consumption of fish meals during pregnancy was investigated.[58,59] The children were tested at the age of four, using the Denver Developmental Screening Test (DDST), which encompasses four major function sectors: gross motor, fine motor, language, and personal-social. The prevalence of developmental delay was 52% in children whose mothers had been exposed to high levels of mercury, compared to 17% in the reference group.

In a follow-up study, at the age of 6, each child was tested using the Test of Language Development, the Wechsler Intelligence Scale for Children, and the McCarthy Scale of Children's Abilities.[59] Although high prenatal methylmercury exposure decreased performance in these tests, it contributed little to the variation in test results, because ethnic background and social class showed greater influence.

5.6.3.4 The Seychelles

In the Seychelles Islands, the developmental effects of *in utero* methylmercury exposure from consumption of marine fish by mothers have been studied (the pilot study).[60] An association between *in utero* methylmercury exposure was found for when abnormal plus questionable scores were combined.[61] Maternal hair mercury concentration during pregnancy was negatively associated with four endpoints: The McCarthy General Cognitive Index, Perceptual Performance subscale, Preschool Language Scale Total Language, and Auditory Comprehension subscale. When statistically determined outliers and points considered to be influential were removed from the analyses, statistical significance of the association remained only for Auditory Comprehension.

The main study, which was designed to be prospective and involved 779 mother–child pairs, followed the above mentioned study.[62] In this study, children were evaluated at 6.5, 19, 26, and 66 months of age. No association between the maternal hair mercury level and the test results were found in the children tested at 6.5 months. No effects of mercury exposure were seen at 19 months. Investigation at 66 months did not reveal the deviation typically associated with prenatal methylmercury exposure for the following tests: McCarthy Scales of Children's Abilities in General Cognitive Index, Preschool Language Scale, Letter-Word Recognition of Woodcock- Johnson (W-J) Tests of Achievement, Applied Problems of W-J Tests of Achievement, Bender Gestalt test, and Total T score from the Child Behavior Checklist. The analysis was adjusted for possible confounding factors, including birth weight, the rank of birth, sex, medical records of the infants, age of the mother, alcohol consumption and smoking habits during pregnancy, and socioeconomic status.

The overall conclusion of the studies in the Seychelles Islands is that it is currently unclear whether an association exists between low level prenatal methylmercury exposure and neurologic deficits in the child.

The study in the Seychelles Islands was continued when the cohort subjects reached 9 years old.[63] Two of 21 endpoints were associated with prenatal methylmercury exposure; one association involved diminished performance (grooved pegboard non-dominant hand in males only), and the other an enhancement (hyperactivity index of the Connors teacher rating scale). The conclusion is, however, that both these outcomes are probably due to chance.

In a review of the studies in the Seychelles Islands,[64] the authors concluded that "Our primary analyses have so far identified only one adverse association with prenatal exposure". They also pointed out consideration of the potential for adverse effects of prenatal methylmercury exposure at maternal hair levels above 10–12 ppm, although the numbers of observations in that exposure range are limited. They planned continuing longitudinal data collection in the Seychelles Islands cohort to determine whether late effects of prenatal exposure would appear. Evaluation at age 16 years has been conducted under the hypothesis that if prenatal exposure to low methylmercury concentrations (<12 ppm in maternal hair) does incur adverse effects, they may be apparent only in higher order cognitive functions that develop with maturity.

5.6.3.5 The Faroe Islands

Another large study has been conducted in the Faroe Islands since 1986.[39] Increased methylmercury exposure was largely attributed to the eating of pilot whale.[65] The subjects consisted of a group of approximately 1000 children. They were evaluated for their neurophysiological and neuropsychological performances at 7 years of age. Mercury in maternal hair and cord blood was analyzed, and a subset of cords was analyzed for PCBs.[39] Although the neurophysiological tests showed no indication of mercury-associated dysfunction, significant negative associations were observed in several neuropsychological tests. Even with inclusion of covariates with uncertain influence, multiple regression analysis indicated that 9 out of 20 measurements showed mercury related decrements. The authors concluded that *in utero* exposure to methylmercury affects several domains of cerebral function.

At the age of 14 years, investigations were repeated. As described in Section 5.5.1.3, a change in cardiovascular autonomic nervous functions was reported.

Brainstem auditory evoked potentials were measured. Latencies of brainstem resulted in an increase of around 0.012 ms in peaks II and V when the cord blood mercury concentration doubled.[66] As seen at age 7 years, this effect appeared mainly within the I–III interpeak interval. Despite lower postnatal exposures, the child's hair mercury level at age 14 years was associated with prolonged III–V interpeak latencies. The authors concluded that a change in vulnerability to methylmercury toxicity is suggested by the apparent sensitivity of the peak III–V component to recent methylmercury exposure.

At age 14 years, indicators of prenatal methylmercury exposure were significantly associated with deficits in finger tapping speed, reaction time on a continued performance task, and cued naming.[67] Postnatal methylmercury exposure had no discernible effect. An analysis of the test score difference between results at 7 and 14 years suggested that mercury-associated deficits had not changed between the two examinations. The authors concluded that the effects of prenatal methylmercury exposure on brain function appear to be permanent.

The results of these studies are controversial, especially when comparing those of the Seychelles and Faroe Islands. In both studies, doses were principally indicated by the mothers' hair mercury concentration and the difference between the dose in each case is small. The study designs and test-batteries were similar but not identical. The main difference between the two studies was the source of methylmercury exposure, in the Seychelles by consumption of ocean fish, and in the Faroe Islands, meat and blubber (fat) of pilot whales. One possible explanation is that contamination by PCBs may confound the results of the Faroe island study.

5.6.3.6 Japan

A recent study simultaneously evaluated exposures to both methylmercury and PCBs and their early postnatal effects.[41] In a total of 498 mother-neonate pairs, the total mercury level (median, 1.96 $\mu g\ g^{-1}$) in maternal hair at parturition and the PCB level (45.5 $ng\ g^{-1}$ lipid) in cord blood were analyzed, and maternal seafood intake was estimated using a semi-quantitative food frequency questionnaire. The Neonatal Behavioral Assessment Scale examination was conducted 3 days after birth. A negative relationship between hair mercury level and motor cluster was observed, even after adjusting for PCBs, maternal seafood intake, and possible confounders. The PCB level was negatively correlated with the motor cluster, but this association was attenuated after adjusting for mercury and the confounders. A positive association was observed between maternal seafood intake and the motor cluster when considering the effects of mercury and PCBs. The authors concluded that the data suggests prenatal exposure to methylmercury adversely affects neonatal neurobehavioral function; in contrast, maternal seafood intake appears to be beneficial. The neurobehavioral effect of prenatal exposure to PCBs remains unclear, perhaps because the concentration of PCBs is too low to produce substantial effects.

It is considered that seafood intake appears to be beneficial, because fish consumption during gestation can provide the fetus with long-chain polyunsaturated fatty acids (LCPUFAs) and other nutrients essential for growth and development of the brain.[68] However, fish consumption also brings about methyl mercury exposure. In the Seychelles Child Development Nutrition Study, Psychomotor Developmental Index (PDI) of Bayley Scales of Infant Development II at ages 9 months was positively associated with total omega-3 LCPUFA and negatively associated with the ratio of omega-6/omega-3 LCPUFA. These associations were stronger in models adjusted for prenatal methylmercury exposure. There were significant adverse associations between prenatal methylmercury and the 30 month PDI when the LCPUFA measures were included in the regression analysis. These data support the potential importance to child development of prenatal availability of omega-3 LCPUFA present in fish. Furthermore, they indicate that the beneficial effects of LCPUFA can obscure the determination of adverse effects of prenatal methylmercury exposure in longitudinal observational studies.

5.7 Aging and Toxicity of Mercury

5.7.1 Minamata Disease Patients

Kinjo *et al.* (1993)[69] surveyed 1144 Minamata Disease patients aged 40 or over, living in the Minamata area. Fetal Minamata Disease patients were not included. Together with the same number of neighbor(hood) controls matched for age and sex, they were investigated by questionnaire with regard to subjective complaints and activities of daily living (ADL). It was found that Minamata Disease patients had significantly higher response rates of all 18 complaints than controls did. The odds ratio of weakness was highest at 29.0 (19.4–43.9; 95% confidence interval). The odds ratios of difficulty of speaking, tremor, hypoesthesia, dysesthesia *etc.* were 10–20. These complaints were related to neurological signs and symptoms of Minamata Disease. The age-specific differences in prevalence of the complaints between Minamata Disease patients and the control group were large in younger (40–50 years) groups and relatively small in older (70–80 years) groups. ADL analysis revealed that the difference in the ADL disability between Minamata Disease patients and controls significantly increased with age and that ADL disability in Minamata Disease patients was aggravated by aging.

The conclusion was different to that of Liu *et al.*, mentioned previously (section 5.5.1.2). It is noteworthy that the subjects of the study by Liu *et al.* was fetal Minamata Disease patients with the average age of approximately 45 years old and the range of the subject age was narrow. Their age might not be great enough for aggravate ADL.

5.7.2 Residual or Remote Effects Among Workers Exposed to Mercury Vapor

5.7.2.1 Mercury Miners

Residual effects due to previous exposure to mercury vapor have become a concern. Among ex-mercury miners in Japan, neurobehavioral disorders related to previous exposure that ceased more than 17 years ago have been reported.[70]

Neurobehavioral tests were carried out on ex-mercury miners around 18 years after the end of mercury exposure. Seventy-six male ex-mercury miners who had been exposed to high concentrations of mercury vapor (over $1.0\,mg\,m^{-3}$) and with a history of mercury intoxication were compared with controls matched for age (within 3 years), sex, and education. The extent of the symptoms, caused by mercury poisoning (*erethismus merculialis*) decreased considerably after the end of exposure. But matched paired comparison showed significantly deteriorated performances of motor coordination, simple reaction time, and short term memory in the exposed group. The duration of exposure correlated with poorer performance in hand-eye coordination, tapping, and a color card reading test. Those in job categories classified as having exposure to mercury also exhibited deteriorated performances. The length of time (years) after the end of exposure had a significant correlation with better performance of reaction time and digit span. On the other hand, the history of intoxication itself had no significant association with any of the current neurobehavioral performances. In multiple linear regression analysis, the interaction term of age × history of mercury intoxication showed a significant correlation with deteriorating performance of hand eye coordination (aiming), pegboard, and block design test. The subjects 65 years of age and older showed a larger differences between those with histories of mercury poisoning and control subjects than younger age groups.

5.7.2.2 Mercury Workers

To identify potential exposure-related neurological abnormalities in workers, aged 20 to 35 years, previously exposed to mercury vapor, workers completed occupational and medical questionnaires, with the assistance of a trained interviewer, and underwent neurological examination.[71] They were exposed to mercury vapor in the production of the isotope lithium-6. Few significant differences existed between exposed (n = 247) and unexposed (n = 255) subjects. However, multiple linear regression analysis demonstrated several significant correlations between declining neurological function and increasing exposure as determined by urine mercury measurements. Subjects who showed urine mercury peak levels above 0.6 mg L^{-1} during the work that involved exposure demonstrated significantly decreased strength, decreased coordination, increased tremor, decreased sensation, and increased prevalence of Babinski and snout reflexes when compared with those with mercury levels below 0.6 mg L^{-1}. Although exposure was not age dependent, several neurological measures showed significant age–mercury level interaction. Subjects 70 years of age and older demonstrated the most significant differences in several neurological impairments between high- and low-exposure, compared to control subjects.

5.7.2.3 Aging and Mercury Vapor Exposure

These results suggest that there are slight but persistent effects on neurobehavioral function, especially motor coordination, among mercury miners, even more than 20 years after the end of exposure. At the same time age x exposure interaction was also observed, although it is not known whether the mercury exposure accelerated aging or the natural neuronal attrition unmasked prior exposure-related subclinical abnormalities.

5.7.3 Age-Related Increase in Auditory Impairment

Age-related increase in auditory impairment in monkeys exposed *in utero* and postnatally to methylmercury has been reported.[72] Monkeys (*Macaca fascicularis*) were exposed, throughout gestation and postnatally until 4 years of age, to 0, 10, 25, or 50 μg kg^{-1} per day mercury as methylmercuric chloride. Pure-tone detection thresholds were determined when the subjects were 11 and 19 years of age. At 19 years of age, all five methylmercury-exposed monkeys exhibited elevated pure-tone thresholds compared with controls. Impairment was generally observed across the full range of frequencies. Comparisons of performance at 11 and 19 years revealed relatively greater deterioration in function in the treated monkeys compared with the control monkeys. Although these results provide evidence for acceleration of impairment of auditory function during aging as a consequence of developmental methylmercury exposure, it is not clear from this experiment whether *in utero* or postnatal exposure has a greater effect on the acceleration of impairment.

5.8 Effects of Mercury Vapor Exposure During the Perinatal Period

Compared with methylmercury, studies concerning effects of mercury vapor exposure during the prenatal period have been extremely scarce in both human cases and animal experiments.[73] Since little mercury is transfered to the fetus *via* the placenta after maternal exposure to mercury vapor, it is plausible that fetuses should not been readily affected. But recently, postnatal behavioral effects have been reported. Furthermore, effects of coexposure to mercury vapor and methylmercury during gestation have been investigated.

5.8.1 Effects of Prenatal Mercury Vapor Exposure

Danielsson *et al.* (1993)[74] reported the effects of inhalation of metallic mercury vapor (Hg^0)— approximately at 1.8 mg m^{-3} for 1 or 3 hours during days 11–14 and 17–20 of gestation—on pregnant rats. The developmental and behavioral effects on the offspring were studied. Maturation milestones, such as surface righting, negative geotaxis, pinna unfolding, and tooth eruption, revealed no differences between Hg^0-treated offspring and controls. Spontaneous motor activity showed that the Hg^0-treated offspring were hypoactive at 3 months of age but hyperactive at 14 months. The exposed offspring showed retarded acquisition in the radial arm maze but no differences in the circular swim maze. A simple test of habituation to a novel environment (habituation ratios were calculated as the quotient of the second 30-min period to the first 30-min period for locomotion, rearing, rearing time, and total activity parameters) indicated, for the exposed offspring, a reduced ability to adapt. Mercury concentration in the brains of offspring exposed for 1 or 3 hours was 0.005 or 0.012 mg Hg kg^{-1} respectively at day 2–3 postpartum. Whereas in non-exposed offspring, 0.001 mg Hg kg^{-1} was reported.

Since sample collection was carried out after the cessation of exposure, and the brain, in terms of weight, rapidly develops, it is expected that mercury concentration might decrease drastically. But considerably low concentrations of mercury in the brain of fetuses could cause postnatal behavioral changes.

Behavioral consequences of *in utero* exposure to mercury vapor were studied in the offspring of pregnant squirrel monkeys exposed to 0.5 or 1.0 mg m^{-3} of mercury vapor during the last 2–3 month of gestation or later.[75] The estimated cumulative doses were 1304 to 4305 μg. The monkeys' lever pressing was maintained under various Concurrent Random-Interval Random-Interval schedules of reinforcement. No difference in sensitivity to reinforcer ratios was identified in the steady state, but there was much more variability in the steady-state performance of exposed monkeys, as indicated by the standard deviation of the regression, than in controls. Exposed monkeys were found to produce smaller or slower transitions than controls. One monkey's exposure began during the third week of gestation (earlier than any of the others), and the behavior of this monkey was so erratic that some of the analyses could not be accomplished. No data on mercury concentration in the brain was available.

Evaluation of sensory evoked potentials in Long Evans rats gestationally exposed to 4 mg m^{-3} mercury vapor revealed no changes in responses evoked from peripheral nerves, or the somatosensory, auditory, or visual modalities (Herr *et al.*, 2004).[76] Dams were placed in cylindrical holding tubes during nose-only exposure to either conditioned air or 4 mg m^{-3} mercury vapor for 2 h/day for 10 consecutive days from gestational day (GD) 6 through to GD15. No data on mercury concentration in the offspring's brains was available in this report. A previous report employing the same exposure protocol described mercury concentration in the fetal brain.[77] The mercury concentration in the fetal brain on GD15 was 49 ± 5 ng g^{-1}, while in the maternal brain was approximately 7 μg g^{-1} (by visual inspection of the figure). The observed maternal toxicity was decrease of body weight gain during late pregnancy at this dose.

Yoshida *et al.* (2005)[78] compared postnatal neurobehavioral toxicity of prenatal mercury vapor exposure between metallothionein-null (MT-null) and wild-type mice. Pregnant mice of both strains were repeatedly exposed at 0.50 mg m^{-3} for 6 h/day until GD18. Locomotor activity in the open field, learning ability in the passive avoidance response, and spatial learning ability in the Morris water maze were evaluated at 12 weeks of age. The exposed MT-null mice showed a significant decrease in total locomotor activity in males, and a learning disability in the passive avoidance response and a retarded acquisition in the Morris water maze in females, as compared with non-exposed controls. In contrast, the exposed wild-type mice did not differ from controls in the three behavioral measurements. The results indicate that MT-null mice were more susceptible than wild-type mice to the behavioral neurotoxicity of prenatal mercury exposure. Mercury concentrations in the brains of both strains were slightly higher (8–11 ng g^{-1}) in the exposed group than in the control group (5–7 ng g^{-1}) 12 weeks after the cessation of the exposure. Lack of MT in the brain may increase vulnerability to mercury vapor exposure.

5.8.2 Effects of Neonatal Mercury Vapor Exposure

Fredriksson *et al.* (1992)[79] examined the effect of neonatal exposure of rats to mercury vapor, at the concentration of 0.05 mg m^{-3} for 1 h (low dose) or 4 h (high dose), on their behavior in adulthood. Exposure occurred on days 11–17 (the period of rapid brain growth). Tests for spontaneous motor activity were performed at the ages of 2 and 4 months. Rats exposed to the high dose mercury vapor showed a marked increase in locomotion and total activity but a decrease for rearing when tested at 2 months of age. At 4 months of age, these rats showed a marked hypoactivity with respect to all 3 variables. Rats exposed to the low dose showed no significant differences at 2 months compared to controls. However, at the age of 4 months, increase in locomotion and total activity, but a decrease for rearing, already observed at 2 months in the high dose group, was observed. In the radial arm maze and circular swim maze, neonatally exposed pups showed a retarded acquisition to the radial arm maze, while there was no difference compared to controls in the circular swim maze. These data indicate that neonatal exposure to mercury vapor results in similar behavior changes to those reported in offspring prenatally exposed to mercury vapor or methylmercury. Brain mercury concentrations were reported as 0.017

and 0.063 mg kg^{-1} for the low and high dose group respectively, at 25 days of age. Whereas in the non-exposed control group, 0.002 mg kg^{-1} was reported.

5.8.3 Effects of Coexposure to Mercury Vapor and Methylmercury During Gestation

The predominant species of mercury exposure among the general population is methylmercury from consumption of fish and seafood. In addition, mercury vapor generated from dental amalgam is also considered to be a significant source in the countries where the mercury amalgam is still in use. Therefore, animal studies to simulate coexposure to methylmercury and mercury vapor have been conducted.

Fredriksson *et al.* (1996)[80] conducted the following experiment: Pregnant rats were 1) administered methylmercury (MeHg) by gavage (2 mg kg^{-1} per day during GDs 6–9; 2) exposed by inhalation to mercury vapor (Hg^0, 1.8 mg m^{-3} in air for 1.5 h per day) during GDs 14–19; and 3) exposed to both MeHg by gavage and mercury vapor by inhalation (MeHg + Hg^0); or 4) were given combined vehicle administration for each of the two treatments (control). Clinical observations and developmental markers up to weaning showed no differences among any of the groups. Behavioral function was examined between 4 and 5 months of age and included spontaneous motor activity, spatial learning in a circular bath, and instrumental maze learning for food reward. Offspring of dams exposed to Hg^0 showed hyperactivity in the motor activity test chambers over all three parameters: locomotion, rearing, and total activity; this effect was potentiated in the animals of the MeHg + Hg^0 group. In the swim maze test, the MeHg + Hg^0 and Hg^0 groups evidenced longer latencies before reaching a submerged platform compared to either the control or MeHg groups. In the modified, enclosed radial arm maze, both the MeHg + Hg^0 and Hg^0 groups showed longer latencies and made more errors in acquiring all eight pellets. The results indicate that prenatal exposure to Hg^0 causes alterations to both spontaneous and learned behaviors, suggesting some deficit in adaptive functions. Coexposure to MeHg, which by itself did not alter these functions at the dose given in this study, served to significantly aggravate the changes. The mercury concentration in the brain of offspring 2–3 days post parturition was 4, 5, and 12 ng g^{-1} for MeHg, Hg^0 and MeHg + Hg^0 respectively.

More recently, mercury vapor of a much lower concentration was applied in a coexposure experiment. Yoshida *et al.* (2011)[81] exposed pregnant mice to Hg^0 at a mean concentration of 0.030 mg m^{-3} for 6 h/day during gestation period. The methylmercury was supplied with food containing 5 ppm of MeHg from GD1 to postnatal day 10. The coexposure group was exposed to both Hg^0 vapor and MeHg, according to the procedure described. The offspring reached the age of 8 weeks and then underwent behavioral analyses. Open field tests showed an increase and decrease in voluntary activity in male and female mice respectively in the MeHg exposure group. The results of open field test in the Hg^0 + MeHg exposure group were similar to those in the MeHg exposure group in both males and females. The results in the Hg^0 exposure group did not significantly differ from those in the control group. Passive avoidance tests revealed no significant differences in avoidance latency in the retention trial between the Hg^0, MeHg, or Hg^0 + MeHg exposure group and the control group in males or females. Morris water maze tests showed a delay to reach the platform in the MeHg and Hg^0 + MeHg exposure groups compared with the control group in males but no significant differences between the Hg^0, MeHg, or Hg^0 + MeHg exposure group and the control group in females.

Apparently, effects of mercury vapor exposure were not observed due to the low concentration. The brain mercury concentration at 10 days postpartum was 3.0 ± 0.3, 340 ± 91, and $652 \pm 33\,ng\,g^{-1}$ for the male Hg^0, MeHg, and MeHg + Hg^0 group respectively, and 3.2 ± 0.6, 380 ± 89, and $341 \pm 69\,ng\,g^{-1}$ for the female Hg^0, MeHg or MeHg + Hg^0 group respectively. The control group showed 1.7 ± 0.4 or $2.1 \pm 0.4\,ng\,g^{-1}$ for males and females respectively. Although the exposure to mercury vapor ceased at parturition, and the exposure to methylmercury continued until 10 days after birth, the difference in concentrations between the two species of mercury is two orders of magnitude. Mercury concentration in the brain of offspring with mercury vapor exposure was similar to that of the control group.

Animal experiments to elucidate the toxicokinetics of mercury after prenatal mercury vapor exposure support the fact described previously (low concentration of mercury in the offspring's brain).

Morgan *et al.* (2006)[82] exposed pregnant rats to 1, 2, or $4\,mg\,Hg^0\,m^{-3}$ or air (controls) for 2 h/day from GD6 through to GD15. On the day of birth, the brain mercury concentration, by visual inspection of the figure, was approximately 20, 10, 8, and $1\,ng\,g^{-1}$ in the groups of 4, 2, and1 $mg\,Hg^0\,m^{-3}$, and air, respectively. The concentration decreased from postnatal day 1 to postnatal day14; thereafter the decrease was slow. The amount of mercury in the whole brain however, was rather stable between birth and weaning, indicating no elimination of mercury. After weaning, the amount of mercury in the brain of the control group abruptly increased to the levels of the mercury vapor exposure group. This elevation was attributed to consumption of a diet containing trace levels of mercury.

Female Long Evans hooded rats were exposed to methylmercury (0, 3, 6, or 9 ppm as a drinking solution), mercury vapor (0, 300, or $1{,}000\,\mu g\,m^{-3}$ for 2 h/day), or a combination of these, from 30 days before breeding through to GD18.[83] On postnatal day 4, organic and inorganic mercury concentrations in the offspring brain were analyzed by cold vapor atomic absorption spectrometry. Statistical analysis using linear mixed effects models showed that dose was the primary determinant of both organic and inorganic brain mercury levels. Mercury concentration in the offspring brains was $20–30\,ng\,g^{-1}$ for non-exposed controls and $30–50\,ng\,g^{-1}$ for the 300 or $1000\,\mu g\,m^{-3}$ exposed group.

These data indicate that after prenatal mercury vapor exposure, the brain mercury concentration increase by up to tens of $ng\,g^{-1}$ at most. One experiment[76] described corresponding maternal brain mercury concentration of $7\,\mu g\,g^{-1}$. Therefore, it is concluded that a small amount of mercury is transfered to the fetal brain after prenatal mercury vapor exposure. It is surprising that behavioral effects were observed in the animal with such a low concentration of mercury in the brain.

On the contrary, methylmercury exposure employed in animal experiments to date has caused substantial elevation of offspring brain mercury concentration (of the order of $\mu g\,g^{-1}$), with the exception of the study by Fredriksson *et al.* (1996).[80] In their experiment, methylmercury was given by gavage during GDs 6–9, and the brain was sampled for chemical analysis at 2–3 days after birth. Therefore, elimination of methylmercury from the brain and dilution of methylmercury concentration due to rapid growth in brain volume during late gestational and early postnatal periods possibly lowered mercury concentration in the offspring's brain. It is surprising however, in the experiment by Fredriksson *et al.* (1996),[80] that the brain mercury concentration after prenatal methylmercury exposure showed extremely low mercury concentration, such as 4 or $12\,ng\,g^{-1}$ for MeHg and MeHg + Hg^0, respectively. This needs to be confirmed.

5.9 Conclusions

5.9.1 Prenatal Methylmercury Exposure in Humans

It is evident that prenatal mercury exposure causes postnatal neurobehavioral effects in offspring. Human cases have been typically represented by fetal Minamata Disease patients. They developed neurological disorders after birth and the disorders have persisted until today, at their middle age. Observations of their ADL over a 15 year period did not reveal exacerbation among fetal Minamata Disease patients. Minamata Disease patients with adult exposure however, showed that the difference in ADL disability between Minamata Disease patients and controls significantly increased with age and that ADL disability in Minamata Disease patients was aggravated by aging. It should be considered that the ages of the two populations are different; fetal Minamata Disease patients were at middle age when studied, but the adult Minamata Disease patients were middle aged to elderly.

Cardiac autonomic nervous function was affected by methylmercury exposure, during both fetal and adult periods. It seems that this consequence has been permanent for fetal exposure, whereas the effect caused by exposure in adulthood was temporary. It is plausible that perturbation during fetal (and/or early postnatal) development may result in permanent (or long lasting at least) changes, indicating vulnerability of fetuses.

5.9.2 Prenatal Methylmercury Exposure in Animal Experiments

In animal experiments studies, neurobehavioral effects of fetal methylmercury exposure have been reported in mice, rats, and non-human primates. Maternal animals were not affected by methylmercury exposure; it is considered that fetal animals are much more sensitive than maternal animals. It is also evident that neurobehavioral effects are still observed after substantial time has passed, indicating long-lasting effects of prenatal exposure.

It is, however, not known whether prenatal exposure to methylmercury results in acceleration of aging. One experiment employing monkeys only showed age-related increase in auditory impairment.

5.9.3 Mercury Vapor Exposure and Aging in Exposed Miners and Workers

Mercury miners who experienced mercury poisoning 18 years previously exhibited deteriorated performances of motor coordination, simple reaction time, and short term memory compared with age matched controls. Moreover, subjects 65 years of age and older showed larger differences between those with histories of mercury poisoning and control subjects than did the younger age groups. Among the workers who were exposed to mercury vapor in plants 20 to 35 years previously, subjects 70 years of age and older demonstrated the most significant differences in several neurological impairments between high- (peak urinary mercury concentration $>0.6\,\mathrm{mg\,L^{-1}}$) and low-exposure or control subjects. From these results, effects of mercury vapor exposure persists for a long time, and previous exposure substantially exacerbates neurobehavioral performance in the elderly, though such exacerbation was not obvious in younger age. Therefore, it is possible that mercury vapor exposure accelerates aging.

5.9.4 Prenatal Mercury Vapor Exposure in Animal Experiments

Not only methylmercury, but also mercury vapor exposures resulted in postnatal effects without overt toxic signs and symptoms in either maternal or offspring animals. The postnatal neurobehavioral changes last for a long time (months or years, depending on the life span of the animals).

Of interest is the concentration of mercury in the brain of fetuses or offspring that causes such neurobehavioral changes. In the case of methylmercury exposure, concentration of the order of $\mu\mathrm{g\,g^{-1}}$ in the brain was reported from animal experiments. In contrast, the concentration was tens of $\mathrm{ng\,g^{-1}}$ or $\mathrm{ng\,g^{-1}}$, smaller by 2 or 3 orders of the magnitude, of methylmercury. Since in these experiments the offspring brain was sampled after parturition on various days, depending on each experimental protocol, the peak concentration could not be detected. Only one toxicokinetic study[77] revealed mercury concentration in fetal brain samples collected on the same day of the last exposure. The concentration was $49 \pm 5\,\mathrm{ng\,g^{-1}}$ after 10 consecutive exposures from GD6 to GD15 at $4\,\mathrm{mg\,Hg\,m^{-3}}$ for 2 h/day. Maternal brain mercury concentration was approximately $7\,\mu\mathrm{g\,g^{-1}}$ on GD15. Therefore, it is not likely that mercury concentration in fetal brain is elevated drastically by maternal mercury exposure to mercury vapor.

It is surprising that such low concentrations of mercury from mercury vapor exposures during gestation or neonatal period, presumably in the mercuric form in the brain after oxidation in the tissue, cause neurobehavioral changes. Is mercuric mercury derived from mercury vapor so toxic to fetal or neonatal brain tissue? Or does mercury vapor exposure have an unknown action that causes a disturbance in brain development? It is also possible that the toxic species of mercury is not methylmercury but inorganic mercury derived from decomposition of methylmercury. This hypothesis should be examined.

References

1. M. Berlin, R. K. Zalups and B. A. Fowler in *Handbook on the Toxicology of Metals*, 3rd edition, eds. G. Nordberg, B. A. Fowler, M. Nordberg and L. Friberg, Academic Press, Inc., 2007, pp. 675–729.
2. M. Berlin, J. Fazackerley and G. Nordberg, *Arch. Environ. Health*, 1969, **18**, 719.
3. J. B. Hursh, T. W. Clarkson, E. F. Miles and L. A. Goldsmith, *Arch. Environ. Health*, 1989, **44**, 120.
4. T. W. Clarkson, J. Gatzy and C. Dalton in *Atomic Energy Commission Research and Development Report UR-582*, 1961.
5. S. Halbach and T. W. Clarkson, *Biochimica et biophysica acta*, 1978, **523**, 522.
6. M. Berlin, L. G. Jerksell and H. von Ubisch, *Arch. Environ. Health*, 1966, **12**, 33.
7. T. W. Clarkson, L. Magos and M. R. Greenwood, *Biol. Neonate*, 1972, **21**, 239.
8. M. Yoshida, Y. Yamamura and H. Satoh, *Arch.* Toxicol., 1986, **58**, 225.
9. T. Clarkson and A. Rothstein, *Health Physics*, 1964, **10**, 1115.
10. J. B. Hursh, M. G. Cherian, T. W. Clarkson, J. J. Vostal and R. V. Mallie, *Arch. Environ. Health*, 1976, **31**, 302.
11. L. Kosta, A. R. Byrne and V. Zelenko, *Nature*, 1975, **254**, 238.
12. L. C. Rossi, G. F. Clemente and G. Santaron, *Arch. Environ. Health*, 1976, **31**, 160.
13. R. Garnier, J. M. Fuster, F. Conso, B. Dautzenberg, C. Sors and E. Fournier, *Toxicol. Eur. Res.*, 1981, **3**, 77.
14. L. Friberg and G. F. Nordberg in *Mercury in the Environment*, eds. L. Friberg and J. Vostal, CRC Press, Boca Raton, 1972, pp. 113–139.
15. S. Langworth, C. G. Elinder, K. G. Sundquist and O. Vesterberg, *Br. J. Ind. Med.*, 1992, **49**, 394.
16. J. K. Miettinen in *Mercury, Mercurials and Mercaptans*, eds. M. W. Miller and T. W. Clarkson, Charles C Thomas, Springfield, 1973, pp. 233–243.

17. K. Kostial, D. Kello, S. Jugo, I. Rabar and T. Maljkovic, *Environ. Health Perspect.*, 1978, **25**, 81.
18. L. Friberg, E. Skog and J. E. Wahlberg, *Acta Derm.-Venereol.*, 1961, **41**, 40.
19. H. Satoh, T. Suzuki, T. Nobunaga, A. Naganuma and N. Imura, *J. Pharmacobio-Dyn.*, 1981, **4**, 191.
20. A. Shimada, E. Yamamoto, T. Morita, M. Yoshida, J. S. Suzuki, M. Satoh and C. Tohyama, *Toxicol. Pathol.*, 2004, **32**, 519.
21. H. Satoh and T. Suzuki, *Arch. Toxicol.*, 1979, **42**, 275.
22. Y. Sugata and T. W. Clarkson, *Biochem. Pharmacol.*, 1979, **28**, 3474.
23. J. D. Dunn, T. W. Clarkson and L. Magos, *Science*, 1981, **213**, 1123.
24. J. R. Wands, S. W. Weiss, J. H. Yardley and W. C. Maddrey, *Am. J.Med.*, 1974, **57**, 92.
25. D. Hunter, *The Diseases of Occupations*, The English Universities Press Ltd., London, 1962.
26. D. W. Nierenberg, R. E. Nordgren, M. B. Chang, R. W. Siegler, M. B. Blayney, F. Hochberg, T. Y. Toribara, E. Cernichiari and T. Clarkson, *New Engl. J. Med.*, 1998, **338**, 1672.
27. T. Suzuki and K. Yoshino, *Ind. Med. J.*, 1969, **11**, 21.
28. M. Aschner, *Pharmacol. Toxicol.*, 1989, **65**, 17.
29. Y. Kajiwara, A. Yasutake, T. Adachi and K. Hirayama, *Arch. Toxicol.*, 1996, **70**, 310.
30. B. Aberg, L. Ekman, R. Falk, U. Greitz, G. Persson and J. O. Snihs, *Arch. Environ. Health*, 1969, **19**, 478.
31. J. H. Koeman, W. H. Peeters, C. H. Koudstaal-Hol, P. S. Tjioe and J. J. de Goei, *Nature*, 1973, **245**, 385.
32. I. R. Rowland, R. D. Robinson and R. A. Doherty, *Arch. Environ. Health*, 1984, **39**, 401.
33. F. Bakir, S. F. Damluji, L. Amin-Zaki, M. Murtadha, A. Khalidi, N. Y. al-Rawi, S. Tikriti, H. I. Dahahir, T. W. Clarkson, J. C. Smith and R. A. Doherty, *Science*, 1973, **181**, 230.
34. M. Shimada, K. Nakai, N. Tatsuta, K. Yaginuma, N. Kurokawa, H. Satoh and H. Akagi, *Nihon eiseigaku zasshi (Japanese journal of hygiene)*, 2011, **60**, 404.
35. T. Suzuki, T. Miyama and H. Katsunuma, *Ind. Health*, 1970, **8**, 39.
36. K. Yaginuma-Sakurai, K. Murata, M. Iwai-Shimada, K. Nakai, N. Kurokawa, N. Tatsuta and H. Satoh, *J.Toxicol. Sci.*, 2012, **37**, 123.
37. H. Al-Shahristani, K. Shihab and I. K. Al-Haddad, *Bull. W.H.O.*, 1976, **53**(Suppl, 105).
38. D. Marsh, G. Myers, T. Clarkson, L. Amin-Zaki, S. Tikriti and M. Majeed, *Annal. Neurol.*, 1980, **7**, 348.
39. P. Grandjean, P. Weihe, R. F. White, F. Debes, S. Arak, K. Yokoyama, K. Murata, N. Sorensen, I. R. Dah and P. J. Jorgensen, *Neurotox. Teratol.*, 1997, **19**, 417.
40. E. Oken, R. O. Wright, K. P. Kleinman, D. Bellinger, C. J. Amarasiriwardena, H. Hu, J. W. Rich-Edwards and M. W. Gillman, *Environ. Health Perspect.*, 2005, **113**, 1376.

41. K. Suzuki, K. Nakai, T. Sugawara, T. Nakamura, T. Ohba, M. Shimada, T. Hosokawa, K. Okamura, T. Sakai, N. Kurokawa, K. Murata, C. Satoh and H. Satoh, *Environ. Res.*, 2010, **110**, 699.
42. D. A. Spyker and J. M. Spyker, *Toxicol. Appl. Pharmacol.*, 1977, **40**, 511.
43. M. Harada, *Crit.Rev.Toxicol.*, 1995, **25**, 1.
44. R. Doi, *Nihon Koshu Eisei Zasshi*, 2002, **49**, 73.
45. X. J. Liu, M. Sakamoto, T. Kato, M. Okamoto and K. Arimura, *Nihon eiseigaku zasshi (Japanese journal of hygiene)*, 2007, **62**, 905.
46. T. Oka, M. Matsukura, M. Okamoto, N. Harada, T. Kitano, T. Miike and M. Futatsuka, *Tohoku J. Exp. Med.*, 2002, **8**, 15.
47. K. Yaginuma-Sakurai, K. Murata, M. Shimada, K. Nakai, N. Kurokawa, S. Kameo and H. Satoh, *Neurotoxicol.Teratol.*, 2010, **32**, 240.
48. H. Satoh, *Tohoku J. Exp. Med.*, 2003, **201**, 1.
49. J. M. Spyker, S. B. Sparber and A. M. Goldberg, *Science*, 1972, **177**, 621.
50. B. Weiss and J. M. Spyker, *Pediatrics*, 1974, **53**, 851.
51. S. Shimai and H. Satoh, *J. Toxicol. Sci.*, 1985, **10**, 199.
52. C. Watanabe and H. Satoh, *Environ. Health Perspect.*, 1996, **104**(Suppl. 2), 367.
53. L. Amin-Zaki, M. A. Majeed, T. W. Clarkson and M. R. Greenwood, *Br. Med. J.*, 1978, **1**, 613.
54. L. Amin-Zaki, M. A. Majeed, M. R. Greenwood, S. B. Elhassani, T. W. Clarkson and R. A. Doherty, *J. Appl. Toxicol.*, 1981, **1**, 210.
55. C. Cox, D. Marsh, G. Myers and T. Clarkson, *Neurotoxicology*, 1995, **16**, 727.
56. C. Cox, T. W. Clarkson, D. O. Marsh, L. Amin-Zaki, S. Tikriti and G. J. Myers, *Environ. Res.*, 1989, **49**, 318.
57. WHO in *Environmental health criteria 101, Methylmercury*, World Health Organization, Geneva, 1990, pp. 11–17.
58. T. Kjellstrom, P. Kennedy, S. Wallis and C. Mantell, Report 3080, National Swedish Environmental Protection Board Solna, Sweden, 1986.
59. T. Kjellstrom, P. Kennedy, S. Wallis and C. Mantell, Report 3642, National Swedish Environmental Protection Board Solna, Sweden, 1989.
60. D. Marsh, T. Clarkson, G. Myers, P. Davidson, C. Cox, E. Cernichiari, M. Tanner, W. Lednar, C. Shamlaye, O. Choisy, C. Hoareau and M. Berlin, *Neurotoxicology*, 1995, **16**, 583.
61. G. Myers, P. Davidson, C. Cox, C. Shamlaye, M. Tanner, O. Choisy, J. Sloane-Reeves, D. Marsh, E. Cernichiari, A. Choi, M. Berlin and T. Clarkson, *Neurotoxicology*, 1995, **16**, 639.
62. G. Myers, D. Marsh, P. Davidson, C. Cox, C. Shamlaye, M. Tanner, A. Choi, E. Cernichiari, O. Choisy and T. Clarkson, *Neurotoxicology*, 1995, **16**, 653.
63. G. J. Myers, P. W. Davidson, C. Cox, C. F. Shamlaye, D. Palumbo, E. Cernichiari, J. Sloane-Reeves, G. E. Wilding, J. Kost, L.-S. Huang and T. W. Clarkson, *Lancet*, 2003, **361**, 1686.
64. P. W. Davidson, G. J. Myers, B. Weiss, C. F. Shamlaye and C. Cox, *Neurotoxicology*, 2006, **27**, 1106.

65. P. Grandjean, P. Weihe, P. Jorgensen, T. Clarkson, E. Cernichiari and T. Videro, *Arch. Environ. Health*, 1992, **47**, 185.
66. K. Murata, P. Weihe, E. Budtz-Jorgensen, P. J. Jorgensen and P. Grandjean, *J. Pediatr.*, 2004, **144**, 177.
67. F. Debes, E. Budtz-Jorgensen, P. Weihe, R. F. White and P. Grandjean, *Neurotoxicol, Teratol.*, 2006, **28**, 363.
68. J. J. Strain, P. W. Davidson, M. P. Bonham, E. M. Duffy, A. Stokes-Riner, S. W. Thurston, J. M. W. Wallace, P. J. Robson, C. F. Shamlaye, L. A. Georger, J. Sloane-Reeves, E. Cernichiari, R. L. Canfield, C. Cox, L. S. Huang, J. Janciuras, G. J. Myers and T. W. Clarkson, *Neurotoxicology*, 2008, **29**, 776.
69. Y. Kinjo, H. Higashi, A. Nakano, M. Sakamoto and R. Sakai, *Environ. Res.*, 1993, **63**, 241.
70. R. Kishi, R. Doi, Y. Fukuchi, H. Satoh, T. Satoh, A. Ono, F. Moriwaka, K. Tashiro, N. Takahata, H. Sasatani, H. Shirakashi, T. Kamada and K. Nakagawa, *Occup. Environ. Med.*, 1994, **51**, 35.
71. J. Albers, L. Kallenbach, L. Fine, G. Langolf, R. Wolfe, P. Donofrio, A. Alessi, K. Stolp-Smith and M. Bromberg, *Annal. Neurol.*, 1988, **24**, 651.
72. D. C. Rice, *Toxicol. Sci.*, 1998, **44**, 191.
73. M. Yoshida, *Tohoku J. Exp. Med.*, 2002, **196**, 79.
74. B. R. Danielsson, A. Fredriksson, L. Dahlgren, A. T. Gardlund, L. Olsson, L. Dencker and T. Archer, *Neurotoxicol. Teratol.*, 1993, **15**, 391.
75. M. C. Newland, K. Warfvinge and M. Berlin, *Toxicol. Appl. Pharmacol.*, 1996, **139**, 374.
76. D. W. Herr, S. M. Chanda, J. E. Graff, S. S. Barone, R. P. Beliles and D. L. Morgan, *Toxicol. Sci.*, 2004, **82**, 193.
77. D. L. Morgan, S. M. Chanda, H. C. Price, R. Fernando, J. Liu, E. Brambila, R. W. O'Connor, R. P. Beliles and S. Barone, *Toxicol. Sci.*, 2002, **66**, 261.
78. M. Yoshida, C. Watanabe, K. Horie, M. Satoh, M. Sawada and A. Shimada, *Toxicol. Lett.*, 2005, **155**, 361.
79. A. Fredriksson, L. Dahlgren, B. Danielsson, P. Eriksson, L. Dencker and T. Archer, *Toxicology*, 1992, **74**, 151.
80. A. Fredriksson, L. Dencker, T. Archer and B. R. Danielsson, *Neurotoxicol. Teratatol.*, 1996, **18**, 129.
81. M. Yoshida, M. Suzuki, M. Satoh, A. Yasutake and C. Watanabe, *J. Toxicol. Sci.*, 2011, **36**, 73.
82. D. L. Morgan, H. C. Price, R. Fernando, S. M. Chanda, R. W. O'Connor, S. S. Barone, D. W. Herr and R. P. Beliles, *Environ. Health Perspect.*, 2006, **114**, 735.
83. H. Ishitobi, S. Stern, S. W. Thurston, G. Zareba, M. Langdon, R. Gelein and B. Weiss, *Environ. Health Perspect.*, 2010, **118**, 242.

CHAPTER 6

Manganese

ROBERTO G LUCCHINI,[a] DONALD R. SMITH[b] AND RONALD B TJALKENS[c]

[a] Department of Preventive Medicine, Mount Sinai School of Medicine, New York, NY 10029 and Occupational Medicine, University of Brescia, Italy; [b] Department of Microbiology and Environmental Toxicology, University of California, Santa Cruz, CA 95064, USA; [c] Department of Environmental and Radiological Health Sciences, Colorado State University, Fort Collins, CO 80523, USA
*E-mail: roberto.lucchini@mssm.edu

6.1 Introduction

It is clear that the aged are at greater risk of and more susceptible to the deleterious effects from exposure to environmental agents compared to younger adults.[60,13] Moreover, there is emerging evidence that early life exposure to environmental agents increases risk of neurologic disease and toxicity late in life.[18,71] In particular, there is clear evidence of health impacts of occupational and environmental manganese (Mn) exposure in adults, with implications in the elderly,[31,95,106] and evidence from animal studies that exposure to manganese during early life stages may contribute to disease risk later in life.[87,123] These studies build upon evidence linking transition metal dyshomeostasis and the accumulation of transition metals, most notably iron, in brain regions most commonly affected in neurodegenerative diseases.[12,31,81,96] Notably, the well-described interactions between manganese and cellular iron regulation and dyshomeostasis,[35,92,139,168,169] suggest that manganese may contribute to neurological dysfunction in the aged *via* multiple

Issues in Toxicology No. 16
Aging and Vulnerability to Environmental Chemicals: Age-related Disorders and their Origins in Environmental Exposures
Edited by Bernard Weiss

Published by the Royal Society of Chemistry, www.rsc.org

direct and indirect mechanisms. Here, we briefly review the physiologic and toxicologic properties of manganese, exposure sources, and evidence—molecular, animal model, and clinical—supporting a likely role of manganese in neurologic disease in the aged.

6.2 Environmental Occurrence of Manganese and Exposure Sources

Manganese is the 5th most abundant metal and 12th most abundant element, accounting for 0.1% of the earth's crust. Natural weathering processes result in the ubiquitous presence of manganese in soil, dust, and water, and in ambient air containing suspended particles. Overall enrichment of manganese in soil in developed regions is gradually increasing due to industrial emission.[76] Current estimates of world manganese reserves, including high grade ores (defined as having more than 44% manganese content), are in the range of 680 million tons of ore, situated in the southern hemisphere, with Australia, Brazil, Gabon, and South Africa, supplying over 90% of the international market. Ghana and India, both large suppliers in the past, are now exporting only limited quantities of low or medium grade ore. The ore mined in Mexico is mostly for use within that country. The CIS, which as the USSR was the largest supplier of manganese ore at the beginning of the century, is now left with low grade ore reserves. Low or medium grade manganese ore deposits are widely distributed in China.

Anthropogenic uses of manganese are largely in metallurgical processes. About 90% of industrially processed manganese is used in steel manufacture as a deoxidizing and desulfurizing additive, and as an alloying constituent. Most manganese ore is smelted in electric furnaces to produce ferromanganese, widely used in the production of steel. Metallic manganese (ferromanganese) is used principally in steel production to improve hardness, stiffness, and strength. It is used in carbon steel, stainless steel, high-temperature steel, and tool steel, along with cast iron and super alloys.[79] Manganese is also a minor but indispensable component of welding consumables. Most welding consumables contain less than 6% manganese. The chemical forms in which it is used include ferromanganese, silico-manganese and manganese carbonate.

The most important non-metallurgical application of manganese is in the form of manganese dioxide, which is used as a depolarizer in dry-cell batteries. Manganese dioxide is also used in the manufacture of matches, fireworks, porcelain, glass-bonding materials, and amethyst glass, and as the starting material for production of many other manganese compounds. Manganese sulfate is used primarily as a fertilizer and as a livestock supplement where soils are deficient in manganese, as well as in some glazes, varnishes, ceramics, and fungicides. Potassium permanganate, due to its oxidizing power, is used as a disinfectant, an anti-algal agent, for metal cleaning, tanning and bleaching, and as a preservative for fresh flowers and fruits, as well as in water and waste-treatment plants for water purification purposes.[79] Other uses of manganese compounds are in textile bleaching, for linseed oil driers, in dyeing, in tanning of leather, and as an oxidizing agent for electrode coating in welding roads. Another important material is manganese ferrite, a soft ferrite widely used in electronics. Large amounts are consumed in the manufacture of television circuit boards.

Manganese is also used as a constituent in a number of organometallic compounds. Perhaps most notable is the organic manganese compound MMT (methylcyclo-pentadienyl manganese tricarbonyl), which has received considerable attention as a potential airborne exposure source of manganese.[162] MMT is an octane booster or anti-knock additive in gasoline. It was introduced in Canada in 1976 and had completely replaced tetraethyl lead in gasoline by 1990. In 1977, MMT was banned by the Environmental Protection Agency (EPA) as an additive in unleaded gasoline in the US.[42] In 1995, the ban was lifted, and a court decision ordered the EPA to register the product for use as a fuel additive again, although testing for health effects continues. The Afton (former Ethyl) Corporation, the manufacturer of MMT, has been marketing MMT since late 1995. Nevertheless, MMT is currently used only sparsely in the developed world.[162] The major refiners in Canada have voluntarily stopped using MMT, out of concern for the impact of MMT on advanced vehicles, and as a result, as much as 95% of Canadian gasoline is now MMT-free.[83] In Europe, MMT is used in Greece,[59,160] in a couple of the Eastern countries, and perhaps by one small refiner in Belgium.[11] The EU Fuel Quality legislation in April 2012 set a limit of 6 mg L^{-1} manganese in gasoline, falling to 2 mg L^{-1} from 2014, based on a risk assessment that is due to the EU Commission by the end of 2012. China is following the same requirements as Europe (Michael Walsh, personal communication).

Another potentially important class of organomanganese compounds is the fungicides, including maneb (ethylene-bisdithiocarbonate) and mancozeb (a polymeric mixture of maneb and a zinc salt); both contain ~20% manganese by weight.[79] There is limited evidence that use of these fungicides contributes to increased environmental manganese loading, though a recent study in the agricultural Salinas Valley (California, USA), where maneb and mancozeb are regularly applied, reported an association between manganese floor dust loadings in the homes of agricultural workers and manganese levels in shed deciduous teeth in resident children[4] (see section 6.3).

6.3 Essential and Toxicological Roles of Manganese in Humans

Manganese is an essential element for humans and animals and is needed for normal prenatal and neonatal bone mineralization, protein and energy metabolism, metabolic regulation, cellular protection from damaging free radical species, and the formation of glycosaminoglycans, among other things. Mitochondrial superoxide-dismutase (Mn-SOD), pyruvate carboxylase, and liver arginase are some of the known manganese metalloenzymes. In astrocytes, a large portion of intracellular manganese occurs as a cofactor in the enzyme glutamine synthetase.[8] Manganese has also been shown to stimulate the synthesis of chondroitin sulfate, an important constituent of the cartilage and connective tissue.[100]

As an essential element, manganese exhibits a classic inverted 'U' shaped dose–optimum heath response curve, with deleterious health impacts from physiologic deficiency as well as over exposure when the homeostatic range is exceeded. Oral intake *via* the normal diet is the physiological absorption route for manganese, and inhalation is the typical route for occupational and environmental exposure. In healthy adults, tight homeostatic control regulates gastrointestinal absorption and systemic uptake to about 3% of ingested manganese. The US Food and Nutrition Board of the National Research Council established Estimated Safe and Adequate Daily Dietary Intake (ESADDI) levels as follows: 0.3–0.6 mg per day for infants from birth to 6 months; 0.6–1.0 mg per day for infants from 6 months to 1 year; 1.0–1.5 mg per day for children from 1 to 3 years; 1.0–2.0 mg per day for children from 4 to 10 years; and 2.0–5.0 mg per day for adolescents (>11 years) and adults.[130] We are not aware of any comparable estimates specific to the elderly, though it is reasonable to consider that ESADDI values would differ from those of younger adults.

Emerging literature shows neurotoxic effects from airborne particles, especially of ultrafine dimension, carried through the olfactory tract. Therefore the role of olfactory transport and brain deposition of manganese mandates further research to assess the impacts on brain functions like olfaction.[170] Once absorbed in the body, manganese is rapidly distributed to various organs and tissues, including the bone and the brain.[151] In the circulation, manganese binding to blood proteins, such as α_2-macroglobulin and transferrin, is important in mediating the distribution within the body and target organs such as the brain.[34,38,84,119] In the brain, manganese accumulates in the caudate-putamen, globus pallidus, substantia nigra, and subthalamic nuclei,[5] though recent studies have suggested that following occupational exposures, manganese may accumulate more broadly across the brain than previously believed.[32]

6.4 Manganese Toxicity in Adults and the Elderly

Studies have shown clear health impacts of elevated manganese in occupationally exposed adults.[33,145] Prolonged occupational exposure to manganese, such as may occur in welders, miners, smelters, and other industrial workers that are exposed to high levels of manganese in fumes, may lead to irreversible neurological damage resulting in the disorder of manganism. Initially, manganism presents with psychiatric disturbances that are later followed by ataxia and an extrapyramidal syndrome. These symptoms resemble somewhat the progression of Parkinson's disease.[8] However, recent studies have indicated important differences in the signatures of brain dysfunction in occupational manganese neurotoxicity *versus* Parkinson's disease. For example, in asymptomatic welders at risk for developing manganism, positron emission tomography (PET) imaging has shown reduced FDOPA uptake in the nigrostriatal pathway, with the pattern of affected brain areas as the caudate > anterior putamen > posterior putamen, which is the exact opposite brain regional pattern of dysfunction in symptomatic idiopathic Parkinson's disease.[33]

Neuromotor, neurosensory and cognitive effects have been observed in welders with relatively low manganese exposures.[15,41] These findings are similar to those observed in other manganese-exposed populations, such as workers in battery production,[145,146] ferroalloy production,[106,117] and ore-processing.[127,132] Early evidence of pre-clinical neuropsychological alteration includes reduced performance on neuropsychological testing, poor eye-hand coordination and hand steadiness, reduced reaction time, reduced cognitive flexibility, and poor postural stability.[97] Other symptoms commonly reported include: headache, weakness, memory loss, sleep disturbance, irritability, anxiety disorders, and gait disturbance. These effects have been associated with manganese deposition in the brain, as measured with magnetic resonance imaging in otherwise normal (*i.e.*, asymptomatic) occupational populations.[90] Recent literature also indicates the impairment of cognitive abilities in adults with occupational and environmental exposure to manganese.[147] Chronic manganese exposure in non-human primates has been shown to produce neurodegenerative changes, diffuse A-beta plaques and alpha-synuclein aggregation in the frontal cortex. These changes support the observation of cognitive and working memory deficits observed in these animals.[62]

While there is compelling justification for special consideration of the elderly as a population particularly susceptible to the deleterious effects of environmental exposures,[142] few studies have investigated manganese pathophysiology in the elderly as a specific sensitive population. Elevated environmental manganese exposure may also affect non-occupational populations living in the vicinities of elevated manganese emissions. Studies have shown increased risk for Parkinson disease or parkinsonian disturbances in older adults living in areas with elevated environmental manganese.[106,107,164] Indeed, manganese exposure may play a role in the development of idiopathic Parkinson's disease by acting as an environmental trigger, able to accelerate the onset of neurodegenerative damage.[112] Welders have been studied for a possible increase of Parkinsonism due to manganese exposure. An increased frequency of parkinsonian disturbances has been shown in case control studies on large groups of welders in the US. The parkinsonian features in welders do not appear to be different from idiopathic Parkinson's disease (PD), except for a younger age of onset and a tendency to familiarity. Epidemiological studies conducted in Norway, Italy, and Canada have shown increased prevalence of Parkinson's disease and Parkinsonism in the vicinity of industrial sites causing emission of manganese dust.[108] The differences between manganism and manganese-induced parkinsonism may be interpreted. Relatively short term exposure to high concentrations of manganese appear to target the *globus pallidus*, sparing the *substantia nigra pars compacta* and resulting in the typical features of classical manganism, as described by Couper in 1837,[30] only 20 years after sir James Parkinson's description of the "shaking palsy". Prolonged and lifetime exposure to much lower levels of manganese, that may still exceed the homeostatic range, can target the entire area of the basal ganglia. This may explain the increased frequency of parkinsonism among elderly people with prolonged environmental exposure to manganese.[109,164] Welders may represent a particular at-risk group, where a combination of both manganism and manganese-induced parkinsonism takes place, according to the different levels of interaction between intensity and duration of manganese exposure.

6.5 Early Life Exposure to Manganese and Adult Disease

There is a compelling need to understand the extent to which early life exposure to elevated manganese may contribute to increased risk of disease in the elderly. Emerging evidence from studies of other environmental agents, such as air pollution and lead, support the concept of health effects in adults who suffered exposures as children.[18,71] However, currently, there are no comparable human data we are aware of linking early life manganese exposure with adult disease. Notably, the developing brain is more sensitive to manganese than the adult brain, due to enhanced absorption of the metal, relatively lower biliary excretion, and the continued development of synapses throughout childhood until adolescence, particularly in the prefrontal cortex. All of these factors increase the potential for neurological injury from excessive exposures.[6,136] During development, manganese readily crosses the placenta and can accumulate in the brain, and neonates receiving total parental nutrition (TPN) can accumulate over 200% more manganese in the brain compared to children not receiving TPN.[50] However, information addressing toxicity from oral exposure in children has only recently emerged. Except for recent reports of impairment in motor skills and odor identification,[110] health effects associated with elevated manganese exposure in children have been impairment of cognitive functions, with decrements in memory, verbal learning, and intelligence.[14,115,141,157,163,165]

These studies reported that neurotoxicity occurs in children drinking water with high (>1000 $\mu g\ L^{-1}$) concentrations of manganese,[70,88] and a potential association has been reported between ingestion of elevated levels of manganese and learning problems, based upon data indicating that manganese levels in hair are higher in learning-disabled and hyperactive children than in normal functioning children.[29,135] Several epidemiological studies have examined the relationship between elevated manganese levels in water and toxic effects in children. A study conducted in the Chinese province of Shanxi compared 92 children aged 11 to 13 whose drinking water was contaminated with elevated levels of manganese (241–346 $\mu g\ L^{-1}$) to children whose drinking water had low levels of manganese (30–40 μg L^{-1}).[73] The exposed children performed more poorly in school and on neurobehavioral exams than control students ($p<0.01$), with deficits noted in manual dexterity and rapidity, short-term memory, and visual identification. A second study, conducted in Bangladesh, showed that manganese may affect intellectual function, resulting in lower IQ.[163] This study examined a cross-section of 142 10-year old children whose well water supply was contaminated with a mean concentration of 793 μg Mn L^{-1}. The data indicated that manganese exposure was significantly associated with reduced Full-Scale, Performance and Verbal raw scores on the Wechsler Intelligence Scale for Children in a dose-response fashion. Additionally, a study conducted in Quebec, Canada, examined the relationship between exposure to chronic levels of manganese and hyperactive behavior in children.[13] Hair manganese concentration was correlated with hyperactive and oppositional behaviors, with the high exposure group having significantly greater levels of manganese in hair and a stronger association with hyperactive behaviors. Likewise, inhaled manganese was negatively associated with intellectual function in school aged children living near a manganese mining and processing facility.[141] Collectively, these data suggest that high levels of manganese in drinking water directly affect neurobehavioral function in children. Considered alongside recent findings that mice exposed to manganese during juvenile development experience greater neuroinflammatory injury and behavioral dysfunction upon exposure to manganese as adults than mice without juvenile exposure,[122,123] a background of manganese exposure, particularly during critical developmental years, could render individuals more susceptible, later in life, to neurotoxic insults which may predispose them to neurological disease.

6.6 Biological Markers of Manganese Exposure in Humans

While elevated manganese exposures are clearly associated with neurological deficits in humans, details of the exposure–effect relationships across occupational and environmental exposures are still being .[82,118,152] In part, this may be due to the challenges of accurately characterizing exposure over the lifetime or life stage of susceptibility, and to the fact that there are no well-recognized and validated biological markers of manganese exposure to better define dose–effect relationships, as there are for some other well-studied metal toxicants such as lead.[131] The identification and validation of exposure biomarkers is fundamental to human toxicology and risk assessment, and the assessment of a dose–response relationship is essential for the demonstration of cause and effect relationships, according to Hill's criteria of causation.[77]

Ideally, biological markers of exposure should reflect an integration of the internalized dose over time. Studies in occupationally-exposed adults have reported that blood manganese was associated with exposure and neurotoxic outcomes,[2,15,104,105,116,117,127,128,144] while studies in environmentally-exposed children have reported that hair manganese,[13,165] manganese in the exposure medium (*e.g.*, water[163]), or tooth manganese levels,[4,43] but *not* blood manganese, were predictors of exposure and/or neurotoxic outcomes. The reasons for these discrepancies in the predictive value of various manganese exposure biomarkers across pediatric environmental and adult occupational exposure studies are not known. The toxicokinetics of manganese suggests that exposure biomarkers such as blood and urine may best at best reflect recent exposure (*i.e.*, days), while hair and teeth may integrate or reflect longer-term exposure (*e.g.*, weeks –months or longer).[82,118,152]

These studies evidence the challenges associated with the identification and validation of biomarkers for manganese exposure and effect. Contributing to this challenge is the fact that manganese is an essential element; normally, concentrations in the body are controlled by homeostatic mechanisms regulating absorption, disposition, and excretion. These processes also play an important role in manganese toxicokinetics, different from many other non-essential toxic metals like mercury and lead. In the latter case, the relationship between lead exposures from environmental and occupational sources and biological indicators of exposure and effect, such as the significant associations between blood lead levels and toxic outcomes, have been well established over years of study.[93,131]

Analytical challenges associated with the accurate and precise measurement of manganese concentrations in various biological media (*e.g.*, blood, plasma, hair, urine) may confound assessment of suitable biomarkers of exposure. The existing literature suggests substantial variability in blood and hair manganese levels in environmentally or occupationally exposed subjects,[14,15,104,115,117,128,144] but the role of analytical variability in these differences has not been addressed. Unlike the significant efforts devoted to improving blood lead measurements,[53,131] there has been little recognition of potential sample contamination during collection, processing, and analyses of biological samples for manganese concentrations, even though manganese is a relatively common constituent of environmental media, such as soil and dust.[143]

To date, only a few studies have measured manganese in cross sections of shed deciduous teeth as a means of assessing prenatal and early postnatal exposure.[4,43] Ericson and colleagues reported a significant association between tooth manganese and hyperactivity/behavioral outcomes.[43] Arora and colleagues found a significant association between manganese in prenatally formed tooth dentine and floor dust manganese loadings in the homes of agricultural workers in regions where the manganese-containing fungicides maneb and mancozeb are routinely applied.[4] Measurement of manganese in teeth may offer several strengths as an exposure biomarker and predictor of adverse health effects. As a biologic analog to calcium, manganese [as Mn(II)] is incorporated directly into developing dentine. And, modern analytical methods, such as laser ablation ICP-mass spectrometry, allow detailed manganese measurements along histological transects contemporaneous with fetal and neonatal development.

6.7 Animal Studies - Dosimetry

Animal model studies have been crucial for elucidating the relationship between manganese dose, resultant target tissue manganese levels, and the resultant functional, cellular and sub-cellular effects of elevated exposure.[6,8] As an essential element, manganese homeostasis is physiologically regulated in adults, though regulatory processes may be overwhelmed with excessive exposure, depending on the exposure magnitude and frequency. This is well illustrated with data from a rodent study we conducted to determine whether manganese exposure and resultant toxic outcomes are a function of the magnitude of the nominal dose, the duration of the treatment, or a combination of both. Adult female Sprague-Dawley rats (age 9 months) were treated with nominal manganese doses of 0, 1.6, 4.8 and 9.6 mg kg^{-1} *via* intraperitoneal (IP) injection three times per week for either 5 weeks or 15 weeks (the latter dose for only 5 weeks; $n = 10$–14 per treatment). Blood, plasma, and brain manganese concentrations were significantly associated with the nominal dose, but not the cumulative dose of exposure (Figure 6.1), indicating there was no substantial accumulation of manganese with time in the circulation or the brain beyond the 5 week exposure duration, within a nominal dose treatment. This is best illustrated by the essentially identical blood manganese levels in animals who received the relatively modest nominal dose of 1.6 mg kg^{-1} for 5 weeks (blood $Mn = 53.0$ ng mL^{-1}) or 15 weeks (blood $Mn = 53.2$ ng mL^{-1}), even though the total cumulative manganese doses for these two groups differed by three-fold (24 and 72 mg kg^{-1} respectively). In contrast, animals who received the same cumulative dose of 72 mg kg^{-1} over a total exposure duration of either 5 weeks (4.8 mg kg^{-1} nominal dose) or 15 weeks (1.6 mg kg^{-1} nominal dose) exhibited blood manganese levels that differed by more than four-fold [*i.e.*, 236 ng mL^{-1} *versus* 53.2 ng mL^{-1}, Figure 6.1(a)], consistent with the difference in nominal dose between these treatment groups.

More recently, a study by Schroeter *et al.*[151] reported the use of a multi-route physiologically-based pharmacokinetic model for manganese to evaluate dose-dependent neurological effects, drawing exclusively on data from non-human primate studies. Applying the model across studies that used a variety of exposure routes (inhalation, oral, intravenous, intraperitoneal, and subcutaneous) and exposure durations (several weeks to over two years), their results support the hypothesis that the dose–response relationship for the neurotoxic effects of manganese is independent of exposure route. Their results also support the use of target tissue manganese concentration or cumulative target tissue manganese levels as an internal exposure measure predictive of neurological effects. This is consistent with the suggestion of Gwiazda *et al.* [68] that cumulative manganese dose is a predictor of significant health effects. This underscores the importance of understanding both the frequency and magnitude of exposure relative to the rate of body manganese elimination, a suggestion that has clear implications for human exposures as well.[6]

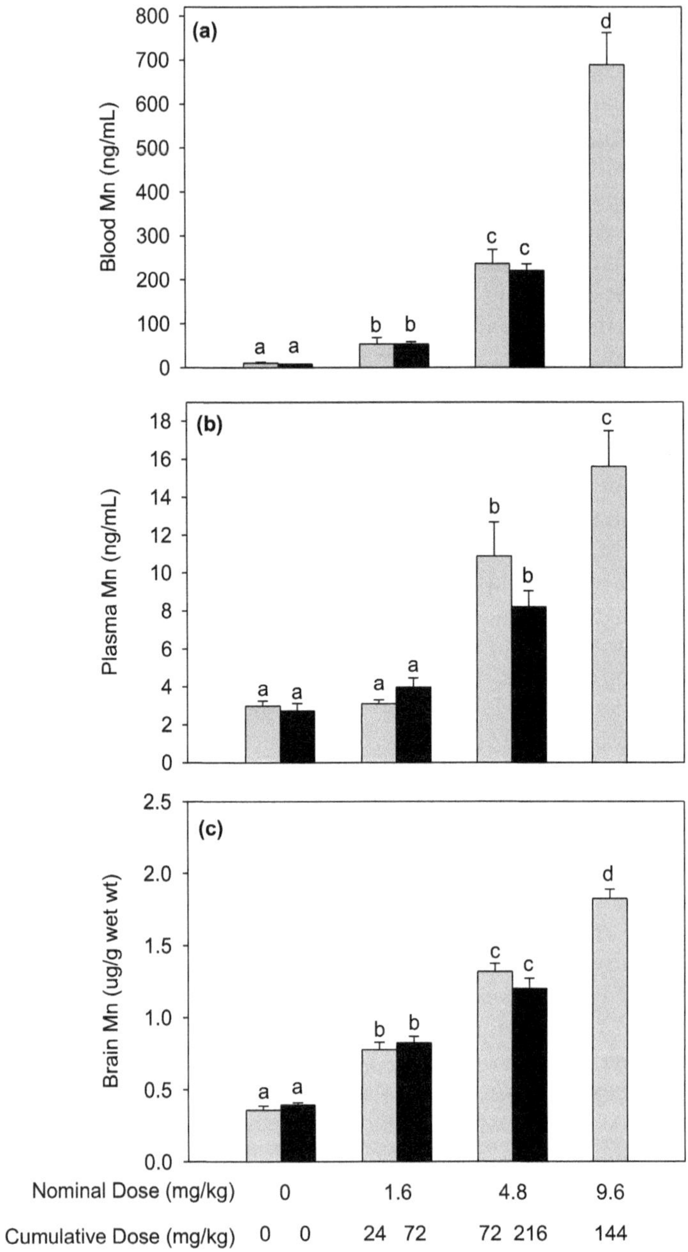

Figure 6.1 (a) Blood, (b) plasma, and (c) brain manganese concentrations in adult Sprague-Dawley rats (mean $\pm$ SE, n = 8 – 14/bar) exposed to manganese *via* IP injection (3 injections/week) for 5 weeks (grey) or 15 weeks (black). The x-axis shows nominal dose for each IP injection in mg Kg^{-1} body weight, or the total cumulative dose of manganese administered over the entire 5 or 15 week exposure period. Within a tissue, bars with different superscript letters were statistically different ($p < 0.05$), based on Tukey *post hoc* analyses.

6.8 Animal Studies - Early Life Manganese Exposure as a Determinant of Late Onset Disease

Animal model studies have also proven invaluable in specifically evaluating the impacts of exposure to agents suffered during discrete life stages, including the extent that insults suffered during early life may increase the risk of dysfunction and disease late in life. While studies have shown that increased iron intake in neonatal mice resulted in a Parkinson-like neurodegeneration as aged adults,[85] few studies have specifically evaluated the persistence of functional defects into adulthood as a result of early life exposure to manganese.[87,113,122,123,140] In one study, Kern and Smith[87] showed that rats exposed to manganese in early life showed an increased spontaneous motor activity response as adults (postnatal day, PND ~100) to a D-amphetamine challenge (D-amphetamine is a catacholamine agonist that produces increased levels of dopamine in the synaptic cleft). Consistent with this, dopamine D2 receptor levels were increased to a significant ~500–800% of controls in the prefrontal cortex, while D1 receptor levels were increased to ~160% of control in the nucleus accumbens of these adult rats exposed to manganese in early life. These data provide evidence of lasting alteration of the dopamine synaptic environment in adults following early life manganese exposure. Moreover, Moreno and colleagues recently reported that mice exposed to manganese during juvenile development experienced greater neuroinflammatory injury and behavioral dysfunction upon exposure to manganese as adults than mice without juvenile exposure.[122,123] Collectively, these animal studies further support the hypothesis that early life manganese exposures in humans may increase susceptibility to dysfunction in aged individuals.

6.9 Mechanisms of Manganese Toxicity

The dominant mechanisms of manganese toxicity are believed to include: mitochondrial dysfunction,[56–58] free radical production and oxidative stress,[39] disruption of cellular antioxidant defense mechanisms (such as glutathione, catalase, and glutathione peroxidase), manganese-mediated disruptions to intracellular calcium and Fe metabolism,[35,91,92,167,169] and activation of proinflammatory pathways.[51,124,159]

Manganese is a redox-active transition metal and a biologic analogue to iron(III), as Mn(III), and Ca(II), as Mn(II).[37] Within eukaryotic cells, manganese is predominantly in the Mn(II) oxidation state.[66,67,137] though is believed to undergo rapid redox activity in oxidizing environments or if not suitably stabilized by coordination with molecular ligands.[37,66] As such, manganese may exhibit both prooxidant and antioxidant properties, depending upon the local environment. Manganese is taken up into cells *via* a number of mechanisms, including the divalent metal transporter 1 (DMT1), transferrin receptor, and Ca^{2+} uniporter.[5,8,55] In contrast, comparatively little is known about cellular manganese efflux mechanisms, though recent studies have suggested that the golgi transmembrane proteins SPCA-1 and golgi phosphoprotein IV play important roles in cellular manganese homeostatsis and efflux.[125] DMT1 is highly expressed in the basal ganglia, which is a target area for both Parkinsonism and manganese toxicity,[80] and certain DMT1 polymorphisms have been related to Parkinson's disease[74] and neurodegeneration in animals models.[150] Additionally, rats exposed to manganese welding fumes mimicking occupational exposure have shown increased DMT1 mRNA expression related to neurodegeneration.[155] A role for DMT-1 in enhanced manganese olfactory transport, especially in anemic animals,[158] has also been observed.

6.9.1 Manganese Induces Oxidative Stress and Mitochondrial Dysfunction

Manganese is widely regarded as a prooxidant that contributes to heightened oxidative stress within cells.[1,5,91,138,139] Experimental evidence suggests that prooxidant activity of Mn^{2+} is dependent on trace amounts of Mn^{3+}. Superoxide produced in the mitochondrial electron transport chain may catalyze this transition through a set of reactions similar to those mediated by superoxide dismutase and thus lead to the increased oxidant capacity of the metal. Manganese may enhance the auto oxidation or turnover of various intracellular catecholamines, such as dopamine, leading to an increased production of free radicals, reactive oxygen species, and other cytotoxic metabolites.[3,39,103] It has also been shown to impair cellular antioxidant defense mechanisms. Oxidative stress generated through mitochondrial dysfunction due to manganese may be a key event in the injury of targeted central nervous system cells.

The mitochondrion is an important intracellular target of elevated manganese, with numerous studies demonstrating impaired function of the mitochondria or mitochondrial components with elevated exposures. Numerous studies have shown that elevated manganese exposure impairs mitochondrial function and energy production,[56–58,171,172] and specifically targets mitochondrial enzymes, including aconitase,[34,167] and components of the electron transport chain.[54] As manganese alters ATP production and glutamate uptake in astrocytes, basal ganglia neurons could be susceptible to excitotoxic damage. Changes in glutamic acid decarboxylase (GAD) and GABA content can be found as a consequence of manganese exposure.[52,69] It has been proposed that loss of GAD-positive cells in the striatum and globus pallidus of manganese-treated rats may be caused by the loss of chemical, electrical, or physical support because of neurite dysfunction encountered in mesencephalic cultures exposed to manganese (resulting in profound changes in the cytoskeleton and neurite length), or may be an independent neurotoxic event. Long-term manganese-intoxication effects are similar to those produced by other substances that also affect the mitochondria in the same brain structures, for instance carbon monoxide (CO) and cyanide. Parkinsonism and dystonia are common sequelae of manganese, cyanide, and carbon monoxide intoxications. Why manganese is able to produce the same effects as these substances is not known, but there may be common mechanisms of injury; for example, all of them are able to produce alterations in oxidative phosphorylation, and both manganese and CO induce mPT and ROS production.[8]

6.9.2 Manganese Causes Dysregulation of Cellular Iron Homeostasis

There is compelling *in vitro*, *in vivo*, and epidemiological evidence supporting the hypothesis that elevated manganese exposures lead to alteration of cellular iron metabolism.[35,40,91,92,120,139,148,167,168,169] and that polymorphisms of iron metabolism genes are associated with blood manganese levels in humans.[75] In mammalian cells, cellular iron metabolism is controlled primarily post-transcriptionally by the coordinated translation of proteins critical to iron uptake (transferrin receptor, TfR and divalent metal transporter-1, DMT-1), storage (ferritins), and utilization (m-aconitase and erythroid 5-aminolevulinate synhetase).[133] Translation of these proteins is controlled by iron regulatory proteins (IRPs), which interact with stem-loop structures (iron responsive elements, IREs) located in mRNAs coding for the above proteins. Two distinct IRPs have been identified: IRP-1 and IRP-2. IRP-1 is a bifunctional protein, exhibiting (cytosolic) aconitase activity in its holo form (containing a [4Fe-4S] cluster), and IRE binding activity in its apo-form (*i.e.*, loss of the [4Fe-4S] cluster). Because of its aconitase activity, IRP-1 in its holo from is also known as cytosolic aconitase (c-aconitase). In contrast, IRP-2, which does not contain an Fe–S cluster and lacks aconitase activity, regulates IRE binding activity through changes in its intracellular abundance.

Recent evidence suggests that manganese exposure produces an iron response akin to iron deficiency, leading to increased iron uptake, reduced storage of cellular iron, and increased labile cellular iron levels.[35,91,92,98,138,139,169] Since manganese can inhibit the enzymatic activity of aconitase,[26,35,161,167] it has been suggested that manganese may alter iron homeostasis *via* a direct interaction with c-aconitase/IRP1. However, there is compelling evidence that IRP-2 binding activity in cells is also strongly altered by manganese and in fact may be the predominant IRP mediating the manganese effect on iron dysregulation.[35,91,92] In light of (i) laboratory data indicating that misregulation of iron leads to increased redox cycling of iron complexes, increased oxidative stress, reduced antioxidant capabilities, and lipid and protein oxidation in the basal ganglia and other affected brain regions; (ii) suggestions that these effects are likely both cell type and brain region-specific, and also likely exacerbated with ageing; and (iii) the growing body of evidence indicating that iron toxicity may play an important role in many neurodegenerative diseases, including Alzheimer's, Parkinson's, and Huntington's disease,[96] it is quite likely that manganese-induced dysregulation of cellular iron homeostasis is an important mechanism of cellular toxicity.

6.9.3 Manganese Targets Dopaminergic and Glutamatergic Systems

There is clear evidence that manganese exposure in animal models, at levels below those that produce overt toxicity or neurodegeneration, alters dopamine system function, including reduced striatal dopamine release, reduced striatal dopamine transporter protein expression, and enhanced D2 receptor.[86,87,113,140] Similarly, in one of the few studies to report D2 receptor activity/expression, Calabresi *et al.*[19] showed that exposure of *post-weanling* rats to manganese significantly enhanced striatal D2 receptor activity compared to controls, based on electrophysiological measurements in brain slices treated with the D2 receptor agonist quinpirole. Comparable studies in *adult* non-human primates have similarly shown that elevated manganese exposure alters DA function. Guilarte *et al.*[64] used PET imaging in adult primates exposed to weekly IV. injections of manganese (3.3–4.9 mg kg^{-1} weekly injection for ~40 weeks) to show that manganese exposure resulted in reduced amphetamine-stimulated dopamine release in the striatum. Eriksson *et al.*[44,45] used PET imaging and quantitative autoradiography in adult non-human primates to show that chronic adult manganese exposure (200 mg SC injection every 2 months for 16–26 months) produced a 60–75% reduction in dopamine transporter levels in the striatum. Earlier studies in adult primates have shown that chronic manganese exposure also decreased tissue dopamine levels in the striatum.[10,46]

Changes in olfactory perception may be caused by a dopaminergic dysregulation, possibly related to changes at the level of dopamine receptors. Being actively transported through the olfactory tract, manganese can cause impairment of olfactory function and motor coordination. Odor and motor changes are interrelated and may be caused by a manganese-induced dopaminergic dysregulation affecting both functions. The interconnection between manganese and dopaminergic toxicity through changes in DMT1 expression warrant further research on the possible role of manganese exposure as a pathogenetic factor for Parkinsonism. Manganese exposure has shown to both increase and decrease serum prolactin levels in rats[111,139] and humans, including children,[121] as further support of changes in the dopaminergic system.

There is similar though less complete evidence from adult animal and cellular studies showing that manganese exposure disrupts glutamate (Glu) function.[24,36,47,65,126] For example, Erikson *et al.* showed that chronic respiratory $MnSO_4$ exposure in juvenile monkeys (≥ 0.3 mg m^{-3} for 65 days) decreased levels of GLT-1 and GLAST protein in the caudate, globus pallidus, olfactory cortex, and cerebellum, though total tissue Glu levels were unchanged compared to controls.[47] Centonze *et al.* found that manganese exposure in post-weanling rats (20 mg mL^{-1} in drinking water for 10 weeks) increased the frequency and amplitude of spontaneous striatal excitatory postsynaptic potentials, but did not change the sensitivity of striatal neurons to Glu AMPA and NMDA receptor stimulation, suggesting that the abnormal excitation of striatal neurons in this manganese dose range was due to hyperactivity of corticostriatal neurons.[24] These findings in animal models are accompanied by findings in cell model studies. Collectively, these support the theory that manganese exposure may disrupt Glu function through altered Glu release and/or activity, or decreased astrocytic Glu uptake, possibly potentiating the effects of increased cortical excitatory input.[17,27,36,48,49,52,72,153]

6.9.4 Glial Activation and Nitrosative Stress in Manganese Neurotoxicity

Inducible expression of multiple inflammatory genes in glia is regulated by the transcription factor NF-κB, which is under intense study as a therapeutic target for blocking neuroinflammation in neurodegenerative disease.[21] Multiple stress and inflammatory signals activate NF-κB through the IκB Kinase (IKK) complex.[129] Mitogen activated protein (MAP) kinase cascades are one of the pathways central to activation of IKK, and recent studies reported that manganese directly stimulates cGMP-dependent activation of NF-κB in astrocytes *via* MAPK signaling that potentiates the effects of inflammatory cytokines on expression of nitric oxide synthase (NOS2).[124] These data help to explain how low levels of manganese can potentiate inflammatory signaling in glial cells and suggest a mechanism by which manganese may act on NF-κB in concert with factors such as TNFα and IL-1β to promote a neuroinflammatory phenotype in glia.

The broader functional significance of NF-κB-dependent regulation of inflammatory genes in the basal ganglia was highlighted in recent studies demonstrating that the orphan nuclear receptor, Nurr1 normally inhibits NF-κB-regulated neuroinflammatory genes in astrocytes, and its deficiency causes loss of dopaminergic neurons.[149] Active Nurr1, as well as selected other nuclear receptors, stabilizes constitutively bound nuclear corepressor proteins and prevents NF-κB-induced NOS2 expression in astrocytes and microglia. Interestingly, deficiency in expression of Nurr1 is also associated with a late-onset form of Parkinson's disease,[61,94] suggesting that nuclear regulators of NF-κB are linked to glial inflammatory activation and neuronal injury within the basal ganglia. Supporting the importance of these nuclear regulatory mechanisms to neuroinflammatory injury, transgenic animals containing microglial- and astroglial-specific gene deletion of NF-κB are protected in diverse models of inflammatory neurodegeneration.[16,28] Thus, the capacity of manganese to stimulate a damaging inflammatory phenotype in glia may not only promote neuronal injury during exposure, but may also render selected populations of neurons more vulnerable to secondary neurotoxic insult later in life.

6.9.5 Neuroinflammation may Link Between Early Life Exposure to Manganese and Susceptibility to Late Onset Neurological Disease

The most prominent neuropathologic findings in human manganism are neuronal loss and reactive gliosis in the globus pallidus and substantia nigra

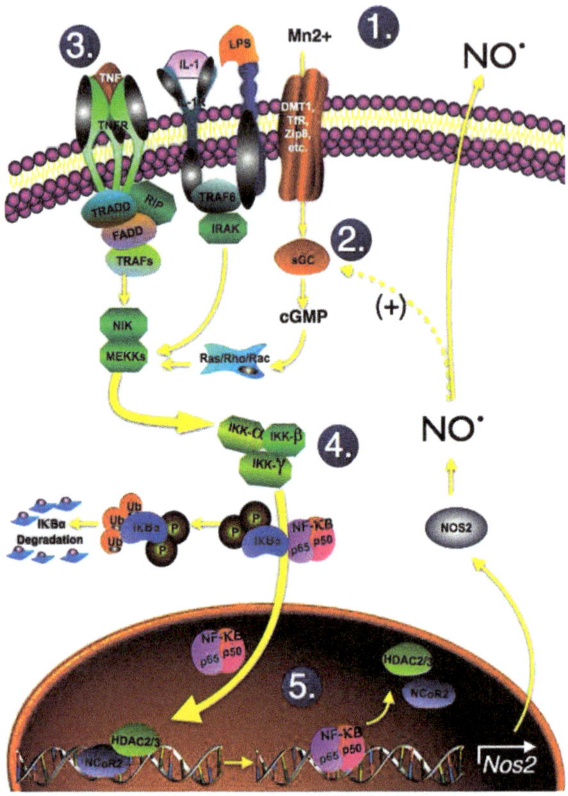

Figure 6.2 Manganese potentiates NF-κB signaling in astrocytes, leading to increased expression of neuroinflammatory genes. Until recently, it was unclear how manganese could potentiate inflammatory signaling in astrocytes through multiple pro-inflammatory pathways. The studies of Tjalkens and colleagues revealed that manganese uptake into astrocytes (**1**) results in rapid increases in cGMP through soluble guanylate cyclase (**2**), which activates MEKK/ERK signaling (likely through Rho/Rac family kinases) and the IKK/NF-κB signaling complex. (**3**) Diverse inflammatory signals such as TNFα and LPS activate IKK/NF-κB signaling through intracellular receptor-associated protein (MEK) complexes and the NF-κB-interacting kinase (NIK), resulting in a convergence of stimuli that magnifies otherwise low-level inflammatory activation (**4**). Activated NF-κB translocates to the nucleus, where chromatin remodeling occurs by removal of transcriptional co-repressors such as NCoR2 and (likely) other factors such as histone deacetylase (HDAC) proteins, permitting binding of p65 to NF-κB enhancer elements (**5**). Increased expression of NOS2 elevates levels of NO, which may further increase intracellular cGMP levels, as well as magnify neuronal protein nitration and injury.

pars reticulata (SNpr).[166] Gliosis in the striatum (caudate nucleus and putamen) and subthalamic nucleus has also been reported and, less frequently, the substantia nigra pars compacta (SNpc).[20] A key feature of the reactive gliosis observed in human and experimental manganism is the presence of

Alzheimer type II astrocytosis, although ultrastructural studies also report reactive microglia surrounding degenerating neurons that contain increased numbers of large secondary lysosomes, indicative of an active phagocytic process.[9,63,134] Additionally, it has been reported that manganese induces astrogliosis in the pre-frontal cortex of exposed Cynomolgus macaques, with activated astrocytes in this model occurring proximal to degenerating neurons that express Amyloid-β precursor-like protein 1.[63] Previous studies in juvenile and adult mice indicate that adult mice pre-exposed to manganese as juveniles have a more severe neuroinflammatory phenotype and greater neurological dysfunction when re-exposed to manganese as adults, compared to mice without prior exposure.[122,123] This suggests that glial activation may represent a type of 'memory' within the CNS that sensitizes affected brain regions to

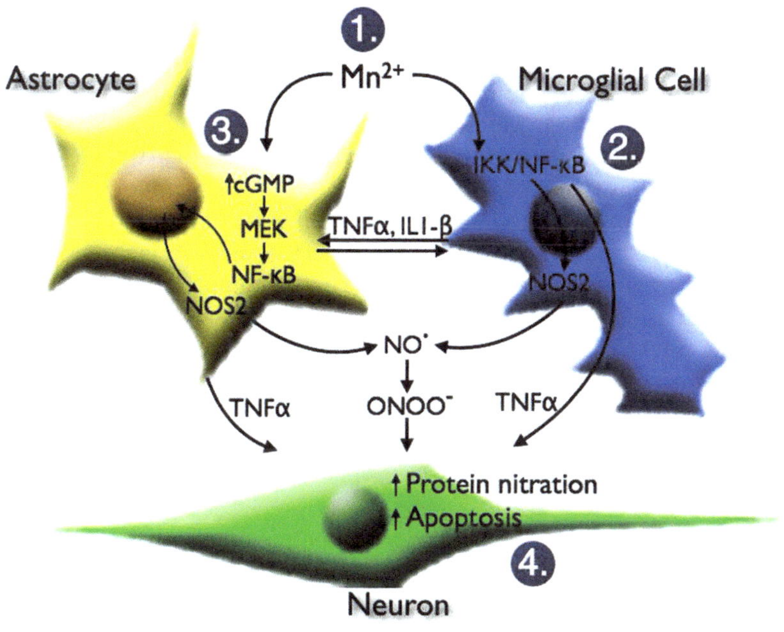

Figure 6.3 Microglial-astrocyte interactions promote a neuroinflammatory phenotype following exposure to manganese during development. Developmental exposure to manganese stimulates intercellular signaling between microglia and astrocytes, which results in a persistent inflammatory phenotype that can enhance neurological dysfunction during aging. (**1**) Manganese directly affects both microglia and astrocytes, stimulating NF-κB-dependent gene expression in microglia (**2**), which enhances production of pro-inflammatory factors such as TNFα and IL-1β, leading to inflammatory priming of astrocytes. Manganese accumulation in astrocytesstimulates cGMP/MAPK/IKK-mediated activation of NF-κB, potentiating expression of neuroinflammatory genes (**3**), which further stimulate microglial cells and cause neuronal protein nitration and injury through release of inflammatory mediators including NO and TNFα (**4**).

neurological dysfunction from manganese and that might also promote a more severe neuroinflammatory phenotype later in life upon exposure to manganese or other environmental or endogenous neurotoxicants.

Less is known regarding the role of microglial activation in manganese neurotoxicity, or about interactions between microglia and astrocytes that may promote persistent astrogliosis. Microglia are not uniformly distributed in the brain and are enriched in several regions, including the basal ganglia.[89] Activated microglia and astrocytes produce pro-inflammatory mediators such as nitric oxide (NO), prostaglandins, TNFα, and IL-1β, that are associated with neuronal injury in multiple neurodegenerative disorders.[22,78,114] Increased expression of inducible NOS2 and overproduction of NO is also associated with neuroinflammatory injury in manganism,[7,154] but the relative contributions of microglia and astrocytes to NOS2 expression in glia and subsequent induction of nitrosative stress in neurons following exposure to manganese *in vivo* are not well understood. Manganese enhances the release of the inflammatory cytokines interleukin-6 and TNFα from microglial cells,[23,51] which can promote activation of astrocytes and subsequent release of prostaglandin E2 and NO.[25,99] Manganese increases neuronal protein nitration in developing[123] and adult[101] mice, and inhibition of NOS2 in astrocytes protects co-cultured neurons from manganese toxicity.[102,159] This supports a causative role for NO in manganese-induced neuronal injury, as do recent studies indicating that NOS2 knockout mice are protected against manganese neurotoxicity during juvenile development.[156] Thus a complex interplay between microglia and astrocytes mediates the neuroinflammatory phenotype observed in manganese toxicity, and a better understanding of the underlying signaling pathways is necessary to identify critical interactions between glial cells that determine neuronal injury.

6.10 Conclusion

Manganese is an essential element and also a potentially hazardous element, in full accordance with Paracelsus' motto "*dosis facit venenum*" (the dose makes the poison). For manganese, the dose *per se* is not the only important factor; the integration between dose and exposure frequency and duration can determine different types of toxicity. "*Dosis et tempus faciunt venerum*" would have been Paracelsus' definition for manganese. The time variable entails "when" and "how long" exposure takes place, pointing out the most vulnerable windows of pre and post-natal life. Time is also important in terms of exposure duration. Short time exposure to high doses can cause the classical features of manganism, whereas lifetime exposure to very low doses can result in neurodegenerative changes identifiable as parkinsonism.

Long term neurotoxicity of manganese has been extensively studied for the impact on motor coordination, but cognitive functions are also impacted and further studies are required to elucidate the mechanisms of toxicity. The elderly may be particularly susceptible to manganese as a product of long term exposure, impacting both motor and cognitive functionality. This suggestion builds upon evidence linking transitional metal dyshomeostasis and the accumulation of transition metals like iron in brain regions most commonly affected in neurodegenerative diseases. Manganese-induced dysregulation of cellular iron homeostasis appears to be a key factor of neuronal damage.

Glial activation induced by pre-exposure to manganese in juvenile animals may represent a "memory" able to promote neuroinflammation and neurological dysfunction in older age, especially upon further exposure to manganese or other neurotoxic agents. Neuroinflammation is also based on the interaction between microglia and astrocytes, which needs further study to better elucidate the role of glial cells in neuronal injury. Persistent neuroinflammation may be one of the reasons neurological symptoms worsen over time in individuals with high level exposure to manganese, and why damage to multiple brain regions and cell types is triggered by long term exposure to lower doses. Future research that integrates these diverse mechanisms of injury will be important both for development of better therapeutic interventions and for identifying populations that are most at risk from exposure to manganese.

References

1. S. F. Ali, H. M. Duhart, G. D. Newport, G. W. Lipe and W. Slikker, Jr., *Neurodegeneration*, 1995, **4**(3), 329–324.
2. P. Apostoli, R. Lucchini and L. Alessio, *Am J. Ind. Med.*, 2000, **37**, 283–290.
3. F. S. Archibald and C. Tyree, *Arch. Biochem. Biophys.*, 1987, **256**, 638–650.
4. M. Arora, A. Bradman, C. Austin, M. Vedar, N. Holland, B. Eskenazi and D. R. Smith., *Environ. Sci. Technol.*, 2012, **46**(9), 5118–5125.
5. J. L. Aschner and M. Aschner, Nutritional aspects of manganese homeostasis, *Mol. Aspects Med.*, 2005, **26**(4-5), 353–362.
6. M. Aschner, K. M. Erikson and D. C. Dorman, Manganese dosimetry: species differences and implications for neurotoxicity, *Crit. Rev. Toxicol.*, 2005, **35**, 1–32.
7. M. Aschner, K. M. Erikson, E. Herrero Hernández, E. H. Hernández and R. Tjalkens, Manganese and its role in Parkinson's disease: from transport to neuropathology, *Neuromolecular Med.*, 2009, **11**, 252–266.
8. ATSDR. Toxicological profile for Manganese (Draft for Public Comment). 2008; Atlanta, GA (U.S. Department of Health and Human Services, Public Service).
9. T. Z. Bikashvili, A. A. Shukakidze and G. I. Kiknadze, Changes in the ultrastructure of the rat cerebral cortex after oral doses of manganese chloride, *Neurosci. Behav. Physiol.*, 2001, **31**, 385–389.
10. E. D. Bird, A. H. Anton and B. Bullock, The effect of manganese inhalation on basal ganglia dopamine concentrations in rhesus monkey, *Neurotoxicology*, 1984, **5**(1), 59–65.

11. Blumberg, K. and Walsh, M. P. (2004) Status report concerning the use of MMT in gasoline International Council on Clean Transportation (ICCT). Available on line, http://www.healthandcleanair.org/mmt/icct.pdf.
12. D. J. Bonda, H. G. Lee, J. A. Blair, X. Zhu, G. Perry and M. A. Smith, Role of metal dyshomeostasis in Alzheimer's disease, *Metallomics*, 2011 Mar, **3**(3), 267–270.
13. M. Bouchard, F. Laforest, L. Vandelac, D. Bellinger and D. Mergler, Hair manganese and hyperactive behaviours: pilot study of school-age children exposed through tap water, *Environ Health Perspect*, 2007, **115**(1), 122–127.
14. M. F. Bouchard, S. Sauve, B. Barbeau, M. Legrand, M. E. Brodeur, T. Bouffard, E. Limoges, D. C. Bellinger and D. Mergler, Intellectual impairment in school-age children exposed to manganese from drinking water, *Environ Health Perspect*, 2011, **119**(1), 138–143.
15. R. Bowler, H. Roels, S. Nakagawa, M. Drezgic, E. Diamond, R. Park, W. Koller, R. Bowler, D. Mergler, D. Smith, R. Gwiazda and R. Doty, Dose-effect relations between manganese exposure and neurological, neuropsychological, and pulmonary function in confined space bridge welders, *J. Occup. Environ. Med.*, 2007, **64**(3), 167–177.
16. R. Brambilla, *et al.*, Transgenic inhibition of astroglial NF-kappa B improves functional outcome in experimental autoimmune encephalomyelitis by suppressing chronic central nervous system inflammation, *J Immunol*, 2009, **182**, 2628–2640.
17. E. P. Brouillet, *et al.*, Manganese injection into the rat striatum produces excitotoxic lesions by impairing energy metabolism, *Exp Neurol*, 1993, **120**(1), 89–94.
18. C. J. Brubaker, V. J. Schmithorst, E. N. Haynes, K. N. Dietrich, J. C. Egelhoff, D. M. Lindquist, B. P. Lanphear and K. M. Cecil, Altered myelination and axonal integrity in adults with childhood lead exposure: a diffusion tensor imaging study, *Neurotoxicology*, 2009 Nov, **30**(6), 867–875.
19. P. Calabresi, *et al.*, A synaptic mechanism underlying the behavioral abnormalities induced by manganese intoxication, *Neurobiol Dis*, 2001, **8**(3), 419–432.
20. D. B. Calne, N. S. Chu, C. C. Huang, C. S. Lu and W. Olanow, Manganism and idiopathic parkinsonism: similarities and differences, *Neurology*, 1994, **44**, 1583–1586.
21. S. Camandola and M. P. Mattson, NF-kappa B as a therapeutic target in neurodegenerative diseases, *Expert Opin Ther Targets*, 2007, **11**, 123–132.
22. E. Carreño-Müller, *et al.*, Thrombin induces in vivo degeneration of nigral dopaminergic neurones along with the activation of microglia, *J Neurochem*, 2003, **84**, 1201–1214.
23. J. Y. Chang and L. Z. Liu, Manganese potentiates nitric oxide production by microglia, *Brain Res Mol Brain Res*, 1999, **68**, 22–28.
24. D. Centonze, *et al.*, Impaired excitatory transmission in the striatum of rats chronically intoxicated with manganese, *Exp Neurol*, 2001, **172**(2), 469–476.

25. C.-J. Chen, *et al.*, Manganese modulates pro-inflammatory gene expression in activated glia, *Neurochem. Int*, 2006, **49**, 62–71.
26. J. Y. Chen, G. C. Tsao, Q. Zhao and W. Zheng, "Differential cytotoxicity of Mn(II) and Mn(III): special reference to mitochondrial [Fe-S] containing enzymes.", *Toxicol Appl Pharmacol*, 2001, **175**(2), 160–168.
27. C. J. Chen and S. L. Liao, Oxidative stress involves in astrocytic alterations induced by manganese, *Exp Neurol*, 2002, **175**(1), 216–225.
28. I.-H. Cho, *et al.*, Role of microglial IKKbeta in kainic acid-induced hippocampal neuronal cell death, *Brain*, 2008, **131**, 3019–3033.
29. P. J. Collipp, S. Y. Chen and S. Maitinsky, Manganese in infant formulas and learning disability, *Ann. Nutr. Metab.*, 1983, **27**, 488–494.
30. J. Couper, On the effects of black oxide of manganese when inhaled into the lungs, *Br Ann Med Pharmacol*, 1837, **1**, 41–42.
31. J. P. Covy, B. I. Giasson. α-Synuclein, leucine-rich repeat kinase-2, and manganese in the pathogenesis of Parkinson disease. *Neurotoxicology*. 2011 Oct, **32**(5), 622–629.
32. S. R. Criswell, J. S. Perlmutter, J. L. Huang, N. Golchin, H. P. Flores, A. Hobson, M. Aschner, K. M. Erikson, H. Checkoway and B. A. Racette, Basal ganglia intensity indices and diffusion weighted imaging in manganese-exposed welders, *Occup Environ Med*, 2012 Jun, **69**(6), 437–443.
33. S. R. Criswell, J. S. Perlmutter, T. O. Videen, S. M. Moerlein, H. P. Flores, A. M. Birke and B. A. Racette, Reduced uptake of [^{18}F]FDOPA PET in asymptomatic welders with occupational manganese exposure, *Neurology*, 2011 Apr 12, **76**(15), 1296–1301.
34. J. W. Critchfield and C. L. Keen, Manganese +2 exhibits dynamic binding to multiple ligands in human plasma, *Metabolism*, 1992, **41**, 1087–1092.
35. D. Crooks, M. Ghosh, M. Braun-Sommargren, T. Rouault and D. R. Smith, Manganese targets m-aconitase and activates iron regulatory protein 2 in AF5 GABAergic cells, *J. Neurosci. Res.*, 2007, **85**, 1797–1809.
36. D. Crooks, N. Welch and D. Smith, Low-level manganese exposure alters glutamate metabolism in GABAergic AF5 cells, *Neurotoxicology*, 2007, **28**(3), 548–554.
37. J. J. R. F. da Silva and R. J. P. Williams. The biological chemistry of the elements: the inorganic chemistry of life. Second Edition. Oxford University Press, Oxford England, New York. 2001, 575 pp.
38. L. Davidsson, B. Lonnerdal, B. Sandstrom, C. Kunz and C. L. Keen, Identification of transferrin as the major plasma carrier protein for manganese introduced orally or intravenously or after in vitro addition in the rat, *J Nutr*, 1989, **119**, 1461–1464.
39. J. Donaldson, Involvement of manganese in physiological and biochemical processes: an overview, *Neurotoxicology*, 1984 Spring, **5**(1), 1–3.
40. D. G. Ellingsen, E. Haug, R. J. Ulvik and Y. Thomassen, "Iron status in manganese alloy production workers." *J Appl Toxicol*, 2003, **23**(4), 239–247.

41. D. G. Ellingsen, R. Konstantinov, R. Bast-Pettersen, L. Merkurjeva, M. Chashchin, Y. Thomassen and V. Chashchin, A neurobehavioral study of current and former welders exposed to manganese, *Neurotoxicol*, 2008, **29**, 48–59.
42. EPA. U.S. (1978) Environmental Protection Agency. Federal Register 43: 41424–41429.
43. J. E. Ericson, F. M. Crinella, K. A. Clarke-Stewart, V. D. Allhusen, T. Chan and R. T. Robertson, Prenatal manganese levels linked to childhood behavioral disinhibition, *Neurotoxicol Teratol*, 2007, **29**(2), 181–187.
44. H. Eriksson, *et al.*, Receptor alterations in manganese intoxicated monkeys, *Arch Toxicol*, 1992, **66**(5), 359–364.
45. H. Eriksson, *et al.*, Manganese induced brain lesions in Macaca fascicularis as revealed by positron emission tomography and magnetic resonance imaging, *Arch Toxicol*, 1992, **66**(6), 403–407.
46. H. Eriksson, *et al.*, Effects of manganese oxide on monkeys as revealed by a combined neurochemical, histological and neurophysiological evaluation, *Arch Toxicol*, 1987, **61**(1), 46–52.
47. K. M. Erikson, *et al.*, Manganese inhalation by rhesus monkeys is associated with brain regional changes in biomarkers of neurotoxicity, *Toxicol Sci*, 2007, **97**(2), 459–466.
48. K. Erikson and M. Aschner, Manganese causes differential regulation of glutamate transporter (GLAST) taurine transporter and metallothionein in cultured rat astrocytes, *Neurotoxicology*, 2002, **23**(4-5), 595–602.
49. K. M. Erikson, R. L. Suber and M. Aschner, Glutamate/aspartate transporter (GLAST), taurine transporter and metallothionein mRNA levels are differentially altered in astrocytes exposed to manganese chloride, manganese phosphate or manganese sulfate, *Neurotoxicology*, 2002, **23**(3), 281–288.
50. J. M. Fell, *et al.*, Manganese toxicity in children receiving long-term parenteral nutrition, *Lancet*, 1996, **347**, 1218–1221.
51. N. M. Filipov, R. F. Seegal and D. A. Lawrence, Manganese potentiates in vitro production of proinflammatory cytokines and nitric oxide by microglia through a nuclear factor kappa B-dependent mechanism, *Toxicol Sci*, 2005, **84**, 139–148.
52. V. A. Fitsanakis, *et al.*, The effects of manganese on glutamate, dopamine and gamma-aminobutyric acid regulation, *Neurochem Int*, 2006, **48**(6-7), 426–433.
53. A. R. Flegal and D. R. Smith, Current needs for increased accuracy and precision in measurements of low levels of lead in blood, *Environ Res*, 1992, **58**, 125–133.
54. P. Galvani, P. Fumagalli and A. Santagostino, Vulnerability of mitochondrial complex I in PC12 cells exposed to manganese, *Eur J Pharmacol*, 1995, **293**, 377–383.
55. M. D. Garrick, K. G. Dolan, C. Horbinski, A. J. Ghio, D. Higgins, M. Porubcin, E. G. Moore, L. N. Hainsworth, J. N. Umbreit,

M. E. Conrad, L. Feng, A. Lis, J. A. Roth, S. Singleton and L. M. Garrick, DMT1: a mammalian transporter for multiple metals, *Biometals*, 2003, **16**, 41–54.

56. C. E. Gavin, K. K. Gunter and T. E. Gunter, "Manganese and calcium efflux kinetics in brain mitochondria. Relevance to manganese toxicity.", *Biochem J*, 1990, **266**(2), 329–334.
57. C. E. Gavin, K. K. Gunter and T. E. Gunter, "Mn2+ sequestration by mitochondria and inhibition of oxidative phosphorylation.", *Toxicol Appl Pharmacol*, 1992, **115**(1), 1–5.
58. C. E. Gavin, K. K. Gunter and T. E. Gunter, "Manganese and calcium transport in mitochondria: implications for manganese toxicity.", *Neurotoxicology*, 1999, **20**(2-3), 445–453.
59. S. Geivanidis, P. Pistikopoulos and Z. Samaras, Effect on exhaust emissions by the use of methylcyclopentadienyl manganese tricarbonyl (MMT) fuel additive and other lead replacement gasolines, *Sci. Total Environ*, 2003, **305**, 129–141.
60. A. M. Geller and H. Zenick, Aging and the environment: a research framework, *Environ Health Perspect*, 2005 Sep, **113**(9), 1257–1262.
61. D. A. Grimes, *et al.*, Translated mutation in the Nurr1 gene as a cause for Parkinson's disease, *Mov Disord*, 2006, **21**, 906–909.
62. T. R. Guilarte, APLP1, Alzheimer's-like pathology and neurodegeneration in the frontal cortex of manganese-exposed non-human primates, *Neurotoxicology*, 2010 Sep, **31**(5), 572–574.
63. T. R. Guilarte, *et al.*, Increased APLP1 expression and neurodegeneration in the frontal cortex of manganese-exposed non-human primates, *J Neurochem*, 2008, **105**, 1948–1959.
64. T. R. Guilarte, *et al.*, Nigrostriatal dopamine system dysfunction and subtle motor deficits in manganese-exposed non-human primates, *Exp Neurol*, 2006, **202**(2), 381–390.
65. T. R. Guilarte, *et al.*, Impairment of nigrostriatal dopamine neurotransmission by manganese is mediated by pre-synaptic mechanism(s): implications to manganese-induced parkinsonism, *J Neurochem*, 2008, **107**(5), 1236–1247.
66. K. K. Gunter, M. Aschner, L. M. Miller, R. Eliseev, J. Salter, K. Anderson and T. E. Gunter. "Determining the oxidation states of manganese in NT2 cells and cultured astrocytes." *Neurobiol Aging*, 2005.
67. K. K. Gunter, M. Aschner, L. M. Miller, R. Eliseev, J. Salter, K. Anderson, S. Hammond and T. E. Gunter, "Determining the oxidation states of manganese in PC12 and nerve growth factor-induced PC12 cells.", *Free Radic Biol Med*, 2005, **39**(2), 164–181.
68. R. Gwiazda, R. Lucchini and D. R. Smith, Adequacy and consistency of animal studies to evaluate the neurotoxicity of chronic low level manganese exposure in humans, *J Toxicol Env Health*, 2007, **70**, 594–605.
69. R. G. Gwiazda, D. Lee, J. Sheridan and D. R. Smith, Low cumulative manganese exposure affects striatal GABA but not dopamine, *Neurotoxicology*, 2002, **95**, 1–8.

70. D. Hafeman, P. Factor-Litvak, Z. Cheng, A. van Geen and H. Ahsan, Association between manganese exposure through drinking water and infant mortality in Bangladesh, *Environ Health Perspect*, 2007, **115**, 1107–1112.
71. R. Harding and G. Maritz, Maternal and fetal origins of lung disease in adulthood, *Semin Fetal Neonatal Med*, 2012 Apr, **17**(2), 67–72.
72. A. S. Hazell and M. D. Norenberg, Manganese decreases glutamate uptake in cultured astrocytes, *Neurochem Res*, 1997, **22**(12), 1443–1447.
73. P. He, D. H. Liu and G. Q. Zhang, [Effects of high-level-manganese sewage irrigation on children's neurobehavior], *Zhonghua Yu Fang Yi Xue Za Zhi*, 1994, **28**, 216–218.
74. Q. He, T. Du, X. Yu, A. Xie, N. Song, Q. Kang, J. Yu, L. Tan, J. Xie and H. Jiang, DMT1 polymorphism and risk of Parkinson's disease, *Neurosci Lett*, 2011, **501**(3), 128–131.
75. B. C. Henn, J. Kim, M. Wessling-Resnick, M. M. Téllez-Rojo, I. Jayawardene, A. S. Ettinger, M. Hernandez-Avila, J. Schwartz, D. C. Christiani, H. Hu and R. O. Wright, Associations of iron metabolism genes with blood manganese levels: a population-based study with validation data from animal models, *Environ Health*, 2011, **10**, 97.
76. E. M. Herndon, L. Jin and S. L. Brantley, Soils reveal widespread manganese enrichment from industrial inputs, *Environ Sci Technol*, 2011, **45**(1), 241–247.
77. A. B. Hill, The environment and disease: Association or causation?, *Proceed Roy Soc Medicine – London*, 1965, **58**, 295–300.
78. E. C. Hirsch and S. Hunot, Neuroinflammation in Parkinson's disease: a target for neuroprotection?, *Lancet Neurol*, 2009, **8**, 382–397.
79. HSDB, Hazardous Substances Data Bank. (1998) National Institutes of Health, National Library of Medicine, Bethesda, MD.
80. E. Huang, W. Y. Ong and J. R. Connor, Distribution of divalent metal transporter-1 in the monkey basal ganglia, *Neuroscience*, 2004, **128**(3), 487–496.
81. X. Huang, R. D. Moir, R. E. Tanzi, A. I. Bush and J. T. Rogers, Redox-active metals, oxidative stress, and Alzheimer's disease pathology, *Ann N Y Acad Sci*, 2004 Mar, **1012**, 153–163.
82. H. K. Hudnell, Effects from environmental Mn exposures: a review of the evidence from non-occupational exposure studies, *Neurotoxicology*, 1999, **20**(2-3), 379–397.
83. Inside fuels. (2004) "As MMT gasoline additive use in Canada plummets, use in U.S. may be spreading". *Inside fuels & Vehicles*. Vol. 3, no. 13. Inside Washington Publishers, Washington, DC.
84. T. Jursa and D. R. Smith, Ceruloplasmin alters the tissue disposition and neurotoxicity of manganese, but not its loading onto transferrin, *Toxicol Sci*, 2009 Jan, **107**(1), 182–193.
85. D. Kaur, J. Peng, S. J. Chinta, S. Rajagopalan, D. A. Di Monte, R. A. Cherny and J. K. Andersen, Increased murine neonatal iron intake

results in Parkinson-like neurodegeneration with age, *Neurobiol Aging*, 2007 Jun, **28**(6), 907–913.

86. C. Kern, G. Stanwood and D. R. Smith, Pre-weaning manganese exposure causes hyperactivity, disinhibition, and spatial learning and memory deficits associated with altered dopamine receptor and transporter levels, *Synapse*, 2010, **64**, 363–378.
87. C. Kern and D. R. Smith, Pre-weaning Mn exposure leads to prolonged astrocyte activation and lasting effects on the dopaminergic system in adult male rats, *Synapse*, 2011, **65**(6), 532–544.
88. Khan, K. *et al.* Manganese Exposure from Drinking Water and Children's Classroom Behavior in Bangladesh. Environ Health Perspect (2011). doi:10.1289/ehp.1003397.
89. W. G. Kim, *et al.*, Regional difference in susceptibility to lipopolysaccharide-induced neurotoxicity in the rat brain: role of microglia, *J Neurosci*, 2000, **20**, 6309–6316.
90. Y. Kim, K. S. Jeong, H. J. Song, J. J. Lee, J. H. Seo, G. C. Kim, H. J. Lee, H. J. Kim, J. H. Ahn, S. J. Park, S. H. Kim, Y. J. Kwon and Y. Chang, Altered white matter microstructural integrity revealed by voxel-wise analysis of diffusion tensor imaging in welders with manganese exposure, *Neurotoxicol*, 2011, **32**(1), 100–109.
91. C. L. Kwik-Uribe, S. Reaney, Z. Zhu and D. Smith, "Alterations in cellular IRP-dependent iron regulation by in vitro manganese exposure in undifferentiated PC12 cells.", *Brain Res*, 2003, **973**(1), 1–15.
92. C. Kwik-Uribe and D. R. Smith, Temporal responses in the disruption of iron regulation by manganese, *J. Neurosci. Res.*, 2006, **83**, 1601–1610.
93. B. P. Lanphear, R. Hornung, J. Khoury, K. Yolton, P. Baghurst, D. C. Bellinger, R. L. Canfield, K. N. Dietrich, R. Bornschein, T. Greene, S. J. Rothenberg, H. L. Needleman, L. Schnaas, G. Wasserman, J. Graziano and R. Roberts, Low-level environmental lead exposure and children's intellectual function: an international pooled analysis, *Environ Health Perspect*, 2005, **13**(7), 894–899.
94. W. Le, *et al.*, Decreased NURR1 gene expression in patients with Parkinson's disease, *J. Neurol. Sci*, 2008, **273**, 29–33.
95. B. K. Lee and Y. Kim. Relationship between blood manganese and blood pressure in the Korean general population according to KNHANES 2008. Environ Res. 2011 Aug, 111(6), 797–803. Epub 2011 May 23.
96. D. W. Lee and J. K. Andersen, Iron elevations in the aging Parkinsonian brain: a consequence of impaired iron homeostasis?, *J Neurochem*, 2010 Jan, **112**(2), 332–339.
97. B. S. Levy and W. J. Nassetta, Neurologic effects of manganese in humans: a review, *Int J Occup Environ Health*, 2003, **9**, 153–163.
98. G. J. Li, Q. Zhao and W. Zheng, "Alteration at translational but not transcriptional level of transferrin receptor expression following manganese exposure at the blood-CSF barrier in vitro.", *Toxicol Appl Pharmacol*, 2005, **205**(2), 188–200.

99. G. T. Liberatore, *et al.*, Inducible nitric oxide synthase stimulates dopaminergic neurodegeneration in the MPTP model of Parkinson disease, *Nat Med*, 1999, **5**, 1403–1409.
100. A. C. Liu, B. S. Heinrichs and R. M. Leach, Jr. Influence of manganese deficieny on the characteristics of proteoglycans of avian epiphyscal growth plate cartilage, *Poult-Sci*, 1994, **73**(5), 663–669.
101. X. Liu, K. A. Sullivan, J. E. Madl, M. Legare and R. B. Tjalkens, Manganese-induced neurotoxicity: the role of astroglial-derived nitric oxide in striatal interneuron degeneration, *Toxicol Sci*, 2006, **91**, 521–531.
102. X. Liu, *et al.*, NF-kappaB-dependent production of nitric oxide by astrocytes mediates apoptosis in differentiated PC12 neurons following exposure to manganese and cytokines, *Brain Res Mol Brain Res*, 2005, **141**, 39–47.
103. R. V. Lloyd, Mechanism of the manganese-catalyzed autoxidation of dopamine, *Chem Res Toxicol*, 1995, **8**, 111–116.
104. R. Lucchini, L. Selis, D. Folli, P. Apostoli, A. Mutti, O. Vanoni, A. Iregren and L. Alessio, Neurobehavioral effects of manganese in workers from a ferroalloy plant after temporary cessation of exposure, *Scand J Work Environ Health*, 1995, **21**(2), 143–149.
105. R. Lucchini, E. Bergamaschi, A. Smargiassi, D. Festa and P. Apostoli, Motor function, olfactory threshold, and hematological indices in manganese-exposed ferroalloy workers, *Environ Res*, 1997, **73**(1-2), 175–180.
106. R. Lucchini, P. Apostoli, C. Perrone, D. Placidi, E. Albini, P. Migliorati, D. Mergler, M. P. Sassine, S. Palmi and L. Alessio, Long-term exposure to "low levels" of manganese oxides and neurofunctional changes in ferroalloy workers, *Neurotoxicology*, 1999, **20**(2-3), 287–297.
107. R. Lucchini, L. Benedetti, S. Borghesi, S. Garattini, G. Parrinello and L. Alessio, Exposure to neurotoxic metals and prevalence of parkinsonian syndrome in the area of Brescia, *G Ital Med Lav Ergon*, 2003, **25**(Suppl(3)), 88–89.
108. R. G. Lucchini, and Y. Kim (2009) Health effects of manganese. In: M. Vojtisek, R. Prakash (eds) Metals and Neurotoxicity. JALGAON: Society for science and environment, ISBN/ISSN: 81-85543-09-7, pp. 119–147.
109. R. G. Lucchini, C. J. Martin and B. C. Doney, From manganism to manganese-induced parkinsonism: a conceptual model based on the evolution of exposure, *Neuromolecular Med*, 2009, **11**(4), 311–321.
110. R. G. Lucchini, S. Guazzetti, S. Zoni, F. Donna, S. Peter, A. Zacco, M. Salmistraro, E. Bontempi, N. J. Zimmerman, and D. R. Smith. Tremor, olfactory and motor changes in Italian adolescents exposed to historical ferro-manganese emission. *Neurotoxicology*. 2012 Jan 31. [Epub ahead of print].
111. A. P. Marreilha Dos Santos, M. Lopes Santos, M. C. Batoréu and M. Aschner, Prolactin is a peripheral marker of manganese neurotoxicity, *Brain Res*, 2011 Mar, **25**(1382), 282–290.

112. C. Martin, Manganese neurotoxicity: Connecting the dots along the continuum of dysfunction, *Neurotoxicol*, 2006, **27**, 347–349.
113. S. A. McDougall, *et al.*, Postnatal manganese exposure alters dopamine transporter function in adult rats: Potential impact on nonassociative and associative processes, *Neuroscience*, 2008, **154**(2), 848–860.
114. P. McLaughlin, *et al.*, Proteomic analysis of microglial contribution to mouse strain-dependent dopaminergic neurotoxicity, *Glia*, 2006, **53**, 567–582.
115. J. A. Menezes-Filho, O. Novaes Cde, J. C. Moreira, P. N. Sarcinelli and D. Mergler, Elevated manganese and cognitive performance in school-aged children and their mothers, *Environ Res*, 2011, **111**(1), 156–163.
116. D. Mergler, *et al.*, Manganese neurotoxicity, a continuum of dysfunction: results from a community based study, *Neurotoxicology*, 1999, **20**(2-3), 327–342.
117. D. Mergler, G. Huel, R. Bowler, A. Iregren, S. Belanger, M. Baldwin, R. Tardif, A. Smargiassi and L. Martin, Nervous system dysfunction among workers with long-term exposure to manganese, *Environ Res*, 1994, **64**(2), 151–180.
118. D. Mergler and M. Baldwin, Early manifestations of manganese neurotoxicity in humans: An update, *Env Res*, 1997, **73**, 92–100.
119. D. B. Milne, R. L. Sims and N. V. Ralston, Manganese content of the cellular components of blood, *Clin Chem*, 1990, **36**, 450–452.
120. R. M. Molina, S. Phattanarudee, J. Kim, K. Thompson, M. Wessling-Resnick, T. J. Maher and J. D. Brain, Maternal Ingestion of Mn and Pbby rats during and after pregnancy alters iron metabolism and behavior in offspring, *Neurotoxicology*, 2011, **32**, 413–422.
121. S. Montes, A. Schilmann, H. Riojas-Rodriguez, Y. Rodriguez-Agudelo, R. Solis-Vivanco, S. L. Rodriguez-Dozal, L. A. Tristan-López and C. Rios, Serum prolactin rises in Mexican school children exposed to airborne manganese, *Environ Res*, 2011, **111**(8), 1302–1308.
122. J. A. Moreno, *et al.*, Age-dependent susceptibility to manganese-induced neurological dysfunction, *Toxicological Sciences*, 2009, **112**, 394–404.
123. J. A. Moreno, K. M. Streifel, K. A. Sullivan, M. E. Legare and R. B. Tjalkens, Developmental exposure to manganese increases adult susceptibility to inflammatory activation of glia and neuronal protein nitration, *Toxicological Sciences*, 2009, **112**, 405–415.
124. J. A. Moreno, K. A. Sullivan, D. L. Carbone, W. H. Hanneman and R. B. Tjalkens, Manganese potentiates nuclear factor-kappaB-dependent expression of nitric oxide synthase 2 in astrocytes by activating soluble guanylate cyclase and extracellular responsive kinase signaling pathways, *J Neurosci Res*, 2008, **86**, 2028–2038.
125. Mukhopadhyay S, Bachert C, Smith DR, Linstedt AD. Manganese-induced trafficking and turnover of the cis-Golgi glycoprotein GPP130. *Mol Biol Cell* 21: 1282–1292, 2010 (E-pub: Feb 3, 2010).
126. L. Mutkus, *et al.*, The in vitro uptake of glutamate in GLAST and GLT-1 transfected mutant CHO-K1 cells is inhibited by manganese, *Biol Trace Elem Res*, 2005, **107**(3), 221–230.

127. J. E. Myers, J. teWaterNaude, M. Fourie, H. B. Zogoe, I. Naik, P. Theodorou, H. Tassel, A. Daya and M. L. Thompson, Nervous system effects of occupational manganese exposure on South African manganese mineworkers, *Neurotoxicology*, 2003 Aug, **24**(4-5), 649–656.
128. J. E. Myers, M. L. Thompson, I. Naik, P. Theodorou, E. Esswein, H. Tassell, A. Daya, K. Renton, A. Spies, J. Paicker, T. Young, M. Jeebhay, S. Ramushu, L. London and D. J. Rees, The utility of biological monitoring for manganese in ferroalloy smelter workers in South Africa, *Neurotoxicology*, 2003, **24**(6), 875–883.
129. H. Nakano, *et al.*, Differential regulation of IkappaB kinase alpha and beta by two upstream kinases, NF-kappaB-inducing kinase and mitogen-activated protein kinase/ERK kinase kinase-1, *Proc Natl Acad Sci USA*, 1998, **95**, 3537–3542.
130. National Research Council (1989) Recommended dietary allowances. National Research Council. Washington DC. pp. 231–235.
131. National Research Council. Measuring Lead Exposure in Infants, Children, and Other Sensitive Populations; National Academy Press: Washington D.C., 1993.
132. G. Nelson, S. R. Criswell, J. Zhang, J. Murray, and B. A. Racette. Research capacity development in South African manganese mines to bridge exposure and neuropathologic outcomes. Neurotoxicology. 2012 Jan 31. [Epub ahead of print].
133. K. Pantopoulos, "Iron metabolism and the IRE/IRP regulatory system: an update.", *Ann N Y Acad Sci*, 2004, **1012**, 1–13.
134. A. Pentschew, F. F. Ebner and R. M. Kovatch, Experimental manganese encephalopathy in monkeys. A preliminary report, *J Neuropathol Exp Neurol*, 1963, **22**, 488–499.
135. R. O. Pihl and M. Parkes, Hair element content in learning disabled children, *Science*, 1977, **198**, 204–206.
136. J. L. Rapoport and N. Gogtay, Brain neuroplasticity in healthy, hyper-active and psychotic children: insights from neuroimaging, *Neuropsychopharmacology*, 2008, **33**, 181–197.
137. S. Reaney, C. Kwik-Uribe and D. Smith, Manganese Oxidation State and Its Implications for Toxicity, *Chem. Res. Toxicol.*, 2002, **15**, 1119–1126.
138. S. H. Reaney and D. R. Smith, Manganese oxidation state mediates toxicity in PC12 cells, *Toxicol. Appl. Pharmacol.*, 2005, **205**(3), 271–281.
139. S. Reaney, G. Bench and D. Smith, Brain accumulation and toxicity of Mn(II) and Mn(III) exposures, *Tox. Sci*, 2006, **93**(1), 114–124.
140. C. M. Reichel, *et al.*, Postnatal manganese exposure attenuates cocaine-induced locomotor activity and reduces dopamine transporters in adult male rats, *Neurotoxicology and Teratology*, 2006, **28**(3), 323–332.
141. H. Riojas-Rodriguez, R. Solis-Vivanco, A. Schilmann, S. Montes, S. Rodriguez, C. Rios and Y. Rodríguez-Agudelo, Intellectual function in Mexican children living in a mining area and environmentally exposed to manganese, *Environ Health Perspect*, 2010, **118**(10), 1465–1470.

142. J. F. Risher, G. D. Todd, D. Meyer and C. L. Zunker, The elderly as a sensitive population in environmental exposures: making the case, *Rev Environ Contam Toxicol*, 2010, **207**, 95–157.
143. H. Rollin, A. Mathee, J. Levin, P. Theodorou and F. Wewers, Blood manganese concentrations among first-grade schoolchildren in two South African cities, *Env Res*, 2005, **97**(1), 93–99.
144. H. Roels, R. Lauwerys, J. P. Buchet, P. Genet, M. J. Sarhan, I. Hanotiau, M. de Fays, A. Bernard and D. Stanescu, Epidemiological survey among workers exposed to manganese: effects on lung, central nervous system, and some biological indices, *Am J Ind Med*, 1987, **11**(3), 307–327.
145. H. A. Roels, P. Ghyselen, J. P. Buchet, E. Cculemans and R. R. Lauwerys, Assessment of the permissible exposure level to manganese in workers exposed to manganese dioxide dust, *Br J Ind Med*, 1992, **49**(1), 25–34.
146. H. A. Roels, M. I. Ortega Eslava, E. Ceulemans, A. Robert and D. Lison, Prospective study on the reversibility of neurobehavioral effects in workers exposed to manganese dioxide, *Neurotoxicology*, 1999 Apr-Jun, **20**(2-3), 255–71.
147. H. A. Roels, R. M. Bowler, Y. Kim, B. Claus Henn, D. Mergler, P. Hoet, V. V. Gocheva, D. C. Bellinger, R. O. Wright, M. G. Harris, Y. Chang, M. F. Bouchard, H. Riojas-Rodriguez, J. A. Menezes-Filho and M. M. Téllez-Rojo, Manganese exposure and cognitive deficits: A growing concern for manganese neurotoxicity, *Neurotoxicology*, 2012 Apr, 3. [Epub ahead of print].
148. J. A. Roth and M. D. Garrick, Iron interactions and other biological reactions mediating the physiological and toxic actions of manganese, *Biochem Pharmacol*, 2003, **66**, 1–13.
149. K. Saijo, *et al.*, A Nurr1/CoREST pathway in microglia and astrocytes protects dopaminergic neurons from inflammation-induced death, *Cell*, 2009, **137**, 47–59.
150. J. Salazar, N. Mena, S. Hunot, A. Prigent, D. Alvarez-Fischer, M. Arredondo, C. Duyckaerts, V. Sazdovitch, L. Zhao, L. M. Garrick, M. T. Nunez, M. D. Garrick, R. Raisman-Vozari and E. C. Hirsch, Divalent metal transporter 1 (DMT1) contributes to neurodegeneration in animal models of Parkinson's disease, *Proc Natl Acad Sci U S A*, 2008, **105**(47), 18578–18583.
151. J. Schroeter, D. Dorman, M. Yoon, A. Nong, M. Taylor, M. E. Andersen and H. Clewell, Application of a Multi-Route Physiologically-Based Pharmacokinetic Model for Manganese to Evaluate Dose-Dependent Neurological Effects in Monkeys, *Toxicol Sci*, 2012 Jun, 21. [Epub ahead of print].
152. D. R. Smith, R. Gwiazda, H. Roels, R. Park, R. Bowler, P. Apostoli and R. Lucchini, Biomarkers of Mn exposure in humans, *Am. J. Ind. Med.*, 2007, **50**(11), 801–811.
153. F. Spadoni, *et al.*, Selective vulnerability of pallidal neurons in the early phases of manganese intoxication, *Exp Brain Res*, 2000, **135**(4), 544–51.

154. M. Spranger, *et al.*, Manganese augments nitric oxide synthesis in murine astrocytes: a new pathogenetic mechanism in manganism?, *Exp Neurol*, 1998, **149**, 277–283.
155. K. Sriram, G. X. Lin, A. M. Jefferson, J. R. Roberts, R. S. Chapman, B. T. Chen, J. M. Soukup, A. J. Ghio and J. M. Antonini, Dopaminergic neurotoxicity following pulmonary exposure to manganese-containing welding fumes, *Arch Toxicol*, 2010, **84**(7), 521–540.
156. K. M. Streifel, J. A. Moreno, W. H. Hanneman, M. E. Legare and R. B. Tjalkens, Gene Deletion of nos2 Protects Against Manganese-Induced Neurological Dysfunction in Juvenile Mice, *Toxicological Sciences*, 2012, **126**, 183–192.
157. L. Takser, D. Mergler, G. Hellier, J. Sahuquillo and G. Huel, Manganese, monoamine metabolite levels at birth, and child psychomotor development, *Neurotoxicol*, 2003, **24**(4-5), 667–674.
158. K. Thompson, R. M. Molina, T. Donaghey, J. E. Schwob, J. D. Brain and M. Wessling-Resnick, Olfactory uptake of manganese requires DMT1 and is enhanced by anemia, *FASEB J*, 2007, **21**, 223–230.
159. R. B. Tjalkens, *et al.*, The peroxisome proliferator-activated receptor-gamma agonist 1,1-bis(3'-indolyl)-1-(p-trifluoromethylphenyl)methane suppresses manganese-induced production of nitric oxide in astrocytes and inhibits apoptosis in cocultured PC12 cells, *J Neurosci Res*, 2008, **86**, 618–629.
160. G. Tsivgoulis, I. Heliopoulos, K. Vadikolias, P. Argyropoulou and C. Piperidou, Ingestion of gasoline in a suicide attempt: an uncommon cause of bilateral basal ganglia T1 hyperintensities, *Neurol Sci*, 2011, **32**(4), 739–740.
161. J. J. Villafranca and A. S. Mildvan, "The mechanism of aconitase action. II. Magnetic resonance studies of the complexes of enzyme, manganese(II), iron(II), and substrates.", *J Biol Chem*, 1971, **246**(18), 5791–5798.
162. M. P. Walsh, The global experience with lead in gasoline and the lessons we should apply to the use of MMT, *Am J Ind Med*, 2007, **50**(11), 853–860.
163. G. A. Wasserman, X. Liu, F. Parvez, H. Ahsan, D. Levy, P. Factor-Litvak, J. Kline, A. van Geen, V. Slavkovich, N. J. LoIacono, Z. Cheng, Y. Zheng and J. H. Graziano, Water manganese exposure and children's intellectual function in Araihazar, Bangladesh, *Environ Health Perspect*, 2006, **114**(1), 124–129.
164. A. W. Willis, B. A. Evanoff, M. Lian, A. Galarza, A. Wegrzyn, M. Schootman and B. A. Racette, Metal emissions and urban incident Parkinson disease: a community health study of Medicare beneficiaries by using geographic information systems, *Am J Epidemiol*, 2010 Dec 15, **172**(12), 1357–1363.
165. R. O. Wright, C. Amarasiriwardena, A. D. Woolf, R. Jim and D. C. Bellinger, Neuropsychological correlates of hair arsenic, manganese, and cadmium levels in school-age children residing near a hazardous waste site, *Neurotoxicology*, 2006, **27**(2), 210–216.

166. M. Yamada, *et al.*, Chronic manganese poisoning: a neuropathological study with determination of manganese distribution in the brain, *Acta Neuropathol*, 1986, **70**, 273–278.
167. W. Zheng, S. Ren and J. H. Graziano, "Manganese inhibits mitochondrial aconitase: a mechanism of manganese neurotoxicity." *Brain Res*, 1998, **799**(2), 334–342.
168. W. Zheng, Q. Zhao, V. Slavkovich, M. Aschner and J. H. Graziano, Alteration of iron homeostasis following chronic exposure to manganese in rats, *Brain Res*, 1999, **833**(1), 125–132.
169. W. Zheng and Q. Zhao, Iron overload following manganese exposure in cultured neuronal, but not neuroglial cells, *Brain Res*, 2001, **897**(1–2), 175–179.
170. S. Zoni, G. Bonetti and R. G. Lucchini, Olfactory functions at the intersection between environmental exposure to manganese and parkinsonism, *J Trace Elem Med Biol*, 2012, **26**(2-3), 179–182.
171. C. Zwingmann, D. Leibfritz and A. S. Hazell, "Energy metabolism in astrocytes and neurons treated with manganese: relation among cell-specific energy failure, glucose metabolism, and intercellular trafficking using multinuclear NMR-spectroscopic analysis." *J Cereb Blood Flow Metab*, 2003, **23**(6), 756–771.
172. C. Zwingmann, D. Leibfritz and A. S. Hazell, "Brain energy metabolism in a sub-acute rat model of manganese neurotoxicity: an ex vivo nuclear magnetic resonance study using [1-13C]glucose." *Neurotoxicology*, 2004, **25**(4), 573–587.

CHAPTER 7

The Role of Persistent Organic Pollutants and Plastic-Associated Chemicals in Cardiovascular Disease and Metabolic Syndrome

LARS LIND[a] AND P. MONICA LIND*[b]

[a] Dept of Medical Sciences, Uppsala University, University Hospital Uppsala 751 85, Sweden; [b] Occupational and Environmental Medicine, Uppsala University, Ulleråkersvägen 40 Uppsala 751 85, Sweden
*E-mail: Monica.Lind@medsci.uu.se

7.1 Introduction

Cardiovascular (CV) diseases are the main cause of death in high-income countries. As previously low-income countries like China and India become industrialized, the incidence rates of CV diseases are rising. Among CV diseases, the major killers are myocardial infarction, stroke, and heart failure. All of these diseases are mainly encountered in the elderly.

The incidence rate for myocardial infarction peaked in the 1970s, and thereafter a decline has been noted in high-income countries.[1,2] This has been attributed to a reduction in LDL-cholesterol levels and a drop in smoking prevalence in the last few decades. A reduction in stroke incidence has also been seen in the high-income countries,[3,4] although this is less than the decline seen

Issues in Toxicology No. 16
Aging and Vulnerability to Environmental Chemicals: Age-related Disorders and their Origins in Environmental Exposures
Edited by Bernard Weiss

Published by the Royal Society of Chemistry, www.rsc.org

for myocardial infarction. The major risk factor for stroke is hypertension, which is more recognized today than some decades ago.

Regarding heart failure, community-based cohorts have presented conflicting results. Data from the Framingham study suggests that the incidence of heart failure may be declining among women, but not men.[5] In contrast, an analysis of data from Olmsted County, Minnesota, implied that the incidence of heart failure has remained stable during the past 20 years in both men and women and that men and patients aged 70 years or younger have experienced disproportionate gains in survival.[6] More recently, even an increase in incidence was observed in an elderly, community-based, managed-care population followed from the early 1970s to the early 1990s.[7] Previous myocardial infarction and hypertension are the major risk factors for heart failure.

Clustering of several CV risk factors in the same individual is nowadays generally denoted metabolic syndrome (MetS). Although described in general terms as early as the 1930s, the MetS was described in its present form by separate groups, including us, in 1988.[8,9] Several definitions of the MetS exist, but in epidemiology, the NCEP/ATP III-criteria are the most commonly used.[10] By this definition, a subject with the MetS should show at least three deviations out of five in visceral obesity, blood pressure, high triglyceride levels, low HDL, and impaired glucose tolerance. This is generally seen in 15–30% of populations in Europe and the US.[11] Although the role of insulin resistance as the underlying pathophysiological driver of metabolic syndrome was emphasized in the past,[9] it is today generally believed that visceral accumulation of adipose tissue is the main driver of metabolic syndrome. The usefulness of metabolic syndrome as a separate entity has been questioned. This is because it has been shown that the magnitude of risk of future cardiovascular events associated with having metabolic syndrome is not greater than the sum of the risks associated with the individual components of the syndrome.[12,13] Thus, although metabolic syndrome does not include any unique information in terms of risk prediction, it is useful as a descriptive term for patients with multiple risk factors.

As the prevalence of the MetS is increasing in both high and low-income countries, it is anticipated that the incidence rates of myocardial infarction and heart failure will start to increase again due to the higher burden of risk factors that will accompany the obesity epidemic seen worldwide.

The number of man-made chemicals used in our environment has increased dramatically during recent decades. More than 100 000 chemical substances are registered in the EU (http://www.echa.europa.eu/). Although the toxicity of certain pollutants, like lead and arsenic, has been known for years, potential deleterious health effects of most other substances are largely unknown.

One area of major concern is that several of the high-volume produced chemicals could interfere with the basal hormonal systems governing fundamental homeostatic systems in our bodies. Therefore, the term, "endocrine disruption" has been coined to describe this general action of some environmental contaminants. Actions of environmental contaminants on the reproductive system, the glucocorticoid hormones and thyroid hormones have been described, and have resulted in the ban of dichlorodiphenyltrichloroethane (DDT) and polychlorinated biphenyls (PCBs) in many parts of the world during the 1970s and 1980s.

Many of the compounds regarded as endocrine disruptors are highly lipophilic chemicals that accumulate in adipose tissues, resulting in a long half-life. They are collectively named persistent organic pollutants (POPs), and a number of these chemicals have been identified as deleterious to health and have been listed at the Stockholm convention. Amongst those listed are organochlorine pesticides, such as hexachlorobenzene (HCB) and DDT, various chlordanes, PCBs, dioxins, brominated flame retardants, and fluorinated compounds.

A group of less persistent organic chemicals that has received attention in recent years is plastic associated compounds (PACs). Amongst these, the health effects of bisphenol A (BPA) have been highlighted, as well as that of different phthalates. These chemicals have a considerably shorter half-life than the POPs, but could nevertheless act as endocrine disrupters. Since humans are exposed to these chemicals on a daily basis, measurable circulating levels of BPA, as well as phthalate metabolites, are seen in most individuals.[14] However, since analytic capacity for large-scale measurements of PACs has only been available for a few years, data on PACs are limited compared to data on POPs.

The present review will focus on evidences in humans of a relationship between POP and PAC exposure and metabolic syndrome and cardiovascular disease. We will mainly consider data from cross-sectional and longitudinal studies and population-based studies, but will also consider evidences from occupational studies, geographical studies, and accidents, if appropriate. A more extensive review on this topic has recently been published.[15]

7.2 Metabolic Syndrome

The term, 'metabolic syndrome' is a descriptive term regarding subjects with a clustering of cardio-metabolic risk factors. Although described by a couple of groups in 1988,[8,9] the first uniform definition of the syndrome came in a WHO report in 1998.[16] This definition of the syndrome was much governed by the thought that insulin resistance is the driver of the syndrome. Consequently, insulin resistance was amongst the major criteria of that definition. Since insulin resistance is very seldom evaluated in clinical practice, this definition of the syndrome has never been frequently used.

In 2001, the NCEP/ATPIII panel suggested a different definition of the syndrome, based on the idea that visceral obesity is the main driver of the syndrome[10] (See Table 7.1).

This definition uses five criteria commonly used in clinical practice: blood pressure, fasting blood glucose, serum triglycerides, HDL-cholesterol, and waist circumference; metabolic syndrome is considered to be present if a subject

Table 7.1 Definition of the metabolic syndrome using the NECP/ATP III criteria (NECP 2001). The metabolic syndrome is considered to be present if 3 or more of the 5 criteria presented in the table are present.

Blood pressure	>130/85 mm Hg or antihypertensive treatment
Fasting blood glucose	>5.6 mmol L^{-1}
Serum triglycerides	>1.7 mmol L^{-1}
Waist circumference	>102 cm in men and >88 cm in women
HDL-cholesterol	<1.0 mmol L^{-1} in men and <1.3 L^{-1} in women

shows deviations in three or more of these five criteria (see Table 7.1 for details regarding cut-off limits). This definition of metabolic syndrome has been used extensively in clinical research. Although other definitions have been proposed, the so-called NCEP-definition was widely accepted following some minor modifications.

Only a couple of studies have evaluated whetehr POPs or PACs are related to metabolic syndrome. Both of these studies used the US-based National Health and Nutrition Examination Survey (NHANES) study as the evaluated sample. The NHANES is a program of studies designed to assess the health and nutritional status of adults and children in the US. For more than a decade, the survey has examined a nationally representative sample of about 5000 persons each year. These persons are located in counties across the country, 15 of which are visited each year. NHANES is a cross-sectional survey and does not include follow-up data on future diseases.

Lee and co-workers studied the relationships between POPs and the prevalence of metabolic syndrome in the NHANES 1999–2002 examination cycles.[17] They used data on 19 different POPs in 721 subjects who were free from diabetes in a cross-sectional fashion. The POPs were divided into 5 classes: polychlorinated dibenzo-p-dioxins (PCDDs), polychlorinated dibenzofurans (PCDFs), dioxin-like PCBs, non-dioxin-like PCBs, and OC pesticides. Almost a quarter (24%) of the population showed metabolic syndrome. The most striking association between POPs and metabolic syndrome was seen for the OC pesticides. In this case, subjects in the fourth quartile of OC pesticide levels showed more than a five-fold increased risk of having metabolic syndrome compared to subjects with the lowest levels [OR 5.3 (95% CI 2.5–11.3), $p<0.01$] following adjustment for multiple confounding variables (age, sex, race, poverty index, cigarette smoking, serum cotinine, alcohol consumption, and exercise). Additional adjustment for BMI only marginally affected the risk. Associations between metabolic syndrome and dioxin-like PCBs and non-dioxin-like PCBs were also observed, although the increased risk was lower for these POPs (OR 2.0–2.2). One striking finding for the PCBs was that the maximal risk was generally not found in the highest quartile but rather in the 3rd quartile. Especially for the non-dioxin PCBs, the risk was not increased in those with the highest levels, suggesting non-monotonic relationships.

The authors also investigated how the five different components of the syndrome were related to the POP levels. An increased waist circumference was mainly related to non-dioxin PCBs and OC pesticides. Increased serum triglyceride levels were mainly related to dioxin-like PCBs and OC pesticides, while only OC pesticide levels were related to low HDL-cholesterol. Elevated blood pressure was only related to PCDFs, while increased fasting glucose was mainly related to non-dioxin PCBs and OC pesticides.

Thus this important study disclosed that POPs are related to metabolic syndrome, that different components of metabolic syndrome might be associated with different types of POPs, and that the relationships might not always be linear, suggesting that low-dose effects of POPs might be present.

The same research team also conducted a case-control study of 50 subjects with metabolic syndrome and 50 age and sex-matched healthy controls randomly selected from a health survey conducted in South Korea.[18] Eight OC pesticides were evaluated. Significantly higher levels of beta-hexachlorocyclohexane and heptachlor epoxide were found in the subjects with metabolic syndrome compared to the controls ($p<0.01$). Also, trans-nonachlor tended to be elevated amongst the subjects with metabolic syndrome, while no major differences were seen for DDT, DDE or hexachlorobenzene. Beta-hexachlorocyclohexane was mainly related to elevated blood pressure, while heptachlor epoxide levels were related to all of the five components of metabolic syndrome. In this case, the associations were no longer significant when adjusted for BMI.

Originating from the same research group, a report regarding the associations between brominated flame retardants and metabolic syndrome using data from the NHANES 2003–2004 examination cycle has also been published.[19] They used 637 subjects in this cross-sectional analysis, and studied six different brominated flame retardants: polybrominated biphenyl 153 (PBB 153) and the polybrominated diphenyl ethers 28 (PBDE 28), 47, 99, 100, and 153. In the sample, 37% showed metabolic syndrome and mean age was 50 years. PBB 153 levels were associated with an increased risk of having metabolic syndrome (OR 3.1 (95% CI 1.4–6.5), $p<0.01$) following adjustment for age, sex, race, poverty index, cigarette smoking, serum cotinine, alcohol consumption, and exercise. Also, PBDE 153 levels showed a similar relationship, although not as powerful (OR 2.5). Just as observed for some of the POPs, non-monotonic relationships were seen for both of these brominated compounds, with increased risk already at very modest increased levels, suggesting low-dose effects.

When PBB 153 and PBDE 153 levels were related to the different components of metabolic syndrome, relationships were found mainly in relation to elevated serum triglyceride levels. However, when related to prevalent diabetes, both increased PBB 153 and PBDE 153 levels were associated with an increased risk of prevalent diabetes with ORs in the range of 1.9–2.7.

The only other research group that has paid attention to the relationship between metabolic syndrome and environmental contaminants is a Japanese team.[20] In a health survey conducted in different parts of Japan, 1374 subjects not occupationally exposed to dioxins and related compounds were investigated. It was found that 12% of the population showed metabolic syndrome using a modified version of the NCEP criteria. The investigators calculated the toxic equivalents (TEQs) for a total of 29 PCDDs, PCDFs, and dioxin-like PCBs. Belonging to the upper quartile of total TEQ was associated with a 5.3 increased risk of having metabolic syndrome (95% CI 2.3–13, $p<0.01$), following adjustment for age, sex, smoking, alcohol habits, regional area, and survey year. Also, when TEQ was calculated separately for the three different groups of compounds (PCDDs, PCDFs, and dioxin-like PCBs), the TEQs for each of these groups were all related to the risk of metabolic syndrome (OR 3.2–4.8). Similar results were obtained if diabetics were excluded from the analysis.

When the five components of metabolic syndrome were related to TEQ values, all components of metabolic syndrome, except the modified obesity criteria using BMI instead of waist circumference ($p=0.07$), were significantly related to total TEQ. Only for dioxin-like PCBs was TEQ related to the obesity criteria. In general, for all three groups of compounds (PCDDs, PCDFs, and dioxin-like PCBs), TEQ was related to the four other components of metabolic syndrome (with the exception of TEQ for PCDFs and low HDL-cholesterol). In most cases, monotonic relationships between TEQ values and prevalent metabolic syndrome were observed.

While most of the PCDDs and PCDFs investigated were related to the risk of having metabolic syndrome, a striking difference was seen between different PCB congeners. PCB 126, 105, 114, 118, 123, and 167 were all significantly related to prevalent metabolic syndrome, with ORs in the 4.1 to 9.1 range for the highest *versus* lowest quartile. The PCBs 156, 157, 169, and 189 were far from being related to metabolic syndrome. Thus, although the TEQs for the dioxin-like PCBs were related to the risk of metabolic syndrome, it is evident that not all PCBs are similar in this respect.

As previously discussed, metabolic syndrome is a combination of the common cardiovascular risk factors, dyslipidemia, diabetes, hypertension, and abdominal obesity. Of those risk factors, diabetes is the condition most frequently studied. Five prospective studies have uniformly shown that high levels of the OC pesticide, *p,p′*-DDE are related to future diabetes.[21–25] Most, but not all, of these studies also show that high levels of PCBs increase the risk of incident diabetes.[21,24,25] The five studies are very different with respect to the age at inclusion of the samples, the duration of the follow-up, and the calendar time when the measurements were performed. These discrepancies make them hard to compare. In our own cohort study, the Prospective Investigation of the Vasculature in Uppsala Seniors (PIVUS) study, we measured 19 POPs in almost 1000 subjects, all aged 70 years, and followed the development of diabetes in 5 years.[25] During this period, 36 incident diabetes cases emerged. Subjects in the highest quintile of a summary measure of the 16 evaluated PCBs showed a 7.5-fold increase in the risk of future diabetes (95% CI 1.4–38.8, $p<0.01$), following adjustment for sex, BMI, cigarette smoking, exercise, alcohol consumption, triglycerides, and total cholesterol. The corresponding

OR for those with the highest levels of a summary measure of three OC pesticides were 3.4 (1.0–11.7, $p = 0.03$). A point of note is that PCB levels were a more powerful predictor of future diabetes than BMI (or waist circumference), even following adjustment for BMI. This is quite remarkable since obesity is regarded to be the major predictor of diabetes development in the elderly.

Several cross-sectional or case-control studies support the view that PCBs and OC pesticides are related to diabetes.[26–36] Furthermore, other types of studies—such as investigations of US Vietnam veterans who had been spraying the dioxin-containing compound, "Agent Orange",[37–42] victims from a PCB accident in Taiwan,[43] and a geographical study of individuals living close to POP-contaminated waste sites in New York[44]—also support the view that POPs could be involved in the development of diabetes.

Regarding hypertension, data are scarce compared to diabetes. There is however, an investigation using NHANES-data,[45] and a study from a POP contaminated in Aniston in the US, showing relationships between POPs and hypertension.[46] Furthermore, the Vietnam veterans studies[41] and the geographical study from New York[47] also support the view that POP exposure is related to hypertension.

Lipid disturbances and obesity are harder to study in terms of POP exposure than hypertension and diabetes, since POPs are highly lipid soluble, being transported by lipoproteins, and accumulate in the adipose tissue. Thus, if lipid parameters or obesity measures are used as outcomes, it is not evident whether or not the circulating levels used to determine exposure are affected by the outcome in a major way, and how this will affect the analysis of the relationship between the POP levels and lipids or obesity. A large fat mass will "protect" the circulation from POPs by binding the compounds to the adipose tissue for a certain period in relation to the metabolism of the individual compounds. Thus, if a population is exposed to a certain amount of a POP at a certain time-point, a lean subject will initially have higher circulating levels of that POP than an obese subject, due to the lipid soluble character of the POP. During this initial phase, a negative relationship between the POP levels and BMI would be seen. However, due to the more rapid metabolism of the POP in the lean subjects, the circulating levels (and also the adipose tissue levels) will decline faster in the lean subjects and at some time point, estimated to be 2–3 times half-lives of the POP, the former negative relationship between BMI and the POP will turn into a positive relationship, as nicely illustrated by Wolff and co-workers.[48] This change in the sign of the relationship between POP levels and obesity will take place earlier for compounds with a shorter half-life compared with substances with a long half-life. This toxicokinetic pattern does, however, presume no further exposure of the POP and a constant fat mass, two prerequisites that are hard to achieve in real life.

Despite these problems with the evaluation of relationships between POP levels and lipid disturbances and obesity, several papers have been published on these topics. Using occupational exposure to high levels of dioxins and other POPs, some studies have been able to show increased levels of lipids, like cholesterol and triglycerides, in exposed subjects.[6,49–51] Furthermore, a geographical study comparing subjects living in contaminated areas with matched non-contaminated areas have pointed in the same direction.[52]

Also, a number of studies have investigated relationships between POP levels and obesity in adults. Some of these studies have found positive relationships between POP levels and various obesity measurements,[24,53] but in the PIVUS study, we found that PCBs with a short half-life showed positive relations in relation to waist circumference or fat mass, while PCBs with a long half-life showed negative relationships.[54] The same pattern was seen regardless of whether we used a cross-sectional approach to analyze the data,[54] or we evaluated incident cases of abdominal obesity during a five year follow-up period.[55] It is likely that the toxicokinetic problems discussed contributed to these discrepancies between different PCBs. It is therefore likely that study of environmental "obesogens" is better carried out in mother–child cohorts than in adult and elderly cohorts if the compounds to be studied are highly lipid-soluble.

Amongst the POPs, the perfluorinated compounds are not highly lipid-soluble and are therefore not subject to the same problems as the majority of POPs. In a large US cross-sectional population-based study, an association was found between PFOS/PFOA levels and serum cholesterol.[56] Also, in a cross-sectional study of 1025 active workers with potential exposure to PFOA, circulating levels of this compound were associated with LDL-cholesterol.[57]

No studies on the relationships between plastic associated chemicals (PACs) and metabolic syndrome exist. However, some studies exist on the associations in relation to different components of the syndrome. Using data on 1455 subjects included in the 2003–2004 examination cycle of the NHANES study, Lang and co-workers showed that urinary levels of BPA were increased in relation both to diabetes prevalence and to BMI.[58] One increase in standard deviation of measured BPA levels was associated with a 1.39 times increased risk of prevalent diabetes, following adjustment for age, sex , race, education, income, smoking, BMI, and waist circumference (95% CI 1.21–1.60, $p<0.001$). They also showed that obese subjects excreted almost double the amount of BPA compared to lean subjects. BPA has a half-life of only a few hours and almost all BPA is excreted within 24h following a single dose. However, in a similar analysis of the NHANES 2005–2006 cycle, the associations between urinary BPA and diabetes was less evident.[59]

We have also recently shown that circulating levels of BPA is related to LDL-cholesterol in the PIVUS study.[60]

Due to the very high abundance of phthalates in the environment, including the laboratory, it is hardly possible to measure the parent phthalate compounds. Instead, the mono- metabolites not present in the environment are measured.

Urinary levels of several phthalate metabolites were determined in the NHANES 2003–2004 examination cycle. Several of these metabolites were significantly related to measures of obesity, such as BMI and waist circumference.[61,62] A similar pattern was seen in the PIVUS study, where especially the serum levels of the phthalate metabolite mono-isobutyl phthalate (MiBP) was positively related to fat accumulation, measured by both dual-energy X-ray absorptiometry (DXA)-scan and abdominal magnetic resonance imaging (MRI), but in women only.[63]

In a small study carried out in Mexican women, high levels of some phthalate metabolites in the urine were related to prevalent diabetes.[64] In the PIVUS study, we have recently shown that circulating levels of especially the phthalate metabolites monomethyl phthalate (MMP), MiBP, and monoethyl phthalate were related to prevalent diabetes.[65] Moreover, we found that some of the phthalate metabolites were related to measures of insulin resistance and insulin secretion, the two cornerstones in glucose control. We have also recently shown that the phthalate MMP is related to LDL-cholesterol levels.[60]

Thus a picture is starting to emerge; plastic-associated compounds are related to different cardiovascular risk factors, although the number of studies are small compared to the literature on POPs and prospective studies are lacking.

7.3 Cardiovascular Disease

Some of the first evidences that POPs could be involved in cardiovascular disease came from occupational studies. When those studies pooled their data into the IARC international cohort, consisting of 36 cohorts from 13 countries, including 21 863 workers followed for >20 years, it was a very consistent finding that exposure to dioxin was related to future coronary heart disease (RR 1.67, 95% CI 1.23–2.26).[66] Also, studies in Vietnam veterans spraying the dioxin-contaminated Agent Orange showed the same pattern with a 52% increased risk of future cardiovascular risk during 30 years follow-up.[41]

Also, a couple of accidents might also support the idea that exposure to POPs could induce cardiovascular disease. In 1979, an industrial plant in Seveso in northern Italy exploded and contaminated the surrounding area with dioxins. In a follow-up some 25 years later, an increased mortality rate in cardiovascular diseases was found in the population living in the contaminated area compared to a non-contaminated neighborhood. It is of interest to note that it was only during the first 10 years of follow-up that an increased mortality rate due to cardiovascular diseases could be noted. The peak in risk was seen in the 5–10 year follow-up interval (RR 1.84, 95% CI 1.09–3.12).[67]

In an accident with PCB-contaminated rice in Yucheng, a non-significant tendency for a higher incidence rate of cardiovascular diseases was observed during a 24 year follow-up period (OR 1.50, 95% CI 0.8–2.7).[43]

Also, geographical studies support the idea of a role of environmental contaminants in cardiovascular diseases. Individuals living close to a POP contaminated waste site in New York showed an increased risk for both myocardial infarction (RR 1.20, 95% CI 1.03–1.39)[47] and stroke (RR 1.15, 95% CI, 1.05–1.26)[68] compared to those not living close to a contaminated waste site.

The first report using measured concentrations of POPs in a population-based study and investigated the relationship between POP levels and cardiovascular diseases used the NHANES 1999–2002 examination cycle.[69] The sample consisted of 889 individuals, 108 of which reported a history of cardiovascular disease (coronary heart disease or stroke). A total of 21 POPs were evaluated, divided into 5 classes: PCDDs, PCDFs, dioxin-like PCBs, non-dioxin-like PCBs and OC pesticides. When the POPs were divided into quartiles, high levels of dioxin-like PCBs were associated with an increased risk of cardiovascular diseases (OR 5.0, 95% CI 1.2–20.4, $p<0.01$ for highest *versus* lowest quartile). Also, the non dioxin-like PCBs and the OC pesticides showed similar associations, although not as strong (OR 3.8, 95%CI 1. 1–12.8, $p=0.02$ for non dioxin-like PCBs and OR 4.0, 95% CI 1.0–17.1, $p=0.03$ for the OC pesticides). One point to note is that these significant associations between POP exposure and prevalent cardiovascular diseases were seen in women only. In men, the corresponding ORs were in the 1.7–2.2 range and far from significant.

When the individual contaminants were analyzed, PCB 74, PCB 118, PCB 138, PCB 153, PCB 156, PCB 170, oxychlordane, and trans-Nonachlor were all significantly related to prevalent cardiovascular diseases in women. For PCB 138, PCB 153, and PCB 156, subjects in the highest quartile showed a more than 10-fold increased risk for prevalent cardiovascular diseases in women following adjustment for age, race, poverty index, BMI, cigarette smoking, serum cotinine, alcohol consumption, exercise, HDL-cholesterol, total cholesterol, triglycerides, hypertension, and C-reactive protein.

In an analysis of NHANES data from 1999–2004, Min and co-workers analyzed associations between OC pesticide exposure and peripheral artery disease, defined as an ankle-brachial index <0.9.[70] Amongst the 2032 participants, 143 were considered to have peripheral artery disease. Five OC pesticides were investigated: *p,p'*-DDE, trans-nonachlor, oxychlordane, dieldrin and beta-HCH. When the sum of these five OC pesticides was evaluated, an interaction in relation to obesity was found in that the sum of these five OC pesticides was only related to peripheral artery disease in the obese subjects (OR 1.28, 95% CI 1.04–1.57 in the obese group and 0.95, 95% CI 0.70–1.28 in the non-obese group) following adjustment for age, sex, race, education, income, cigarette smoking, serum cotinine, alcohol consumption, total cholesterol, triglycerides, and diabetes. When the five OC pesticides were analyzed individually, *p,p'*-DDE, trans-nonachlor, and oxychlordane were significantly related to prevalent peripheral artery disease in the obese only.

Thus, despite the fact that some evidence from these cross-sectional evaluations of NHANES data points towards an association between some POPs and cardiovascular disease prospective data on POP exposure and cardiovascular disease are still lacking in the population-based setting.

Using data on 1455 subjects included in the 2003–2004 examination cycle of the NHANES study, Lang and co-workers showed that urinary levels of BPA were increased in relation to prevalent cardiovascular disease ($n=79$).[58] One SD increase in BPA levels was associated with a 1.39 times increased risk of prevalent cardiovascular disease following adjustment for age, sex, race, education, income, smoking, BMI, and waist circumference (95% CI 118–1.63, $p<0.001$). A similar risk was seen when only cases with heart attack were considered. On the other hand, no association between BPA and stroke ($n=40$) was found (OR 0.97, 95% CI 0.74–1.27, $p<0.001$).

When the same research group performed a similar analysis using data from the 2005–2006 NHANES cycle, the relationships between urinary BPA levels and cardiovascular disease were generally weaker and no longer significant for the combined end-point cardiovascular disease (OR 1.21, 95% CI 0.92–1.59, $p=0.16$).[59] However, heart attack was still significantly associated with urinary BPA levels in 2005–2006 (OR 1.31, 95% CI 1.03–1.68, $p=0.036$), and when pooling data from the two examination cycles, the combined end-point cardiovascular disease was related to BPA levels in a highly significant fashion (OR 1.26, 95% CI 1.11–1.43, $p=0.001$).

The same research group has recently published the first prospective study on environmental contaminants and future coronary heart disease.[71] They used a nested case-control design to study 758 incident cases of coronary heart disease and 861 controls from a >10 year long follow-up of the European Prospective Investigation of Cancer, Norfolk, UK. It was found that one standard deviation increase in urinary bisphenol levels was associated with an 11% increased risk of coronary heart disease (95% CI 1.02–1.24, $p=0.017$). Following adjustment for age, sex, education, social class, BMI, blood pressure, lipids and exercise, the OR was not affected.

7.4 Atherosclerosis

The major underlying cause of cardiovascular diseases like coronary heart disease, stroke, and peripheral artery disease is atherosclerosis. Regarding coronary heart disease and stroke, the most likely mechanism is rupture of a lipid-rich atherosclerotic plaque, which will trigger a thrombus formation that will occlude the vessel and thereby create an ischemic damage. Only a couple of studies originated from the PIVUS cohort have investigated whether POPs or PACs are linked to atherosclerosis. We used ultrasound to quantify whether plaques were present in the carotid arteries and examined the grey scale intensity of the vascular wall and plaques to determine the degree of lipid infiltration. We have previously shown that subjects with an echolucent (dark) vascular wall have an increased risk of future cardiovascular death.[72]

We found that subjects with elevated levels of PCBs had an increased risk of having carotid artery atherosclerotic plaques,[73] even following adjustment for sex, blood pressure, lipids, diabetes, smoking, and BMI (OR 1.03, 95% CI 1.01–1.05, $p=0.002$). Several of the PCBs evaluated were significantly related to plaque occurrence in the carotid arteries. Some of the highly chlorinated PCBs and PCB126 were also related to an echolucent vascular wall, suggesting not only an effect on plaque formation, but also on the lipid infiltration in the vascular wall, an early step in the atherosclerotic process.

In another report from the PIVUS study, we investigated the role of plastic associated chemicals.[74] We found MMP to be related to carotid plaques in an inverted U-shaped manner. This pattern was significant after adjustment for gender, body mass index, blood glucose, blood pressure, HDL and

LDL-cholesterol, serum triglycerides, smoking, antihypertensive treatment, and statin use ($p = 0.004$). High levels of BPA, MiBP and MMP were associated with an echogenic (white) vascular wall, while high levels of mono-2-ethylhexylphthalat were associated with an echolucent (dark) vascular wall ($p < 0.0001$after adjustment).

Thus both PCBs and plastic associated chemicals are related to plaque occurrence in the carotid artery, as well as to lipid infiltration in the vascular wall, independently of traditional cardiovascular risk factors, suggesting the these compounds might have a direct vascular effect.

7.5 Mechanisms of Action

For the POPs, the basic mechanism discovered for some of the compounds, such as dioxin and dioxin-like PCBs, is an activation of the aryl hydrocarbon (Ah)-receptor (AHR). This activation leads to up-regulation of some enzymes known to be involved in the detoxification process (CYP1A1, CYP 1A2, and CYP 1B1). Activation of these P450-enzymes has also been associated with formation of reactive oxygen spices and inflammation as two of the major results.[75,76] Also, alterations in apoptosis rate and cell cycling following activation of the AHR has been described.[77–80]

Some of the OC pesticides are known to activate the androgen receptor (AR). The endogenous ligand testosterone is known to have an influence on cardiovascular disease.

BPA was originally synthesized as an estrogenic compound\z and activates the estrogen receptors. Before menopause, women are known to be protected against atherosclerotic complications and have a more favorable risk factor profile compared with women post-menopause. However, the value of estrogen supplementation following menopause in terms of cardiovascular disease is debated. How the relatively weak estrogen BPA fits into the balance between endogenous estrogen and its receptors is largely unknown.

The phthalates are known to be PPAR-agonists.[81] Activation of PPAR-gamma promotes differentiation of adipocytes and storage of fat in adipose tissue. Thus, phthalates are important candidates for actions on obesity and related traits, such as metabolic syndrome and diabetes.

7.6 Conclusions

Today there is mounting evidences that both POPs and PACs could be involved in both metabolic syndrome and its different components, such as obesity, diabetes, dyslipidemia, and hypertension, as well as in the development of atherosclerosis and cardiovascular disease. However, since epidemiology never can prove causality, a combination of concordant prospective large-scale cohort studies, together with concordant experimental data, is needed to definitively confirm that both POPs and PACs could be involved in cardiovascular disease. The data accumulated today definitely suggests that this as an area to further explore.

References

1. E. S. Ford, U. A. Ajani, J. B. Croft, J. A. Critchley, D. R. Labarthe, T. E. Kottke, W. H. Giles and S. Capewell, "Explaining the decrease in U.S. deaths from coronary disease, 1980–2000", *N Engl J Med*, 2007, **356**(23), 2388–2398.
2. H. C. Wijeysundera, M. Machado, F. Farahati, X. Wang, W. Witteman, G. van der Velde, J. V. Tu, D. S Lee, S. G. Goodman, R. Petrella, M. O'Flaherty, M. Krahn and S. Capewell, "Association of temporal trends in risk factors and treatment uptake with coronary heart disease mortality, 1994–2005." *JAMA*, 2010, **303**(18): 1841–1847.
3. S. C. Johnston, S. Mendis and C. D. Mathers, "Global variation in stroke burden and mortality: estimates from monitoring, surveillance, and modelling", *Lancet Neurol*, 2009, **8**(4), 345–354.
4. S. Kinlay, "Changes in stroke epidemiology, prevention, and treatment", *Circulation*, 2011, **124**(19), e494–496.
5. D. Levy, S. Kenchaiah, M. G. Larson, E. J. Benjamin, M. J. Kupka, K. K. Ho, J. M. Murabito and R. S. Vasan, "Long-term trends in the incidence of and survival with heart failure", *N Engl J Med*, 2002, **347**(18), 1397–1402.
6. V. L. Roger, S. A. Weston, M. M. Redfield, J. P. Hellermann-Homan, J. Killian, B. P. Yawn and S. J. Jacobsen, "Trends in heart failure incidence and survival in a community-based population", *JAMA*, 2004, **292**(3), 344–350.
7. W. H. Barker, J. P. Mullooly and W. Getchel, "Changing incidence and survival for heart failure in a well-defined older population, 1970–1974 and 1990–1994", *Circulation*, 2006, **113**(6), 799–805.
8. L. Lind, S. Jakobsson, H. Lithell, B. Wengle and S. Ljunghall, "Relation of serum calcium concentration to metabolic risk factors for cardiovascular disease", *BMJ*, 1988, **297**(6654), 960–963.
9. G. M. Reaven, "Banting lecture 1988. Role of insulin resistance in human disease", *Diabetes*, 1988, **37**(12), 1595–1607.
10. NECP, "Executive summary of the third report of the international cholesterol education program (NECP) expert panel on detection, education and treatment of high blood cholesterol in adults (ATP III)", *Journal of the American Medical Association*, 2001, **285**, 2486–2497.
11. L. Lind, B. Vessby and J. Sundstrom, "The apolipoprotein B/AI ratio and the metabolic syndrome independently predict risk for myocardial infarction in middle-aged men", *Arterioscler Thromb Vasc Biol*, 2006, **26**(2), 406–410.
12. J. Sundstrom, U. Riserus, L. Byberg, B. Zethelius, H. Lithell and L. Lind, "Clinical value of the metabolic syndrome for long term prediction of total and cardiovascular mortality: prospective, population based cohort study", *BMJ*, 2006, **332**(7546), 878–882.
13. J. Sundstrom, E. Vallhagen, U. Riserus, L. Byberg, B. Zethelius, C. Berne, L. Lind and E. Ingelsson, "Risk associated with the metabolic syndrome versus the sum of its individual components", *Diabetes Care*, 2006, **29**(7), 1673–1674.

14. L. Olsen, E. Lampa, D. A. Birkholz, L. Lind and P. M. Lind, "Circulating levels of bisphenol A (BPA) and phthalates in an elderly population in Sweden, based on the Prospective Investigation of the Vasculature in Uppsala Seniors (PIVUS)", *Ecotoxicol Environ Saf*, 2012, **75**(1), 242–248.
15. L. Lind and P. M. Lind, "Can persistent organic pollutants and plastic-associated chemicals cause cardiovascular disease?", *J Intern Med*, 2012.
16. K. G. Alberti and P. Z. Zimmet, "Definition, diagnosis and classification of diabetes mellitus and its complications. Part 1: diagnosis and classification of diabetes mellitus provisional report of a WHO consultation", *Diabet Med*, 1998, **15**(7), 539–553.
17. D. H. Lee, I. K. Lee, M. Porta, M. Steffes and D. R. Jacobs, Jr., "Relationship between serum concentrations of persistent organic pollutants and the prevalence of metabolic syndrome among non-diabetic adults: results from the National Health and Nutrition Examination Survey 1999–2002", *Diabetologia*, 2007, **50**(9), 1841–1851.
18. S. K. Park, H. K. Son, S. K. Lee, J. H. Kang, Y. S. Chang, D. R. Jacobs and D. H. Lee, "Relationship between serum concentrations of organochlorine pesticides and metabolic syndrome among non-diabetic adults", *J Prev Med Public Health*, 2010, **43**(1), 1–8.
19. J. S. Lim, D. H. Lee and D. R. Jacobs, Jr., "Association of brominated flame retardants with diabetes and metabolic syndrome in the U.S. population 2003–2004", *Diabetes Care*, 2008, **31**(9), 1802–1807.
20. H. Uemura, K. Arisawa, M. Hiyoshi, A. Kitayama, H. Takami, F. Sawachika, S. Dakeshita, K. Nii, H. Satoh, Y. Sumiyoshi, K. Morinaga, K. Kodama, T. Suzuki and M. Nagai, "Prevalence of metabolic syndrome associated with body burden levels of dioxin and related compounds among Japan's general population", *Environ Health Perspect*, 2009, **117**(4), 568–573.
21. O. Vasiliu, L. Cameron, J. Gardiner, P. Deguire and W. Karmaus, "Polybrominated biphenyls, polychlorinated biphenyls, body weight, and incidence of adult-onset diabetes mellitus", *Epidemiology*, 2006, **17**(4), 352–359.
22. A. Rignell-Hydbom, J. Lidfeldt, H. Kiviranta, P. Rantakokko, G. Samsioe, C. D. Agardh and R. Rylander, "Exposure to p,p′-DDE: a risk factor for type 2 diabetes", *PLoS One*, 2009, **4**(10), e7503.
23. M. Turyk, H. Anderson, L. Knobeloch, P. Imm and V. Persky, "Organochlorine exposure and incidence of diabetes in a cohort of Great Lakes sport fish consumers", *Environ Health Perspect*, 2009, **117**(7), 1076–1082.
24. D. H. Lee, M. W. Steffes, A. Sjodin, R. S. Jones, L. L. Needham and D. R. Jacobs, Jr., "Low dose of some persistent organic pollutants predicts type 2 diabetes: a nested case-control study", *Environ Health Perspect*, 2010, **118**(9), 1235–1242.
25. D. H. Lee, P. M. Lind, D. R. Jacobs, Jr., S. Salihovic, B. van Bavel and L. Lind, "Polychlorinated biphenyls and organochlorine pesticides in plasma predict development of type 2 diabetes in the elderly: the prospective investigation of the vasculature in Uppsala Seniors (PIVUS) study", *Diabetes Care*, 2011, **34**(8), 1778–1784.

26. L. Rylander, A. Rignell-Hydbom and L. Hagmar, "A cross-sectional study of the association between persistent organochlorine pollutants and diabetes", *Environ Health*, 2005, **4**, 28.
27. D. H. Lee, I. K. Lee, K. Song, M. Steffes, W. Toscano, B. A. Baker and D. R. Jacobs, Jr., "A strong dose-response relation between serum concentrations of persistent organic pollutants and diabetes: results from the National Health and Examination Survey 1999–2002", *Diabetes Care*, 2006, **29**(7), 1638–1644.
28. N. Codru, M. J. Schymura, S. Negoita, R. Rej and D. O. Carpenter, "Diabetes in relation to serum levels of polychlorinated biphenyls and chlorinated pesticides in adult Native Americans", *Environ Health Perspect*, 2007, **115**(10), 1442–1447.
29. S. Cox, A. S. Niskar, K. M. Narayan and M. M. Marcus, "Prevalence of self-reported diabetes and exposure to organochlorine pesticides among Mexican Americans: Hispanic health and nutrition examination survey, 1982–1984", *Environ Health Perspect*, 2007, **115**(12), 1747–1752.
30. A. Rignell-Hydbom, L. Rylander and L. Hagmar, "Exposure to persistent organochlorine pollutants and type 2 diabetes mellitus", *Hum Exp Toxicol*, 2007, **26**(5), 447–452.
31. M. E. Jorgensen, K. Borch-Johnsen and P. Bjerregaard, "A cross-sectional study of the association between persistent organic pollutants and glucose intolerance among Greenland Inuit", *Diabetologia*, 2008, **51**(8), 1416–1422.
32. H. Uemura, K. Arisawa, M. Hiyoshi, H. Satoh, Y. Sumiyoshi, K. Morinaga, K. Kodama, T. Suzuki and M. Nagai, "Associations of environmental exposure to dioxins with prevalent diabetes among general inhabitants in Japan", *Environ Res*, 2008, **108**(1), 63–68.
33. M. Turyk, H. A. Anderson, L. Knobeloch, P. Imm and V. W. Persky, "Prevalence of diabetes and body burdens of polychlorinated biphenyls, polybrominated diphenyl ethers, and p,p′-diphenyldichloroethene in Great Lakes sport fish consumers", *Chemosphere*, 2009, **75**(5), 674–679.
34. C. J. Everett and E. M. Matheson, "Biomarkers of pesticide exposure and diabetes in the 1999–2004 national health and nutrition examination survey", *Environ Int*, 2010, **36**(4), 398–401.
35. H. K. Son, S. A. Kim, J. H. Kang, Y. S. Chang, S. K. Park, S. K. Lee, D. R. Jacobs, Jr. and D. H. Lee, "Strong associations between low-dose organochlorine pesticides and type 2 diabetes in Korea", *Environ Int*, 2010, **36**(5), 410–414.
36. J. Ukropec, Z. Radikova, M. Huckova, J. Koska, A. Kocan, E. Sebokova, B. Drobna, T. Trnovec, K. Susienkova, V. Labudova, D. Gasperikova, P. Langer and I. Klimes, "High prevalence of prediabetes and diabetes in a population exposed to high levels of an organochlorine cocktail", *Diabetologia*, 2010, **53**(5), 899–906.
37. G. L. Henriksen, N. S. Ketchum, J. E. Michalek and J. A. Swaby, "Serum dioxin and diabetes mellitus in veterans of Operation Ranch Hand", *Epidemiology*, 1997, **8**(3), 252–258.

38. M. P. Longnecker and J. E. Michalek, "Serum dioxin level in relation to diabetes mellitus among Air Force veterans with background levels of exposure", *Epidemiology*, 2000, **11**(1), 44–48.
39. K. Steenland, G. Calvert, N. Ketchum and J. Michalek, "Dioxin and diabetes mellitus: an analysis of the combined NIOSH and Ranch Hand data", *Occup Environ Med*, 2001, **58**(10), 641–648.
40. J. Michalek, J. Robinson, K. Fox *et al.*, "Air Force Health Study – An Epidemiologic Investigation of Health Effects in Air Force Personnel Following Exposure to Herbicides: 2002 Follow-up Examination Results May 2002 to March 2005", *SCIENCE APPLICATIONS INTERNATIONAL CORP RESTON VA*, 1994.
41. H. K. Kang, N. A. Dalager, L. L. Needham, D. G. Patterson, Jr., P. S. Lees, K. Yates and G. M. Matanoski, "Health status of Army Chemical Corps Vietnam veterans who sprayed defoliant in Vietnam", *Am J Ind Med*, 2006, **49**(11), 875–884.
42. J. E. Michalek and M. Pavuk, "Diabetes and cancer in veterans of Operation Ranch Hand after adjustment for calendar period, days of spraying, and time spent in Southeast Asia", *J Occup Environ Med*, 2008, **50**(3), 330–340.
43. S. L. Wang, P. C. Tsai, C. Y. Yang and Y. Leon Guo, "Increased risk of diabetes and polychlorinated biphenyls and dioxins: a 24-year follow-up study of the Yucheng cohort", *Diabetes Care*, 2008, **31**(8), 1574–1579.
44. M. Kouznetsova, X. Huang, J. Ma, L. Lessner and D. O. Carpenter, "Increased rate of hospitalization for diabetes and residential proximity of hazardous waste sites", *Environ Health Perspect*, 2007, **115**(1), 75–79.
45. M. H. Ha, D. H. Lee, H. K. Son, S. K. Park and D. R. Jacobs, Jr., "Association between serum concentrations of persistent organic pollutants and prevalence of newly diagnosed hypertension: results from the National Health and Nutrition Examination Survey 1999–2002", *J Hum Hypertens*, 2009, **23**(4), 274–286.
46. A. Goncharov, M. Bloom, M. Pavuk, I. Birman and D. O. Carpenter, "Blood pressure and hypertension in relation to levels of serum polychlorinated biphenyls in residents of Anniston, Alabama", *J Hypertens*, 2010, **28**(10), 2053–2060.
47. A. V. Sergeev and D. O. Carpenter, "Hospitalization rates for coronary heart disease in relation to residence near areas contaminated with persistent organic pollutants and other pollutants", *Environ Health Perspect*, 2005, **113**(6), 756–761.
48. M. S. Wolff, H. A. Anderson, J. A. Britton and N. Rothman, "Pharmacokinetic variability and modern epidemiology – the example of dichlorodiphenyltrichloroethane, body mass index, and birth cohort", *Cancer Epidemiol Biomarkers Prev*, 2007, **16**(10), 1925–1930.
49. G. M. Calvert, K. K. Willie, M. H. Sweeney, M. A. Fingerhut and W. E. Halperin, "Evaluation of serum lipid concentrations among U.S. workers exposed to 2,3,7,8-tetrachlorodibenzo-p-dioxin", *Arch Environ Health*, 1996, **51**(2), 100–107.

50. S. W. Hu, T. J. Cheng, G. P. ChangChien and C. C. Chan, "Association between dioxins/furans exposures and incinerator workers' hepatic function and blood lipids", *J Occup Environ Med*, 2003, **45**(6), 601–608.
51. D. Pelclova, Z. Fenclova, P. Urban, P. Ridzon, J. Preiss, K. Kupka, J. Malik, Z. Dubska and T. Navratil, "Chronic health impairment due to 2,3,7,8-tetrachloro-dibenzo-p-dioxin exposure", *Neuro Endocrinol Lett*, 2009, **30**(Suppl 1), 219–224.
52. P. Langer, "The impacts of organochlorines and other persistent pollutants on thyroid and metabolic health", *Front Neuroendocrinol*, 2010, **31**(4), 497–518.
53. M. A. Elobeid, M. A. Padilla, D. W. Brock, D. M. Ruden and D. B. Allison, "Endocrine disruptors and obesity: an examination of selected persistent organic pollutants in the NHANES 1999–2002 data", *Int J Environ Res Public Health*, 2010, **7**(7), 2988–3005.
54. M. Ronn, L. Lind, B. van Bavel, S. Salihovic, K. Michaelsson and P. M. Lind, "Circulating levels of persistent organic pollutants associate in divergent ways to fat mass measured by DXA in humans", *Chemosphere*, 2011, **85**(3), 335–343.
55. D. H. Lee, L. Lind, D. R. Jacobs, Jr., S. Salihovic, B. van Bavel and P. M. Lind, "Associations of persistent organic pollutants with abdominal obesity in the elderly: The Prospective Investigation of the Vasculature in Uppsala Seniors (PIVUS) study", *Environ Int*, 2012, **40**, 170–178.
56. B. D. Kerger, T. L. Copeland and A. P. DeCaprio, "Tenuous dose-response correlations for common disease states: case study of cholesterol and perfluorooctanoate/sulfonate (PFOA/PFOS) in the C8 Health Project", *Drug Chem Toxicol*, 2011, **34**(4), 396–404.
57. C. J. Sakr, K. H. Kreckmann, J. W. Green, P. J. Gillies, J. L. Reynolds and R. C. Leonard, "Cross-sectional study of lipids and liver enzymes related to a serum biomarker of exposure (ammonium perfluorooctanoate or APFO) as part of a general health survey in a cohort of occupationally exposed workers", *J Occup Environ Med*, 2007, **49**(10), 1086–1096.
58. I. A. Lang, T. S. Galloway, A. Scarlett, W. E. Henley, M. Depledge, R. B. Wallace and D. Melzer, "Association of urinary bisphenol A concentration with medical disorders and laboratory abnormalities in adults", *JAMA*, 2008, **300**(11), 1303–1310.
59. D. Melzer, N. E. Rice, C. Lewis, W. E. Henley and T. S. Galloway, "Association of urinary bisphenol a concentration with heart disease: evidence from NHANES 2003/06", *PLoS One*, 2010, **5**(1), e8673.
60. L. Olsen, L. Lind and P. M. Lind, "Associations between circulating levels of bisphenol A and phthalate metabolites and coronary risk in the elderly", *Ecotoxicol Environ Saf*, 2012.
61. R. W. Stahlhut, E. van Wijngaarden, T. D. Dye, S. Cook and S. H. Swan, "Concentrations of urinary phthalate metabolites are associated with increased waist circumference and insulin resistance in adult U.S. males", *Environ Health Perspect*, 2007, **115**(6), 876–882.

62. E. E. Hatch, J. W. Nelson, M. M. Qureshi, J. Weinberg, L. L. Moore, M. Singer and T. F. Webster, "Association of urinary phthalate metabolite concentrations with body mass index and waist circumference: a cross-sectional study of NHANES data 1999–2002", *Environ Health*, 2008, **7**, 27.
63. P. M. Lind, V. Roos, M. Ronn, L. Johansson, H. Ahlstrom, J. Kullberg and L. Lind, "Serum concentrations of phthalate metabolites related to abdominal fat distribution two years later in elderly women", *Environ Health*, 2012, **11**(1), 21.
64. K. Svensson, R. U. Hernandez-Ramirez, A. Burguete-Garcia, M. E. Cebrian, A. M. Calafat, L. L. Needham, L. Claudio and L. Lopez-Carrillo, "Phthalate exposure associated with self-reported diabetes among Mexican women", *Environ Res*, 2011, **111**(6), 792–796.
65. P. M. Lind, and B. Zethelius. "Circulating Levels of Phthalate Metabolites Are Associated With Prevalent Diabetes in the Elderly", *Diabetes Care*, 2012.
66. J. Vena, P. Boffetta, H. Becher, T. Benn, H. B. Bueno-de-Mesquita, D. Coggon, D. Colin, D. Flesch-Janys, L. Green, T. Kauppinen, M. Littorin, E. Lynge, J. D. Mathews, M. Neuberger, N. Pearce, A. C. Pesatori, R. Saracci, K. Steenland and M. Kogevinas, "Exposure to dioxin and nonneoplastic mortality in the expanded IARC international cohort study of phenoxy herbicide and chlorophenol production workers and sprayers", *Environ Health Perspect*, 1998, **106**(Suppl 2), 645–653.
67. D. Consonni, A. C. Pesatori, C. Zocchetti, R. Sindaco, L. C. D'Oro, M. Rubagotti and P. A. Bertazzi, "Mortality in a population exposed to dioxin after the Seveso, Italy, accident in 1976: 25 years of follow-up", *Am J Epidemiol*, 2008, **167**(7), 847–858.
68. I. Shcherbatykh, X. Huang, L. Lessner and D. O. Carpenter, "Hazardous waste sites and stroke in New York State", *Environ Health*, 2005, **4**, 18.
69. M. H. Ha, D. H. Lee and D. R. Jacobs, "Association between serum concentrations of persistent organic pollutants and self-reported cardiovascular disease prevalence: results from the National Health and Nutrition Examination Survey 1999–2002", *Environ Health Perspect*, 2007, **115**(8), 1204–1209.
70. J. Y. Min, J. S. Cho, K. J. Lee, J. B. Park, S. G. Park, J. Y. Kim and K. B. Min, "Potential role for organochlorine pesticides in the prevalence of peripheral arterial diseases in obese persons: results from the National Health and Nutrition Examination Survey 1999–2004", *Atherosclerosis*, 2011, **218**(1), 200–206.
71. D. Melzer, N. J. Osborne, W. E. Henley, R. Cipelli, A. Young, C. Money, P. McCormack, R. Luben, K. T. Khaw, N. J. Wareham and T. S. Galloway, "Urinary bisphenol A concentration and risk of future coronary artery disease in apparently healthy men and women", *Circulation*, 2012, **125**(12), 1482–1490.
72. M. Wohlin, J. Sundstrom, B. Andren, A. Larsson and L. Lind, "An echolucent carotid artery intima-media complex is a new and independent

predictor of mortality in an elderly male cohort", *Atherosclerosis*, 2009, **205**(2), 486–491.
73. P. M. Lind, B. van Bavel, S. Salihovic and L. Lind, "Circulating levels of persistent organic pollutants (POPs) and carotid atherosclerosis in the elderly", *Environ Health Perspect*, 2012, **120**(1), 38–43.
74. P. M. Lind and L. Lind, "Circulating levels of bisphenol A and phthalates are related to carotid atherosclerosis in the elderly", *Atherosclerosis*, 2011, **218**(1), 207–213.
75. A. Puga, A. Hoffer, S. Zhou, J. M. Bohm, G. D. Leikauf and H. G. Shertzer, "Sustained increase in intracellular free calcium and activation of cyclooxygenase-2 expression in mouse hepatoma cells treated with dioxin", *Biochem Pharmacol*, 1997, **54**(12), 1287–1296.
76. H. G. Shertzer, D. W. Nebert, A. Puga, M. Ary, D. Sonntag, K. Dixon, L. J. Robinson, E. Cianciolo and T. P. Dalton, "Dioxin causes a sustained oxidative stress response in the mouse", *Biochem Biophys Res Commun*, 1998, **253**(1), 44–48.
77. D. N. Sadhu, M. Merchant, S. H. Safe and K. S. Ramos, "Modulation of protooncogene expression in rat aortic smooth muscle cells by benzo[a]pyrene", *Arch Biochem Biophys*, 1993, **300**(1), 124–131.
78. D. W. Nebert, A. L. Roe, M. Z. Dieter, W. A. Solis, Y. Yang and T. P. Dalton, "Role of the aromatic hydrocarbon receptor and [Ah] gene battery in the oxidative stress response, cell cycle control, and apoptosis", *Biochem Pharmacol*, 2000, **59**(1), 65–85.
79. E. A. Thackaberry, Z. Jiang, C. D. Johnson, K. S. Ramos and M. K. Walker, "Toxicogenomic profile of 2,3,7,8-tetrachlorodibenzo-p-dioxin in the murine fetal heart: modulation of cell cycle and extracellular matrix genes", *Toxicol Sci*, 2005, **88**(1), 231–241.
80. K. Y. Kim, D. S. Kim, S. K. Lee, I. K. Lee, J. H. Kang, Y. S. Chang, D. R. Jacobs, M. Steffes and D. H. Lee, "Association of low-dose exposure to persistent organic pollutants with global DNA hypomethylation in healthy Koreans", *Environ Health Perspect*, 2010, **118**(3), 370–374.
81. B. Desvergne, J. N. Feige and C. Casals-Casas, "PPAR-mediated activity of phthalates: A link to the obesity epidemic?", *Mol Cell Endocrinol*, 2009, **304**(1–2), 43–48.

CHAPTER 8

Obesity and Diabetes: Role of Environmental Chemical Exposures

THADDEUS T. SCHUG,[a] SARAH G. HOWARD,[b] KYLA W. TAYLOR[c] AND JERROLD J. HEINDEL*[a]

[a] National Institute of Environmental Health Sciences, Division of Extramural Research and Training, Research Triangle Park, USA; [b] Collaborative on Health and the Environment, PO Box 316, Bolinas, CA 94924, USA; [c] National Institute of Environmental Health Sciences, Office of Health Assessment and Translation, Division of National Toxicology Program, Research Triangle Park, NC, USA
*E-mail: heindelj@NIEHS.NIH.GOV

8.1 Background

The world is experiencing an alarming increase in the rate of obesity, diabetes and metabolic syndrome. In 2008, the World Health Organization estimated that 1.5 billion adults aged 20 and over were overweight, and nearly 500 million shared body mass index readings are above 30 kg m^{-2}, which is considered the threshold of obesity. Currently, in the United States, approximately 27% of adults and 17% of children and adolescents are obese. Moreover, one in four adults in the United States and estimated 2.1 billion people worldwide suffer from diseases associated with metabolic syndrome, such as glucose intolerance, insulin resistance, and raised blood pressure, which increases the risk of cardiovascular disease and diabetes.

Issues in Toxicology No. 16
Aging and Vulnerability to Environmental Chemicals: Age-related Disorders and their Origins in Environmental Exposures
Edited by Bernard Weiss

Published by the Royal Society of Chemistry, www.rsc.org

Worldwide, the number of people with diabetes increased from 153 million to 347 million between 1980 and 2008. Approximately 70% of this growth is attributable to population growth and aging, while the remaining 30% is attributable to a rise in age-specific prevalence.[1] The global health expenditure on diabetes was expected to total $376 billion USD in 2010, and rise to 490 billion USD in 2030, representing 12% of all per capita health care expenditures.[2]

Among US adults, diabetes incidence increased by 41% between 1997 and 2003 in all age groups. This increase was highest (65%) in people 65–79 years of age, and only includes those diagnosed with diabetes.[3] Almost 6% of US adults over age 65 have undiagnosed diabetes. When both diagnosed and undiagnosed diabetes cases are included, almost 1 in 4 Americans over age 65 have diabetes, a number expected to increase rapidly in the coming decades.[4] Alarmingly, children are beginning to develop type 2 diabetes, even before age 10.[5] The economic and social burdens that diabetes places on societies are already significant, and are growing rapidly.

The incidence of type 1 diabetes is increasing in children worldwide, especially in the youngest children, under age 5.[6,7] Type 1 diabetes incidence trends among adults, especially older adults, are not well documented, although some surveys show an increasing incidence in younger adults.[8] In industrialized countries, childhood type 1 diabetes incidence began to increase around the 1950s.[9]

8.2 Comorbidities and Complications

Why do we care if someone is overweight or obese? There are several classifications of obesity, and indeed some obese individuals appear quite healthy. However, the overwhelming majority of obese individuals have multiple comorbidity factors that result in poor health. These include significant risk of diabetes, gall bladder disease, sleep apnea, high blood pressure, insulin resistance, inflammation, breathlessness and, when pregnant, gestational diabetes, metabolic syndrome and nonalcoholic fatty liver disease (NAFLD). Obese individuals also have increased risk of coronary heart disease and stroke, osteoarthritis and gout, impaired fertility, increased risk of cancers, cataracts and back problems.[10]

The long term consequences of diabetes can also be severe. Type 2 diabetes carries with it increased morbidity and mortality, largely due to complications. Long-term microvascular complications include neuropathy, retinopathy, and nephropathy. Long-term macrovascular complications include cardiovascular disease, cerebrovascular disease, and hypertension.[11] In addition to these complications, older adults with diabetes have a higher risk for a variety of other geriatric conditions, including falls, fractures, cognitive impairment, physical disability, and depression.[4] Type 2 diabetes is also associated with other conditions, such as NAFLD[12] and cancer.[13]

Chronic hyperglycemia is associated with the microvascular long-term complications of diabetes.[11] Numerous studies have also found associations between hemoglobin A1c (HbA1c, a long term marker of average blood glucose levels) and cardiovascular disease incidence.[14] Longer disease duration and severity of disease (higher HbA1c or insulin-dependence) are associated with a higher risk of most of the geriatric age-related complications.[4] And yet most clinical trials have not found that intensive glucose control improves cardiovascular outcomes[14] or geriatric outcomes[4] in people with type 2 diabetes. Intensive glucose control in elderly patients may in fact cause more harm than good.[15]

When type 2 diabetes is diagnosed during childhood/adolescence, the development and progression of micro and macrovascular diabetes complications may be especially rapid. Microvascular complications, including nephropathy and retinopathy, are usually diagnosed at an early age and are often already present by the time of diagnosis. Onset of type 2 diabetes during adolescence is associated with an overall risk for complications similar to that of adults with type 2, and a rate of progression higher than that of adolescents with type 1 diabetes.[16]

The microvascular complications associated with type 1 diabetes are similar to those of type 2 diabetes and include retinopathy, nephropathy, and neuropathy. Macrovascular complications are also similar and include cardiovascular disease and stroke.[17,18] Intensive glucose control reduces the development and progression of these microvascular complications.[19] Increased insulin resistance, on the other hand, increases the subsequent risk of both micro and macrovascular complications in people with type 1 diabetes.[20]

Additional autoimmune diseases—especially celiac disease, thyroid disease, and Addison's disease (hypoadrenalism)—are common in people with type 1 diabetes, and at diagnosis, one third of children with type 1 diabetes test positive for the antibodies associated with these diseases.[21] Bone mineral density is lower in adults with type 1 diabetes, although higher in adults with type 2. Both type 1 and type 2 patients however, have a higher risk of bone fracture.[22]

In addition to the health problems associated with obesity and diabetes, there is a tremendous burden, in term of both time and money, placed on our health care systems and governmental agencies. Obesity is now more costly than any other preventive cause of death, with costs estimated to be 17% of all US medical costs each year.[23] It is clear that individuals that were obese or overweight as adolescents are highly likely to be obese adults, and to develop cardiovascular disease, colon cancer, and arthritis, even if they loseweight later in life.[24] Furthermore, obese children at age 12, and who remain overweight, will have direct medical expenses of an estimated $6.24B associated with their excess weight throughout their lives.[24] Thus there are enormous health and health care costs associated with obesity and diabetes.

8.3 Genetics and Obesity and Diabetes

Evidence for a genetic basis for obesity comes mainly from studies of resemblance and differences among family members, twins, and adoptees.[25] A few studies have reported that specific genes or genetic polymorphisms account for higher rates of obesity in certain populations. For instance, linkage studies in humans and animal models have uncovered some rare obesity causing genes, such as leptin and its receptor, as well as mutations in the melanocortin 4 receptor gene.[26] The genome-wide association studies utilizing massive populations have uncovered some 40 novel single-nucleotide polymorphisms that while robustly associating with BMI, even together only explain less than 5% of the observed variation.[27] Numerous genetic alleles—more than 40—have been associated with type 2 diabetes, but their overall effect remains small; the heritability of type 2 diabetes is usually estimated to be around 25%.[28] As with obesity, the rapidly increasing diabetes incidence cannot be attributed to genetic susceptibility. However, the relative paucity of direct genetic evidence suggests that other factors play a major role in obesity.

The genes associated with type 2 diabetes act in conjunction with various recognized environmental factors, including aging, pregnancy, physical inactivity, nutrition, puberty, and weight to contribute to disease.[29] More than 50 genetic susceptibility loci have been identified for type 1 diabetes to date. Compared to childhood-onset type 1, a lower frequency of high-risk alleles are found in people with adult-onset type 1.[30] In fact, both type 1 and type 2 associated genes have been associated in adult-onset type 1.[31,32] A number of analyses have confirmed that the highest risk genotype has been decreasing in new onset type 1 diabetes cases over recent decades; those with a lower or moderate risk of disease are now more likely to develop type 1 diabetes. This finding suggests that some environmental change that increases disease penetrance in those with lower risk geneotypes plays a role in the increasing incidence of disease.[33] High genetic risk is neither necessary nor sufficient for the development of type 1 diabetes.

In summary, there is no doubt that genetics plays an important role in both obesity and type 1 and 2 diabetes. It is clear however, that genetics is not the only factor and that environmental factors also play an important role. Obesity and diabetes, like all complex diseases, are the result of gene-environment interactions. To really understand the etiology of these diseases, one must focus not just on genetics but on the interaction of genetic background with environmental effects. The myopic focus on genetics as the only or primary cause of these diseases is not likely to be a fruitful endeavor, especially in light of the significant increases in disease incidence and prevalence over the last 40 years, during which there has been little change in genetics but drastic changes in the environment.

8.4 Endocrine Mechanisms Controlling Weight Gain

Feeding behavior, satiety, energy metabolism, and blood glucose levels are all controlled by a complex, interactive endocrine system that consists of the brain, adipose tissue, GI tract, muscle, liver, pancreas, and hormones and adipokines that circulate between these endocrine organs (Figure 8.1). There are two main pathways controlling food intake, the homeostatic system and the brain reward

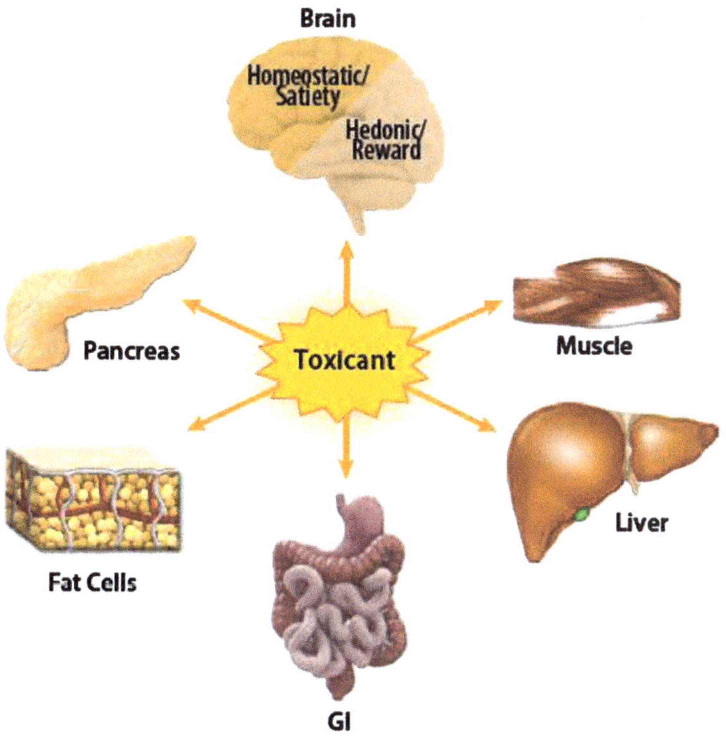

Figure 8.1 The two main pathways controlling food intake, the homeostatic system and brain reward (hedonic) system, both of which are centered in the brain. Feeding behavior, satiety, energy metabolism, and blood glucose levels are all controlled by a complex interacting endocrine system that consists of the brain, adipose tissue, GI tract, muscle, liver, pancreas, and also hormones and adipokines that circulate between these endocrine organs.

(hedonic) system, both of which are centered in the brain. One of the primary functions of the brain during periods of food scarcity or surplus is to prioritize behavioral output to procure and consume food, thereby maintaining a homeostatic energy balance. The hypothalamus is the brain region responsible for controlling food intake and satiety via a series of homeostatic pathways and mechanisms. It acts by sensing glucose, fatty acids and proteins as well as integrating signals from leptin, cholecystokinin, ghrelin, insulin, and neuropeptide Y, to control food intake[34–37] (Table 8.1).

In addition to homeostatic energy systems, reward systems also have key roles in regulating feeding behavior.[38] The brain reward systems control learning about the palatable (hedonic) properties of food and thus regulate the incentive value of food or environmental stimuli that predict the availability of food rewards. These areas are regulated by dopamine, cannabinoids, opiods, and serotonin, along with input from homeostatic mechanisms.[39,40] Hormonal regulators of energy homeostasis can also act on brain reward circuits, most

Table 8.1 Hormonal control of appetite and metabolism.

Hormone	*Site of Production*	*Effect*
Leptin	Adipose tissue	Reduces food intake
Ghrelin	Stomach	Stimulates food intake
Cholycystekinin/GLP-1	Intestine	Inhibits food intake
Insulin	Pancreas	Inhibits food intake
Cortisol	Adrenal gland	Stimulates food intake
NPY/AGRP	Brain	Stimulates food intake
Orexin	Brain	Stimulates food intake
Seratonin/5HT	Brain	Inhibits food intake
Alpha MSH/POMC	Brain	Inhibits food intake/increase
Energy expenditure		
Dopamine System	Brain	Controls food reward

[a]Selected examples, not a complete list.

notably on the dopamine system,[41] to increase or decrease the incentive value of food depending on energy requirements. However, stimulation of brain areas that regulate food reward can trigger binge-like overeating, even in recently fed animals in which homeostatic satiety signals have been engaged.[42,43] This suggests that obtaining the pleasurable effects of food is a powerful motivating force that can override homeostatic satiety signals, leading individuals to consume food with greater frequency and in greater portions.[44] And since a single meal of increased portion size can trigger increased food intake over several days, hedonic stimulated overeating is likely to be an important contributor to weight gain and the development of obesity.[38] In addition, certain foods, for example those high in sugars and fat, stimulate the reward pathways, leading to increased consumption even when not hungry. Thus, in many respects, these reward pathways are similar to addiction pathways.

In summary, there is neither an independent hunger center nor pleasure center; complex interactions among multiple tissues and organs are involved in all aspects of food intake and metabolism. The homeostatic regulatory system (control of hunger) is easily overturned by the reward (hedonic) system (control of food craving), resulting in weight gain. Similarly, the homeostatic system defends against weight loss such that weight gained is not easily lost.[45]

8.5 Causes of Obesity

The prevailing hypothesis for the obesity epidemic is that people simply overeat and under-exercise. We live in a world surrounded by highly processed foods containing a high fat and sugar content. Indeed it is clear that technological advances in agriculture and food processing have enhanced the nature and variety of food available to people, thus increasing the likelihood of overeating. The ease of access to highly palatable food increases a person's desire to eat and thus it requires a strong physiologic system to overcome these food urges. Interestingly, only a subset of individuals overeat and gain weight, and have what some researchers refer to as a "food addiction". This specificity raises the question of why, when individuals are exposed to the same basic environment, do only some overeat and become obese? In other words, does the simple availability of highly palatable foods cause us to eat more and become obese? Or are there other underlying differences between individuals who remain lean and those that overeat that predisposes some to overeating and obesity? As described, genetics clearly plays a role, but it is also clear that genetics can only account for a small portion of obesity and diabetes and not for the increase over past decades. Thus the environment, more specifically environmental chemicals, must play an important role in susceptibility to obesity and diabetes.

We postulate that early life environmental events are likely to be a contributing cause of the obesity epidemic due to disruption of perinatal and prenatal metabolic programming events, which leads to increased risks of obesity later in life. It is plausible that individuals at risk for weight gain may have been subject to altered programming events early in life, which makes them more susceptible to "food addiction" and overeating. Since obesity is controlled by homeostatic mechanisms that regulate both hunger and satiety, as well as reward pathways that control desire for food and conditioning to food cues, changes at any point in this circuitry could predispose individuals to weight gain. Perhaps we can learn more about obesity by asking the question: What are the fundamental differences between lean and obese individuals aside from genetics? And, why do some people become obese whilst others do not when exposed to the same foods?

Table 8.2 illustrates that there are many different behavioral patterns between lean individuals and obese individuals. Overweight individuals view food differently; they have a higher preference for high fat and sugar foods, crave foods, are emotional eaters, will work harder for food, and overeat despite the negative consequences. Obese individuals have increased desire for certain foods when they attempt to abstain from eating, and have withdrawal symptoms, such as agitation or anxiety, when they stop eating certain foods.[46] These differences are not just psychological, but in fact can be traced to actual

Table 8.2 Differences between obese and lean individuals.

Characteristics and behaviors	*Obese compared to lean*
Food preferences and behaviors	Preference for high fat and high sugar foods
Food satiety	Higher desire and anticipation for food Delayed state of satiation (delayed satiety signals)
Emotional links to food	Increased eating in response to anxiety, depression, mood swings
Food satisfaction	Greater reward from food intake
Brain activity	Increased dopamine receptors in brain and pleasure sensation
Hormones	Higher insulin levels, impaired leptin signaling
Receptors	Decreased striatal dopamine (DR2) receptors
Acquisition of food	Work harder to obtain food

differences in brain chemistry. On the other hand, lean individuals eat primarily to sustain life and can stop eating mid-meal, when they perceive they are "full".

8.6 Metabolic Programming, Epigenetics and Obesity

Metabolic programming during prenatal and perinatal development has become an active area of research in the study of obesity. The developmental origins of health and disease (DOHaD) hypothesis, first proposed by David Barker in 1997, showed that poor *in utero* nutrition resulted in high rates of disease—including obesity—later in life.[47] More recent studies have linked higher maternal pre-pregnancy BMI and higher gestational weight gain with increased birth weight and fat mass at birth. Maternal diabetes is also associated with increased birth weight as well as childhood overweight and obesity. Interestingly, paternal nutrition has also been traced to ill-fated health outcomes in offspring. For instance, reports have shown that paternal obesity is associated with a disruption in insulin secretion and glucose tolerance in offspring. Paradoxically, children and adults born small for their gestational age also have an increased risk of obesity, which may be mediated by rapid compensatory postnatal growth. Thus there are significant data linking developmental nutritional status to obesity later in life.

The concept of disruptions in developmental programming has now been extended to include non-nutritional early life exposures that have been shown to alter the body's physiology. Focus on the fetus and/or neonate is of primary concern since developing organisms are extremely sensitive to perturbation by chemicals with hormone-like activity, *e.g.* endocrine disruptors. Adverse effects may occur at concentrations of the chemical that are far below levels that would be considered harmful in the adult.[48] Some reasons for this increased sensitivity are that the protective mechanisms available to the adult—such as DNA repair mechanisms, a competent immune system, detoxifying enzymes, liver metabolism, and the blood/brain barrier—are not fully functional in the fetus or newborn. In addition, the developing organism has an increased metabolic rate as compared to an adult which, in some cases, may result in increased toxicity.[48] Finally, prenatal exposure to environmental factors can modify normal cellular and tissue development and function through developmental programming, such that individuals may have a higher risk of reproductive pathologies and metabolic and hormonal disorders later in life. Thus exposures during critical windows of perinatal development may not manifest until much later in life. While fetal development is commonly known to be a period of increased sensitivity to chemical insult, childhood and adolescence are also marked by continued maturation of key endocrine systems, and are therefore susceptible to chemical exposure.[49]

Of special concern are man-made hormone mimicking chemicals capable of evading defense mechanisms and misdirecting developmental decisions. Recent studies document detectable quantities of a variety of endocrine disrupting chemicals (EDCs)—such as persistent organic pesticides (POPs), phthalates, polybrominated diphenyl ethers, polycyclic aromatic hydrocarbons, and bisphenol A (BPA)—in pregnant women, fetuses, newborns, young children, and adolescents.[50–55] Since each organ system has a different developmental trajectory, and the sensitive window for exposures to cause toxicity changes during tissue development, the effects of exposures are dependent not only on the type and dose of the chemical, but also on when the exposure occurs.[56] These studies illustrate that the *in utero* developmental period is a critically sensitive window of vulnerability. Disruptions during this time-frame can lead to subtle functional changes that may not emerge until later in life.[56] Evidence now suggests that early life exposures to toxic chemicals can be directly associated with subsequent increases in the prevalence of the most common diseases in the last 20 years (Figure 8.2). Table 8.3 shows diseases that have been demonstrated, in animal studies, to result from exposure to environmental chemicals during development, *e.g.* due to altered programming. Note that obesity and diabetes are among the diseases/dysfunctions that result from altered developmental programming by environmental chemicals.

There are several important principles that demonstrate how early life environmental exposures contribute to increased risks of adult disease. Firstly, chemical exposures can have both tissue-specific and time-specific consequences on growth and development. As long as tissue is developing, it is susceptible to disruptions from environmental exposures. These disruptions can result from

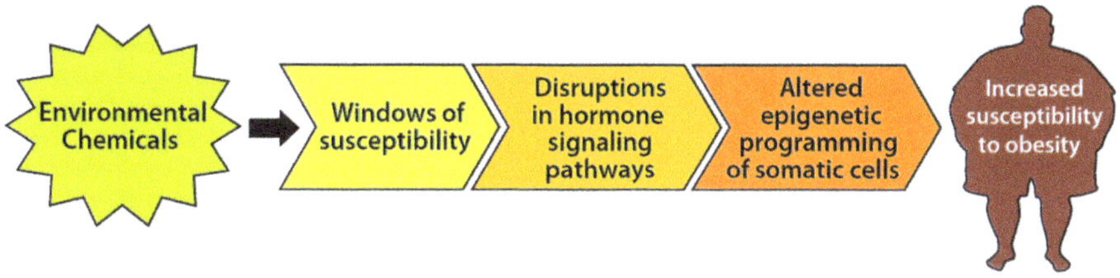

Figure 8.2 Model illustrating early life exposures may cause functional changes at cellular levels that lead to changes in physiological status, and ultimately increased susceptibility to obesity later in life.

Table 8.3 Diseases/dysfunctions in animals that can be traced to alterations in developmental programming caused by exposure to environmental chemicals.

Disease/dysfunction	*References*
Learning and behavioral problems	[58–61]
Early puberty	[62–64]
Infertility	[65, 66]
Breast and prostate cancer	[67, 68]
Parkinson's disease	[69, 70]
Obesity and diabetes	[71–73]
Asthma	[74, 75]
Heart disease/hypertension	[76, 77]
Neurodegenerative diseases	[78]

changes in gene expression, protein activity, cell communication, or other mechanisms. Secondly, the initiating *in utero* exposure may act alone or in concert with other environmental stressors. That is, the risk of developing disease in adulthood can be due to the combined insults over a lifetime. Thirdly, the pathophysiology may be manifested in a disease that otherwise might not have occurred, and disease progression may have variable latent periods. Fourthly, there is a latent period between exposure and disease which could range from months to decades. Finally, the effects of environmental chemical exposures can be transgenerational, thus affecting future generations (Figure 8.3).[57]

It seems likely that at least of part of the developmental programming of disease/dysfunction is the result of alterations in the epigenetic control of gene expression during development. Epigenetic mechanisms of gene regulation, such as DNA methylation and histone modifications (*e.g.* methylation, acetylation, ubiquitination) regulate gene expression during development and are thus responsible for normal tissue and organ development.[79,80] During this critical time period, the epigenome cycles through a series of precisely timed methylation changes, designed to ensure proper development. The appropriate timing and extraordinary accuracy of methylation in the gametes and following fertilization makes this system particularly vulnerable to interference from environmental exposures.[81] The highly orchestrated processes that occur

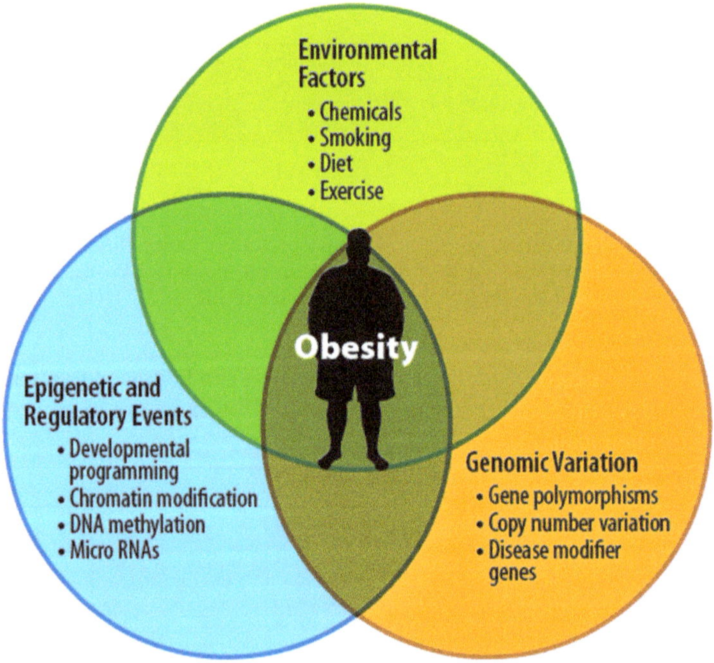

Figure 8.3 Illustration of the complex interactions between environmental factors, epigenetic regulatory events, and genomic variations that can lead to increased risk of obesity.

during these critical developmental periods give rise to concerns about vulnerability during the early stages of life. Indeed it is now clear that the epigenetic system is responsive to environmental stimuli, such as drugs of abuse, diet, or chemical exposures. Recent reports have identified epigenetic modifications in the central nervous system in response to altered diet, particularly in the prenatal or early postnatal time period, when brain development is particularly vulnerable to perturbations.[80] For example, consumption of a palatable high-fat diet increases DNA and histone methylation and decreases histone acetylation status in the promoter region of the opioid receptor mu 1 (MOR1) gene, which correlates with decreased MOR expression.[80] Thus changes in DNA methylation patterns and chromatin remodeling in response to nutritional status *in utero* or during early postnatal development can affect dietary preference and metabolism.[5]

8.7 The Obesogen Hypothesis

Chemicals that give rise to obesity have been referred to as "obesogens".[82] These chemicals are found in a wide variety of products, and most are categorized as endocrine disruptors due to their hormone mimicking abilities. Like hormones, these chemicals exert their effects at very low concentrations and often operate in a non-linear dose response manner. Moreover, if these hormonal disruptions occur during critical developmental periods, life-long functional changes can occur. These properties—low concentrations, tissue specificity, non-linear dose responses, and disruptions at precise time periods—make it difficult to assess the role of environmental chemicals in causing obesity and diabetes. Nonetheless, there are now close to 20 chemicals, including organophosphate pesticides, carbamates, and antithyroid drugs, that have been linked to obesity or diabetes in animals. In addition, there are chemicals , such as anabolic steroids and the estrogenic drug diethylstilbestrol (DES), that have been used for decades to promote fattening and growth of farm animals.[83,84] Here, we review selected examples associating chemical exposure to the development of obesity.

8.8 Animal Studies

8.8.1 Bisphenol A

Recently, there has been a great deal of interest in BPA because of its high production volume and its potential for widespread commercial use. Numerous studies have shown a link between BPA exposure and increased body weight and adiposity in animal models.[85–90] BPA exposure during gestation and lactation accelerated adipogenesis or increased fat pad weights at the time of, or soon after, weaning.[90–92] A recent study in rats confirmed an increase in the expression of adipogenic genes in adipose tissue at the time of weaning in BPA exposed animals.[91] Some evidence suggests that the increases in body weight are sex specific, but timing and dose may contribute to the complexity of these findings.[89,91,92] Thus far changes in body weight have been reported in animals exposed to BPA during gestation, during the gestation and throughout lactation, and in one study, BPA exposure continued through PND 30 when animals were sacrificed.[93] To date, no studies have continued BPA exposure throughout life, and few have followed measurements of body weight and adiposity through adulthood and to later ages. Far more investigation is needed in order to understand the effects of BPA exposure on body weight and adiposity prepubertally later in life, and the mechanisms through which BPA may be acting.[94]

8.8.2 Organotins

Organotins are used in plasticizers, slimicides, fungicides, antifoulants, catalysts, and stabilizers. Tributyl tin (TBT) and triphenyl tinare retinoid X receptor and PPARγ agonists.[95,96] Peripubertal exposure to TBT increases both body and fat mass. Neonatal male and female mice exposed to TBT *in utero* had greater Oil Red O staining (indicative of lipid droplets) in their livers, testis, and adipose tissues at birth and 20% increased adipose mass over controls in adulthood.[96] *In utero* exposure of mice to TBT caused multipotent stem cells to differentiate into adipocytes when collected from adult mice, compared with similarly collected *ex vivo* cells from vehicle-treated mice.[97] This resulted in a greater lipid accumulation within stem cells-turned-adipocytes from mice prenatally exposed to TBT, compared with vehicle-treated mice.[97] Further, the stem cells from mice exposed to TBT *in utero* had a greater propensity to become lipid-filled adipocytes when exposed to more TBT or the diabetes drug rosiglitizone, another PPARγ agonist. This increased adipogenic capacity may have resulted in a TBT-induced shift in cell population.[97,98] Male mice exposed to TBT during puberty had increased body mass, associated with increased relative fat mass.[98,99] In rats exposed to TBT beginning *in utero* and continuing throughout adulthood, the trend of body mass and fat is less consistent than that observed for other TBT developmental exposure studies; male rats had a small decrease in body mass, whereas 2 other studies found opposite effects of TBT exposure on the body weights of female rats.[98,100] Thus the animal data are conclusive for the role of TBT and other tin analogs as obesogens. Unfortunately there are no human data on developmental exposures to TBT and weight gain and few data on human exposures.

8.8.3 Cigarette Smoke/Nicotine

When mice were exposed to cigarette smoke while pregnant, the influence of the cigarette smoke on the body weights of their offspring was gender-dependent and diet-dependent.[101] Adult female offspring fed a normal diet had significantly increased body weights if exposed to cigarette *smoke in utero*, compared with unexposed females, but cigarette smoke did not impact body weights of females fed a high fat diet for 2 weeks.[102] Adult male offspring exposed to cigarette smoke *in utero* had a higher body weight than control-treated males if fed a high fat diet, but there was no cigarette smoking effect on male body weight if males ate a normal diet.[102] Male rats exposed to nicotine *in utero* had significantly increased body mass and white adipose tissue mass at weaning and throughout adulthood.[101] There was also evidence of adipocyte hypertrophy in the white adipose tissue mass at weaning. *In utero* nicotine exposure did not change food intake or energy expenditure. However, nicotine exposure was associated with higher food efficiency (food intake relative to body weight increase), decreased physical activity, decreased brown adipose tissue mass, and decreased thermogenesis.[101] None of these *in utero* nicotine effects were evident in female offspring.[101] Adult male mice (females were not tested) exposed to the cigarette smoke and diesel exhaust constituent, benzo[a]pyrene had increased body weights and weight gain compared with unexposed mice.[101] In another study, the longer that adult male rats were exposed to diesel exhaust, the greater the increase in their body weights.[103] These effects have not been reproduced in cell culture, where differentiation of 3T3-L1 preadipocytes, as well as their lipid accumulation, was decreased dose-dependently up to exposure equivalent to 1 pack of cigarettes.[98,104]

8.8.4 Polyfluoroalkynes (PFOAs)

Perfluorooctanoic acid (PFOA), also known as C8 or perfluorooctanoate, is a synthetic, stable, perfluorinated carboxylic acid and fluorosurfactant. PFOAs are used as surfactants in the emulsion polymerization of fluoropolymers, such as in the manufacture of prominent consumer goods like Teflon and Gore-Tex. PFOA has been manufactured in industrial quantities since the 1940s. It is also formed by the degradation of precursors such as some fluorotelomers. PFOAs are persist indefinitely in the environment. It is a toxicant and carcinogen in animals. PFOAs have been detected in the blood of more than 98% of the general US population in the low and sub-parts per billion range, and levels are higher in chemical plant employees and surrounding subpopulations.[105]

Mice exposed to low levels of PFOAs *in utero* had significantly increased body mass by 10 weeks old, which persisted through to midlife.[106] Interestingly, when these mice reached 18 months of age, there was an inverse and direct dose–response relationship between *in utero* PFOA doses and abdominal white and brown adipose tissue masses respectively.[106] However, mice exposed to high doses of PFOAs during gestation had decreased body mass.[106–108] In line with observations of adult human exposure to PFOAs, mice exposed to PFOAs as adults experienced no change in body mass or fat mass across PFOA doses and ages.[106]

8.9 Human Studies

8.9.1 Maternal Smoking

The epidemiological data strongly support a positive and likely causal association between maternal smoking and increased risk of obesity or

Reference	Study Description (n)	Risk Estimate adjOR (95% CI)	Exposure
Gorog et al. 2009	Europe (6 countries) CESAR, 9-12y, ♂♀ (8,926)	1.26 (1.03, 1.55)	yes/no
Toschke et al. 2002	Germany (Bavaria) 5-6.9y (1997), ♂♀ (8,365)	1.92 (1.29, 2.86)	yes/no
Toschke et al. 2003	Germany (Bavaria) 5-6y (2001/2002), ♂♀ (4,974)	2.22 (1.33, 3.69)	yes/no
Toschke et al. 2007	Germany (Bavaria) 5-6y (2001/2002), ♂♀ (5,472)	1.75 (1.25, 2.43)	yes/no
Von Kries 2002	Germany (Bavaria) 5-6.9y, ♂♀ (6,483)	2.06 (1.31, 3.23)	yes/no
Von Kries 2008	Germany (Bavaria) 5-6.9y, ♂♀ (5,899)	1.9 (1.3, 2.7)	yes/no
Ino et al. 2011	Japan (Kumagaya) 9-10y, ♂♀ (2,508)	1.55 (0.67, 3.57) [crude prevOR]	yes/no
Koshy et al. 2011	UK (Merseyside) 5-11y, ♂♀ (3,038)	1.61 (1.19, 2.18)	yes/no
Raum et al. 2011	Germany (Aachen) 6y, ♂♀ (1,954)	1.51 (0.99, 2.28)	yes/no
Toschke et al. 2002	Germany (Bavaria) 5-6.9y (1997), ♂♀ (8,365)	1.58 (1.23, 2.04)	yes/no
Toschke et al. 2003	Germany (Bavaria) 5-6y (2001/2002), ♂♀ (4,974)	1.52 (1.14, 2.01)	yes/no
Toschke et al. 2007	Germany (Bavaria) 5-6y (2001/2002), ♂♀ (5,472)	1.32 (1.10, 1.61)	yes/no
Von Kries 2002	Germany (Bavaria) 5-6.9y, ♂♀ (6,483)	1.43 (1.07, 1.90)	yes/no
Von Kries 2008	Germany (Bavaria) 5-6.9y, ♂♀ (5,899)	1.3 (1.1, 1.7)	yes/no
Al Mamum 2006	Australia (Brisbane, Queensland) 14y, ♂♀ (3,253)	1.40 (1.01, 1.94)	yes/no
Bergmann et al. 2003	Germany (multi-site) 6y, ♂♀ (918)	2.3 (1.2, 4.6)	yes/no
Dubois and Girard 2006	Canada (Quebec) 4.5y, ♂♀ (2,103)	1.8 (1.2, 2.8)	yes/no
Durmus et al. 2011	Netherlands (Gen R) 4y, ♂♀ (5,342)	1.61 (1.03, 2.53)	yes/no
Montgomery and Ekbom 2002	UK (nat'l) NCDS, 33y, ♂♀ (4,917)	1.38 (1.06, 1.79)	heavy vs no
Power and Jefferis 2002	UK (England, Scotland, Wales) 1958 BBC, 33y, ♀ (2,921)	1.45 (1.13, 1.87)	yes/no, >4 month
Power and Jefferis 2002	UK (England, Scotland, Wales) 1958 BBC, 33y, ♂ (2,918)	1.55 (1.19, 2.00)	yes/no, >4 month
Power et al. 2010	UK (England, Scotland, Wales) 1958 BBC, 45y, ♂♀ (8,815)	1.40 (1.25, 1.56)	yes/no, >4 month
Reilly et al. 2005	UK (multi-site) ALSPAC 7y, ♂♀ (7,758)	1.80 (1.01, 3.99)	1-9 cig/d vs 0
Rooney et al. 2010	US (3 midwestern states) 9-14y, ♂♀ (777)	2.15 (1.22, 3.78)	yes/no
Salsberry and Reagan 2005	US (nat'l) NLSY Child-Mother, 6-7y, ♂♀ (3,022)	1.74 (1.32, 2.29)	yes/no
Salsberry and Reagan 2007	US (nat'l) NLSY Child-Mother, 12-13y, ♂♀ (3,368)	1.41 (1.08, 1.84)	yes/no
Suzuki et al. 2009	Japan (Koshu City) 9-10y, ♂♀ (1,644)	2.56 (1.02, 6.38)	current vs none/former
Al Mamum 2006	Australia (Brisbane, Queensland) 14y, ♂♀ (3,253)	1.3 (1.1, 1.6)	yes/no
Bergmann et al. 2003	Germany (multi-site) 6y, ♂♀ (918)	2.08 (1.19, 3.63)	yes/no
Boerschmann et al. 2010	Germany (multi-site) GDM offspring study 2y, ♂♀ (1,420)	2.2 (0.6, 8.3)	≥1 cig/d vs 0
Boerschmann et al. 2010	Germany (multi-site) GDM offspring study 11y, ♂♀ (1,420)	22.7 (1.9, 2.8)	≥1 cig/d vs 0
Braun et al. 2010	US (Cincinnati, OH) 3y, ♂♀ (389)	1.9 (0.6, 6.1)	yes/no
Chen et al. 2006	US (multi-site) CPP 8y, ♀ (14,612)	1.37 (1.19, 1.58)	active vs never
Chen et al. 2006	US (multi-site) CPP 8y, ♂ (14,486)	1.21 (1.05, 1.39)	current vs never
Durmus et al. 2011	Netherlands (Gen R) 4y, ♂♀ (5,342)	1.00 (0.78, 1.28)	yes/no
Gillman et al. 2008	US (Boston, MA) Project Viva, 3y, ♂♀ (1,110)	1.71 (0.90, 3.25)	yes/no
Iliadou et al. 2010	Sweden (nat'l) milt. serv. registry 17-24y, ♂ (124,203)	1.41 (1.34, 1.49)	1-9 cig/d vs 0
Koupil et al. 2008	Sweden (nat'l) registries, 18y, ♂ (6,535)	1.71 (1.21, 2.43)	yes/no
Kuhle et al. 2010	Canada (Nova Scotia) CLASS 5th grade, ♂♀ (3,426)	1.43 (1.17, 1.75)	>0-5 packs/d vs none
Mizutani et al. 2007	Japan (Enzan City) Project Enzan, 5y, ♂♀ (1417)	2.15 (1.12, 4.11)	yes/no, early pregnancy
Oken et al. 2005	US (Boston, MA) Project Viva, 3y, ♂♀ (2,218)	2.2 (1.2, 3.9)	yes/no, early pregnancy
Tome et al. 2007	Brazil (Ribeirao) 8-10y, ♂♀ (2,797)	1.07 (0.84, 1.37)	yes/no
Wideroe et al. 2003	Norway/Sweden (Trondheim/Bergen) 5y, ♂♀ (482)	3.8 (2.1, 7.2)	yes/no
Sharma et al. 2008	US (multi-site) PedNSS (Asia/Pacific) 2-4y, ♂♀ (4,740)	0.85 (0.35, 2.07)	yes/no
Sharma et al. 2008	US (multi-site) PedNSS (Am. Ind./AK Nat.) 2-4y , ♂♀ (2,228)	1.01 (0.71, 1.44)	yes/no
Sharma et al. 2008	US (multi-site) PedNSS (Hispanic) 2-4y, ♂♀ (34,378)	1.11 (0.95, 1.31)	yes/no
Sharma et al. 2008	US (multi-site) PedNSS (Black) 2-4y, ♂♀ (31,704)	1.32 (1.17, 1.50)	yes/no
Sharma et al. 2008	US (multi-site) PedNSS (White) 2-4y, ♂♀ (82,361)	1.59 (1.5, 1.68)	yes/no
Whitaker 2004	US (OH) WIC, 4y, ♂♀ (8,494)	1.21 (1.01, 1.45)	yes/no
Adams et al. 2005	US (WI) Amer. Ind./WIC program, 3y, ♂♀ (252)	2.16 (1.05, 4.47)	yes/no

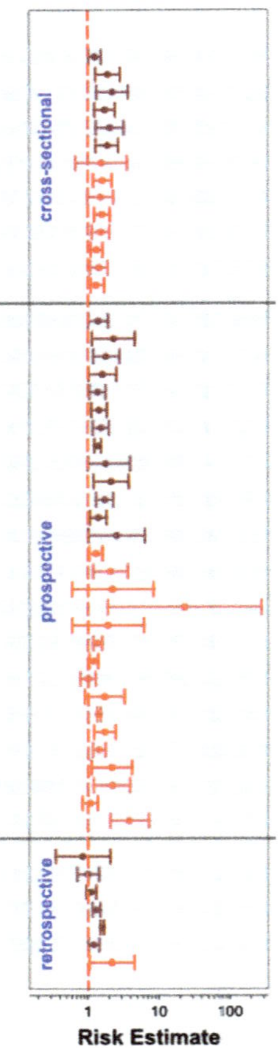

overweight
obesity

⊢ upper 95th confidence limit ⊣ lower 95th confidence limit ● risk estimate

overweight in offspring. This conclusion was based on the very consistent pattern of overweight/obesity observed in the children of mothers' who smoked during pregnancy, along with findings from laboratory animals exposed to nicotine during development.[71] Approximately 20 epidemiological studies have examined the impact of maternal smoking during pregnancy and body weight on offspring during childhood or adulthood. These studies show a consistent association between maternal smoking during pregnancy and increased risk of overweight/obesity in the offspring (Figure 8.4). This literature was evaluated in two recent meta-analyses.[109,110] The pooled OR estimate in Oken *et al.*[109] for elevated risk of overweight was 1.50 (95% CI: 1.35–1.65) based on 14 studies. The pooled OR in Ino[110] for obesity (BMI>95th percentile) was 1.64 (1.42–1.90) based on 16 studies.

Both meta-analyses used funnel plot methods to ascertain publication bias and concluded that there was some evidence for publication bias, but not enough to negate the overall conclusion of increased risk. Adjusted pooled ORs that considered publication bias were still significant: OR (95% CI) = 1.40 (1.26–1.55)[109] and 1.52 (1.36–1.70).[110]

8.9.2 Persistent Organic Pollutants

As mentioned earlier, the prevalence of obesity is reaching epidemic proportions worldwide and the increasing prevalence of obesity in young children is alarming. Early environmental influences may be a large contributor to this problem as children may be especially sensitive to the effects of endocrine-disrupting chemicals, such as POPs, when exposed prenatally and/or postnatally. Unfortunately, the human literature on POPs and childhood obesity is very limited and results are not consistent. Some studies have reported that exposure to pesticides (*e.g.* DDE) and organochlorines (*e.g.* PCBs) are associated with increased BMI during childhood[111,112] and in adulthood.[113] One study found that children with higher levels of hexachlorobenzene (HCB) have an elevated risk of 1.69 (95% CI: 1.05, 2.72) and 2.02 (95% CI: 1.06, 3.85) of being overweight and obese.[114] However, there is also

Figure 8.4 Human studies on maternal smoking during pregnancy and risk for childhood overweight and obesity. Abbreviations: Amer. Ind – American Indian; ALSPAC – Avon Longitudinal Study of Parents and Children; adjOR – adjusted odds ratio; BBC – British Birth Cohort; BMI – body mass index; CESAR – Central European Study on Air Pollution and Respiratory Health; CLASS – Children's Lifestyle and School Performance study; CPP – Collaborative Perinatal Project; GDM – gestational diabetes mellitus; Gen R – Generation R study; NCDS – National Child Development Study; NLSY – National Longitudinal Survey of Youth; PedNSS – Pediatric Nutrition Surveillance System; WIC – Women, Infants, and Children program; RR– relative risk; wt. – weight; ref. – referent group. Risk estimates for bracketed statistics, *i.e.*, [crudeRR] calculated based on data presented in the paper using an open source epidemiology statistics programs, OpenEpi (http://www.openepi.com/menu/openEpiMenu.htm)

Reference	*Study Design*	*Study Description (n)*	*Health Outcome*	*Chemical*	*Exposure*	*Statistic adjOR (95% CI)*
Lin 2009	cross-sectional	US (NHANES 99-00, 03-04) 12-20y, ♂♀, (474)	waist circumference	PFHxS	0.95[avg] log ng/mL (serum)	0.64 (0.45, 0.91) per 1-unit ↑
Lin 2009	cross-sectional	US (NHANES 99-00, 03-04) 12-20y, ♂♀, (474)	waist circumference	PFNA	−0.35[avg] log ng/mL (serum)	1.09 (0.61, 1.95) per 1-unit ↑
Lin 2009	cross-sectional	US (NHANES 99-00, 03-04) 12-20y, ♂♀, (474)	waist circumference	PFOA	1.51[avg] log ng/mL (serum)	0.58 (0.34, 1) per 1-unit ↑
Lin 2009	cross-sectional	US (NHANES 99-00, 03-04) 12-20y, ♂♀, (474)	waist circumference	PFOS	3.11[avg] log ng/mL (serum)	0.37 (0.16, 0.82) per 1-unit ↑
Lin 2009	cross-sectional	US (NHANES 99-00, 03-04) >20y, ♂♀, (969)	waist circumference	PFHxS	0.6[avg] log ng/ml (serum)	0.8 (0.58, 1.1) per 1-unit ↑
Lin 2009	cross-sectional	US (NHANES 99-00, 03-04) >20y, ♂♀, (969)	waist circumference	PFNA	−0.21[avg] log ng/ml (serum)	1.34 (0.93, 1.92) per 1-unit ↑
Lin 2009	cross-sectional	US (NHANES 99-00, 03-04) >20y, ♂♀, (969)	waist circumference	PFOA	1.48[avg] log ng/ml (serum)	0.97 (0.65, 1.46) per 1-unit ↑
Lin 2009	cross-sectional	US (NHANES 99-00, 03-04) >20y, ♂♀, (969)	waist circumference	PFOS	3.19[avg] log ng/ml (serum)	0.91 (0.59, 1.41) per 1-unit ↑
Smink 2008	prospective	Spain (Menorca) 6.5y, ♂♀, (405)	obese	HCB	≥0.46 vs <0.46 log ng/mL (serum, mat. cord)	2.02 (1.06, 3.85)
Smink 2008	prospective	Spain (Menorca) 6.5y, ♂♀, (405)	overweight	HCB	≥0.46 vs <0.46 log ng/mL (serum, mat. cord)	1.69 (1.05, 2.72)

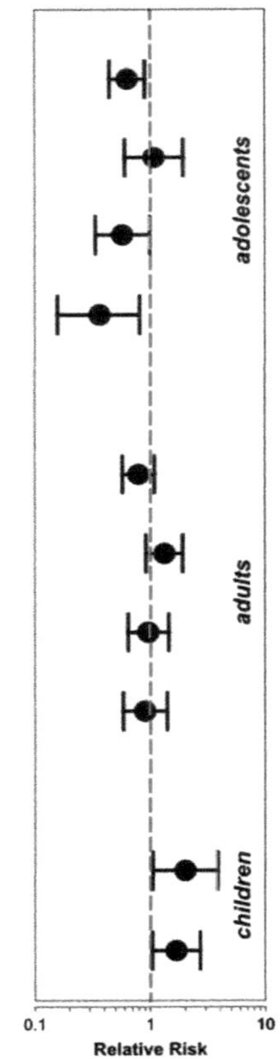

⊢ Lower 95% CL ⊣ Upper 95% CL ● Relative Risk

evidence of inverse associations between some POPs and childhood growth,[115] meaning there is still much research needed before any causal inferences can be made (Figures 8.5 and 8.6).

8.10 Type 2 diabetes

8.10.1 Background

Type 1 diabetes (formerly known as juvenile, or insulin-dependent diabetes) is caused by autoimmune destruction of the pancreatic beta cells, resulting in deficient or absent insulin production, and can occur at any age. Type 2 diabetes (formerly known as adult-onset, or non-insulin-dependent diabetes), accounts for 90–95% of diabetes cases, and is characterized by increased insulin resistance, as well as pancreatic beta cell dysfunction. The third most common type of diabetes, gestational diabetes, appears during pregnancy and resolves afterwards. Gestational diabetes complicates about 7% of all pregnancies, and increases the mother's later risk of type 2 diabetes. Pre-diabetes is an intermediate step (in all types of diabetes), defined by impaired glucose tolerance (post-meal) or impaired fasting blood glucose levels that are above normal but not high enough to qualify as diabetes.[11]

Increased insulin resistance (equivalent to decreased insulin sensitivity) occurs when the body's cells fail to respond effectively to circulating insulin. In an insulin resistant state, the ability of insulin to promote glucose uptake in the fat, muscle, and liver cells is reduced, and/or the ability of insulin to inhibit the liver's production of glucose is reduced.[109] In type 2 diabetes, insulin resistance may occur many years before diabetes develops, in conjunction with hyperinsulinemia (excess circulating insulin).[29] It is not known whether hyperinsulinemia preceeds insulin resistance in the progression of type 2 diabetes, or *vice versa*.[109] It is thought however, that during pre-diabetes, the beta cells hypersecrete insulin in an attempt to maintain normal blood glucose levels during a state of high insulin resistance. This hyperinsulinemia produces excess insulin signaling and can lead to hypertension and high triglyceride levels.[110] Eventually, when the pancreatic beta cells are no longer able to secrete adequate insulin to compensate for the increased demands of insulin resistance, impaired glucose tolerance results, finally progressing to type 2 diabetes.[29] In addition to its association with insulin resistance, type 2 diabetes is also characterized by beta cell failure, which involves both a deterioration in beta cell function and a loss of beta cell mass.[111]

Figure 8.5 Human studies on POPs exposure and risk for childhood overweight and obesity. Abbreviations: NHANES – National Health and Nutrition Examination Survey; HCB – Hexachlorobenzene; PFOS – perfluorooctane sulfonate; PFOA – perfluorooctanoic acid; PFNA – perfluorononanoic acid; PFHxS – perfluorohexane sulfonate; adjOR – adjusted odds ratio; avg – average; mat. cord – maternal cord.

Reference	Study Design	Health Outcome	Chemical	Exposure	Statistic adjB (95% CI)
Cupul-Uicab et al. 2010	Mexico (Chiapas) infant (median age 1.5y), ♂, (787)	BMI SDS, Δ	DDE, p,p'	>9.00 vs ≤3.00 µg/g lipid (serum, maternal)	[0.073 (−0.15, 0.297)]
Karmaus et al. 2009	US (MI) adult, ♀ of fish-eating moms, (267)	BMI	DDE	>2.9 vs <1.5 µg/L (serum, maternal)	[adjβ (SE): 2.88 (1.96, 3.8)]
Ribas-Fita et al. 2006	US (multi-site) Collaborative Perinatal Project, 7y, ♂♀, (1,371)	height	DDE, -p,p' (mat.)	≥60 vs <15 µg/L (serum, maternal)	[adjβ (SE): −2.19 (−2.65, −1.73)]
Verhulst et al. 2009	Belgium (Flanders) mother-infant pairs, 1-3y, ♂♀	BMI SDS 1-3y	DDE	212 (24-1,816) [avg (range)] ng/g lip. (serum, mat. cord)	[β (SE): −0.002 (± 0.001)]
Burns et al. 2011	Russia (Chapaevsk) Russian Children's Study, 8-9y, ♂, (461)	BMI	PCBs	152-209 (Q2) vs 62-151 (Q1) ng/g lipid (serum)	[−0.81 (−1.14, −0.48)]
Burns et al. 2011	Russia (Chapaevsk) Russian Children's Study, 8-9y, ♂, (461)	BMI	PCDD/PCDF/PCB	265-329 (Q2) vs 123-264 (Q1) pg/g lipid (serum)	[0.46 (−0.79, −0.12)]
Burns et al. 2011	Russia (Chapaevsk) Russian Children's Study, 8-9y, ♂, (461)	BMI	total TEQ	12.7-18.5 (Q2) vs 4.0-12.6 (Q1) pg TEQ/g lipid (serum)	[−0.53 (−0.86, −0.19)]
Karmaus et al. 2009	US (MI) adult, ♀ of fish-eating moms, (267)	BMI	PCBs	>1.94 vs <0.05 µg/L (serum, maternal)	[adjβ (SE): 1.28 (0.1, 2.46)]
Smink et al. 2008	Spain (Menorca) 6.5y, ♂♀ (405)	BMI	HCB	0.68 (0.46-1.03)[median (25th-27th)] ng/mL (serum, maternal cord)	[adjβ (SE): 0.51 (0.32, 0.70)]
Verhulst et al. 2009	Belgium (Flanders) mother-infant pairs, 1-3y, ♂♀	BMI SDS 1-3y	PCBs	117 (9-442) [avg (range)] ng/g lip. (serum, mat. cord)	[β (SE): 0.003 (±0.001)]
Andersen et al. 2010	Denmark (nat'l) Nat'l Birth Cohort, 1y, ♂♀ (1,026)	BMI	PFOS	33.4 (6.4-106.7)[median (range)] ng/m/ (serum, maternal)	[−0.011 (−0.019, 0.003) per 1-ng/ml ↑
Andersen et al. 2011	Denmark (nat'l) Nat'l Birth Cohort, 1y, ♂♀ (1,026)	BMI	PFOA	5.21 (0.5-21.9)[median (range)] ng/m/ (serum, maternal)	[−0.042 (−0.086, 0.002)] per 1-ng/ml ↑

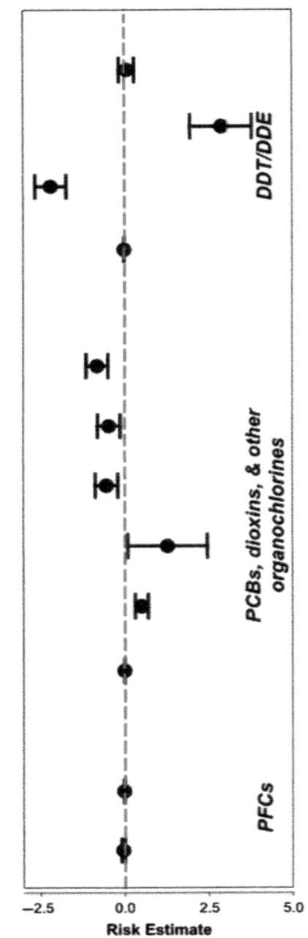

⊢ Lower 95% Confidence Interval ⊣ Upper 95% Confidence interval ● Adjusted Beta Coefficients

Whether this reduction in beta cell mass is a cause or consequence of disease is debated. Pancreatic beta cells originate from ductal cell precursors *in utero* and expand during early infancy. Around 97% of human beta cells are established by age 20.[112] In rodents, beta cells can adapt to an increased insulin requirement (due to pregnancy, obesity, *etc.*) by increasing beta cell mass. In humans, beta cell mass is somewhat increased during pregnancy and obesity, although not to the extent seen in rodents. Human beta cells can also significantly increase their secretory capacity to compensate for insulin resistance. During their first year of life, rodents can respond to beta cell damage with beta cell proliferation. In humans, beta cell replication is also highest in early life, and may not occur at all over age 30.[112]

Type 2 diabetes incidence and prevalence increases with age.[4,113] Whether or not insulin resistance increases and/or beta cell function declines simply due to age is not clear. Beta cell proliferation does decline with age, as apoptosis increases.[12] Glucose tolerance also declines with age, although the mechanisms vary by sex. In elderly men, defects in insulin secretion and insulin action, with increased glucose uptake by the liver, leads to this impaired glucose tolerance. In elderly women however, insulin secretion and insulin action do not differ from that of younger women.[114]

Obesity alone is not necessary or even sufficient to cause type 2 diabetes. In a US-wide survey, while obesity was clearly associated with type 2 diabetes, 20% of adults with diabetes were neither overweight nor obese, and 57% of obese individuals did not have type 2 diabetes.[115] Overweight and obesity can, however, contribute to insulin resistance *via* several pathways, including an imbalance in hormones (leptin, adiponectin, glucagon) and inflammatory signals [29].

8.10.2 Control of Blood Glucose Levels

Diabetes is a disease of high blood glucose (hyperglycemia). Like control of weight and metabolism, the control of blood glucose is controlled by a complex endocrine system. The body control of blood glucose is simpler than control of food intake and metabolism. The main regulators are insulin and glucagon, with involvement of sex hormones, thyroid hormones, glucocorticoids, and numerous other hormonal systems. Blood glucose levels are controlled primarily with two hormones, insulin and glucagon. Insulin signals fat, muscle,

---

Figure 8.6 Human studies on POPs exposure and risk for childhood overweight and obesity (beta estimates). Beta estimates are adjusted β's except for studies by Verhulst *et al.* Abbreviations: PCB – polychlorinated biphenyls; DDT– dichlorodiphenyltrichloroethane; DDE – dichlorodiphenyldichloroethylene; HCB – Hexachlorobenzene; PFCs- perfluorinated compounds; PFOS – perfluorooctane sulfonate; PFOA – perfluorooctanoic acid; PCDD – polychlorinated dibenzodioxins; PCDF – polychlorinated dibenzofurans; adjβ – adjusted Beta Coefficient; nat'l – national; BMI – body mass index; SDS– standard deviation score; mat. – maternal; TEQ – toxic equivalent; avg. – average; MI – Michigan; Q1 – 1st quartile; Q2 – 2th quartile.

and liver cells to take up and store glucose from the blood, reducing blood glucose levels. Glucagon raises blood glucose levels by signaling to the liver to synthesize and release glucose into the blood. Insulin is produced and secreted by the beta cells of the pancreas, stimulated directly by high glucose levels in the blood. Glucagon is produced and secreted by the alpha cells of the pancreas, in response to low glucose levels in the blood. Insulin secretion by beta cells depends primarily on glucose levels, but is complemented by various other hormonal signals, as well as fatty acids and amino acids.[111]

Estrogens are involved in blood glucose regulation. At normal, physiological levels, estrogens help maintain proper glucose control, and protect beta cell function. At high or low levels however, estrogens may promote type 2 diabetes and insulin resistance. Low estrogen levels, due to menopause or ovariectomy, are associated with impaired glucose tolerance and insulin resistance, which are counteracted by hormone replacement therapy. High estrogen levels, due to pregnancy, are also associated with impaired glucose tolerance and increased insulin resistance. During pregnancy, beta cells increase insulin secretion to adapt to this insulin resistance, and estrogen probably plays a role in this adaptation, by promoting insulin secretion. (If the beta cells fail to adequately adapt, gestational diabetes results). When adult male mice are given estradiol, their beta cells increase insulin production and secretion, and they develop insulin resistance, as if they are pregnant. This artificially-induced high insulin secretion overstimulates beta cells and, over time, may contribute to their failure. Excessive insulin signaling can lead to glucose intolerance in fat cells and promote insulin resistance in the liver and muscle. In combination, the effects of estradiol in male mice could contribute to the development of type 2 diabetes.[110]

8.10.3 Developmental Programming, Environmental Exposures and Type 2 Diabetes

Many of the chemicals discussed affect the beta cells, disrupting beta cell function and mechanisms of insulin production and secretion (Table 8.4).[116,118] Many of the chemicals discussed can also cause insulin resistance in animals, or are associated with insulin resistance in humans. Many are also linked to hyperglycemia, impaired glucose intolerance, or gestational diabetes. These chemicals are not all estrogenic, but most are EDCs. Aside from estrogen, other hormones also play a role in glucose metabolism. Androgens can affect insulin sensitivity and glucose tolerance; various chemicals can act as androgen agonists or antagonists, and may thus disrupt glucose homeostasis. Chemicals that disrupt the thyroid, glucocorticoid, or AhR hormone receptors may also have diabetogenic effects.[117]

In addition to endocrine disruption, other mechanisms may play a role in the diabetogenic effect of chemicals. For example, metals, including mercury, cadmium, and nickel, may affect beta cells or glucose regulation *via* oxidative stress. Beta cells are susceptible to oxidative stress, and reactive oxygen species have been shown to promote the progression of beta cell dysfunction.[118]

Table 8.4 Chemical associations with various types of diabetes (including impaired glucose tolerance and/or insulin resistance) in epidemiological or animal studies. The strengths of the associations differ. Abbreviations: Dev = developmental exposure; Ad = adult exposure; Dev + Ad = developmental through adulthood exposure; Dev, Ad = both developmental and adult exposures; IGT = impaired glucose tolerance.

Human	*Animal*
Type 2 or unspecified diabetes	***Insulin resistance or hyperglycemia***
Agricultural pesticides (Ad) [136]	Air pollutants (Ad) [185]
Air pollution (Ad) [137, 186–189]	Arsenic (Dev + Ad, Ad) [190, 191]
Arsenic (Ad) [191]	Atrazine (Ad) [192]
BPA (Ad) [11, 138, 141]	BPA (Dev, Ad) [193, 194]
Brominated flame retardants (Ad) [127]	Cadmium (Ad) [133]
Cadmium (Ad) [133]	Nitrosamines (Dev) [195]
Dioxin (Ad) [196]	Organophosphorous pesticides (Dev) [197]
Phthalates (Ad) [142]	Phthalates (Dev, Ad) [198, 199]
POPs: DDE, PCBs, HCB, organochlorine pesticides (Ad) [125, 129–131, 191, 200–202]	POPs: DDT, farmed salmon oil (Ad) [203, 204]
Insulin resistance	***IGT or insulin resistance during pregnancy***
BPA [205]	BPA (Ad) [194]
Dioxin and mercury (Ad) [206]	***Diabetes***
POPs (Ad) [200]	Nitrite/nitrosamines (Dev) [176]
Phthalates (Ad) [143]	***Autoimmunity***
Gestational diabetes	BPA (Dev, Ad) [178]
Agricultural pesticides (Ad) [144]	Dioxin (Dev) [179]
IGT during pregnancy	Mercury (Ad) [180, 207]
Arsenic (Ad) [145]	Phthalates (Ad) [181]
Type 1 or insulin-dependent diabetes	Tricholorethylene (Dev, Ad) [182, 183, 208]
Air pollutants ozone and sulfate (Dev) [169]	
Arsenic, cadmium, and lead (Ad) [172]	
Nitrite/nitrate/nitrosamines (Dev) [167, 168]	
PCBs (Ad) [171]	
Autoimmunity	
Mercury (Ad) [209]	
Tricholorethylene (Ad) [208]	

The effects of estradiol on male mice, namely insulin resistance and hyperinsulinemia, are mimicked by the estrogenic actions of the widespread endocrine disrupting compound BPA.[110] Both estradiol and BPA promote insulin secretion from beta cells and cause hyperinsulinemia, insulin resistance, and impaired glucose tolerance in mice. Since high insulin levels can in itself cause insulin resistance, chemicals that increase insulin secretion may contribute to insulin resistance.[109] BPA (and estradiol) can also disrupt signaling in pancreatic alpha cells, interfering with the release of glucagon from alpha cells in response to low blood glucose levels.[119]

Gestational diabetes alone increases the risk of glucose abnormalities in the offspring. In animal experiments, developmental exposure to hyperglycemia/maternal diabetes is clearly linked to later metabolic dysfunction in the offspring, including disruption of beta cell function and insulin secretion, and abnormal insulin signaling.[120]

The bottom line is that it is likely that type 2 diabetes, like obesity, starts during development, both *in utero* and in early childhood. Thus the developmental origins of disease paradigm also holds true for type 2 diabetes.

In contrast to obesity where the majority of the supporting data comes from animal studies, in type 2 diabetes, the majority of the data comes from human studies, which we review here.

8.10.4 Developmental Exposures in Humans

To date, there have been no epidemiological studies on developmental exposures to environmental chemicals and the later development of type 2 diabetes. However, other non-chemical developmental exposures have long been linked to later type 2 diabetes. Individuals whose mothers suffered through the Dutch winter famine during pregnancy had impaired glucose tolerance in their 50s. The effect does not appear to progress more rapidly with increasing age.[121] Low birth weight is also associated with the development of type 2 diabetes in adulthood.[122] Fetal exposure to maternal diabetes is associated with a higher risk of impaired glucose tolerance and insulin resistance, an effect that can even be transmitted to subsequent generations, implying an epigenetic mechanism.[123] Based on this evidence, it is reasonable to propose that developmental exposures to environmental chemicals may also affect the later development of type 2 diabetes.

8.10.5 Human Adult Exposures

In humans, there is growing evidence that adult exposures to EDCs can contribute to the development of type 2 diabetes. Numerous cross-sectional studies of adults have found associations between diabetes and exposure to various POPs, especially dioxin.[116] While some of these studies were conducted in populations with high exposure levels, cross-sectional studies using the US National Health and Nutrition Examination Survey (NHANES) have found associations between diabetes and various POPs, including dioxin-like PCBs, organochlorine pesticides, and brominated flame retardants at background exposure levels.[124–127] POPs are also associated with insulin resistance in NHANES.[128]

Longitudinal studies have also found associations between POPs and diabetes. The specific POPs and the shapes of the dose–response curves vary, with some dose–response curves showing non-monotonic associations.[129–131] One longitudinal study of Swedish 70 year olds found that exposure POPs, especially PCBs and organochlorine pesticides, was strongly linked to the development of type 2 diabetes 5 years later.[132] In a cohort of 50–59 year old Swedish women, baseline DDE levels were associated with an increased risk of diabetes in the women who developed diabetes more than 6 years after baseline.[130] In a cohort of adult Great Lakes sport fish consumers, DDE was associated with type 2 diabetes development 10 years after baseline.[131] A study of young US adults without diabetes found that baseline levels of DDE and PCBs was linked to higher insulin resistance 18 years later.[132]

Additionally, epidemiological studies have linked cadmium exposure to diabetes.[133]

Agricultural pesticide exposure has been associated with diabetes or mortality rates from diabetes in agricultural workers.[134–136] Cross-sectional studies have found associations between air pollution and type 2 diabetes. One longitudinal study of elderly German women found that traffic-related air pollution was associated with type 2 diabetes.[137]

A number of cross-sectional studies have evaluated BPA levels and diabetes, and most have found associations, although the findings are inconsistent.[11,138–141] Overall, NHANES data from 2003–2004, but not necessarily data from other years or other surveys, show an association between diabetes and BPA. Exposure to phthalates are associated with self-reported diabetes in Mexican women in one cross-sectional study.[142] Increased insulin resistance is also associated with phthalate levels in US adult men.[143] The lack of longitudinal data, or developmental exposure data, on these less persistent chemicals makes it difficult to form conclusions from the existing data.

8.10.6 Exposure During Pregnancy

Exposure to environmental chemicals during pregnancy may increase the risk of gestational diabetes. Pregnant women exposed to agricultural pesticides during their first trimester were more likely to develop gestational diabetes.[144] Arsenic exposure has been associated with impaired glucose tolerance during pregnancy in women with relatively low levels of arsenic exposure.[145] Since gestational diabetes increases the risk of later diabetes in the mother and later glucose abnormalities in the child, the role of environmental chemicals in gestational diabetes should be further investigated.

Environmental chemical exposures may also play a role in diabetes complications. Exposure to organochlorine pesticides is associated with neuropathy in people with diabetes or impaired fasting glucose. The association remained strong even in people with a low HbA1c (below 7%). Exposure to these POPs was also strongly associated with a higher HbA1c. POPs are known to be neurotoxicants, which may be a factor in their association with neuroapathy.[128] Similarly, cadmium is toxic to the kidney and may act together with hyperglycemia to contribute to nephropathy.[133]

8.11 Type 1 Diabetes

8.11.1 Background

While the autoimmune disease type 1 diabetes is often thought to be a disease of childhood, type 1 diabetes can develop at any age. Surveys from Sweden,

Minnesota, Finland, and Denmark have found that incidence peaks in both children and older adults: in children around the time of puberty, and in adults aged 50–80 years.[113] About 10% of adults with presumed type 2 diabetes test positive for type 1-associated GAD or islet cell autoantibodies and actually have a slowly progressive form of autoimmune or type 1 diabetes.[146]

8.11.2 Incidence

A number of environmental factors—including early infant diet, viruses, vitamin D deficiency, excess weight gain, and gut microbiota—are being investigated as potential contributors to an increase in the incidence of type 1 diabetes, although none have been clearly identified.[147] The role of environmental chemicals in this increase remains a largely unexplored area of research.[148]

8.11.3 Endocrine Role and Endocrine Disruption

The immune system interacts extensively with the endocrine system; numerous immune cells have estrogen receptors and androgen receptors for example. Sex hormones are involved in both in the development and progression of autoimmune diseases. In women, hormonal fluctuations (*e.g.* pregnancy, menstrual cycle, oral contraceptives) influence the course of autoimmune disease. Most autoimmune diseases are more common in women than in men, perhaps due to the stimulation of an immune response by estrogen. Yet while estrogens appear to promote many autoimmune diseases, androgens appear to promote others.[149] The role of estrogens in autoimmunity however, depends on the concentration studied, the differing effects of different peripheral estrogen metabolites, and the differing effects on target cells and different receptors.[150] The overall pattern is not clear-cut, since some autoimmune diseases tend to ameliorate during pregnancy, and flare postpartum, while others exhibit the opposite pattern, worsening during pregnancy but improving postpartum.[151,152]

Unlike most other autoimmune diseases, the male/female sex ratio in type 1 diabetes is approximately equal, although this ratio varies by age and by population. Natural hormonal fluctuations may influence the development of type 1 diabetes, since type 1 diabetes incidence is high during puberty and is more likely to appear during pregnancy than in a non-pregnant state (whether these patterns are due to hormonal changes, increased insulin resistance, or both is not known).[153] Pregnancy can influence the appearance and levels of type 1 related autoantibodies; in a group of women without diabetes, most exhibited a decline in type 1 autoantibody levels during the course of pregnancy, while others experienced an increase, and a few converted from antibody negative to positive during pregnancy.[151] Around 10% of gestational diabetes cases are autoimmune and associated with later progression to type 1 diabetes. Women with this "autoimmune gestational diabetes" generally require insulin during pregnancy, experience remission of insulin dependence postpartum, and later progress to type 1 diabetes and insulin dependence.[154]

In women with type 1 diabetes, hormonal fluctuations during the menstrual cycle affect insulin dose, as do fluctuations during puberty and pregnancy. During pregnancy, insulin requirement peaks at week 9, falls until week 16, rises again until week 37, and falls by 50% immediately following delivery. Some pregnant women with long-standing type 1 diabetes even appear to regain some beta cell function during pregnancy, a finding that, in addition to hormone-induced insulin resistance, may also affect insulin dose.[155]

The peak incidence of type 1 diabetes in childhood is during puberty, perhaps due to insulin resistance during that time. In adolescents without diabetes, insulin resistance and insulin secretion increase during puberty, peaking in mid-puberty and returning to prepubertal levels by the end of puberty. The changes in insulin resistance correlate with growth hormone levels and adrenal androgens, but not sex steroid hormones.[156]

Metabolic factors appear to play a role in the development of type 1 diabetes. Higher body weight is associated with type 1 diabetes development, and insulin resistance is a risk factor for progression to type 1 diabetes in people with islet autoimmunity.[157] Beta cells that are stressed by metabolic factors such as obesity and insulin resistance may offer more of a target to the autoimmune attack of type 1 diabetes, accelerating the progression of disease.[158]

Endocrine disrupting chemicals are known to affect the immune system, and promote autoimmunity. These chemicals can also affect beta cells, and contribute to obesity and insulin resistance. These effects may play a role in the initiation or progression of type 1 diabetes. Whether individual chemicals with multiple effects or multiple chemicals acting in concert influence type 1 is not known. Since the antibodies associated with type 1 diabetes may appear very early in life (even *in utero*), followed by diabetes years later, developmental exposures are likely to be important in disease development.[159]

8.11.4 Evidence from Human and Animal Studies

EDCs have not been adequately evaluated in the development or progression of type 1 diabetes. We will briefly review the evidence from human studies first, followed by animal studies. Where evidence on EDCs is lacking, we will include some evidence of other chemicals and other environmental factors.

8.11.4.1 Human Evidence

Early life exposure to a number of environmental factors—including vitamin D deficiency, cow's milk infant formula, and viruses—has been associated with later type 1 diabetes development in humans. For example, in Norway, the risk of type 1 diabetes is more than two-fold higher for the children of mothers who had low levels of vitamin D during pregnancy, as compared to mothers with higher levels.[160] Finnish children given regular vitamin D supplements during infancy had a reduced risk of type 1 diabetes into adulthood.[160] The high incidence of type 1 diabetes in these Scandinavian countries has prompted research into vitamin D deficiency and type 1 diabetes.

Preliminary results from an ongoing double-blind, randomized controlled trial shows that dietary supplementation with hydrolyzed infant formula when breast milk is not available reduces the risk of type 1 associated antibodies in children until age 10, as compared to regular infant formula.[161] Virus exposure in the first year of life, in conjunction with early exposure to cow's milk, is associated with type 1 diabetes-associated autoimmunity, suggesting an interaction between these two factors.[162]

Other developmental factors associated with an increased risk of later type 1 diabetes includes birth by Cesarean section,[163] high birth weight,[164] and advanced maternal age.[165] The congenital rubella syndrome predisposes people to diabetes later in life, although whether this is autoimmune diabetes is not entirely clear since the studies on congenital rubella were carried out before the rubella vaccine, before testing for autoimmunity was well established.[166]

Dietary consumption of nitrates and nitrites may play a role in type 1 diabetes development, although studies are somewhat inconsistent.[167] An early epidemiological study from Iceland found that parents' consumption of Icelandic smoked mutton, a meat cured with nitrites, around the time of conception increased their sons' risk for type 1 diabetes.[168]

Measurements of environmental chemical exposures are largely absent from ongoing studies of type 1 diabetes development. One study however, found that exposure to the air pollutants sulfate and ozone during infancy and childhood increased the risk of type 1 diabetes in children.[169] Another study of *in utero* exposure to POPs however, did not find an association between POP exposure and a later risk of type 1 diabetes.[170]

In adults however, POPs have been associated with type 1 diabetes. In a group of pregnant women, PCB levels in those with type 1 diabetes were 30% higher than in those without diabetes.[171] Similarly, levels of arsenic, cadmium, and lead were higher in insulin-dependent diabetic mothers than in controls without diabetes.[172] Until it was removed from the market, the rodenticide Vacor caused, *via* beta cell toxicity, insulin-dependent diabetes in children and adults who ingested it. Autoantibodies characteristic of type 1 diabetes were found in some of these people.[173]

8.11.4.2 Animal Exposures

A large number of environmental factors—including viruses, vitamin D levels, weight gain, a hydrolyzed diet, a gluten-free diet, probiotics, antibiotics, beta cell rest (including insulin treatment), pharmaceutical drugs (*e.g.* cyclosporin) and beta cell toxins—modulate the development of diabetes in animal models.[174]

Some chemicals promote diabetes in laboratory animals. The beta cell toxin streptozotocin (STZ), given to rodents to induce insulin-dependent diabetes in the lab, also induces insulin-dependent diabetes, accompanied by signs of autoimmunity in young primates.[175] Developmental exposure to nitrites in smoked meat causes diabetes in mice; glucose levels were affected even when parents consumed this meat only up until the time of conception, implying an effect on germ cells.[176]

Laboratory animals prenatally exposed to immunotoxic chemicals show exacerbated autoimmunity. The effects of perinatal exposure may be greater or more persistent than the effects following adult exposure.[177] Numerous chemicals—including BPA,[178] dioxin,[179] mercury,[180] phthalates,[181] and trichloroethylene[182]—have been found to promote autoimmunity in animals following either developmental or adult exposures (see Table 8.4). None of these chemicals have yet been evaluated in type 1 diabetes in humans. Yet some (mercury and trichloroethylene) have different results in non-obese diabetic (NOD) mice (an animal model of type 1 diabetes), showing almost protective effects. The conflicting animal experiments appear to indicate that timing, duration of exposure, and predisposing factors like genetic background are probably important in the development of autoimmunity.[183] These conflicting results may also be due to the peculiarities of NOD mice, in that most interventions prevent diabetes in these mice. NOD mice develop diabetes spontaneously, *via* mechanisms that are not always relevant to humans.[184]

While direct evidence is lacking, preliminary evidence indicates that exposure to environmental chemicals with immunotoxic and/or beta cell toxic effects may exacerbate the development and/or progression of type 1 diabetes. Incorporating measurements of environmental chemical exposures into ongoing developmental studies of type 1 diabetes would likely help fill the gap in knowledge about the role of chemicals in this disease, and their possible interaction with other environmental factors.

8.12 Conclusion

There is growing concern in the scientific community that EDCs may be contributing to the rapidly increasing rates of diabetes and obesity. It is of particular concern that the incidence of both obesity and diabetes are rising rapidly in the young. While it is clear that eating calorie-dense, nutrient-poor food in large portions, combined with lack of exercise, plays an important role, the rapid rise in obesity and diabetes in the young suggests the influence of early life exposures to chemicals may be playing an important role. Indeed the mounting evidence reviewed in this chapter clearly links exposure to EDCs with the incidence of obesity and diabetes. While the precise metabolic pathways targeted by most of these chemicals remain to be discovered, the data linking EDCs with obesity, metabolic syndrome, and diabetes are strong, and the number of studies finding positive association is growing. Understanding the molecular mechanisms involved in the role of epigenetics and early life exposures will provide important insights into the etiology of these chronic disorders and should play an important role in designing effective prevention strategies.

References

1. G. Danaei *et al.*, National, regional, and global trends in fasting plasma glucose and diabetes prevalence since 1980: systematic analysis of health

examination surveys and epidemiological studies with 370 country-years and 2.7 million participants, *Lancet*, 2011, **378**(9785), 31–40.
2. P. Zhang *et al.*, Global healthcare expenditure on diabetes for 2010 and 2030, *Diabetes Res. Clin. Pract.*, 2010, **87**(3), 293–301.
3. L. S. Geiss *et al.*, Changes in incidence of diabetes in U.S. adults, 1997–2003, *Am. J. Prev. Med*, 2006, **30**(5), 371–377.
4. S. Volpato, C. Maraldi and R. Fellin, Type 2 diabetes and risk for functional decline and disability in older persons, *Curr. Diabetes Rev.*, 2010, **6**(3), 134–143.
5. D. Dabelea *et al.*, Incidence of diabetes in youth in the United States, *JAMA*, 2007, **297**(24), 2716–2724.
6. D. P. Group, Incidence and trends of childhood Type 1 diabetes worldwide 1990–1999, *Diabet. Med.*, 2006, **23**(8), 857–866.
7. C. C. Patterson *et al.*, Incidence trends for childhood type 1 diabetes in Europe during 1989–2003 and predicted new cases 2005–20: a multicentre prospective registration study, *Lancet*, 2009, **373**(9680), 2027–2033.
8. G. Bruno *et al.*, The incidence of type 1 diabetes is increasing in both children and young adults in Northern Italy: 1984–2004 temporal trends, *Diabetologia*, 2009, **52**(12), 2531–2535.
9. E. A. Gale, The rise of childhood type 1 diabetes in the 20th century, *Diabetes*, 2002, **51**(12), 3353–3361.
10. K. Calkins and S. U. Devaskar, Fetal origins of adult disease, *Curr Probl Pediatr Adolesc Health Care*, 2011, **41**(6), 158–176.
11. A. Shankar and S. Teppala, Relationship between Urinary Bisphenol A Levels and Diabetes Mellitus, *J. Clin. Endocrinol. Metab.*, 2011.
12. U. Gunasekaran and M. Gannon, Type 2 diabetes and the aging pancreatic beta cell, *Aging (Albany.NY)*, 2011, **3**(6), 565–575.
13. B. Carstensen, D. R. Witte and S. Friis, Cancer occurrence in Danish diabetic patients: duration and insulin effects, *Diabetologia*, 2011.
14. C. S. Fox, Cardiovascular disease risk factors, type 2 diabetes mellitus, and the Framingham Heart Study, *Trends Cardiovasc. Med.*, 2010, **20**(3), 90–95.
15. L. J. Dominguez, G. Paolisso and M. Barbagallo, Glucose control in the older patient: from intensive, to effective and safe, *Aging Clin. Exp. Res.*, 2010, **22**(4), 274–280.
16. O. Pinhas-Hamiel and P. Zeitler, Acute and chronic complications of type 2 diabetes mellitus in children and adolescents, *Lancet*, 2007, **369**(9575), 1823–1831.
17. S. P. Laing *et al.*, Mortality from cerebrovascular disease in a cohort of 23 000 patients with insulin-treated diabetes, *Stroke*, 2003, **34**(2), 418–421.
18. S. P. Laing *et al.*, Mortality from heart disease in a cohort of 23,000 patients with insulin-treated diabetes, *Diabetologia*, 2003, **46**(6), 760–765.
19. The effect of intensive treatment of diabetes on the development and progression of long-term complications in insulin-dependent diabetes mellitus. The Diabetes Control and Complications Trial Research Group. *N. Engl. J. Med.*, 1993, **329**(14), 977–986.

20. E. S. Kilpatrick, A. S. Rigby and S. L. Atkin, Insulin resistance, the metabolic syndrome, and complication risk in type 1 diabetes: "double diabetes" in the Diabetes Control and Complications Trial, *Diabetes Care*, 2007, **30**(3), 707–712.
21. T. M. Triolo *et al.*, One-Third of Patients Have Evidence for an Additional Autoimmune Disease at Type 1 Diabetes Diagnosis, *Diabetes Care*, 2011.
22. V. Carnevale, E. Romagnoli and E. D'Erasmo, Skeletal involvement in patients with diabetes mellitus, *Diabetes Metab. Res. Rev.*, 2004, **20**(3), 196–204.
23. J. Cawley and C. Meyerhoefer, The medical care costs of obesity: An instrumental variables approach, *J Health Econ*, 2011.
24. L. Trasande and Y. Liu, Reducing the staggering costs of environmental disease in children, estimated at $76.6 billion in 2008, *Health Aff (Millwood)*, 2011, **30**(5), 863–870.
25. J. Naukkarinen *et al.*, Causes and consequences of obesity: the contribution of recent twin studies, *Int J Obes (Lond)*, 2011.
26. L. H. Larsen *et al.*, Prevalence of mutations and functional analyses of melanocortin 4 receptor variants identified among 750 men with juvenile-onset obesity, *J Clin Endocrinol Metab*, 2005, **90**(1), 219–224.
27. E. K. Speliotes *et al.*, Association analyses of 249,796 individuals reveal 18 new loci associated with body mass index, *Nat Genet*, 2010, **42**(11), 937–948.
28. M. E. Travers and M. I. McCarthy, Type 2 diabetes and obesity: genomics and the clinic, *Hum. Genet.*, 2011, **130**(1), 41–58.
29. A. A. Tahrani *et al.*, Management of type 2 diabetes: new and future developments in treatment, *Lancet*, 2011.
30. J. M. Howson *et al.*, Genetic Analysis of Adult-Onset Autoimmune Diabetes, *Diabetes*, 2011.
31. S. F. Grant, H. Hakonarson and S. Schwartz, Can the Genetics of Type 1 and Type 2 Diabetes Shed Light on the Genetics of Latent Autoimmune Diabetes in Adults?, *Endocr. Rev.*, 2009.
32. J. Lin *et al.*, From Type 1, through LADA, to type 2 diabetes: a continuous spectrum?, *Ann. N. Y. Acad. Sci.*, 2008, **1150**, 99–102.
33. A. K. Steck *et al.*, Stepwise or linear decrease in penetrance of type 1 diabetes with lower-risk HLA genotypes over the past 40 years, *Diabetes*, 2011, **60**(3), 1045–1049.
34. K. A. Simpson and S. R. Bloom, Appetite and hedonism: gut hormones and the brain, *Endocrinol Metab Clin North Am*, 2010, **39**(4), 729–743.
35. T. H. Moran, Gut peptides in the control of food intake, *Int J Obes (Lond)*, 2009, **33**(Suppl 1), S7–S10.
36. H. C. Greenwood, S. R. Bloom and K. G. Murphy, Peptides and their potential role in the treatment of diabetes and obesity, *Rev Diabet Stud*, 2011, **8**(3), 355–368.
37. A. Gonzalez-Bulnes and C. Ovilo, Genetic Basis, Nutritional Challenges and Adaptive Responses in the Prenatal Origin of Obesity and Type-2 Diabetes, *Curr Diabetes Rev*, 2012.

38. P. J. Kenny, Common cellular and molecular mechanisms in obesity and drug addiction, *Nat Rev Neurosci*, 2011, **12**(11), 638–651.
39. N. D. Volkow and P. Skolnick, New medications for substance use disorders: challenges and opportunities, *Neuropsychopharmacology*, 2012, **37**(1), 290–292.
40. N. D. Volkow *et al.*, Food and Drug Reward: Overlapping Circuits in Human Obesity and Addiction, *Curr Top Behav Neurosci*, 2011.
41. P. J. Kenny, Reward mechanisms in obesity: new insights and future directions, *Neuron*, 2011, **69**(4), 664–679.
42. W. Wyrwicka, C. Dobrzecka and R. Tarnecki, On the instrumental conditioned reaction evoked by electrical stimulation of the hypothalamus, *Science*, 1959, **130**(3371), 336–337.
43. M. J. Will, W. E. Pratt and A. E. Kelley, Pharmacological characterization of high-fat feeding induced by opioid stimulation of the ventral striatum, *Physiol Behav*, 2006, **89**(2), 226–234.
44. M. A. McCrory, V. M. Suen and S. B. Roberts, Biobehavioral influences on energy intake and adult weight gain, *J Nutr*, 2002, **132**(12), 3830S–3834S.
45. H. R. Berthoud, N. R. Lenard and A. C. Shin, Food reward, hyperphagia, and obesity, *Am J Physiol Regul Integr Comp Physiol*, 2011, **300**(6), R1266–R1277.
46. A. Meule, How Prevalent is "Food Addiction"?, *Front Psychiatry*, 2011, **2**, 61.
47. D. J. Barker and P. M. Clark, Fetal undernutrition and disease in later life, *Rev Reprod.*, 1997, **2**(2), 105–112.
48. R. R. Newbold *et al.*, Developmental exposure to endocrine disruptors and the obesity epidemic, *Reprod Toxicol*, 2007, **23**(3), 290–296.
49. L. S. Birnbaum and S. E. Fenton, Cancer and developmental exposure to endocrine disruptors, *Environ Health Perspect*, 2003, **111**(4), 389–394.
50. M. K. Skinner, M. Manikkam and C. Guerrero-Bosagna, Epigenetic transgenerational actions of environmental factors in disease etiology, *Trends Endocrinol Metab*, 2010, **21**(4), 214–222. Epub 2010 Jan 14.
51. N. C. Whitelaw and E. Whitelaw, Transgenerational epigenetic inheritance in health and disease, *Curr Opin Genet Dev*, 2008, **18**(3), 273–279. Epub 2008 Aug 12.
52. J. A. McLachlan *et al.*, Reduced fertility in female mice exposed transplacentally to diethylstilbestrol (DES), *Fertil Steril*, 1982, **38**(3), 364–371.
53. R. R. Newbold *et al.*, Proliferative lesions and reproductive tract tumors in male descendants of mice exposed developmentally to diethylstilbestrol, *Carcinogenesis*, 2000, **21**(7), 1355–1363.
54. L. Titus-Ernstoff *et al.*, Offspring of women exposed in utero to diethylstilbestrol (DES): a preliminary report of benign and malignant pathology in the third generation, *Epidemiology*, 2008, **19**(2), 251–257.
55. M. D. Anway, S. S. Rekow and M. K. Skinner, Comparative anti-androgenic actions of vinclozolin and flutamide on transgenerational

adult onset disease and spermatogenesis, *Reprod Toxicol*, 2008, **26**(2), 100–106. Epub 2008 Aug 13.
56. D. C. Dolinoy, D. Huang and R. L. Jirtle, Maternal nutrient supplementation counteracts bisphenol A-induced DNA hypomethylation in early development, *Proceedings of the National Academy of Sciences of the United States of America*, 2007, **104**(32), 13056–13061.
57. T. T. Schug *et al.*, Endocrine disrupting chemicals and disease susceptibility, *J Steroid Biochem Mol Biol*, 2011, **127**(3-5), 204–215.
58. E. Jasarevic *et al.*, Disruption of adult expression of sexually selected traits by developmental exposure to bisphenol A. *Proc Natl Acad Sci U S A*, 2011, **108**(28), 11715–11720.
59. J. Cao *et al.*, Neonatal Bisphenol A exposure alters sexually dimorphic gene expression in the postnatal rat hypothalamus, *Neurotoxicology*, 2012, **33**(1), 23–36.
60. S. M. Dickerson *et al.*, Endocrine disruption of brain sexual differentiation by developmental PCB exposure, *Endocrinology*, 2011, **152**(2), 581–594.
61. W. N. Jefferson, H. B. Patisaul and C. Williams, Reproductive consequences of developmental phytoestrogen exposure, *Reproduction*, 2012.
62. I. Ceccarelli *et al.*, Estrogenic chemicals at puberty change ERalpha in the hypothalamus of male and female rats, *Neurotoxicol Teratol*, 2007, **29**(1), 108–115.
63. S. E. Fenton, C. Reed and R. R. Newbold, Perinatal environmental exposures affect mammary development, function, and cancer risk in adulthood (*), *Annu Rev Pharmacol Toxicol*, 2012, **52**, 455–479.
64. G. Rasier *et al.*, Female sexual maturation and reproduction after prepubertal exposure to estrogens and endocrine disrupting chemicals: a review of rodent and human data, *Mol Cell Endocrinol,*, 2006, **254–255**, 187–201.
65. D. C. Luccio-Camelo and G. S. Prins, Disruption of androgen receptor signaling in males by environmental chemicals, *J Steroid Biochem Mol Biol*, 2011, **127**(1-2), 74–82.
66. R. R. Newbold, W. N. Jefferson and E. Padilla-Banks, Prenatal exposure to bisphenol a at environmentally relevant doses adversely affects the murine female reproductive tract later in life, *Environ Health Perspect*, 2009, **117**(6), 879–885.
67. N. J. Cabaton *et al.*, Perinatal exposure to environmentally relevant levels of bisphenol A decreases fertility and fecundity in CD-1 mice, *Environ Health Perspect*, 2011, **119**(4), 547–552.
68. G. S. Prins *et al.*, Serum bisphenol A pharmacokinetics and prostate neoplastic responses following oral and subcutaneous exposures in neonatal Sprague-Dawley rats, *Reprod Toxicol*, 2011, **31**(1), 1–9.
69. Y. Masuo and M. Ishido, Neurotoxicity of endocrine disruptors: possible involvement in brain development and neurodegeneration, *J Toxicol Environ Health B Crit Rev*, 2011, **14**(5-7), 346–369.
70. M. C. Keifer and J. Firestone, Neurotoxicity of pesticides, *J Agromedicine*, 2007, **12**(1), 17–25.

71. K. A. Thayer *et al.*, Role of Environmental Chemicals in Diabetes and Obesity: A National Toxicology Program Workshop Report, *Environ Health Perspect*, 2012.
72. F. S. Vom Saal *et al.*, The estrogenic endocrine disrupting chemical bisphenol A (BPA) and obesity, *Mol Cell Endocrinol*, 2012.
73. A. Janesick and B. Blumberg, Endocrine disrupting chemicals and the developmental programming of adipogenesis and obesity, *Birth Defects Res C Embryo Today*, 2011, **93**(1), 34–50.
74. R. J. Dearman *et al.*, Butyl benzyl phthalate: effects on immune responses to ovalbumin in mice, *J Appl Toxicol*, 2009, **29**(2), 118–25.
75. T. Kato *et al.*, Endocrine disruptors that deplete glutathione levels in APC promote Th2 polarization in mice leading to the exacerbation of airway inflammation, *Eur J Immunol*, 2006, **36**(5), 1199–209.
76. S. M. Belcher *et al.*, Rapid estrogen receptor-mediated mechanisms determine the sexually dimorphic sensitivity of ventricular myocytes to 17beta-estradiol and the environmental endocrine disruptor bisphenol a, *Endocrinology*, 2012, **153**(2), 712–720.
77. S. Yan *et al.*, Bisphenol A and 17beta-estradiol promote arrhythmia in the female heart via alteration of calcium handling, *PLoS. One*, 2011, **6**(9), e25455.
78. D. A. Drechsel and M. Patel, Role of reactive oxygen species in the neurotoxicity of environmental agents implicated in Parkinson's disease, *Free Radic Biol Med*, 2008, **44**(11), 1873–1886.
79. Z. Vucetic *et al.*, Maternal high-fat diet alters methylation and gene expression of dopamine and opioid-related genes, *Endocrinology*, 2010, **151**(10), 4756–4764.
80. Z. Vucetic *et al.*, Early life protein restriction alters dopamine circuitry, *Neuroscience*, 2010, **168**(2), 359–370.
81. S. K. Murphy and R. L. Jirtle, Imprinting evolution and the price of silence, *BioEssays*, 2003, **25**(6), 577–588.
82. B. Grun F Fau - Blumberg, and B. Blumberg, Perturbed nuclear receptor signaling by environmental obesogens as emerging factors in the obesity crisis. (1389-9155 (Print)).
83. C. V. Bishop and F. Stormshak, Non-genomic actions of progesterone and estrogens in regulating reproductive events in domestic animals, *Vet J*, 2008, **176**(3), 270–280.
84. J. M. Carter *et al.*, Steer responses to feeding soybean hulls and steroid hormone implantation on toxic tall fescue pasture, *J Anim Sci*, 2010, **88**(11), 3759–3766.
85. H. Ashby J Fau - Tinwell, J. Tinwell H Fau - Haseman and J. Haseman, Lack of effects for low dose levels of bisphenol A and diethylstilbestrol on the prostate gland of CF1 mice exposed in utero. (0273-2300 (Print)).
86. O. Takai Y Fau - Tsutsumi *et al.*, Preimplantation exposure to bisphenol A advances postnatal development. (0890-6238 (Print)).
87. A. Honma S Fau - Suzuki *et al.*, Low dose effect of in utero exposure to bisphenol A and diethylstilbestrol on female mouse reproduction. (0890-6238 (Print)).

88. K. Nikaido Y Fau - Yoshizawa *et al.*, Effects of maternal xenoestrogen exposure on development of the reproductive tract and mammary gland in female CD-1 mouse offspring. (0890-6238 (Print)).
89. M. K. Rubin Bs Fau - Murray *et al.*, Perinatal exposure to low doses of bisphenol A affects body weight, patterns of estrous cyclicity, and plasma LH levels. (0091-6765 (Print)).
90. A. M. Ryan Kk Fau - Haller *et al.*, Perinatal exposure to bisphenol-a and the development of metabolic syndrome in CD-1 mice. (1945-7170 (Electronic)).
91. V. M. Somm E Fau - Schwitzgebel *et al.*, Perinatal exposure to bisphenol a alters early adipogenesis in the rat. (1552-9924 (Electronic)).
92. K. Miyawaki J Fau - Sakayama *et al.*, Perinatal and postnatal exposure to bisphenol a increases adipose tissue mass and serum cholesterol level in mice. (1340-3478 (Print)).
93. S. Tian Yh Fau - Hwan Kim *et al.*, Lactational and postnatal exposure to polychlorinated biphenyls induces sex-specific anxiolytic behavior and cognitive deficit in mice offspring. (1098-2396 (Electronic)).
94. B. S. Rubin, Bisphenol A: an endocrine disruptor with widespread exposure and multiple effects. (1879-1220 (Electronic)).
95. A. Makita Y Fau - Tanaka *et al.*, Effects of simultaneous administration of tributyltin (TBT) and p,p(')-DDE on female offspring of Wistar rats. (1528-7394 (Print)).
96. H. Grun F Fau - Watanabe *et al.*, Endocrine-disrupting organotin compounds are potent inducers of adipogenesis in vertebrates. (0888-8809 (Print)).
97. T. Kirchner S Fau - Kieu *et al.*, Prenatal exposure to the environmental obesogen tributyltin predisposes multipotent stem cells to become adipocytes. (1944-9917 (Electronic)).
98. L. S. La Merrill M Fau - Birnbaum, and L. S. Birnbaum, Childhood obesity and environmental chemicals. (1931–7581 (Electronic)).
99. S. Zuo Z Fau - Chen *et al.*, Tributyltin causes obesity and hepatic steatosis in male mice. (1522-7278 (Electronic)).
100. H. Cooke Gm Fau - Tryphonas *et al.*, Oral (gavage), in utero and postnatal exposure of Sprague-Dawley rats to low doses of tributyltin chloride. Part 1: Toxicology, histopathology and clinical chemistry. (0278-6915 (Print)).
101. V. M. Somm E Fau - Schwitzgebel *et al.*, Prenatal nicotine exposure alters early pancreatic islet and adipose tissue development with consequences on the control of body weight and glucose metabolism later in life. (0013-7227 (Print)).
102. D. J. Ng Sp Fau - Conklin *et al.*, Prenatal exposure to cigarette smoke induces diet- and sex-dependent dyslipidemia and weight gain in adult murine offspring. (1552-9924 (Electronic)).
103. A. Tsukue N Fau - Kato *et al.*, Acute effects of diesel emission from the urea selective catalytic reduction engine system on male rats. (1091-7691 (Electronic)).

104. N. Shimada T Fau - Hiramatsu *et al.*, Dual suppression of adipogenesis by cigarette smoke through activation of the aryl hydrocarbon receptor and induction of endoplasmic reticulum stress. (0193-1849 (Print)).
105. A. B. Lindstrom, M. J. Strynar and E. L. Libelo, Polyfluorinated compounds: past, present, and future, *Environ Sci Technol*, 2011, **45**(19), 7954–7961.
106. S. S. Hines Ep Fau - White *et al.*, Phenotypic dichotomy following developmental exposure to perfluorooctanoic acid (PFOA) in female CD-1 mice: Low doses induce elevated serum leptin and insulin, and overweight in mid-life. (1872-8057 (Electronic)).
107. Y. S. Yang C Fau - Tan *et al.*, Differential effects of peripubertal exposure to perfluorooctanoic acid on mammary gland development in C57Bl/6 and Balb/c mouse strains. (1873-1708 (Electronic)).
108. S. E. Wolf Cj Fau - Fenton *et al.*, Developmental toxicity of perfluorooctanoic acid in the CD-1 mouse after cross-foster and restricted gestational exposures. (1096-6080 (Print)).
109. P. Alonso-Magdalena *et al.*, Bisphenol-A: a new diabetogenic factor? *Hormones.(Athens.)*, 2010, **9**(2), 118–126.
110. A. Nadal *et al.*, The pancreatic beta-cell as a target of estrogens and xenoestrogens: Implications for blood glucose homeostasis and diabetes, *Mol. Cell Endocrinol.*, 2009, **304**(1-2), 63–68.
111. D. M. Muoio and C. B. Newgard, Mechanisms of disease: molecular and metabolic mechanisms of insulin resistance and beta-cell failure in type 2 diabetes, *Nat. Rev. Mol. Cell Biol.*, 2008, **9**(3), 193–205.
112. M. Cnop *et al.*, Longevity of human islet alpha- and beta-cells, *Diabetes Obes. Metab.*, 2011, **13**(Suppl 1), 39–46.
113. M. Thunander *et al.*, Incidence of type 1 and type 2 diabetes in adults and children in Kronoberg, Sweden, *Diabetes Res. Clin. Pract.*, 2008, **82**(2), 247–255.
114. R. Basu *et al.*, Effects of age and sex on postprandial glucose metabolism: differences in glucose turnover, insulin secretion, insulin action, and hepatic insulin extraction, *Diabetes*, 2006, **55**(7), 2001–2014.
115. N. T., Nguyen *et al.*, Relationship Between Obesity and Diabetes in a US Adult Population: Findings from the National Health and Nutrition Examination Survey, 1999–2006. *Obes. Surg.*, 2010.
116. T. L. Hectors *et al.*, Environmental pollutants and type 2 diabetes: a review of mechanisms that can disrupt beta cell function, *Diabetologia*, 2011, **54**(6), 1273–1290.
117. B. A. Neel and R. M. Sargis, The paradox of progress: environmental disruption of metabolism and the diabetes epidemic, *Diabetes*, 2011, **60**(7), 1838–1848.
118. Y. W. Chen *et al.*, Heavy metals, islet function and diabetes development, *Islets*, 2009, **1**(3), 169–176.
119. P. Alonso-Magdalena *et al.*, Low doses of bisphenol A and diethylstilbestrol impair Ca2+ signals in pancreatic alpha-cells through a

nonclassical membrane estrogen receptor within intact islets of Langerhans, *Environ. Health Perspect.*, 2005, **113**(8), 969–977.
120. L. Poston, Developmental programming and diabetes - The human experience and insight from animal models, *Best. Pract. Res. Clin. Endocrinol. Metab.*, 2010, **24**(4), 541–552.
121. R. de *et al.*, Glucose tolerance at age 58 and the decline of glucose tolerance in comparison with age 50 in people prenatally exposed to the Dutch famine, *Diabetologia*, 2006, **49**(4), 637–643.
122. P. H. Whincup *et al.*, Birth weight and risk of type 2 diabetes: a systematic review, *JAM*, 2008, **300**(24), 2886–2897.
123. L. S. Fetita *et al.*, Consequences of fetal exposure to maternal diabetes in offspring, *J. Clin. Endocrinol. Metab.*, 2006, **91**(10), 3718–3724.
124. C. J. Everett and E. M. Matheson, Biomarkers of pesticide exposure and diabetes in the 1999-2004 National Health and Nutrition Examination Survey, *Environ. Int.*, 2010.
125. D. H. Lee *et al.*, A strong dose–response relation between serum concentrations of persistent organic pollutants and diabetes: results from the National Health and Examination Survey 1999–2002, *Diabetes Care*, 2006, **29**(7), 1638–1644.
126. D. H. Lee *et al.*, Extended analyses of the association between serum concentrations of persistent organic pollutants and diabetes, *Diabetes Care*, 2007, **30**(6), 1596–1598.
127. J. S. Lim, D. H. Lee and D. R. Jacobs, Jr., Association of brominated flame retardants with diabetes and metabolic syndrome in the U.S. population, 2003-2004, *Diabetes Care*, 2008, **31**(9), 1802–1807.
128. D. H. Lee, D. R. Jacobs, Jr. and M. Steffes, Association of organochlorine pesticides with peripheral neuropathy in patients with diabetes or impaired fasting glucose, *Diabetes*, 2008, **57**(11), 3108–3111.
129. D. H. Lee *et al.*, Low dose of some persistent organic pollutants predicts type 2 diabetes: a nested case-control study, *Environ. Health Perspect.*, 2010, **118**(9), 1235–1242.
130. A. Rignell-Hydbom *et al.*, Exposure to p,p'-DDE: a risk factor for type 2 diabetes, *PLoS. One*, 2009, **4**(10), e7503.
131. M. Turyk *et al.*, Organochlorine exposure and incidence of diabetes in a cohort of Great Lakes sport fish consumers, *Environ. Health Perspect.*, 2009, **117**(7), 1076–1082.
132. D. H. Lee *et al.*, Polychlorinated Biphenyls and Organochlorine Pesticides in Plasma Predict Development of Type 2 Diabetes in the Elderly: The Prospective Investigation of the Vasculature in Uppsala Seniors (PIVUS) Study, *Diabetes Care*, 2011.
133. J. R. Edwards and W. C. Prozialeck, Cadmium, diabetes and chronic kidney disease, *Toxicol. Appl. Pharmacol.*, 2009, **238**(3), 289–293.
134. D. M. Schreinemachers, Perturbation of lipids and glucose metabolism associated with previous 2,4-D exposure: a cross-sectional study of NHANES III data, 1988–1994., *Environ. Health*, 2010, **9**, 11.

135. J. Beard *et al.*, Health impacts of pesticide exposure in a cohort of outdoor workers, *Environ. Health Perspect.*, 2003, **111**(5), 724–730.
136. M. P. Montgomery *et al.*, Incident diabetes and pesticide exposure among licensed pesticide applicators: Agricultural Health Study, 1993–2003, *Am. J. Epidemiol.*, 2008, **167**(10), 1235–1246.
137. U. Kramer *et al.*, Traffic-related air pollution and incident type 2 diabetes: results from the SALIA cohort study, *Environ. Health Perspect.*, 2010, **118**(9), 1273–1279.
138. I. A. Lang *et al.*, Association of urinary bisphenol A concentration with medical disorders and laboratory abnormalities in adults, *JAMA*, 2008, **300**(11), 1303–1310.
139. D. Melzer *et al.*, Association of urinary bisphenol a concentration with heart disease: evidence from NHANES 2003/06, *PLoS. One*, 2010, **5**(1), e8673.
140. G. Ning *et al.*, Relationship of Urinary Bisphenol A Concentration to Risk for Prevalent Type 2 Diabetes in Chinese Adults: A Cross-sectional Analysis, *Ann. Intern. Med.*, 2011, **155**(6), 368–374.
141. M. K. Silver *et al.*, Urinary Bisphenol A and Type-2 Diabetes in U.S. Adults: Data from NHANES 2003-2008, *PLoS. One*, 2011, **6**(10), e26868.
142. K. Svensson *et al.*, Phthalate exposure associated with self-reported diabetes among Mexican women, *Environ. Res.*, 2011.
143. R. W. Stahlhut *et al.*, Concentrations of urinary phthalate metabolites are associated with increased waist circumference and insulin resistance in adult U.S. males, *Environ. Health Perspect.*, 2007, **115**(6), 876–882.
144. T. M. Saldana *et al.*, Pesticide exposure and self-reported gestational diabetes mellitus in the Agricultural Health Study, *Diabetes Care*, 2007, **30**(3), 529–534.
145. A. S. Ettinger *et al.*, Maternal arsenic exposure and impaired glucose tolerance during pregnancy, *Environ. Health Perspect.*, 2009, **117**(7), 1059–1064.
146. S. Fourlanos *et al.*, Latent autoimmune diabetes in adults (LADA) should be less latent, *Diabetologia*, 2005, **48**(11), 2206–2212.
147. K. Vehik and D. Dabelea, The changing epidemiology of type 1 diabetes: why is it going through the roof?, *Diabetes Metab Res. Rev.*, 2011, **27**(1), 3–13.
148. S. G. Howard and D. H. Lee, What is the role of human contamination by environmental chemicals in the development of type 1 diabetes?, *J. Epidemiol. Community Health*, 2011.
149. D. A. Gonzalez *et al.*, Sex hormones and autoimmunity, *Immunol. Lett.*, 2010, **133**(1), 6–13.
150. M. Cutolo *et al.*, The immunomodulatory effects of estrogens: clinical relevance in immune-mediated rheumatic diseases, *Ann. N. Y. Acad. Sci.*, 2010, **1193**, 36–42.
151. S. R. Lindehammer *et al.*, Seroconversion to islet autoantibodies between early pregnancy and delivery in non-diabetic mothers, *J. Reprod. Immunol.*, 2011, **88**(1), 72–79.

152. M. Ostensen *et al.*, Pregnancy and reproduction in autoimmune rheumatic diseases, *Rheumatology.(Oxford)*, 2011, **50**(4), 657–664.
153. E. A. Gale and K. M. Gillespie, Diabetes and gender, *Diabetologia*, 2001, **44**(1), 3–15.
154. H. Wucher, J. Lepercq and J. Timsit, Onset of autoimmune type 1 diabetes during pregnancy: Prevalence and outcomes, *Best. Pract. Res. Clin. Endocrinol. Metab.*, 2010, **24**(4), 617–624.
155. R. Vargas, J. T. Repke and S. H. Ural, Type 1 diabetes mellitus and pregnancy, *Rev. Obstet. Gynecol.*, 2010, **3**(3), 92–100.
156. E. B. Tsai *et al.*, The rise and fall of insulin secretion in type 1 diabetes mellitus, *Diabetologia*, 2006, **49**(2), 261–270.
157. S. Fourlanos, L. C. Harrison and P. G. Colman, The accelerator hypothesis and increasing incidence of type 1 diabetes, *Curr. Opin. Endocrinol. Diabetes Obes.*, 2008, **15**(4), 321–325.
158. G. Dahlquist, Can we slow the rising incidence of childhood-onset autoimmune diabetes? The overload hypothesis, *Diabetologia*, 2006, **49**(1), 20–24.
159. P. Narendran, E. Estella and S. Fourlanos, Immunology of type 1 diabetes, *QJM* , 2005, **98**(8), 547–556.
160. I. M. Sorensen *et al.*, Maternal Serum Levels of 25-Hydroxy-Vitamin D During Pregnancy and Risk of Type 1 Diabetes in the Offspring, *Diabetes*, 2011.
161. M. Knip *et al.*, Dietary Intervention in Infancy and Later Signs of Beta-Cell Autoimmunity, *N. Engl. J. Med.*, 2010, **363**(20), 1900–1908.
162. J. Lempainen *et al.*, Interaction of enterovirus infection and Cow's milk-based formula nutrition in type 1 diabetes-associated autoimmunity, *Diabetes Metab Res. Rev.*, 2011.
163. C. R. Cardwell *et al.*, Caesarean section is associated with an increased risk of childhood-onset type 1 diabetes mellitus: a meta-analysis of observational studies, *Diabetologia*, 2008, **51**(5), 726–735.
164. C. R. Cardwell *et al.*, Birthweight and the risk of childhood-onset type 1 diabetes: a meta-analysis of observational studies using individual patient data, *Diabetologia*, 2010, **53**(4), 641–651.
165. C. R. Cardwell *et al.*, Maternal age at birth and childhood type 1 diabetes: a pooled analysis of 30 observational studies, *Diabetes*, 2010, **59**(2), 486–494.
166. E. A. Gale, Congenital rubella: citation virus or viral cause of type 1 diabetes?, *Diabetologia*, 2008, **51**(9), 1559–1566.
167. S. M. Virtanen and M. Knip, Nutritional risk predictors of beta cell autoimmunity and type 1 diabetes at a young age, *Am. J. Clin. Nutr.*, 2003, **78**(6), 1053–1067.
168. T. Helgason and M. R. Jonasson, Evidence for a food additive as a cause of ketosis-prone diabetes, *Lancet*, 1981, **2**(8249), 716–720.
169. E. H. Hathout *et al.*, Air pollution and type 1 diabetes in children, *Pediatr. Diabetes*, 2006, **7**(2), 81–87.

170. A. Rignell-Hydbom *et al.*, A nested case-control study of intrauterine exposure to persistent organochlorine pollutants in relation to risk of type 1 diabetes, *PLoS. One*, 2010, **5**(6), e11281.
171. M. P. Longnecker *et al.*, Polychlorinated biphenyl serum levels in pregnant subjects with diabetes, *Diabetes Care*, 2001, **24**(6), 1099–1101.
172. N. F. Kolachi *et al.*, Status of Toxic Metals in Biological Samples of Diabetic Mothers and Their Neonates, *Biol. Trace Elem. Res.*, 2010.
173. J. H. Karam *et al.*, Insulinopenic diabetes after rodenticide (Vacor) ingestion: a unique model of acquired diabetes in man, *Diabetes*, 1980, **29**(12), 971–978.
174. K. Buschard, What causes type 1 diabetes? Lessons from animal models, *APMIS Suppl*, 2011, **119**(132), 1–19.
175. L. Wei *et al.*, Induction of diabetes with signs of autoimmunity in primates by the injection of multiple-low-dose streptozotocin, *Biochem. Biophys. Res. Commun.*, 2011, **412**(2), 373–378.
176. T. Helgason *et al.*, Diabetes produced in mice by smoked/cured mutton, *Lancet*, 1982, **2**(8306), 1017–1022.
177. S. D. Holladay, Prenatal immunotoxicant exposure and postnatal autoimmune disease, *Environ. Health Perspect.*, 1999, **107**(Suppl 5), 687–691.
178. H. Yurino *et al.*, Endocrine disruptors (environmental estrogens) enhance autoantibody production by B1 cells, *Toxicol. Sci.*, 2004, **81**(1), 139–147.
179. A. Mustafa *et al.*, An enhanced postnatal autoimmune profile in 24 week-old C57BL/6 mice developmentally exposed to TCDD, *Toxicol. Appl. Pharmacol.*, 2008, **232**(1), 51–59.
180. M. Abedi-Valugerdi, Mercury and silver induce B cell activation and anti-nucleolar autoantibody production in outbred mouse stocks: are environmental factors more important than the susceptibility genes in connection with autoimmunity? *Clin. Exp. Immunol.*, 2009, **155**(1), 117–124.
181. S. Y. Lim and S. K. Ghosh, Autoreactive responses to an environmental factor: 1. phthalate induces antibodies exhibiting anti-DNA specificity, *Immunology*, 2003, **110**(4), 482–492.
182. Blossom, S.J. and J.C. Doss, Trichloroethylene alters central and peripheral immune function in autoimmune-prone MRL(+/+) mice following continuous developmental and early life exposure. *J. Immunotoxicol.*, 2007. **4**(2): 129–141.
183. G. Ravel *et al.*, Trichloroethylene Does Not Accelerate Autoimmune Diabetes in NOD Mice, *J. Immunotoxicol.*, 2004, **1**(3), 141–148.
184. B. O. Roep and M. Atkinson, Animal models have little to teach us about type 1 diabetes: 1. In support of this proposal, *Diabetologia*, 2004, **47**(10), 1650–1656.
185. Y. H. Yan *et al.*, Enhanced insulin resistance in diet-induced obese rats exposed to fine particles by instillation, *Inhal. Toxicol.*, 2011.
186. Z. J. Andersen *et al.*, Diabetes Incidence and Long-Term Exposure to Air Pollution: A cohort study, *Diabetes Care*, 2011.

187. M. B. Dijkema *et al.*, Long-term Exposure to Traffic-related Air Pollution and Type 2 Diabetes Prevalence in a Cross-sectional Screening-study in the Netherlands, *Environ. Health*, 2011, **10**(1), 76.
188. R. C. Puett *et al.*, Are Particulate Matter Exposures Associated with Risk of Type 2 Diabetes?, *Environ. Health Perspect.*, 2010.
189. R. D. Brook *et al.*, The relationship between diabetes mellitus and traffic-related air pollution, *J. Occup. Environ. Med.*, 2008, **50**(1), 32–38.
190. M. E. Davila-Esqueda *et al.*, Low-level subchronic arsenic exposure from prenatal developmental stages to adult life results in an impaired glucose homeostasis, *Exp. Clin. Endocrinol. Diabetes*, 2011, **119**(10), 613–617.
191. C. F. Huang *et al.*, Arsenic and diabetes: Current perspectives, *Kaohsiung. J. Med. Sci.*, 2011, **27**(9), 402–410.
192. S. Lim *et al.*, Chronic exposure to the herbicide, atrazine, causes mitochondrial dysfunction and insulin resistance, *PLoS. One*, 2009, **4**(4), e5186.
193. P. Alonso-Magdalena *et al.*, The estrogenic effect of bisphenol A disrupts pancreatic beta-cell function in vivo and induces insulin resistance, *Environ. Health Perspect.*, 2006, **114**(1), 106–112.
194. P. Alonso-Magdalena *et al.*, Bisphenol A exposure during pregnancy disrupts glucose homeostasis in mothers and adult male offspring, *Environ. Health Perspect.*, 2010, **118**(9), 1243–1250.
195. S. M. de la Monte *et al.*, Nitrosamine exposure exacerbates high fat diet-mediated type 2 diabetes mellitus, non-alcoholic steatohepatitis, and neurodegeneration with cognitive impairment, *Mol. Neurodegener*, 2009, **4**, 54.
196. J. E. Michalek and M. Pavuk, Diabetes and cancer in veterans of Operation Ranch Hand after adjustment for calendar period, days of spraying, and time spent in Southeast Asia, *J. Occup. Environ. Med.*, 2008, **50**(3), 330–340.
197. A. A. Adigun *et al.*, Neonatal organophosphorus pesticide exposure alters the developmental trajectory of cell-signaling cascades controlling metabolism: differential effects of diazinon and parathion, *Environ. Health Perspect.*, 2010, **118**(2), 210–215.
198. N. S. Gayathri *et al.*, Changes in some hormones by low doses of di (2-ethyl hexyl) phthalate (DEHP), a commonly used plasticizer in PVC blood storage bags & medical tubing, *Indian J. Med. Res.*, 2004, **119**(4), 139–144.
199. Y. Lin *et al.*, Developmental Exposure to Di(2-ethylhexyl) Phthalate Impairs Endocrine Pancreas and Leads to Long-term Adverse Effects on Glucose Homeostasis in the Rat, *Am. J. Physiol. Endocrinol. Metab.*, 2011.
200. D. H. Lee *et al.*, Association between serum concentrations of persistent organic pollutants and insulin resistance among nondiabetic adults: results from the National Health and Nutrition Examination Survey 1999–2002, *Diabetes Care*, 2007, **30**(3), 622–628.
201. D. H. Lee *et al.*, Low Dose Organochlorine Pesticides and Polychlorinated Biphenyls Predict Obesity, Dyslipidemia, and Insulin

Resistance among People Free of Diabetes, *PLoS. One*, 2011, **6**(1), e15977.
202. S. L. Wang *et al.*, Increased risk of diabetes and polychlorinated biphenyls and dioxins: a 24-year follow-up study of the Yucheng cohort, *Diabetes Care*, 2008, **31**(8), 1574–1579.
203. S. Takayama *et al.*, Effects of long-term oral administration of DDT on nonhuman primates, *J. Cancer Res. Clin. Oncol.*, 1999, **125**(3-4), 219–225.
204. J. Ruzzin *et al.*, Persistent organic pollutant exposure leads to insulin resistance syndrome, *Environ. Health Perspect.*, 2010, **118**(4), 465–471.
205. T. Wang *et al.*, Urinary Bisphenol A (BPA) Concentration Associates with Obesity and Insulin Resistance, *J. Clin. Endocrinol. Metab.*, 2011.
206. J. W. Chang *et al.*, Simultaneous exposure of non-diabetics to high levels of dioxins and mercury increases their risk of insulin resistance, *J. Hazard. Mater*, 2011, **185**(2-3), 749–755.
207. N. Brenden, H. Rabbani and M. bedi-Valugerdi, Analysis of mercury-induced immune activation in nonobese diabetic (NOD) mice, *Clin. Exp. Immunol.*, 2001, **125**(2), 202–210.
208. G. S. Cooper *et al.*, Evidence of autoimmune-related effects of trichloroethylene exposure from studies in mice and humans, *Environ. Health Perspect.*, 2009, **117**(5), 696–702.
209. J. F. Nyland *et al.*, Biomarkers of Methyl Mercury Exposure Immunotoxicity among Fish Consumers in Amazonian Brazil, *Environ. Health Perspect.*, 2011.

CHAPTER 9

Bisphenol A and Aging

LAURA N. VANDENBERG

Tufts University, Center for Regenerative & Developmental Biology, 200 Boston Ave, Suite 4600, Medford, MA 02155, USA
E-mail: laura.vandenberg@tufts.edu

9.1 Introduction

The plastic monomer bisphenol A (BPA) is one of the highest volume chemicals produced worldwide, with over 6 billion pounds produced each year and over 100 tons released into the atmosphere per year.[1] BPA was first synthesized by A.P. Dianin in 1891 by combining two equivalents of phenol with one equivalent of acetone to produce a product with two phenol groups. It was later investigated in the 1930s as a synthetic estrogen but was never developed for pharmaceutical purposes. In the 1950's, BPA began to be used in the production of polycarbonate plastics and epoxy resins, and production has increased steadily since that time.

9.2 Mechanisms of BPA Action

BPA contains two benzene rings and two (4,4')-OH substituents (Figure 9.1). This simple structure allows the molecule to fit in the estrogen receptor (ER) binding pocket. The majority of natural estrogens are produced by the ovaries or testes and are able to diffuse in and out of all cells in the body.[2] Estrogens are retained by some cells, considered target cells, due to high affinity binding to ERs located in the nucleus. When an estrogen binds to an ER, the receptor then

Issues in Toxicology No. 16
Aging and Vulnerability to Environmental Chemicals: Age-related Disorders and their Origins in Environmental Exposures
Edited by Bernard Weiss

Published by the Royal Society of Chemistry, www.rsc.org

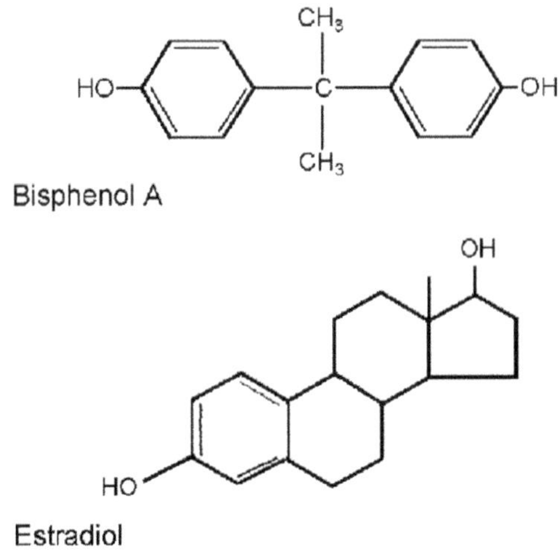

Figure 9.1 Structure of BPA and 17β-estradiol. BPA contains two benzene rings and two (4, 4')-OH substituents. Although BPA only slightly resembles the structures of natural ligands such as 17β-estradiol, its structure allows it to fit in the ER binding pocket. These structures illustrate that chemicals with variable conformations can bind to the estrogen receptors.

binds to specific sites of DNA with high affinity (known as estrogen response elements), modulating transcription of target genes.

BPA binding to the ER is sufficient to trigger many biological responses that are similar to the effects of endogenous estrogens. Biochemical assays indicate that BPA binds both ERα and ERβ, with approximately 10-fold higher affinity for ERβ.[3–5] *In vivo* assays—including the uterotrophic assay, which tests estrogenic responses such as uterine wet weight, luminal epithelial height, and increased expression of lactoferrin, an estrogen-inducible protein—also indicate that BPA has estrogenic activity.[6,7]

Because of its relatively low affinity for the ERs compared to that of natural estrogens, BPA is often referred to as a weak estrogen. However, many studies indicate that BPA can stimulate cellular responses at very low concentrations, below the levels where BPA is expected to bind to the nuclear ERs.[8,9] Instead, these studies indicate that the actions of low doses of BPA can occur *via* binding to membrane receptors, including a membrane-bound form of ERα (mERα), which is similar but not identical to nuclear ERα ,[10,11] and a transmembrane ER called G protein-coupled receptor 30 (GPR30), which is structurally dissimilar to the nuclear ERs.[12,13] Collectively, studies examining the actions of BPA *via* membrane receptors indicate that not only does it have the efficacy of estradiol, but it is also equally potent.[14,15] Additionally, there is evidence that BPA mimics estrogen by binding to estrogen-related receptor γ (ERR-γ),[16] an orphan receptor that behaves as a constitutive activator of transcription.

The majority of mechanistic studies have focused on BPA's actions as an estrogen. However, there is also evidence that BPA binds to thyroid hormone receptors[17] and alters thyroid hormone signaling *in vivo*.[18] Further studies indicate that BPA binds to androgen receptors and may have anti-androgenic activities *in vivo*.[19] Studies have also shown that BPA binds to the ubiquitous aryl hydrocarbon receptor,[20] an orphan receptor that is thought to mediate toxicity following exposure to environmental chemicals. Finally, there may be more targets of BPA action; recent studies indicate that this chemical can bind to the peroxisome proliferator-activated receptor gamma (PPARγ) and can stimulate adipogenesis in pre-adipocyte cell cultures.[21,22]

9.3 BPA Sources

In 1993, a study examining estrogenic substances leaching from laboratory products showed that autoclaving cell culture media in polycarbonate flasks led to the release of an estrogenically active substance which was identified as BPA.[23] Since that time, studies have shown that BPA leaches from polycarbonate baby bottles and other polycarbonate containers intended to be used as reusable food containers.[24] Other items such as polyvinyl chloride stretch films, food-contact papers, and cardboards used as food containers have also been shown to contain BPA, and its transfer to foods from these products has also been demonstrated. In a non-randomized intervention study, college students that consumed all of their cold beverages from a polycarbonate bottle had urinary concentrations of BPA metabolites that were 69% higher than urine samples collected following a wash-out, where all cold beverages were consumed from a BPA-free container.[25] Thus polycarbonate plastics are a plausible source of human exposures.

To protect metallic food cans from rusting and corrosion, an epoxy resin is typically applied to the inner surface; many of these resins are synthesized by the condensation of BPA and epichlorhydrin to create bisphenol A diglycidyl ether (BADGE). BPA leaches from these resins due to incomplete polymerization of the applied BADGE. Several studies have shown that various conditions, including temperature and storage time, can support or enhance BPA migration from the coating of cans,[24] and many studies have shown that detectable levels of BPA are found in specific canned foods, including canned infant formula.[26–29] In another dietary intervention study, urine was collected from individuals consuming their normal diet (containing canned foods), followed by a diet without any canned goods.[30] Urinary metabolites of BPA were significantly reduced when canned goods were removed from the diet and rebounded to pre-intervention levels when typical consumption of canned goods resumed. This study and others indicate that canned goods are a significant source of human exposures to BPA.[31]

Finally, in the last few years, it has been shown that additional consumer products may contribute significantly to human BPA exposures. Many cigarette filters contain BPA, and individuals that smoke have higher levels of BPA metabolites in their urine compared to non-smokers,[32] indicating that this may significantly contribute to total BPA exposures in these individuals. Additionally, thermal papers contain large quantities of BPA,[33] and absorption *via* the skin is strongly suspected.[34,35] Further, these sources and others are thought to contribute to the measurable levels of BPA that have been detected in indoor and outdoor air, dust, water, and landfill leachates.[24]

9.4 Human Exposures

At this time, there is only a limited amount of information available to understand the kinetics of BPA metabolism following exposures. In humans, once BPA enters the body, it is conjugated to form two major metabolites, BPA-glucuronide and BPA-sulfate; this process occurs in the liver. If BPA enters the body *via* the oral route, this is thought to occur soon after exposure in a process referred to as "first pass metabolism".[36] However, toxicokinetic studies clearly indicate that this metabolism is not complete, *i.e.* some BPA is not metabolized, even when exposures are strictly *via* the oral route.[37] Further, when BPA enters the body *via* non-oral routes (*i.e. via* dermal exposures to thermal papers), it can circulate more freely in the body before it is inactivated. Once BPA is conjugated, BPA metabolites are readily removed from the body *via* urine because they are more water-soluble than unconjugated (free) BPA. Importantly, there are factors that can influence the metabolism of BPA; these include age, sex, and physiological status.[37–40] Additionally, there is evidence that BPA metabolites can be deconjugated, and thus returned to the active form of BPA, in certain body tissues.[41–43]

A few studies have examined the disposition and metabolic kinetics of labeled BPA following oral administration. These studies have been used by regulatory agencies to conclude that BPA metabolism is so efficient in humans that unconjugated levels are rarely, if ever, detected in blood samples, and BPA metabolites are cleared from the body within 24–36 hours of exposure.[44,45] Unfortunately, these toxicokinetic studies are extremely limited in their design and interpretation, thus their conclusions have been strongly challenged.[24,46,47] In addition to using inappropriate and insensitive methodologies, these studies did not consider whether BPA metabolism would be affected by constant *versus* acute exposures, or whether non-oral exposures would be metabolized in the same way as oral exposures. Human studies suggest that non-oral exposures significantly contribute to overall exposure profiles.[48]

Biomonitoring studies have been an important source of information about typical human exposures to BPA. In these types of studies, human tissues and fluid samples are collected without any other interventions; BPA concentrations (and concentrations of metabolites) are determined with analytical detection methods and, where sampling numbers permit, relationships between demographic factors and BPA concentrations can be determined. These types of demographic–exposure relationships have been examined in detail using several large studies of reference populations, *i.e.* sampling of groups that are representative of larger populations. These large-scale biomonitoring studies indicate that BPA exposures are widespread in North America, Europe and parts of Asia.[49–51] They also indicate that lifestyle factors and other demographics, including country of residence, significantly influence BPA concentrations in urine.[52]

In addition to these large studies of reference populations, more than thirty additional studies have examined BPA and/or its metabolites in urine samples (for a review, see reference 46). Even though these studies have examined incredibly variable populations, have used a wide variety of analytical methods and have a lot of variability in study size, by and large they report that the majority of individuals sampled have detectable levels of BPA (and BPA metabolites) in their urine. Further, there is remarkable consistency in the concentrations reported from human populations around the world; most studies report levels of 1–3 ng mL^{-1} BPA metabolites in urine.

In addition to these urine studies, approximately two dozen studies have examined BPA concentrations in blood and serum samples collected from pregnant women, non-pregnant adults, and fetal umbilical cords (reviewed in reference 46).These studies specifically focused on determining the concentrations of unconjugated (free) BPA in healthy individuals, and all but two were able to detect this compound in at least some samples. Similar to what has been reported for urine, these studies typically reported blood concentrations in the range of 0.5–2 ng mL^{-1} unconjugated BPA in blood. Additional human tissues and fluids, including amniotic fluid, placenta, breast milk, adipose tissue, and saliva, have been examined for BPA content (reviewed in reference 46). Similar concentrations to those reported for blood have been detected in these samples. Together, it can be concluded that the majority of individuals are exposed to BPA, and that internal exposures are typically in the 1 ng mL^{-1} range.

There are several reasons to be concerned about the levels of BPA and BPA metabolites typically reported in human tissues and fluids. First, reported concentrations of 1ng mL^{-1} are higher than those required to stimulate responses in cultured cells.[53] Second, the reported concentrations in human samples are in the range of concentrations that affect development of rodents and other animals,[54] suggesting that these low levels could influence biological endpoints and development in humans.[55] And finally, several studies have examined BPA metabolism in rodents and non-human primates,[54,56,57] which have remarkably similar metabolic profiles to humans.[58] These studies suggest that relatively large exposures—in the range of hundreds of micrograms per kilogram body weight—are required to produce the levels measured in human samples.[24,54,56]

9.5 Overview of Animal Studies

As discussed earlier in this chapter, many studies of BPA have focused on its estrogenic properties. Much is known about the actions of endogenous estrogens *via* nuclear ERs, including downstream gene expression changes in target cells. Target cells include those in the female reproductive tract (uterus, ovary, vagina, cervix, oviduct), the male reproductive tract (testis, prostate, epididymis, seminal vesicles), the nervous system and brain (including the hypothalamus and pituitary), the mammary gland, the immune system, the cardiovascular system, the metabolic system (including adipose tissue, muscle, the digestive tract, pancreas), and the skeletal system, among others.[59] Hundreds of animal studies, mostly using rodent models, have examined the effects of BPA on these endpoints. The following sections discuss some of these studies, with an emphasis on those findings that are relevant to understanding the influence of BPA on aging.

9.5.1 Determining what is a Low Dose Exposure to BPA

Rodent and other animal studies of BPA have examined a wide range of doses on a considerable number of endpoints. Yet there is significant debate over which doses are truly relevant to inform risk assessments and the human condition in general.[60] In 2001, the National Toxicology Program established guidelines to define "low doses" in studies of environmental chemicals.[61] Two different definitions of "low dose" were proposed: 1) doses in the range of human exposures, and 2) doses below those typically used in traditional toxicology assessments.[62] At a 2006 scientific meeting on BPA organized by the National Institutes of Health (US), an expert panel also defined "low dose" as an administered dose that produces blood concentrations in the range of what has been measured in humans *via* biomonitoring studies.[24] Using these different definitions for "low doses" has important consequences for the analysis of the BPA literature, because each definition produces a widely different cut-off limit, and therefore influences the number of relevant studies (Table 1).

9.5.2 Dealing with Controversy & Conflicting Data in the BPA Literature

Before discussing the literature, it is important to acknowledge the considerable amount of controversy surrounding the study of BPA, and in particular the

Table 9.1 Influence of low dose definition on cut-off level of exposure, number of total studies, and number of studies finding significant effects of BPA.

"Low dose" definition	*Cut-off level of exposure (BPA)*	*Number of studies examining doses at or below low dose cut-off*	*Number of studies finding significant effects at or below low dose cut-off*	*% positive studies*
Doses in the range of (suspected) human exposures	50 μg/kg/day (the US EPA "safe" dose)	124	108	87%
Doses that produce blood concentrations in rodents similar to concentrations measured in environmentally-exposed humans	500 μg kg^{-1} per day	150	134	89%
Doses below those used in traditional toxicology studies	50 mg kg^{-1} per day	~220	~200	91%

study of low doses of BPA. Substantial attention has been given to those studies that were unable to find effects of BPA on any endpoint.[63–66] Some scientists, including those involved in risk assessments, have argued that these 'negative' studies indicate that BPA is safe for humans.[67–70] They have also argued that these 'negative' studies are better designed and implemented than studies that found significant effects of BPA. In response, many scientists have pointed out significant limitations and flaws in these 'negative' studies; these include: inappropriate choice of endpoints, contamination of negative controls, inappropriate choice of positive control substances and doses, and use of insensitive animal strains, among others.[60,71–75] The remainder of this chapter focuses on those studies that have found significant relationships between BPA exposure and age-related diseases.

9.6 BPA & Mammary Cancer

In the rodent, the mammary gland begins to develop about half-way through the period of gestation, and this tissue expresses ERs a few days before birth,[76] making it an important target for BPA and other environmental estrogens.[77] Cells in the gland continue to express ER throughout life, and mammary gland development is significantly enhanced by ovarian production of natural hormones at puberty. In particular, estrogen is responsible for elongation of the mammary ducts and overall development of the gland, allowing the epithelium to fill the stromal compartment in preparation for pregnancy and lactation.[77,78]

Several studies have examined the effects of BPA exposure during perinatal development, stages considered 'critical periods' in the development of the mammary gland.[79] Low levels of BPA during early development can alter developmental parameters of the gland and produce phenotypes that are similar to human risk factors for mammary cancer. One study examining the effects of BPA during the period of exposure reported that it altered development of both the stromal and epithelial compartments at embryonic day 18, accelerating the differentiation of the fat pad and delaying the development of an epithelial lumen, suggesting that BPA exposures affect the organization of the developing gland.[80] Perinatal exposures also affected development of the pubertal gland, with BPA exposed animals displaying altered tissue organization[81–83] and enhanced responses to estradiol[84] and progesterone.[85]

Perhaps even more intriguing are reports showing that perinatal exposure to BPA alters the appearance of the mammary gland in adulthood. In mid and late adulthood, mammary glands from BPA-exposed females had an appearance that resembled glands collected from pregnant females, even though these animals remained sexually naïve.[86] Other studies reported effects of early life BPA exposures on adult mammary gland tissue organization, gene expression, and even the appearance of pre-cancerous lesions.[87,90]

BPA exposures limited to the pre-pubertal period of development can also influence architecture of the mammary gland. Animals exposed at this later period of development had increased numbers of epithelial structures, which may indicate that BPA exposures advance development of the mammary gland, compared to unexposed controls.[91] Finally, adult BPA exposures can also alter organization of the tissue compartments in the adult mammary gland. Following several weeks of low dose exposure, both wildtype females and females with mutations in the BRCA1 gene had abnormalities resembling the effects of perinatal BPA exposure in their mammary gland architectures.[92] Both wildtype and BRCA1 mutant females exposed to BPA had significantly more ductal hyperplasias and increased epithelial proliferation compared to unexposed females. Collectively, these studies link BPA exposure with several human risk factors for breast cancer, including an increase in the number of epithelial structures where cancers are thought to arise,[81,93] increased epithelial density (which may be similar to the human risk factor of increased mammographic density),[94] increased sensitivity to estrogens,[84] and increased numbers of pre-neoplastic lesions.[88,92]

Of course, results showing that BPA increases the appearance of risk factors for mammary cancer are not the same as showing a direct connection between this chemical and cancer itself. Because the rat model of carcinogenesis mimics human breast cancer better than most mouse models,[95,96] experiments to address the link between BPA and mammary cancer have largely used the rat. These studies have shown that BPA can produce neoplastic (cancerous) lesions in the mammary gland, even when no additional hormonal or carcinogen treatments were applied.[89] An additional study using a tumor-prone mouse strain showed that even adult exposures to BPA could promote mammary tumors.[97] Although unexposed females of this mouse strain developed tumors, BPA exposures accelerated their appearance.

BPA exposures during perinatal development changed the response of the mammary gland to chemical carcinogens.[90,98–100] Typically, these carcinogens were administered at doses that produced few, if any, tumors in unexposed animals, yet BPA-exposed females developed significantly more tumors, had a decreased tumor latency, and an increased severity of the tumors' histological grades. Even BPA exposures that were limited to the pubertal period increased the susceptibility of the mammary gland to chemical carcinogens.[101] These findings are supported by subsequent studies which demonstrated that BPA alters gene and protein expression in the mammary gland. Gene expression arrays and proteomic studies indicate that BPA upregulates the expression of genes related to immune function, cell proliferation, cytoskeletal function, and estrogen signaling, and downregulates apoptotic genes.[87,98,99,102] BPA also increased cell proliferation and decreased apoptosis in the gland.[101] Collectively, these studies may shed light on the cellular and molecular mechanisms behind increased susceptibility to mammary cancer.

9.7 BPA & Prostate Cancer

The effects of BPA on the prostate are some of the most contested for this chemical, and for endocrine disruptors as a whole.[103–105] Several regulatory agencies and many scientists have addressed whether low doses of BPA during fetal and perinatal development affect the rodent prostate.[104,106–109] In 1997, the first study to examine the effects of fetal BPA exposure on prostate development showed that exposure during early development significantly increased the weight of the prostate in adulthood compared to prostates collected from age-matched controls.[110] Several subsequent studies have shown similar effects on adult prostate weight following fetal exposures to low doses of BPA.[111–114] BPA has been shown to disrupt tissue organization, protein expression, and cell proliferation in prostate epithelial ducts.[115–118] Low doses of BPA also affect androgen receptor binding activity in the prostate[112] and can alter the volume and size of individual prostatic ducts.[116]

Again, these findings of altered prostate size and expression of proteins in the adult prostate following perinatal BPA exposure are intriguing, but they do not address whether BPA could influence diseases of aging, namely the incidence of prostate cancer. In humans, prostate cancer normally develops when endogenous hormone production is increased.[119] For this reason, many studies examining the influence of environmental chemical exposures examine the incidence of prostate lesions with and without supplemental hormone therapy.[120] Several recent studies have examined whether low doses of BPA influence the incidence of adult-onset prostatic intraepithelial neoplasias (PIN lesions) in male rats. Regardless of how BPA was administered to pups, early life exposures to BPA increased the incidence of PIN lesions in response to a mixture of testosterone and estradiol in adulthood.[121–123] Without this hormone cocktail, no increase in PIN lesions was observed in BPA-exposed males. Studies aimed at understanding the molecular mechanisms behind the response of the prostate to early life BPA exposures have shown that low dose exposures produce permanent epigenetic alterations; prostates isolated from exposed males contained unmethylated sequences in genes are that normally hypermethylated—and therefore silenced—in untreated males.[121,124]

As mentioned, several studies have reported that they were unable to detect any effects of perinatal BPA exposures on the prostate.[63–65,125–130] Importantly, these studies have flaws, including the failure to include a positive control, the use of an inappropriate positive control, an inability to find effects with the positive control, and lack of sensitivity demonstrated by effects of only high doses of the positive control. Even when considering these 'negative' studies, several expert panels have concluded that perinatal BPA exposures can permanently alter the adult prostate.[54,55,131]

9.8 BPA & Metabolic syndrome, Liver Disease & Cardiovascular Disease

In humans, metabolic syndrome comprises a combination of disorders—including a high BMI (including obesity), a concentration of body fat at the center of the body (*i.e.* around the waist), high triglyceride levels, reduced HDL-cholesterol levels, high fasting glucose levels, impaired glucose tolerance, insulin resistance, and/or high blood pressure—that increases the risk of developing cardiovascular disease and diabetes.[132] Genetics and environmental factors, including aging, lifestyle, and endocrine disorders, can contribute to metabolic syndrome. Additionally, recent studies in the field of endocrine disruption have identified a class of chemicals termed 'obesogens', *i.e.* chemicals that can promote the development of adipocytes, alter lipid metabolism, and contribute to obesity.[133,134]

Several of the endpoints observed in human metabolic syndrome have been observed in animal models following exposure to BPA. Low doses of BPA can influence the body weight of offspring exposed during the perinatal period.[135–138] Additionally, the type of food provided to BPA-exposed animals in adolescence and adulthood can significantly impact on whether alterations in body weight are observed.[139,140] In fact, varying composition and estrogenic activity of feed could account for many of the studies that were unable to detect effects of BPA on body weight.[141,142] BPA can also influence the percentage of body weight attributed to adipose tissue and the localization of fat to the viscera.[143]

In one of the more interesting examinations of BPA as an obesogen, Alonso-Magdalena and colleagues administered low doses of BPA to pregnant mice for eight days during pregnancy. Several endpoints were examined in these pregnant females, and the mice were then re-examined 4 months after parturition; the male offspring were also examined 6 months after birth.[144] During pregnancy, the dams were found to have altered glucose tolerance and fasting insulin levels, as well as high circulating levels of leptin and triglycerides after fasting. Four months after delivery, these same females had higher body weights and altered sensitivity to glucose and insulin. Additionally, the male offspring had abnormal blood glucose and fasting insulin levels, glucose intolerance, and abnormal proliferation of pancreatic β-cells.

Other important factors that have been identified in human metabolic syndrome have also been examined in rodents exposed to BPA. Several studies have investigated the influence of early life BPA exposures on liver health later in life. BPA affects the expression of metabolic genes[140] and measures of lipid peroxidation and reduced glutathione in the liver.[145] Finally, only one study has examined heart-related parameters relative to BPA administration, and this study showed that male rats exposed to BPA during early life developed hypertension in adulthood.[143]

Two more studies with plausible relevance to human populations concern BPA exposures prior to *in vitro* fertilization (IVF). In human IVF treatments, embryos are often matured outside of the body prior to implantation. Pre-implantation mouse embryos were exposed to BPA and their rate of development to blastocyst stages was altered, with low doses increasing the number of embryos reaching blastocyst stages and high doses decreasing this number.[146] Additionally, pre-implantation mouse embryos were cultured in 1 nM BPA and then transplanted into unexposed females and allowed to develop; these animals were significantly heavier at weaning compared to mice from embryos that were not cultured with BPA.[147]

9.9 BPA & Infertility

A number of studies have shown that developmental exposures to low doses of BPA alter development of the male and female reproductive tracts[148–153] Several studies clearly indicate that the timing of female reproductive aging is influenced by BPA exposure, starting as early as puberty, with advanced timing of vaginal opening and earlier timing of first estrous.[100,154,155] Alterations were also observed in adult estrous cycles following perinatal exposure.[86,154,156] Another important measure of reproductive aging is the presence of blood-filled ovarian bursae and cystic ovaries; these were observed significantly more often in BPA-exposed females after several months of age compared to age-matched controls.[86,157–159] Finally, females that were developmentally exposed to BPA had significantly more oocytes with meiotic abnormalities, including aneuploidy;[160] when these females were mated, there was a significant increase in the number of aneuploid eggs and embryos.[161] Follow-up studies also suggest that diet plays an important role in this oocyte phenotype.[162,163]

Only a few studies have examined whether BPA influences female fertility and fecundity,[164,165] and only one study has examined the relationships between BPA exposure, fertility/fecundity endpoints and age.[166] Perinatally exposed females were force-bred throughout life to determine the maximum number of litters (a measure of fertility) and the maximum number of pups (a measure of fecundity) they could bear. Interestingly, animals exposed to BPA demonstrated an age-related decline in both fertility and fecundity.

Male fertility has also been investigated with regards to the plausible effects of BPA on this endpoint. As mentioned, developmental exposures to BPA cause malformations of the male reproductive organs. Additionally, relatively high doses of BPA induce measures of oxidative stress and lipid peroxidation in the testes of exposed males.[167–169] But perhaps most important for considering the effects of BPA on fertility are those studies showing that BPA alters sperm characteristics, including sperm number,[114,170–172] sperm morphology,[173,174] and sperm motility.[114,172,173,175] Several of these studies have also shown direct effects on male fertility.[170,172]

9.10 Summary of Animal Studies

This review is focused on an examination of the effects of BPA on aging-related endpoints, including metabolic syndrome, mammary and prostate cancers, and male and female infertility. However, it is important to note that a large number of studies have examined the effects of BPA on other endpoints. Highly significant effects indicating that BPA alters the development of sexually dimorphic regions of the brain and behaviors that are likely controlled by these nuclei have been reported;[176–184] many studies specifically show that BPA alters sex-specific behaviors. Low dose effects of BPA have also been reported with regard to immune responses following antigen exposure[185–187] and serum concentrations of various hormones.[7,164,188,189]

Several researchers have produced models to explain the actions of BPA during early development and how the effects of early hormone exposures can lead to various endocrine-related pathologies (reviewed in references 54, 190, 191, and 192). Typically, these models propose that BPA acts *via* ERs (ERα, ERβ, mER, *etc.*) present in estrogen-target organs. When BPA binds to these ERs, particularly during developmental periods where concentrations of endogenous estrogens are low or absent altogether, this activation of estrogen-signaling pathways permanently alters organ histogenesis and cellular differentiation. Many phenotypes associated with these hormone-related pathologies are observed at puberty and in adulthood, and some syndromes that are associated with aging (cancer incidence, weight gain, infertility) manifest earlier as a consequence of BPA-induced changes. Of course, because different ERs are present in different cell types and at various developmental stages, BPA can have different actions (complementary and opposing) depending on the applied dose, the period of exposure, and various other environmental factors. Because of all of these variables, BPA exposures can produce complex phenotypes, some of which have serious detrimental consequences for the health of the individual.

9.10.1 Overview of Epidemiology Studies

As discussed earlier in this chapter, human exposures to BPA are widespread and there is a general consensus that BPA can be detected in the majority of individuals in many countries.[24,46] Epidemiologists have now begun to collect information about human exposure levels and ask whether there are relationships between circulating levels of BPA, or excreted BPA metabolites, and various health outcomes. These studies are particularly challenging for several reasons: 1) BPA exposures are so widespread that there is no "negative control population" available for study;[193] 2) because BPA itself is ubiquitous, especially in medical and laboratory environments, there are concerns over contamination during the collection and analysis of human samples;[194] 3) most studies examine only single urine samples, but there is wide inter-person variability as well as temporal variability in BPA concentrations;[195–197] 4) most exposure assessments occur in adults, whereas damage inflicted by BPA may occur much earlier in life; and 5) animal studies typically examine single chemical exposures to determine their effects on developing individuals, but humans are exposed to mixtures containing dozens or even hundreds of chemicals.

For these reasons, as well as cost-related issues, only a few epidemiology studies have addressed the role BPA may have in human diseases. Recently, a few of these studies have examined gestational exposures to BPA (*via* sampling of urine from pregnant women) and related these exposures to behavioral outcomes in offspring in the first few years of life.[198,199] These studies are unique in their prospective design, and future studies will likely use a similar strategy to determine any relationships between BPA exposure levels and other health outcomes, including infertility, cancer incidence, metabolic syndrome, and others. Obviously establishing relationships between developmental (perinatal) BPA exposures and adult diseases will take decades to complete.

This review will finish with a brief overview of the few epidemiology studies conducted to date that have examined age-related health outcomes. Although these studies are limited, based on their designs (typically cross-sectional or case-control studies), their results do point to intriguing relationships between BPA and age-related diseases.

9.10.2 BPA & Cancer

Only one study to date has examined whether individuals with higher BPA exposures are at greater risk for developing cancer. In this study, serum BPA concentrations were compared between Korean women with breast cancer and age-matched controls.[200] Although the median exposure levels were higher in the breast cancer patients compared to controls (0.61 ng mL^{-1} *versus* 0.03 ng mL^{-1}), these differences were not significant. Of course, this study was limited by the collection of blood at the time of breast cancer diagnosis/treatment, because these BPA exposures likely do not reflect exposure levels from early life during periods that may be more sensitive to disruption by BPA. Further, these results may be more indicative of the number of medical interventions experienced by the breast cancer patients compared to the healthy controls. Because a large number of medical devices and medical tubing contain and release BPA, these patients may have experienced higher exposures during the treatment period.[9,201]

Studies examining the link between BPA exposures and cancer endpoints are greatly needed in human populations. In studies of diethylstilbestrol (DES), a potent pharmaceutical estrogen, rodents were highly predictive of the effects of this chemical on humans exposed in the womb. Studies showing that DES exposure increased mammary cancer in laboratory animals led to more comprehensive testing of human DES daughters, who were found to have increased risk of breast cancer 25 years after the rodent data was published.[202,203]

9.10.3 BPA, Metabolic Syndrome & Cardiovascular Disease

In contrast to the weak evidence connecting BPA exposures to cancers, perhaps some of the best evidence suggests correlations between BPA and metabolic disorders. Two large studies examining almost 3000 adults in the US found correlations between urinary BPA concentrations and prevalence of self-reported cardiovascular disease.[204,205] Analysis of these same adults also showed correlations between urinary BPA and self-reported incidence of diabetes. Positive correlations between urinary BPA concentrations and serum liver enzymes were also reported. Importantly, these two studies used representative samples from two different populations examined *via* the CDC's National Health and Nutrition Examination Survey (NHANES). Interestingly, associations between these diseases and BPA exposure levels were stronger in the 2003/2004 NHANES compared to the 2005/2006 NHANES. This may be due to the higher BPA concentrations reported in the earlier survey (geometric means: 2.5 *versus* 1.8 ng mL^{-1}).

A subsequent study examined data from both the 2003/2004 and 2005/2006 NHANES studies in order to explore relationships between BPA exposure and obesity. Again using a cross-sectional design, researchers compared urinary BPA concentrations with BMI and waist circumference in almost 3000 adults.[206] Positive correlations were found for both health outcomes; individuals in the upper quartile of BPA exposures were 1.60–1.85 times more likely to be obese and 1.43–1.67 times more likely to have a high waist circumference compared to individuals with the lowest exposures. A second cross-sectional study using only older adults (age 40 and over) from China reported similar relationships between BPA exposures and obesity. Using exposure and health data collected from more than 3000 individuals, the authors indicated that individuals in the top quartile for urinary BPA concentrations were 1.50 times more likely to be obese and 1.37 times more likely to have insulin resistance than individuals with the lowest exposures.[207]

Similar to the limitations discussed for human cancer studies, there are some limitations that must be considered when interpreting these results. Because metabolic syndrome appears to develop over a long period of time, it is unlikely that exposure determinations made after the disease has developed will be informative about exposures preceding the development of the symptoms, especially during critical periods of development. Further, it has been suggested that individuals with these disease characteristics (*i.e.* obesity, high waist circumference, insulin resistance, diabetes, *etc.*) have higher BPA exposures because of lifestyle factors associated with disease prevalence, *i.e.* it is plausible that obese individuals are more likely to eat packaged foods contaminated with BPA. Although this concern cannot be addressed in these cross-sectional studies, it is clear that the human studies conducted to date support findings from rodent studies, which suggest connections between developmental BPA exposures and later life development of metabolic syndrome.

9.10.4 BPA & Male Reproduction

Studies examining the effects of BPA exposure on fertility endpoints in men have generated interesting findings that should be followed-up with larger sample sizes and different demographics. In one of the first epidemiology studies to examine the effects of BPA, workers spraying BPA-containing epoxy resins were compared with unexposed workers.[208] In this cross-sectional study, high BPA exposures were associated with lower levels of FSH. Yet another study, examining men that were not occupationally exposed to BPA, found no relationships between urinary BPA concentrations or FSH,[209] and a third study found a positive relationship between urinary BPA concentrations and FSH levels.[210] Positive relationships between urinary BPA concentrations and serum testosterone levels in men have been reported,[211] which contrasts somewhat with a study showing an inverse relationship between BPA concentrations and free androgen index (the ratio of testosterone to sex hormone binding globulin levels).[210] Clearly these inconsistencies make it difficult to make any conclusions about the relationships between BPA and hormone levels.

BPA has been shown to affect a number of male fertility endpoints in rodents, including aspects of sperm health and receptivity to mating. Human studies have recently examined similar endpoints, focusing on relationships between BPA, sexual function, and semen quality. Several have reported associations between urinary BPA concentrations and one or more measures of reduced semen quality. The first study found that increasing concentrations of urinary BPA were significantly associated with decreased sperm concentration, decreased sperm count, decreased sperm vitality, and decreased sperm mobility,[212] similar to rodents exposed to BPA. A second study, examining men that were recruited *via* an infertility clinic, found associations between BPA concentrations and sperm concentrations, sperm motility, and sperm morphology, although these relationships were not statistically significant.[213] Finally, two studies examining the effects of occupational BPA exposure found associations between urinary BPA concentrations and decreased sexual function in Chinese men.[214,215] One study also found similar negative correlations between urinary BPA concentrations and sexual function in non-occupationally exposed (environmentally exposed) men. Thus these findings may be relevant to the wider population, and not just BPA workers.

9.10.5 BPA & Female Reproduction

In spite of the large animal literature suggesting that BPA can affect development and functionality of the female reproductive tract, only a few epidemiology studies have focused on the effects of BPA exposures on women. Further, those studies that exist are quite small and need to be repeated with larger representative populations. Two studies have examined relationships between BPA exposures and polycystic ovarian syndrome (PCOS). In both, serum BPA concentrations were higher in women with PCOS compared to unaffected women.[216,217] However, both studies used an ELISA method to measure BPA concentrations in serum; this method has some flaws, and although it is unlikely to provide data with a bias related to a disease outcome, replication of these studies using analytical detection methods is needed.

Other studies examining the effects of BPA exposures on women have also focused on fertility-based outcomes. Pregnant women carrying fetuses with an abnormal karyotype had higher serum concentrations of BPA compared to women carrying fetuses with a normal karyotype.[218]Additionally, there were associations between serum BPA concentrations and recurrent miscarriage; women with a history of three or more consecutive miscarriages had serum BPA concentrations that were more than three times higher than those of women without fertility problems.[219] When women with a history of miscarriage then became pregnant and successfully carried to term, they typically had lower BPA concentrations compared to women that became pregnant during the study and miscarried again.

Finally, a recent study of women undergoing IVF treatments found that urinary BPA concentrations were negatively associated with the number of oocytes retrieved during the IVF procedure.[220] Women with high levels of urinary BPA also had decreased concentrations of peak serum estradiol.

9.11 Summary & Conclusions

The epidemiology literature has limitations that have prevented scientists and risk assessors from declaring that BPA is unsafe for human populations. Yet these studies strongly support relationships between levels of BPA exposure and several disease outcomes. In fact, of the approximately two dozen epidemiology studies conducted to date, most of them have found relationships between BPA and an age-related health endpoint. Further, the results obtained from human studies are often supported by mechanistic data from the animal literature; BPA is associated with altered sperm endpoints in both rodents and humans; BPA is associated with altered metabolism and obesity in both rodents and humans; and BPA is associated with female infertility issues in both rodents and humans. Rodents have been exceptionally helpful in dissecting the molecular and cellular mechanisms of BPA action and have been highly predictive for the types of effects that would be observed in human populations.

It has been speculated that increased BPA exposures over the last several decades have contributed to human diseases, including male and female infertility, breast and prostate cancers, and the obesity epidemic. Untangling the relationships between this chemical and human disease is not an easy task, but continued research is dedicated to this undertaking.

References

1. E. Burridge, *ICIS Chemical Business*, 2008, **274**, 48.
2. G. G. Kuiper, B. Carlsson, K. Grandien, E. Enmark, J. Haggblad, S. Nilsson and J. A. Gustafsson, *Endocrinology*, 1997, **138**, 863–870.
3. J. C. Gould, L. S. Leonard, S. C. Maness, B. L. Wagner, K. Conner, T. Zacharewski, S. Safe, D. P. McDonnell and K. W. Gaido, *Mol. Cell. Endocrinol.*, 1998, **142**, 203–214.
4. G. G. Kuiper, J. G. Lemmen, B. Carlsson, J. C. Corton, S. H. Safe, P. T. Van Der Saag, B. van der Burg and J. A. Gustafsson, *Endocrinology*, 1998, **139**, 4252–4263.
5. W. D. Pennie, T. C. Aldridge and A. N. Brooks, *J. Endocrinol.*, 1998, **158**, R11–R14.
6. C. M. Markey, C. L. Michaelson, E. C. Veson, C. Sonnenschein and A. M. Soto, *Environ. Health Perspect.*, 2001, **109**, 55–60.
7. R. Steinmetz, N. A. Mitchner, A. Grant, D. L. Allen, R. M. Bigsby and N. Ben-Jonathan, *Endocrinology*, 1998, **139**, 2741–2747.
8. A. L. Wozniak, N. N. Bulayeva and C. S. Watson, *Environ. Health Perspect.*, 2005, **113**, 431–439.
9. W. V. Welshons, S. C. Nagel and F. S. vom Saal, *Endocrinology*, 2006, **147**, S56–S69.

10. C. S. Watson, N. N. Bulayeva, A. L. Wozniak and R. A. Alyea, *Steroids*, 2007, **72**, 124–134.
11. C. E. Powell, A. M. Soto and C. Sonnenschein, *J. Steroid Biochem. Molec. Biol.*, 2001, **77**, 97–108.
12. P. Thomas and J. Dong, *J. Steroid Biochem. Molec. Biol.*, 2006, **102**, 175–179.
13. P. Thomas, Y. Pang, E. J. Filardo and J. Dong, *Endocrinology*, 2005, **146**, 624–632.
14. C. S. Watson and B. Gametchu, *Proc. Soc. Exp. Biol. Med.*, 1999, **220**, 9–19.
15. C. S. Watson, Y. J. Jeng and M. Y. Kochukov, *Toxicol. Sci.*, 2010, **115**, 1–11.
16. A. Matsushima, Y. Kakuta, T. Teramoto, T. Koshiba, X. Liu, H. Okada, T. Tokunaga, S. Kawabata, M. Kimura and Y. Shimohigashi, *J. Biochem.*, 2007, **142**, 517–524.
17. K. Moriyama, T. Tagami, T. Akamizu, T. Usui, M. Saijo, N. Kanamoto, Y. Hataya, A. Shimatsu, H. Kuzuya and K. Nakao, *J. Clin. Endocrinol. Metab.*, 2002, **87**, 5185–5190.
18. R. T. Zoeller, R. Bansal and C. Parris, *Endocrinology*, 2005, **146**, 607–612.
19. P. Sohoni and J. P. Sumpter, *J. Endocrinol.*, 1998, **158**, 327–339.
20. P. Pocar, B. Fischer, T. Klonisch and S. Hombach-Klonisch, *Reproduction*, 2005, **129**, 379–389.
21. Y. F. Wang, H. R. Chao, C. H. Wu, C. H. Tseng, Y. T. Kuo and T. C. Tsou, *Biotechnol. Lett.*, 2010, **32**, 1789–1796.
22. F. Grun and B. Blumberg, *Rev. Endocr. Metab. Disord.*, 2007, **8**, 161–171.
23. A. V. Krishnan, P. Starhis, S. F. Permuth, L. Tokes and D. Feldman, *Endocrinology*, 1993, **132**, 2279–2285.
24. L. N. Vandenberg, R. Hauser, M. Marcus, N. Olea and W. V. Welshons, *Reprod. Toxicol.*, 2007, **24**, 139–177.
25. J. L. Carwile, H. T. Luu, L. S. Bassett, D. A. Driscoll, C. Yuan, J. Y. Chang, X. Ye, A. M. Calafat and K. B. Michels, *Environ. Health Perspect.*, 2009, **117**, 1368–1372.
26. A. Schecter, N. Malik, D. Haffner, S. Smith, T. R. Harris, O. Paepke and L. Birnbaum, *Environ. Sci. Technol.*, 2010, **44**, 9425–9430.
27. X. L. Cao, J. Corriveau and S. Popovic, *J. Food. Prot.*, 2010, **73**, 1085–1089.
28. J. E. Biles, T. P. McNeal and T. H. Begley, *J. Agric. Food. Chem.*, 1997, **45**, 4697–4700.
29. H.-W. Kuo and W.-H. Ding, *J. Chromatogr. A*, 2004, **1027**, 67–74.
30. R. A. Rudel, J. M. Gray, C. L. Engel, T. W. Rawsthorne, R. E. Dodson, J. M. Ackerman, J. Rizzo, J. L. Nudelman and J. G. Brody, *Environ. Health Perspect.*, 2011, **119**, 914–920.
31. J. L. Carwile, X. Ye, X. Zhou, A. M. Calafat and K. B. Michels, *JAMA*, 2011, **306**, 2218–2220.
32. J. M. Braun, A. E. Kalkbrenner, A. M. Calafat, J. T. Bernert, X. Ye, M. J. Silva, D. B. Barr, S. Sathyanarayana and B. P. Lanphear, *Environ. Health Perspect.*, 2011, **119**, 131–137.

33. T. Mendum, E. Stoler, H. VanBenschoten and J. C. Warner, *Green Chemistry Letters and Reviews*, 2011, **4**, 81–86.
34. D. Zalko, C. Jacques, H. Duplan, S. Bruel and E. Perdu, *Chemosphere*, 2011, **82**, 424–430.
35. S. Biedermann, P. Tschudin and K. Grob, *Anal. Bioanal. Chem.*, 2010, **398**, 571–576.
36. T. Tominaga, T. Negishi, H. Hirooka, A. Miyachi, A. Inoue, I. Hayasaka and Y. Yoshikawa, *Toxicology*, 2006, **226**, 208–217.
37. D. Zalko, A. M. Soto, L. Dolo, C. Dorio, E. Ratahao, L. Debrauwer, R. Faure and J.-P. Cravedi, *Environ. Health Perspect.*, 2003, **111**, 309–319.
38. Y.-H. Kim, C.-S. Kim, S. Park, S. Y. Han, M.-Y. Pyo and M. Yang, *Biochem. Biophys. Res. Commun.*, 2003, **312**, 441–448.
39. H. Mykkanen, J. Tikka, T. Pitkanen and O. Hanninen, *J. Ped. Gastroenterol. Nutr.*, 1997, **25**, 312–316.
40. J. A. Taylor, W. V. Welshons and F. S. vom Saal, *Reprod. Toxicol.*, 2008, **25**, 169–176.
41. M. Nishikawa, H. Iwano, R. Yanagisawa, N. Koike, H. Inoue and H. Yokota, *Environ. Health Perspect.*, 2010, **118**, 1196–1203.
42. C. L. Stowell, K. K. Barvian, P. C. M. Young, R. M. Bigsby, D. E. Verdugo, C. R. Bertozzi and T. S. Widlanski, *Chemistry & Biology*, 2006, **13**, 891–897.
43. H. Sakamoto, H. Yokota, R. Kibe, Y. Sayama and A. Yuasa, *Biochemica et Biophysica Acta*, 2002, **1573**, 171–176.
44. W. Volkel, T. Colnot, G. A. Csanady, J. G. Filsner and W. Dekant, *Chem. Res. Toxicol.*, 2002, **15**, 1281–1287.
45. W. Volkel, N. Bittner and W. Dekant, *Drug Metab. Dispos.*, 2005, **33**, 1748–1757.
46. L. N. Vandenberg, I. Chahoud, J. J. Heindel, V. Padmanabhan, F. J. Paumgartten and G. Schoenfelder, *Environ. Health Perspect.*, 2010, **118**, 1055–1070.
47. L. N. Vandenberg, I. Chahoud, V. Padmanabhan, F. J. R. Paumgartten and G. Schoenfelder, *Environ. Health Perspect.*, 2010, **118**, 1051–1054.
48. R. W. Stahlhut, W. V. Welshons and S. H. Swan, *Environ. Health Perspect.*, 2009, **117**, 784–789.
49. T. Bushnik, D. Haines, P. Levallois, J. Levesque, J. Van Oostdam and C. Viau, *Statistics Canada, Health Reports*, 2010, **21,** Catalogue no. 82-0030-XPE.
50. A. M. Calafat and L. L. Needham, *Int. J. Androl.*, 2008, **31**, 139–143.
51. K. Becker, T. Guen, M. Seiwert, A. Conrad, H. Pick-Fuss, J. Muller, M. Wittassek, C. Schulz and M. Kolossa-Gehring, *Int. J. Hyg. Environ. Health*, 2009, **212**, 685–692.
52. L. N. Vandenberg, *CMAJ*, 2011, **online Feb 22**, doi:10.1503/cmaj.101408.
53. Y. B. Wetherill, B. T. Akingbemi, J. Kanno, J. A. McLachlan, A. Nadal, C. Sonnenschein, C. S. Watson, R. T. Zoeller and S. M. Belcher, *Reprod. Toxicol.*, 2007, **24**, 178–198.

54. C. Richter, L. S. Birnbaum, F. Farabollini, R. R. Newbold, B. S. Rubin, C. E. Talsness, J. G. Vandenbergh, D. R. Walser-Kuntz and F. S. vom Saal, *Reprod. Toxicol.*, 2007, **24**, 199–224.
55. F. S. vom Saal, B. T. Akingbemi, S. M. Belcher, L. S. Birnbaum, D. A. Crain, M. Eriksen, F. Farabollini, L. J. Guillette, Jr., R. Hauser, J. J. Heindel, S. M. Ho, P. A. Hunt, T. Iguchi, S. Jobling, J. Kanno, R. A. Keri, K. E. Knudsen, H. Laufer, G. A. LeBlanc, M. Marcus, J. A. McLachlan, J. P. Myers, A. Nadal, R. R. Newbold, N. Olea, G. S. Prins, C. A. Richter, B. S. Rubin, C. Sonnenschein, A. M. Soto, C. E. Talsness, J. G. Vandenbergh, L. N. Vandenberg, D. R. Walser-Kuntz, C. S. Watson, W. V. Welshons, Y. Wetherill and R. T. Zoeller, *Reprod. Toxicol.*, 2007, **24**, 131–138.
56. J. A. Taylor, F. S. Vom Saal, W. V. Welshons, B. Drury, G. Rottinghaus, P. A. Hunt, P. L. Toutain, C. M. Laffont and C. A. Vandevoort, *Environ. Health Perspect.*, 2011, **119**, 422–430.
57. G. S. Prins, S. H. Ye, L. Birch, S.-M. Ho and K. Kannan, *Reprod. Toxicol.*, 2011, **31**, 1–9.
58. J. A. Taylor, F. S. vom Saal, W. V. Welshons, B. Drury, G. Rottinghaus, P. A. Hunt and C. A. Vandevoort, *Environ. Health Perspect.*, 2011, **119**, 422–430.
59. J. F. Couse and K. S. Korach, *Endocrine Reviews*, 1999, **20**, 358–417.
60. F. S. vom Saal and C. Hughes, *Environ. Health Perspect.*, 2005, **113**, 926–933.
61. NTP, *National Toxicology Program's Report of the Endocrine Disruptors Low Dose Peer Review*, http://ntp.niehs.nih.gov/ntp/htdocs/liason/LowDosePeerFinalRpt.pdf.
62. R. Melnick, G. Lucier, M. Wolfe, R. Hall, G. Stancel, G. Prins, M. Gallo, K. Reuhl, S. M. Ho, T. Brown, J. Moore, J. Leakey, J. Haseman and M. Kohn, *Environ. Health Perspect.*, 2002, **110**, 427–431.
63. R. W. Tyl, C. B. Myers, M. C. Marr, C. S. Sloan, N. P. Castillo, M. M. Veselica, J. C. Seely, S. S. Dimond, J. P. Van Miller, R. N. Shiotsuka, D. Beyer, S. G. Hentges and J. M. Waechter, Jr., *Toxicol. Sci.*, 2008, **104**, 362–384.
64. R. W. Tyl, C. B. Myers, M. C. Marr, B. F. Thomas, A. R. Keimowitz, D. R. Brine, M. M. Veselica, P. A. Fail, T. Y. Chang, J. C. Seely, R. L. Joiner, J. H. Butula, S. S. Dimond, S. Z. Cagen, R. N. Shitsuka, G. D. Stropp and J. M. Waechter, *Toxicol. Sci.*, 2002, **68**, 121–146.
65. K. L. Howdeshell, J. Furr, C. R. Lambright, V. S. Wilson, B. C. Ryan and L. E. Gray, Jr., *Toxicol. Sci.*, 2008, **102**, 371–382.
66. D. G. Stump, M. J. Beck, A. Radovsky, R. H. Garman, L. L. Freshwater, L. P. Sheets, M. S. Marty, J. M. Waechter, Jr., S. S. Dimond, J. P. Van Miller, R. N. Shiotsuka, D. Beyer, A. H. Chappelle and S. G. Hentges, *Toxicol. Sci.*, 2010, **115**, 167–182.
67. EFSA, *The EFSA Journal*, 2006, **428**, 1–75.
68. EFSA, *The EFSA Journal*, 2008, **759**, 1–10.

69. J. E. Goodman, E. E. McConnell, I. G. Sipes, R. J. Witorsch, T. M. Slayton, C. J. Yu, A. S. Lewis and L. R. Rhomberg, *Crit. Rev. Toxicol.*, 2006, **36**, 387–457.
70. J. E. Goodman, R. J. Witorsch, E. E. McConnell, I. G. Sipes, T. M. Slayton, C. J. Yu, A. M. Franz and L. R. Rhomberg, *Crit. Rev. Toxicol.*, 2009, **39**, 1–75.
71. J. P. Myers, F. S. vom Saal, B. T. Akingbemi, K. Arizono, S. Belcher, T. Colborn, I. Chahoud, D. A. Crain, F. Farabollini, L. J. Guillette, T. Hassold, S.-M. Ho, P. A. Hunt, T. Iguchi, S. Jobling, J. Kanno, H. Laufer, M. Marcus, J. A. McLachlan, A. Nadal, J. Oehlmann, N. Olea, P. Palanza, S. Parmigiani, B. S. Rubin, G. Schonfelder, C. Sonnenschein, A. M. Soto, C. E. Talsness, J. A. Taylor, L. N. Vandenberg, J. G. Vandenbergh, S. Vogel, C. S. Watson, W. V. Welshons and R. T. Zoeller, *Environ. Health Perspect.*, 2009, **117**, 309–315.
72. J. P. Myers, R. T. Zoeller and F. S. vom Saal, *Environ. Health Perspect.*, 2009, **117**, 1652–1655.
73. F. S. vom Saal, B. T. Akingbemi, S. M. Belcher, D. A. Crain, D. Crews, L. C. Guidice, P. A. Hunt, C. Leranth, J. P. Myers, A. Nadal, N. Olea, V. Padmanabhan, C. S. Rosenfeld, A. Schneyer, G. Schoenfelder, C. Sonnenschein, A. M. Soto, R. W. Stahlhut, S. H. Swan, L. N. Vandenberg, H. S. Wang, C. S. Watson, W. V. Welshons and R. T. Zoeller, *Toxicol. Sci.*, 2010, **115**, 612–613.
74. F. S. vom Saal and J. P. Myers, *Environ. Health Perspect.*, 2010, **118**, A60.
75. F. S. vom Saal and W. V. Welshons, *Environmental Research*, 2006, **100**, 50–76.
76. J. G. Lemmen, J. L. M. Broekhof, G. G. J. M. Kuiper, J. A. Gustafsson, P. T. Van Der Saag and B. van der Burg, *Mech. Dev.*, 1999, **81**, 163–167.
77. L. Hennighausen and G. W. Robinson, *Genes Dev.*, 1998, **12**, 449–455.
78. M. M. Richert, K. L. Schwertfeger, J. W. Ryder and S. M. Anderson, *J. Mammary Gland Biol. Neoplasia*, 2000, **5**, 227–241.
79. H. A. Bern, K. T. Mills and L. A. Jones, *Proc. Soc. Exp. Biol. Med.*, 1983, **172**, 239–242.
80. L. N. Vandenberg, M. V. Maffini, P. R. Wadia, C. Sonnenschein, B. S. Rubin and A. M. Soto, *Endocrinology*, 2007, **148**, 116–127.
81. C. M. Markey, E. H. Luque, M. Munoz-de-Toro, C. Sonnenschein and A. M. Soto, *Biol. Reprod.*, 2001, **65**, 1215–1223.
82. M. Munoz-de-Toro, C. M. Markey, P. R. Wadia, E. H. Luque, B. S. Rubin, C. Sonnenschein and A. M. Soto, *Endocrinology*, 2005, **146**, 4138–4147.
83. Y. Nikaido, K. Yoshizawa, N. Danbara, M. Tsujita-Kyutoku, T. Yuri, N. Uehara and A. Tsubura, *Reprod. Toxicol.*, 2004, **18**, 803–811.
84. P. R. Wadia, L. N. Vandenberg, C. M. Schaeberle, B. S. Rubin, C. Sonnenschein and A. M. Soto, *Environ. Health Perspect.*, 2007, **115**, 592–598.
85. A. Ayyanan, O. Laribi, S. Schuepbach-Mallepell, C. Schrick, M. Gutierrez, T. Tanos, G. Lefebvre, J. Rougemont, O. Yalcin-Ozuysal and C. Brisken, *Mol. Endocrinol.*, 2011, **Epub 2011 Sep 8**.

86. C. M. Markey, M. A. Coombs, C. Sonnenschein and A. M. Soto, *Evolution and Development*, 2003, **5**, 67–75.
87. R. Moral, R. Wang, I. H. Russo, C. A. Lamartiniere, J. Pereira and J. Russo, *J. Endocrinol.*, 2008, **196**, 101–112.
88. L. N. Vandenberg, M. V. Maffini, C. M. Schaeberle, A. A. Ucci, C. Sonnenschein, B. S. Rubin and A. M. Soto, *Reprod. Toxicol.*, 2008, **26**, 210–219.
89. T. J. Murray, M. V. Maffini, A. A. Ucci, C. Sonnenschein and A. M. Soto, *Reprod. Toxicol.*, 2007, **23**, 383–390.
90. M. Durando, L. Kass, J. Piva, C. Sonnenschein, A. M. Soto, E. H. Luque and M. Munoz-de-Toro, *Environ. Health Perspect.*, 2007, **115**, 80–86.
91. J. B. Colerangle and D. Roy, *J.Steroid Biochem. Molec. Biol.*, 1997, **60**, 153–160.
92. L. P. Jones, A. Sampson, H. J. Kang, H. J. Kim, Y. W. Yi, S. Y. Kwon, J. K. Babus, A. Wang and I. Bae, *Toxicol. Lett.*, 2010, **199**, 261–268.
93. J. Russo and I. H. Russo, *J. Nat. Cancer Inst.*, 1978, **61**, 1451–1459.
94. V. A. McCormack and I. Dos Santos Silva, *Cancer Epidem. Biomar.*, 2006, **15**, 1159–1169.
95. M. Singh, J. N. McGinley and H. J. Thompson, *Lab Invest.*, 2000, **80**, 221–231.
96. S. Nandi, R. Guzman and J. Yang, *Proc. Natl. Acad. Sci. U S A*, 1995, **92**, 3650–3657.
97. S. Jenkins, J. Wang, I. Eltoum, R. Desmond and C. A. Lamartiniere, *Environ. Health Perspect.*, 2011, **119**, 1604–1609.
98. S. Jenkins, N. Raghuraman, I. Eltoum, M. Carpenter, J. Russo and C. A. Lamartiniere, *Environ. Health Perspect.*, 2009, **117**, 910–915.
99. A. M. Betancourt, I. A. Eltoum, R. A. Desmond, J. Russo and C. A. Lamartiniere, *Environ. Health Perspect.*, 2010, **118**, 1614–1619.
100. K. Weber Lozada and R. A. Keri, *Biol. Reprod.*, 2011.
101. C. A. Lamartiniere, S. Jenkins, A. M. Betancourt, J. Wang and J. Russo, *Horm. Mol. Biol. Clin. Investig.*, 2011, **5**, 45–52.
102. A. M. Betancourt, J. A. Mobley, J. Russo and C. A. Lamartiniere, *J. Proteomics*, 2010, **73**, 1241–1253.
103. J. A. Taylor, C. A. Richter, R. L. Ruhlen and F. S. Vom Saal, *J. Steroid Biochem. Mol. Biol.*, 2011.
104. J. W. Owens and J. G. Chaney, *Regul. Toxicol. Pharmacol.*, 2005, **43**, 194–202.
105. H. A. Milman, M. C. Bosland, P. D. Walden and J. E. Heinze, *Regul. Toxicol. Pharmacol.*, 2002, **35**, 338–346.
106. J. Ashby, H. Tinwell, J. Odum and P. Lefevre, *Environ. Health Perspect.*, 2004, **112**, 847–853.
107. F. S. vom Saal, C. A. Richter, R. R. Ruhlen, S. C. Nagel, B. G. Timms and W. V. Welshons, *Birth Defects Res. (Part A)*, 2005, **73**, 140–145.
108. D. M. Sheehan, *Proc. Soc. Exp. Biol. Med.*, 2000, **224**, 57–60.
109. S. A. Vogel, *Am. J. Public Health*, 2009, **99**(Suppl 3), S559–566.

110. S. C. Nagel, F. S. vom Saal, K. A. Thayer, M. G. Dhar, M. Boechler and W. V. Welshons, *Environ. Health Perspect.*, 1997, **105**, 70–76.
111. W. V. Welshons, S. C. Nagel, K. A. Thayer, B. M. Judy and F. S. vom Saal, *Toxicol. Ind. Health*, 1999, **15**, 12–25.
112. C. Gupta, *Proc. Soc. Exp. Biol. Med.*, 2000, **224**, 61 68.
113. B. A. Elswick, F. Welsch and D. B. Janszen, *Reprod. Toxicol.*, 2000, **14**, 359–367.
114. K. C. Chitra, C. Latchoumycandane and P. P. Mathur, *Toxicology*, 2003, **185**, 119–127.
115. J. G. Ramos, J. Varayoud, C. Sonnenschein, A. M. Soto, M. Munoz-de-Toro and E. H. Luque, *Biol. Reprod.*, 2001, **65**, 1271–1277.
116. B. G. Timms, K. L. Howdeshell, L. Barton, S. Bradley, C. A. Richter and F. S. vom Saal, *Proc. Natl. Acad. Sci. U S A*, 2005, **102**, 7014–7019.
117. J. G. Ramos, J. Varayoud, L. Kass, H. Rodrigues, L. Costabel, M. Munoz-de-Toro and E. H. Luque, *Endocrinology*, 2003, **144**, 3206–3215.
118. Y. Ogura, K. Ishii, H. Kanda, M. Kanai, K. Arima, Y. Wang and Y. Sugimura, *Differentiation*, 2007, **75**, 745–756.
119. J. L. Nelles, W. Y. Hu and G. S. Prins, *Expert Rev. Endocrinol. Metab.*, 2011, **6**, 437–451.
120. G. S. Prins, *Endocr. Relat. Cancer*, 2008, **15**, 649–656.
121. S. M. Ho, W. Y. Tang, J. Belmonte de Frausto and G. S. Prins, *Cancer Res.*, 2006, **66**, 5624–5632.
122. G. S. Prins, L. Birch, W. Y. Tang and S. M. Ho, *Reprod. Toxicol.*, 2007, **23**, 374–382.
123. G. S. Prins, S. H. Ye, L. Birch, S.-M. Ho and K. Kannan, *Reprod. Toxicol.*, 2011, **31**, 1–9.
124. G. S. Prins, W. Y. Tang, J. Belmonte and S. M. Ho, *Basic Clin. Pharmacol. Toxicol.*, 2008, **102**, 134–138.
125. T. Ichihara, H. Yoshino, N. Imai, T. Tsutsumi, M. Kawabe, S. Tamano, S. Inaguma, S. Suzuki and T. Shirai, *J. Toxicol. Sci.*, 2003, **28**, 165–171.
126. J. Ashby, H. Tinwell and J. Haseman, *Regul. Toxicol. Pharmacol.*, 1999, **30**, 156–166.
127. S. Z. Cagen, J. M. Waechter, Jr., S. S. Dimond, W. J. Breslin, J. H. Butala, F. W. Jekat, R. L. Joiner, R. N. Shiotsuka, G. E. Veenstra and L. R. Harris, *Toxicol. Sci.*, 1999, **50**, 36–44.
128. S. Z. Cagen, J. M. Wacchter, Jr., S. S. Dimond, W. J. Breslin, J. H. Butala, F. W. Jekat, R. L. Joiner, R. N. Shiotsuka, G. E. Veenstra and L. R. Harris, *Regul. Toxicol. Pharmacol.*, 1999, **30**, 130–139.
129. M. Ema, S. Fujii, M. Furukawa, M. Kiguchi, T. Ikka and A. Harazono, *Reprod. Toxicol.*, 2001, **15**, 505–523.
130. H. Tinwell, J. Haseman, P. A. Lefevre, N. Wallis and J. Ashby, *Toxicol. Sci.*, 2002, **68**, 339–348.
131. R. E. Chapin, J. Adams, K. Boekelheide, L. E. J. Gray, S. W. Hayward, P. S. Lees, B. S. McIntyre, K. M. Portier, T. M. Schnorr, S. G. Selevan, J. G. Vandenbergh and S. R. Woskie, *Birth Defects Res. B Dev. Reprod. Toxicol.*, 2008, **83**, 157–395.

132. S. M. Grundy, H. B. Brewer, Jr., J. I. Cleeman, S. C. Smith, Jr. and C. Lenfant, *Circulation*, 2004, **109**, 433–438.
133. F. Grun and B. Blumberg, *Mol. Cell. Endocrinol.*, 2009, **304**, 19–29.
134. F. Grun and B. Blumberg, *Mol. Endocrinol.*, 2009, **23**, 1127–1134.
135. B. S. Rubin, M. K. Murray, D. A. Damassa, J. C. King and A. M. Soto, *Environ. Health Perspect.*, 2001, **109**, 675–680.
136. S. Honma, A. Suzuki, D. L. Buchanan, Y. Katsu, H. Watanabe and T. Iguchi, *Reprod. Toxicol.*, 2002, **16**, 117–122.
137. K. L. Howdeshell, A. K. Hotchkiss, K. A. Thayer, J. G. Vandenbergh and F. S. vom Saal, *Nature*, 1999, **401**, 763–764.
138. J. Miyawaki, K. Sakayama, H. Kato, H. Yamamoto and H. Masuno, *J. Atheroscler. Thromb.*, 2007, **14**, 245–252.
139. J. Wei, Y. Lin, Y. Li, C. Ying, J. Chen, L. Song, Z. Zhou, Z. Lv, W. Xia, X. Chen and S. Xu, *Endocrinology*, 2011.
140. E. Somm, V. M. Schwitzgebel, A. Toulotte, C. R. Cederroth, C. Combescure, S. Nef, M. L. Aubert and P. S. Huppi, *Environ. Health Perspect.*, 2009, **117**, 1549–1555.
141. F. S. vom Saal, C. A. Richter, J. Mao and W. V. Welshons, *Birth Defects Res. (Part A)*, 2005, **73**, 474–475.
142. J. J. Heindel and F. S. vom Saal, *Environ. Health Perspect.*, 2008, **116**, 389–393.
143. X. Xu, L. Tan, T. Himi, M. Sadamatsu, S. Tsutsumi, M. Akaike and N. Kato, *Neurotoxicol. Teratol.*, 2011.
144. P. Alonso-Magdalena, E. Vieira, S. Soriano, L. Menes, D. Burks, I. Quesada and A. Nadal, *Environ. Health Perspect.*, 2010, **118**, 1243–1250.
145. A. Korkmaz, M. A. Ahbab, D. Kolankaya and N. Barlas, *Food Chem. Toxicol.*, 2010, **48**, 2865–2871.
146. Y. Takai, O. Tsutsumi, Y. Ikezuki, H. Hiroi, Y. Osuga, M. Momoeda, T. Yano and Y. Taketani, *Biochem. Biophys. Res. Commun.*, 2000, **270**, 918–921.
147. Y. Takai, O. Tsutsumi, Y. Ikezuki, Y. Kamei, Y. Osuga, T. Yano and Y. Taketan, *Reprod. Toxicol.*, 2001, **15**, 71–74.
148. J. S. Fisher, K. J. Turner, D. Brown and R. M. Sharpe, *Environ. Health Perspect.*, 1999, **107**, 397–405.
149. J. Wistuba, M. H. Brinkworth, S. Schlatt, I. Chahoud and E. Nieschlag, *Environ. Res.*, 2003, **91**, 95–103.
150. C. M. Markey, P. R. Wadia, B. S. Rubin, C. Sonnenschein and A. M. Soto, *Biol. Reprod.*, 2005, **72**, 1344–1351.
151. S. C. Nagel, J. L. Hagelbarger and D. P. McDonnell, *Endocrinology*, 2001, **142**, 4721–4728.
152. G. Schonfelder, B. Flick, E. Mayr, C. Talsness, M. Paul and I. Chahoud, *Neoplasia*, 2002, **4**, 98–102.
153. G. Schonfelder, K. Friedrich, M. Paul and I. Chahoud, *Neoplasia*, 2004, **6**, 584–594.
154. S. Honma, A. Suzuki, D. L. Buchanan, Y. Katsu, H. Watanabe and T. Igushi, *Reprod. Toxicol.*, 2002, **16**, 117–122.

155. H. B. Adewale, W. N. Jefferson, R. R. Newbold and H. B. Patisaul, *Biol. Reprod.*, 2009, **81**, 690–699.
156. L. Monje, J. Varayoud, M. Munoz-de-Toro, E. H. Luque and J. G. Ramos, *Reprod. Toxicol.*, 2010, **30**, 625–634.
157. R. R. Newbold, W. N. Jefferson and E. Padilla-Banks, *Reprod. Toxicol.*, 2007, **24**, 253–258.
158. P. G. Signorile, E. P. Spugnini, L. Mita, P. Mellone, A. D'Avino, M. Bianco, N. Diano, L. Caputo, F. Rea, R. Viceconte, M. Portaccio, E. Viggiano, G. Citro, R. Pierantoni, V. Sica, B. Vincenzi, D. G. Mita, F. Baldi and A. Baldi, *Gen. Comp. Endocrinol.*, 2010, **168**, 318–325.
159. R. R. Newbold, W. N. Jefferson and E. Padilla-Banks, *Environ. Health Perspect.*, 2009, **117**, 879–885.
160. P. A. Hunt, K. E. Koehler, M. Susiarjo, C. A. Hodges, A. Ilagan, R. C. Voigt, S. Thomas, B. F. Thomas and T. J. Hassold, *Curr. Biol.*, 2003, **13**, 546–553.
161. M. Susiarjo, T. J. Hassold, E. Freeman and P. A. Hunt, *PLoS Genetics*, 2007, **3**, e5.
162. A. Muhlhauser, M. Susiarjo, C. Rubio, J. Griswold, G. Gorence, T. Hassold and P. A. Hunt, *Biol. Reprod.*, 2009, **80**, 1066–1071.
163. P. A. Hunt, M. Susiarjo, C. Rubio and T. J. Hassold, *Biol. Reprod.*, 2009, **81**, 807–813.
164. M. Fernandez, N. Bourguignon, V. Lux-Lantos and C. Libertun, *Environ. Health Perspect.*, 2010, **118**, 1217–1222.
165. J. Varayoud, J. G. Ramos, V. L. Bosquiazzo, M. Lower, M. Munoz-de-Toro and E. H. Luque, *Endocrinology*, 2011, **152**, 1101–1111.
166. N. J. Cabaton, P. R. Wadia, B. S. Rubin, D. Zalko, C. M. Schaeberle, M. H. Askenase, J. L. Gadbois, A. P. Tharp, G. S. Whitt, C. Sonnenschein and A. M. Soto, *Environ. Health Perspect.*, 2011, **119**, 547–552.
167. M. Aydogan, A. Korkmaz, N. Barlas and D. Kolankaya, *Drug Chem. Toxicol.*, 2010, **33**, 193–203.
168. Y. Minamiyama, H. Ichikawa, S. Takemura, H. Kusunoki, Y. Naito and T. Yoshikawa, *Free Radic. Res.*, 2010, **44**, 1398–1406.
169. S. Anjum, S. Rahman, M. Kaur, F. Ahmad, H. Rashid, R. A. Ansari and S. Raisuddin, *Food Chem. Toxicol.*, 2011, **49**, 2849–2854.
170. A. S. Al-Hiyasat, H. Darmani and A. M. Elbetieha, *Eur. J. Oral Sci.*, 2002, **110**, 163–167.
171. F. S. vom Saal, P. S. Cooke, D. L. Buchanan, P. Palanza, K. A. Thayer, S. C. Nagel, S. Parmigiani and W. V. Welshons, *Toxicol. Ind. Health*, 1998, **14**, 239–260.
172. S. Salian, T. Doshi and G. Vanage, *Toxicology*, 2009, **265**, 56–67.
173. H. Aikawa, S. Koyama, M. Matsuda, K. Nakahashi, Y. Akazome and T. Mori, *Cell Tissue Res.*, 2004, **315**, 119–124.
174. Y. Toyama, F. Suzuki-Toyota, M. Maekawa, C. Ito and K. Toshimori, *Arch. Histol. Cytol.*, 2004, **185**, 119–127.

175. K. Kobayashi, K. Ohtani, H. Kubota and M. Miyagawa, *Congenit Anom (Kyoto)*, 2010, **50**, 159–170.
176. R. Carr, F. Bertasi, A. Bentacourt, S. Bowers, B. S. Gandy, P. Ryan and S. Willard, *J. Toxicol. Environ. Health A*, 2003, **66**, 2077–2088.
177. F. Farabollini, S. Porrini and F. Dessi-Fulgheri, *Pharmacol. Biochem. Behav.*, 1999, **64**, 687–694.
178. T. Fujimoto, K. Kubo and S. Aou, *Brain Res.*, 2006, **1068**, 49–55.
179. T. Funabashi, M. Kawaguchi, M. Furuta, A. Fukushima and F. Kimura, *Psychoneuroendocrinology*, 2004, **29**, 475–485.
180. K. Kubo, O. Arai, M. Omura, R. Watanabe, R. Ogata and S. Aou, *Neurosci. Res.*, 2003, **45**, 345–356.
181. K. Kubo, O. Arai, R. Ogata, M. Omura, T. Hori and S. Aou, *Neurosci. Lett.*, 2001, **304**, 73–76.
182. B. S. Rubin, J. R. Lenkowski, C. M. Schaeberle, L. N. Vandenberg, P. M. Ronsheim and A. M. Soto, *Endocrinology*, 2006, **147**, 3681–3691.
183. H. B. Patisaul, A. E. Fortino and E. K. Polston, *Neurotoxicol. Teratol.*, 2006, **28**, 111–118.
184. H. B. Adewale, K. L. Todd, J. A. Mickens and H. B. Patisaul, *Neuro Toxicology*, 2011, **32**, 38–49.
185. M. Goto, Y. Takano-Ishikawa, H. Ono, M. Yoshida, K. Yamaki and H. Shinmoto, *Biosci. Biotechnol. Biochem.*, 2007, **71**, 2136–2143.
186. S. D. Holladay, S. Xiao, H. Diao, J. Barber, T. Nagy, X. Ye and R. M. Gogal, Jr., *Int. J. Environ. Res. Public Health*, 2010, **7**, 2845–2852.
187. T. Midoro-Horiuti, R. Tiwari, C. S. Watson and R. M. Goldblum, *Environ. Health Perspect.*, 2010, **118**, 273–277.
188. A. Okada and O. Kai, *Asian J. Androl.*, 2008, **10**, 271–276.
189. B. T. Akingbemi, C. M. Sottas, A. I. Koulova, G. R. Klinefelter and M. P. Hardy, *Endocrinology*, 2004, **145**, 592–603.
190. A. M. Soto, B. S. Rubin and C. Sonnenschein, in *Endocrine-Disrupting Chemicals*, ed. A. Gore, Humana Press, Totowa, N.J., Editon edn., 2007.
191. L. N. Vandenberg, M. V. Maffini, C. Sonnenschein, B. S. Rubin and A. M. Soto, *Endocrine Reviews*, 2009, **30**, 75–95.
192. B. S. Rubin, *J. Steroid Biochem. Mol. Biol.*, 2011, **127**, 27–34.
193. A. M. Calafat, X. Ye, L. Y. Wong, J. A. Reidy and L. L. Needham, *Environ. Health Perspect.*, 2008, **116**, 39–44.
194. W. Dekant and W. Volkel, *Toxicol. Appl. Pharmacol.*, 2008, **228**, 114–134.
195. S. Mahalingaiah, J. D. Meeker, K. R. Pearson, A. M. Calafat, X. Ye, J. Petrozza and R. Hauser, *Environ. Health Perspect.*, 2008, **116**, 173–178.
196. P. A. Nepomnaschy, D. D. Baird, C. R. Weinberg, J. A. Hoppin, M. P. Longnecker and A. J. Wilcox, *Environ. Res.*, 2009, **109**, 734–737.
197. X. Ye, L. Y. Wong, A. M. Bishop and A. M. Calafat, *Environ. Health Perspect.*, 2011, **119**, 983–988.
198. J. M. Braun, K. Yolton, K. N. Dietrich, R. Hornung, X. Ye, A. M. Calafat and B. P. Lanphear, *Environ. Health Perspect.*, 2009, **117**, 1945–1952.

199. J. M. Braun, A. E. Kalkbrenner, A. M. Calafat, K. Yolton, X. Ye, K. N. Dietrich and B. P. Lanphear, *Pediatrics*, 2011, **128**, 873–882.
200. M. Yang, J. H. Ryu, R. Jeon, D. Kang and K. Y. Yoo, *Arch. Toxicol.*, 2009, **83**, 281–285.
201. A. M. Calafat, J. Weuve, X. Ye, L. T. Jia, H. Hu, S. Ringer, K. Huttner and R. Hauser, *Environ. Health Perspect.*, 2009, **117**, 639–644.
202. A. M. Soto, L. N. Vandenberg, M. V. Maffini and C. Sonnenschein, *Basic Clin. Pharmacol. Toxicol.*, 2008, **102**, 125–133.
203. D. Trichopoulos, *Epidemiology*, 1990, **1**, 95–96.
204. I. A. Lang, T. S. Galloway, A. Scarlett, W. E. Henley, M. Depledge, R. B. Wallace and D. Melzer, *JAMA*, 2008, **300**, 1303–1310.
205. D. Melzer, N. E. Rice, C. Lewis, W. E. Henley and T. S. Galloway, *PLoS ONE*, 2010, **5**, e8673.
206. J. L. Carwile and K. B. Michels, *Environ. Res.*, 2011, **111**, 825–830.
207. T. Wang, M. Li, B. Chen, M. Xu, Y. Xu, Y. Huang, J. Lu, Y. Chen, W. Wang, X. Li, Y. Liu, Y. Bi, S. Lai and G. Ning, *J. Clin. Endocrinol. Metab.*, 2011.
208. T. Hanaoka, N. Kawamura, K. Hara and S. Tsugane, *Occup. Environ. Med.*, 2002, **59**, 625–628.
209. J. Mendiola, N. Jorgensen, A. M. Andersson, A. M. Calafat, X. Ye, J. B. Redmon, E. Z. Drobnis, C. Wang, A. Sparks, S. W. Thurston, F. Liu and S. H. Swan, *Environ. Health Perspect.*, 2010, **118**, 1286–1291.
210. J. D. Meeker, A. M. Calafat and R. Hauser, *Environ. Sci. Technol.*, 2010, **44**, 1458–1463.
211. T. Galloway, R. Cipelli, J. Guralnik, L. Ferrucci, S. Bandinelli, A. M. Corsi, C. Money, P. McCormack and D. Melzer, *Environ. Health Perspect.*, 2010, **118**, 1603–1608.
212. D. K. Li, Z. Zhou, M. Miao, Y. He, J. Wang, J. Ferber, L. J. Herrinton, E. Gao and W. Yuan, *Fertil. Steril.*, 2010.
213. J. D. Meeker, S. Ehrlich, T. L. Toth, D. L. Wright, A. M. Calafat, A. T. Trisini, X. Ye and R. Hauser, *Reprod. Toxicol.*, 2010, **30**, 532–539.
214. D. Li, Z. Zhou, D. Qing, Y. He, T. Wu, M. Miao, J. Wang, X. Weng, J. R. Ferber, L. J. Herrinton, Q. Zhu, E. Gao, H. Checkoway and W. Yuan, *Hum. Reprod.*, 2010, **25**, 519–527.
215. D. K. Li, Z. Zhou, M. Miao, Y. He, D. Qing, T. Wu, J. Wang, X. Weng, J. Ferber, L. Herrinton, Q. Zhu, E. Gao and W. Yuan, *J. Androl.*, 2010.
216. T. Takeuchi and O. Tsutsumi, *Biochem. Biophys. Res. Commun.*, 2002, **291**, 76–78.
217. T. Takeuchi, O. Tsutsumi, Y. Ikezuki, Y. Takai and Y. Taketani, *Endocrine J.*, 2004, **51**, 165–169.
218. H. Yamada, I. Furuta, E. H. Kato, S. Kataoka, Y. Usuki, G. Kobashi, F. Sata, R. Kishi and S. Fujimoto, *Reprod. Toxicol.*, 2002, **16**, 735–739.
219. M. Sugiura-Ogaswara, Y. Ozaki, S.-I. Sonta, T. Makino and K. Suzumori, *Hum. Reprod.*, 2005, **20**, 2325–2329.
220. E. Mok-Lin, S. Ehrlich, P. L. Williams, J. Petrozza, D. L. Wright, A. M. Calafat, X. Ye and R. Hauser, *Int. J. Androl.*, 2009.

CHAPTER 10

Male Reproductive Tract Disorders

JOHN D. MEEKER* AND KELLY K. FERGUSON

Department of Environmental Health Sciences, University of Michigan School of Public Health, Ann Arbor, MI, USA
*E-mail: meekerj@umich.edu

10.1 Introduction

The potential for exposure to environmental chemicals to adversely impact the male reproductive tract has received growing attention over the past several decades. In the late 1970s and early 1980s, the highly publicized case of increased risk of sterility among pesticide production workers exposed to dibromochloropropane led to many new studies investigating whether other occupational exposures adversely affect male fertility. Since the turn of the century, much of the focus has shifted to male reproductive health impacts resulting from lower exposure levels experienced by the general population, as well as the potential for endocrine disrupting chemicals to impair male reproductive tract development *in utero*. The advent of life course epidemiology and concerns for widespread endocrine disruption, combined with trends for delayed family planning and increased life expectancy, have led to increased interest in a new area of inquiry investigating how exposure to chemicals adversely affects health at later life stages. While studies of environmental exposure and men's health among advanced age groups are limited, the overall research conducted thus far on chemicals and male reproductive health will serve to inform those focused on this new line of research.

Issues in Toxicology No. 16
Aging and Vulnerability to Environmental Chemicals: Age-related Disorders and their Origins in Environmental Exposures
Edited by Bernard Weiss

Published by the Royal Society of Chemistry, www.rsc.org

This review describes the state of the human science on the relationship between exposure to environmental chemicals and male reproductive tract disorders. The information has been categorized based on the endpoints that have been most studied to date, including: 1) semen quality and sperm DNA damage, 2) reproductive hormones, 3) thyroid hormones, and 4) cancers of the male reproductive tract. Due to space limitations, the reader is directed toward the individual studies referenced throughout for additional details regarding study design, study populations, covariates considered, and so on.

10.2 Semen Quality and Sperm DNA Damage

The evaluation of semen quality is useful both for assessing male fertility and for indicating effects of exposure to environmental toxicants on the male reproductive tract. Toxicants can effect changes in sperm concentration, motility, and morphology *via* action on the neuroendocrine system (*i.e.* the hypothalamic-pituitary-testis axis), testis (including Sertoli, Leydig, and spermatogenic cells), and post-testicular sites such as the epididymis.[1] They can also induce oxidative stress resulting in sperm DNA damage. Study of the effects of environmental exposures on these measures of male reproductive tract function are particularly important because of recently observed, and unexplained, declines in semen quality in the general population[2,3] as well as among healthy young males.[4] Changes in these parameters are also relevant to older males, as aging is associated with decrease in semen volume and sperm concentration and motility, and increasingly males over 50 are fathering children.[5] Decreased semen quality and increased sperm DNA damage can lead to difficulty in conception, implantation and, potentially, abnormalities in offspring.[5] Additional insults from environmental exposures could consequently compound these declines in semen quality parameters among aging males.

10.3 Persistent Organochlorines

Persistent organochlorines have been widely studied and are associated with a range of adverse health effects, particularly those related to endocrine function.[6] This category of chemicals includes polychlorinated biphenyls (PCBs), used until 1977 in the US as coolants and lubricants in electrical equipment, and organochlorine pesticides (OCs), such as dichlorodiphenyltrichloroethane (DDT), which is no longer used in the US but still employed in developing countries where malaria is prevalent.[7,8] Despite the discontinued use of these materials in the US, exposure continues through contaminated foods and measurable levels are found in the majority of the general population.[9]

A number of studies have investigated associations between OCs and semen quality parameters, both at exposure levels consistent with those observed in the general male population and in instances of accidental high-dose exposure. Beginning in 1986, Bush and colleagues observed an inverse relationship between concentrations of PCB congeners 118, 138 and 153 in semen and sperm motility among oligospermic men.[10] In a study comparing 21 infertile men with poor semen quality with 32 controls with normal semen quality, PCBs were detected in the seminal plasma of infertile men but not control men, and, similarly to the previously mentioned study, total PCB concentrations were inversely correlated with sperm motility ($r = -0.5$), but not with sperm count or normal morphology.[11] This study also showed a positive association between seminal plasma PCB levels and single-stranded DNA in sperm, a marker used frequently in subsequent studies as an indicator of downstream response to oxidative stress.[11] In contrast with these studies, another study comparing men with normal semen quality versus poor semen quality found higher summed PCB metabolites in seminal plasma of men with good sperm quality (0.071 ng mL^{-1} compared to 0.022 ng mL^{-1}, $p = 0.06$).[12] However, these authors did observe an inverse association between summed PCBs and sperm count and progressive motile sperm concentration within men from the good semen quality group. Studies performed on men uncategorized by semen quality have also shown slightly conflicting results. A study of young men ($n = 305$) under conscription for military service found inverse associations between serum PCB 153 and percent motile sperm, but not sperm concentration or total count.[13] In a study examining Swedish fisherman from two different regions, Rignell-Hydborn and colleagues observed that subjects in the highest quintile of PCB 153 exposure had decreased sperm motility compared to men from the lowest quintile of exposure, but there were no differences in sperm concentration.[14] The authors later examined sperm DNA fragmentation in the same population and found that it was positively associated with PCB 153.[15] Both of these findings were confirmed when this study was expanded ($n = 2269$) to four European centers.[16] Lastly, Hauser and colleagues investigated relationships of PCB exposure with semen quality in 212 men who presented with their partners to an infertility clinic at Massachusetts General Hospital in Boston. They observed dose–response relationships between serum PCB 138 and below-reference sperm motility and morphology, but found inconsistent results with PCB 153.[17] They also did not find consistent significant associations between PCBs and DNA integrity in sperm using the neutral comet assay in the same population.[18]

Two groups also investigated the effect of high-dose PCB exposure following a poisoning episode in Taiwan in 1979, where rice oil contaminated with PCBs was ingested. In a study comparing 12 men exposed prenatally with 23 unexposed men, a higher proportion of sperm with abnormal morphology, reduced sperm motility, and reduced rapidly motile sperm in exposed subjects compared to those unexposed was reported.[19] A second study examined 40 men who were directly exposed and compared them to 28 unexposed men, and observed a higher percentage of sperm with abnormal morphology and higher rate of oligospermia in the exposed group.[20]

Although no longer used as a pesticide in the US, DDT is still used for malaria control in several countries. Studies from multiple continents have suggested that exposure to DDT is associated with a decline in semen quality.[16,21,22] There is also evidence for a relationship between DDT exposure and an increase in sperm DNA damage, but the results are inconsistent.[16,18,23]

10.4 Non-Persistent Pesticides

Non-persistent pesticides (also called "contemporary-use pesticides"), including insecticides, herbicides, fungicides and rodenticides, are used commonly in agricultural, commercial, and residential settings. Insecticides, including organophosphates, carbamates, and pyrethroids, have been the most studied. Early research focused on male reproductive effects from occupational exposure. Whorton and colleagues found a greater proportion of oligospermic men among carbaryl-exposed workers in a pesticide production facility compared to other chemical workers.[24] The carbaryl workers also had elevated percentages of abnormal sperm and higher percentages of them were defined as teratopsermics (greater than 60% abnormal sperm) compared to other workers.[25] More recently, another study of exposed carbaryl workers found that subjects with high occupational exposure had elevated percentages of sperm with fragmented DNA compared to internal and external controls, though adjustments were not made for potentially important confounders.[26] Studies of occupational organophosphate exposure have reported similar findings. Padungtod *et al.* observed a reduction in adjusted mean sperm concentration and percentage of motile sperm in 20 Chinese pesticide factory workers exposed to organophosphates, compared to unexposed controls.[27] Also, in a Japanese study, pesticide sprayers exposed primarily to organophosphates and pyrethroids showed season-dependent reductions in motile sperm velocity measures compared to unexposed controls.[28]

There have been several additional studies linking occupational exposure to declines in semen quality, though they have lacked specific information on the types of non-persistent pesticides used. In one analysis of 122 greenhouse workers categorized by low, medium, or high exposure, a higher proportion of abnormal sperm was observed in the high compared to low exposed groups.[29] In another study, men occupationally exposed to pesticides had increased odds for having sperm concentration <1 million mL^{-1} and for having sperm motility $<50\%$, compared to unexposed controls.[30] However, another study observed only marginal differences in the semen quality parameters of 248 Danish farmers who sprayed or did not spray pesticides, although the participation rate in this study was relatively low.[31]

Several studies of environmental (non-occupational) exposure have also been conducted. An early study observed that men with a lower intake of organic food had lower proportions of normally shaped sperm, but no variation in other sperm parameters.[32] In 2003 Swan *et al.* examined male partners of pregnant women in the US Study for Future Families and dichotomized the participants into cases and controls based on semen quality.[33] Urinary measures of the herbicides alachlor and atrazine, and of the insecticide diazinon (2-isoproproxy-4-methyl-pyrimidinol), were associated with increased odds of poorer semen quality, although confidence intervals were wide due to small sample size.[33] In the previously described study of men presenting to an infertility clinic in Boston, an inverse association was observed between sperm concentration and motility and a urinary metabolite of carbaryl, as well as between sperm motility and urinary concentrations of a metabolite of the organophosphate chlorpyrifos.[34] In addition, positive associations were observed between these pesticide biomarkers and sperm DNA damage in the same population.[35] A follow-up to that study also found an inverse relationship between urinary pyrethroid metabolites and sperm concentration, motility, and morphology, as well as a positive relationship between pyrethroid metabolites and sperm DNA damage.[36] The results from this latter study were confirmed by several later analyses in China. Xia *et al.* found an inverse association between non-occupational pyrethroid exposure and sperm concentration.[37] In two additional studies of male partners from infertility clinics, conducted in China and Japan, levels of the pyrethroid metabolite 3-phenoxybenzoic acid in urine were inversely associated with sperm concentration and positively associated with sperm DNA fragmentation.[38,39]

10.5 Heavy Metals

Exposure to heavy metals, such as lead and cadmium, can occur occupationally, but also through environmental pathways, such as the ingestion of contaminated food or water or the inhalation of contaminated air. Importantly, metals can accumulate in the body over time (for example, lead in bone and cadmium in the kidneys). Consequently, aging individuals with increased bone resorption experience an increase in mobilization of lead and are subject to higher circulating blood levels.[40] Studies of lead and cadmium have shown conflicting results with regards to effects on male reproductive parameters; however, calcium and potassium ion channels are susceptible to cadmium and lead respectively which may represent a mechanism for the effect of metals on the testis and spermatozoa.[41]

Several recent non-occupational studies have demonstrated an association between heavy metal exposure and altered semen quality. Hernandez-Ochoa and colleagues found an association between lead measured in spermatozoa or seminal fluid, but not blood, and decreased semen quality parameters in a cross-sectional study in Mexico.[42] Another group observed similar results in men presenting to infertility centers in Spain.[43] In a US population of men presenting to Michigan infertility clinics, a subtle but suggestive association between lead exposure, measured in blood, and decreased semen quality was also found.[44] Some relationships have also been observed in relation to cadmium exposure. Mendiola and colleagues found a positive association between percent immotile sperm and cadmium concentrations measured in seminal plasma, but not in whole blood or blood plasma.[43] These studies seem to indicate that there may be a relationship between exposure to lead and cadmium, especially when levels are measured in seminal fluid, and decreased semen quality; however, several studies have also reported null results.[44–46] The investigation of associations with other metals have been sparse, but there is some evidence for a relationship between decreased semen quality and exposure to manganese, mercury, and molybdenum.[44,47,48]

10.6 Phthalates

Increasing attention has been paid recently to phthalate diesters, chemicals used as plasticizers and solvents in a large number of consumer products. Exposure is widespread, with detectable levels of urinary metabolites observable in the majority of the population.[9] In addition to various other modes of action, certain phthalates have been shown to be anti-androgenic, causing outcomes such as decreased anogenital distance in rats and male infants exposed *in utero*.[49]

Several studies in environmentally exposed adults have indicated an association between phthalate exposure and declines in semen quality, although there has been some variability in results between studies and by phthalate metabolite. In 1987 Murature and colleagues observed an inverse association between di-butyl phthalate (DBP) in cellular fractions of semen and sperm concentration among a small group of university students.[50] Later, another group found an inverse correlation with sperm morphology, but not ejaculate volume, sperm concentration or motility, in a group of infertile men with poor semen quality from India.[11] These two analyses however, may have been subject to contamination as parent phthalate compounds, such as DBP, are found in many products in the laboratory environment. Subsequent studies have primarily used metabolites for assessing individual exposure levels as these measures are less susceptible to contamination.

Duty and colleagues observed significant inverse associations between urinary measures of several phthalate metabolites and semen quality in the previously described cross-sectional study of male partners of subfertile couples recruited through an infertility clinic in Boston.[51] Notably, they also observed a dose-dependent relationship between mono-butyl phthalate (MBP, a metabolite of DBP) and sperm motility and concentration.[51] These results were confirmed several years later in the same study but with a larger sample size.[52] In the same population, the metabolites mono-ethylhexyl phthalate (MEHP, a metabolite of di-ethylhexyl phthalate [DEHP]), mono-benzylbutyl phthalate (MBzP, a metabolite of butylbenzyl phthalate [BBzP]), monoethyl phthalate (MEP, a metabolite of diethyl phthalate [DEP]), monomethyl phthalate (MMP, a metabolite of dimethyl phthalate [DMP]), and MBP showed some suggestive relationships with sperm motion parameters using computer-aided sperm analysis.[53] There were also positive associations between sperm DNA damage measured with the neutral comet assay and MEP and MEHP concentrations in urine, after adjusting for smoking status.[54,55] A subsequent study by Herr and colleagues, in 349 male partners of subfertile couples, reported no associations between urinary DEHP metabolites and sperm concentration, motility, or morphology,[56] which was consistent with results from the US study.

Several additional groups have observed significant relationships between phthalate exposure and decreased semen quality. In a Swedish population of healthy young men at a medical conscript examination ($n = 234$), Jonsson and colleagues found no associations with semen quality and MBP, but observed that subjects in the highest quartile of exposure for MEP had fewer motile sperm and more immotile sperm compared to the those in the lowest quartile.[57] In another study of 150 men recruited through a reproductive institute in China, there was a suggestive positive dose-response relatinoship between MBP exposure tertile and sperm concentration.[58] Relationships with MMP and MEP were not statistically significant, but a positive association was observed between MEP and sperm straight-line velocity.[58] Lastly, a recent analysis that combined an epidemiologic study with an *in vitro* experiment found an inverse association between DEHP and DBP measured in semen and sperm motility in both oligoasthenospermic and asthenospermic men. Additionally, it was foundthat *in vitro* culture of sperm with DEHP and DBP at the maximum concentrations observed in human semen samples, as well as at levels 5- or 10-fold higher, also led to decreased sperm motility.[59] Although the results of these studies are not fully consistent, there is evidence to suggest that phthalate exposure is associated with declines in various semen quality measures.

10.7 Other Environmental Chemicals

Since semen quality represents a useful and, in some instances (*e.g.*, infertility clinics), a relatively convenient marker for studying the effect of exposures on male reproductive health, there are limited studies that have examined semen quality in relation to a wide range of other chemicals to which humans in the workplace or in the general population are environmentally exposed. These include, among others, bisphenol A (BPA), brominated flame retardants such as polybrominated dipheny ethers (PBDEs), organophosphate flame retardants such as triphenyl phosphate (TPP), fluorinated organic compounds such as perfluorooctane octanoate (PFOA) and perfluorooctane sulfonate (PFOS), parabens, and organic solvents such as ethylene glycol. These substances are used in a variety of applications and exposures can occur through multiple routes.

In a recent study of 218 men from four regions of China where high occupational exposures to BPA exist, Li and colleagues found that men with detectable urinary BPA had decreased sperm concentration, total sperm count, sperm vitality, and sperm motility after adjusting for potential confounders.[60] Additionally, in the non-occupational setting, BPA levels in the urine of male partners of infertile couples in the Boston study (n for analysis = 190) were suggestively associated with increased sperm DNA damage.[61] Also suggestive were the relationships observed between BPA and the odds for being below reference for sperm concentration, motility, and morphology, but the results were not statistically significant. Likewise, among 375 male partners of pregnant women in the Study for Future Families, BPA levels in urine were not significantly associated with any semen parameters.[62] More research is necessary to further investigate the effect of BPA on semen quality.

The Boston infertility clinic study also examined urinary parabens, including methyl paraben (MP), propyl paraben (PP), and butyl paraben (BP), in relation to semen quality measures and sperm DNA damage.[63] No relationships were observed for MP or PP, but BP quartiles were significantly and positively associated with sperm DNA damage, and the association remained after adjusting for BPA quartiles.[63] Lack of other findings may be due to the relatively small sample size (n = 190 for semen quality measures, and n = 132 for sperm DNA analysis) and/or substantial temporal variability in paraben concentrations in urine samples, indicating that this area deserves further attention in exposure assessment and epidemiological studies.

Exposure to PBDEs has been suggestively associated with semen quality, but studies have been quite limited in number and sample size. Akutsu and colleagues observed an inverse relationship between serum PBDE concentrations and semen quality and testis size in 10 Japanese males.[64] A study of 52 men visiting an infertility clinic in Quebec reported a negative association between PBDE congeners BDE-47 and BDE-100 and semen motility, but not other semen parameters.[65]

Organic solvents are found primarily in industrial settings and are used in paints, degreasing agents, and other applications. However, environmental contamination can occur, with subsequent human exposure through inhalation of contaminated air or ingestion of contaminated water. Several studies of general organic solvent exposure have shown an association with altered sperm quality. In an infertility clinic in Argentina, researchers found solvent exposure to be associated with increased risk of abnormal sperm motility and morphology in 177 men.[30] Cherry and colleagues also observed a dose-dependent increased risk in abnormal sperm motility in association with high exposure to organic solvents in a study set in a Canadian infertility clinic.[66] In studies of individual solvents, there is evidence for effects of ethylene glycol ethers, trichloroethylene, styrene, benzene, toluene, and xylene on semen quality.[67,68]

There is a range of other exposures that have been explored in relation to semen quality in limited studies. Raymer and colleagues investigated the association between PFOA and PFOS measured in the semen and plasma of 256 men, but no significant relationships were observed with semen volume, sperm concentration, percent motility, swim-up motility, or directional motility in adjusted models.[69] Another study measuring PFOA and PFOS in serum however, observed a significant decline in normal sperm count in Danish males with high exposure levels, as well as suggestive declines in total sperm count and sperm concentration.[70] Meeker and colleagues examined levels of organophosphate flame retardants—including tris(1,2,-dichloro-2-propyl) phosphate (TDCPP) and TPP—in the dust of the houses of 50 men and found levels of TPP to be associated with decreases in sperm concentration.[71] Two groups have investigated associations between exposure to disinfection by-products, such as trihalomethanes (THMs) or haloacetic acids (HAAs), and sperm quality but did not report any significant associations.[72,73] Other exposures associated with changes in semen quality include air pollutants and electromagnetic frequencies emitted from mobile phones.[74] However, because these are not strictly chemical exposures, and exposure assessment methods have generally been less precise for these studies, their potential effects on semen quality are not reviewed here.

10.8 Reproductive Hormones

In addition to a temporal downward trend in semen quality, researchers have observed an age-independent decline in testosterone levels over the last several decades, in men from both the US and Danish populations.[75,76] Decreased testosterone levels in males has been associated with adverse health effects later in life, including increased loss of bone mass and osteoporosis, sexual dysfunction, increased body mass index (BMI) and type 2 diabetes, and increased risk of cardiovascular-related morbidities and mortalities.[77–80] Since aging males are already subject to a steady decline in androgen levels, which may be exaggerated by age-related health problems, older individuals may be more sensitive to changes resulting from environmental insults.[81]

10.8.1 Persistent Organochlorines

Several studies have investigated the effect of OC exposure on male reproductive hormone levels. However, there have been several inconsistencies. Particularly, selection of PCB congeners measured and range of exposure levels in the studied populations have varied greatly. For example, many studies utilized groups of freshwater fisherman who have significantly elevated exposures to PCBs, hexachlorobenzene (HCB), and DDT. In US male sport-caught fish consumers, an inverse relationship between PCB concentrations and steroid hormone-binding globulin (SHGB)-bound testosterone was reported.[82,83] Goncharov and colleagues also observed an inverse relationship between PCB concentrations and total testosterone in a population of 257 Mohawk Native Americans residing along the St. Lawrence River; however, SHBG was not measured in this study.[84]

On the other hand, several groups have observed inverse associations between PCB exposure and free testosterone, as opposed to total testosterone or the bound fraction. In a study of Swedish military conscripts, an inverse relationship was observed between serum PCB-153 and free testosterone, but not bound testosterone.[13] This was also observed in a large 4-center study of European and Inuit men, where a positive association with PCB-153 and LH was also observed.[16] In a population of Latvian and Swedish men, Hagmar and colleagues observed an inverse correlation between summed PCBs and free testosterone, but the relationship was not significant after adjustment for age.[85] They did not find significant associations between individual PCB congeners and other hormones, including follicle-stimulating hormone (FSH), luteinizing hormone (LH), prolactin, SHBG, or total testosterone.[85] However, this could have been due to a limited sample size. Finally, a recent study of men in Norway reported a strong positive association between PCB-153 (a congener that is thought to be representative of cumulative PCB exposure) and SHBG after adjustments for age and BMI.[86] Overall, these findings suggest that PCBs may interact with steroid binding capacity in humans.

In addition to the relationships with testosterone, several groups have observed a link between PCB exposure and other reproductive hormones in males. In an Inuit population in Greenland, Giwercman and colleagues reported a positive association between PCB-153 and LH, although these results were inconsistent with those from other European cohorts examined in the same study.[87] When all cohorts were combined, they observed positive associations between PCB-153 and SHBG, and between dichlorodiphenyldichloroethylene (DDE), a stable metabolite of DDT, and FSH.[87] In another study of a much younger cohort, including 887 15-year-old Flemish males, relationships were observed between total and free testosterone, estradiol and aromatase index, and summed PCBs (including PCB-138, PCB-153 and PCB-180) and hexachlorobenzene (HCB), another OC of interest.[88] They also reported a positive association between estradiol and serum DDE.[88]

10.8.2 Non-Persistent Pesticides

In studies of both agricultural workers and the general population, there is a suggestive relationship between non-persistent pesticide exposure and altered sex hormone levels in men. In a group of agricultural workers, Recio and colleagues reported significant inverse associations between urinary markers of organophosphate pesticides and FSH and LH, and a statistically suggestive inverse association with estradiol.[89] No relationship was observed with testosterone however.[89] The inverse relationship with FSH was consistent with a study of 104 floriculturists in Mexico. Non-specific organophosphate metabolites in urine [dimethylphosphate (DMP), diethylphosphate (DEP), diethylthiophosphate (DETP) and total dialkyl phosphates (DAPs)] were negatively associated with serum FSH, and marginally and positively associated with testosterone.[90] DETP was marginally and negatively associated with LH.[90] A study of Danish greenhouse workers found a suggestive association between exposure to various insecticides and decreased testosterone; however, biomarkers for exposure assessment were not used.[91]

In the population of adult males presenting to a Boston infertility clinic, urinary metabolites of carbaryl and chlorpyrifos were associated with decreased serum testosterone, and the chlorpyrifos metabolite was also inversely associated with estradiol.[92,93] Furthermore, in US and Chinese studies, pyrethroid metabolites have been positively associated with LH and negatively associated with estradiol and inhibin B.[94,95]

10.8.3 Heavy Metals

Heavy metal exposure has been linked to changes in male sex hormone levels in several studies, primarily in instances of occupational exposure. Blood cadmium levels were associated with increased testosterone and LH levels, and decreased prolactin levels, in 149 Croatian industrial workers.[96] In another study of 166 occupationally exposed Chinese men, urinary cadmium levels were similarly associated with an increase in testosterone and LH.[97]

In studies of men exposed environmentally to cadmium, similar results have been reported, although exposure has been measured using several different methods (*e.g.*, using biomarkers in blood, urine and seminal plasma). Using blood cadmium levels, non-occupational exposure in a Croatian population of 123 men was associated with increased serum testosterone, as seen previously, and also with increased FSH and estradiol, after adjustment for confounders.[45] Using urine cadmium as a biomarker of exposure, Zeng and colleagues found that exposure was associated with abnormally high testosterone levels, although they did not observe any relationships with total testosterone, FSH, or LH in multiple regression models.[98] In a large of study of males in the US, utilizing the National Health and Nutrition Examination Survey (NHANES), a positive association was reported between urinary cadmium concentrations and testosterone, estradiol, and SHBG.[99] Using seminal plasma to estimate exposure, one study observed a positive correlation between cadmium and FSH levels, but not with LH or testosterone.[100] Several inverse and null associations have also been reported between cadmium exposure and reproductive hormones. Also utilizing urinary cadmium, Dhooge and colleagues observed an inverse association between cadmium exposure and testosterone, free testosterone, estradiol, and aromatase index after adjustments for confounders in 887 Flemish adolescent males.[88] A smaller study of 64 men from 3 infertility centers in Spain also reported no association between cadmium or other metals in seminal plasma, blood plasma, or whole blood and the hormones testosterone, FSH or LH.[43]

There has also been a range of studies exploring the effects of other metals, particularly with regard to occupational exposures. Blood lead levels in occupationally explosed males have been positively associated with inhibin B, FSH, LH, estradiol, and testosterone.[46,101–103] However, there have also been several studies reporting no evidence of these relationships.[96,104,105] In male welders with inhalational exposure to a variety of compounds, such as hexavalent chromium and stainless steel fumes, some studies have shown exposure to be associated with decreased testosterone levels, increased FSH, and LH, while others have found no association with sex hormones.[106–109] Finally, in magnesium alloy production workers, Elingsen and colleagues reported that manganese exposure was associated with significant increases in prolactin levels.[110]

In non-occupational studies of metals, several relationships with sex hormones in males have been observed as well. Mercury exposure in a small residential population in Cambodia was significantly and positively associated with estradiol levels, although previous studies of occupational mercury exposure did not report similar results.[102,105,111,112] A study of men recruited through Michigan infertility clinics reported inverse relationships between blood molybdenum levels and testosterone.[44] Lastly, there is some evidence for an association between arsenic exposure and decreased circulating testosterone levels, as well as increased risk of erectile dysfunction.[113]

10.8.4 Phthalates

Phthalate exposure has been linked to altered levels of circulating reproductive hormones in several studies. One study of workers in a polyvinyl chloride flooring production facility, where individuals were highly exposed to DEHP and DBP, reported inverse associations between exposure and circulating free testosterone levels.[114] Most other findings have been in relation to environmental phthalate exposure. In the Boston study of 425 men presenting to an infertility clinic, authors reported inverse associations between urinary levels of MEHP and testosterone, estradiol, and free androgen index (FAI, a measure of the ratio of total testosterone to SHBG), as well as a suggestive positive association between MEHP and the ratio of testosterone to estradiol (a measure of aromatase activity).[115] Another analysis among men with proven fertility in the Study for Future Families confirmed the findings for MEHP, observing all DEHP metabolites, including MEHP, mono-2-ethyl-5-hydroxyhexyl phthalate (MEHHP), mono-2-ethyl-5-oxohexyl phthalate (MEOHP), and mono-2-ethyl-5-carboxypentyl phthalate (MECPP), to be inversely correlated with total testosterone, free testosterone, and FAI in crude models.[116] After adjustments for potential covariates, no relationships with total testosterone remained, but several DEHP metabolites were still significantly associated with decreased FAI. In addition, MEHP was correlated with SHBG in this analysis, but there were no significant findings for other combinations of phthalate metabolites and sex hormone levels. In a population of young Swedish men, no relationships were found for MEHP, or other metabolites measured, and FSH, testosterone, estradiol or inhibin B, but a significant negative association was observed between MEP exposure and LH.[57] Lastly, a study of 118 suspected infertile men from a reproductive center in China measured levels of DEHP and DBP in semen and blood serum, and found significant positive associations between prolactin and serum DBP, serum DEHP, and semen DEHP.[117] Positive relationships were also observed between semen DEHP concentrations and estradiol, and between semen DBP and testosterone levels. However, as mentioned previously, exposure measures of parent phthalate compounds are more susceptible to laboratory contamination, and thus results may be unreliable.

10.8.5 Other Environmental Chemicals

Several other compounds have also been studied in relation to reproductive hormone levels in males. BPA in particular has been a focus of recent studies of male endocrine function, as it has been shown to affect the reproductive tract in animals.[118] An initial study of occupational exposure to BPA showed a significant inverse association with serum FSH levels.[119] BPA has also been linked to testosterone levels in several non-occupational studies. One group observed a positive association between urinary BPA levels and serum FSH in the Boston infertility clinic study.[120] They also observed inverse relationships between BPA and inhibin B and the ratio of estradiol to testosterone.[120] In a small group of healthy men and women in Japan, BPA measured in serum was positively associated with circulating total and free testosterone levels.[121] In a prospective population-based study of 715 Italian adults, there was a positive relationship between urinary BPA levels and total serum testosterone after adjustment for covariates.[122] No significant associations were observed, however, with free testosterone, SHBG, or estradiol. Finally, in a study of 375 men from the Study for Future Families, Mendiola and colleagues reported that urinary BPA was significantly and negatively related to serum FAI and FAI/LH ratio, and positively associated with SHBG.[62]

In addition to BPA, several other environmental chemicals of recent interest have demonstrated associations with changes in reproductive hormone levels. Turyk and colleagues found PBDE conger 47 measured in serum to be positively associated with testosterone in a study of 405 adult males.[123] Using concentrations of PBDE in house dust, another US study found that congeners 47, 99, and 100 were inversely related to FAI, LH, and FAI.[124] PFOS and PFOA were examined in two studies. One study reported that PFOA and PFOS in plasma were positively correlated with serum LH levels, but not with other reproductive hormones.[69] The second study, although slightly smaller, did not observe any significant associations with either compound.[125] Finally, the organophosphate compound TDCPP, but not TPP, measured in house dust, was associated with an increase in prolactin levels in 50 men recruited from an infertility clinic.[71] The study also observed a suggestive inverse relationship between TDCPP and FAI, but the association became less clear in adjusted models.

10.9 Thyroid Hormones

Healthy adults have thyroid hormone receptors in almost every tissue, and thyroid hormones and signaling are crucial for maintaining many bodily functions, including energy metabolism, heart rhythm, and bone resorption. Thyroid hormones are also vital to the reproductive system, although connections are less well-established.[126] Thyroid hormones appear to be important for reproductive tract development in males, as Sertoli cells express thyroid hormone receptors, and thyroid hormones themselves may be involved in Leydig cell differentiation and steroidogenesis in the testis of neonates.[127,128] In adults, thyroid hormones may interact with the pituitary to alter the release of LH in response to gonadotropin-releasing hormone (GnRH), leading to a downstream effect on testosterone and estradiol production, and may also be involved in the Leydig cell steroidogenic response to LH.[129,130] Finally, there is some evidence suggesting that thyroid hormone changes could be associated with sperm production and quality, further indicating the importance of studying the influences of environmental exposures on the thyroid system when considering impacts on the male reproductive tract.[131,132] Environmental chemicals have been shown to have adverse effects on thyroid signaling. Hence assessing relationships between these toxicants and markers of altered thyroid signaling in humans is an important aspect of the study of environmental effects on male reproductive function.

10.9.1 Persistent Organochlorines

Perhaps the exposures most studied in relation to thyroid hormones in men have been those of PCBs, DDE, and HCB, which may interact with thyroid hormones by interfering with receptor binding or uptake, or by disrupting hormone transport and metabolism.[133] Although there have been numerous findings in an array of populations exposed at different levels, results have not been fully consistent.[134] In the previously discussed population of Great Lakes fisherman, Persky and colleagues observed an inverse association between PCBs measured in serum and total T4 (thyroxine), but not T3 (triiodothyronine).[82] In a larger follow-up study, additional associations were observed between PCB exposure and T3 and thyroid-stimulating hormone (TSH), and the relationship with T4 was confirmed.[83] Furthermore, there was a suggestive inverse correlation between DDE and T4 in adjusted models, whereas no significant relationships with DDE were detected by Persky and colleagues in the original study.

Two studies of men from North American infertility clinics, with exposure levels more consistent with those observed in the general population, have also investigated these relationships. In 341 men from the Boston study, serum PCBs were inversely associated with total T3 after models were adjusted for covariates.[135] DDE was also significantly related to increased circulating free T4 and total T3 levels, as well as decreased TSH. Furthermore, HCB was inversely associated with total T3 in models adjusting for DDE exposure. In a smaller ($n = 52$) study of men from a clinic in Quebec, summed PCBs and DDE were related to decreased total T4, but not to other thyroid hormones.[65]

10.9.2 Non-Persistent Pesticides

In studies of both occupational and environmental exposure, there is evidence for a link between non-persistent pesticides and circulating thyroid hormone levels in men. In 1997, one group observed an increase in TSH in association with exposure to ethylene-bi(dithiocarbamate) fungicides in Mexican pesticide applicators, but found no change in T4.[136] In another study, among pesticide formulators in India, subjects exposed to a variety of compounds had significantly increased TSH and decreased total T3, as well as suggestively decreased T4, compared to controls.[137] In a longitudinal study of urinary DAP concentrations in Mexican floricultural workers, DMP was related to an increase in serum TSH and T4, and a decrease in total T3.[138] Finally, one study of environmentally exposed males reported an inverse association between biomarkers of carbaryl and chlorpyrifos exposure and free T4 levels.[139]

10.9.3 Heavy Metals and Other Environmental Chemicals

Associations between heavy metals and thyroid hormone levels have primarily been reported in populations of exposed workers, and these reports are inconsistent.[140] However, lead exposure may have an effect on the ability of GnRH to stimulate TSH release in the hypothalamic-pituitary axis, and may also affect the transport and metabolism of thyroid hormones.[141] In support of this hypothesis, a study of adult male automobile mechanics reported that increased exposure to lead was associated with an increase in TSH, but was not associated with alterations in T3 or T4.[142] Another group presented conflicting evidence of decreased levels of T4, but not T3 or TSH, in association with lead exposure among adolescent male auto mechanics.[140] Further analysis, and exploration of other metals, is necessary in order to make a conclusion about the relationship between metals and altered thyroid function.

PBDE exposure appears to have a more decisive relationship with thyroid hormones in humans. Hagmar and colleagues found an inverse relationship between plasma measures of PBDE-47 and TSH after adjustment for age, although no associations were observed with T3 or T4.[85] Another group investigating effects in a population of adult male sports-fishermen confirmed the association with PBDE exposure and decrease in TSH and additionally observed an inverse relationship with total T3 and a positive relationship with free T4.[123] Several other studies also found a link between PBDE exposure and increased free T4 levels.[64,124,143] These results seem to provide substantial evidence for a relationship with PBDE exposure; however, one small longitudinal study was unable to demonstrate statistically significant effects, and more research is necessary to establish causation.[144]

Phthalates may also be associated with altered thyroid hormones in men. In 408 men from the Boston infertility clinic study, urinary MEHP was inversely associated with serum free T4 and total T3, but not TSH, in adjusted models.[145] In a larger population of adults from NHANES ($n = 1346$ adults, male and female), the inverse relationship between MEHP and free T4 was confirmed, and inverse relationships with total T4, total T3, and thyroglobulin were also observed, as was a positive relationship with TSH.[61] More work is necessary to fully understand the mechanism behind the relationship between phthalate exposure and thyroid function.

Lastly, new studies have hypothesized that BPA exposure may also be linked to altered thyroid hormone levels in men. In the Boston infertility clinic study, authors observed a suggestive inverse association between urinary levels of BPA and TSH.[120] In the larger study of adults from the NHANES dataset, this relationship was also observed, as was an inverse association with total T4.[61] More studies on the potential for BPA to alter thyroid signaling are needed.

10.10 Cancers of the Male Reproductive Tract

Of particular concern to the aging population are cancers of the male reproductive tract. Prostate cancer is one of the most common malignancies in men and is expected to increase as the population ages, which represents a significant economic burden.[146] Additionally, although testicular cancer is more common in younger males, approximately 25% of incident cases occur in men over the age of 40.[147] In the last two decades, there has been an increasing trend in the incidence of testicular cancers in the US and Europe, as well as a very rapid increase in Croatia.[148–151] Investigation and prevention of environmental causes of these cancers is therefore particularly important.

Most studies of cancer-inducing effects of chemicals in adult males to date have been performed in agricultural workers occupationally exposed to pesticides. In a cohort of pesticide applicators in Florida, incidence of testicular and prostate cancers between 1975 and 1993 were significantly elevated.[152] This relationship was also observed more recently in British agricultural pesticide users who developed cancers between 1987 and 2004.[153] A larger study of national pesticide users in the US however, did not observe a significant association between exposure and testicular or prostate cancer risk, although there was a relationship with hematopoietic and nervous system cancers.[154]

Effects of non-persistent pesticides have been examined thoroughly in the Agricultural Health Study, an ongoing project that has examined cancer outcomes in commercial pesticide applicators and their families in North Carolina and Iowa since 1994.[155] A recent study has indicated that male participants have a significant excess risk of prostate cancer, despite some limitations in exposure assessment methods.[156–158] Additionally, studies of relationships with prostate cancer and specific pesticide exposures have found links with the organophosphate pesticides terbufos, coumaphos, and others.[159,160] Several of these analyses have not observed significant relationships however, with other common pesticides such as chlorpyrifos.[161] As the study progresses and allows for increased latency times, the effects of some of these compounds will likely become clearer.

Although use has been discontinued, DDE serum levels, representing DDT exposure, have been associated with increased risk of testicular germ cell tumors (TGCT) in several studies among populations in the US, Norway, and Italy.[162–164] However, other studies have reported null relationships between exposure and such cancers.[165,166] These studies have primarily estimated exposure using circulating DDE levels in adults, which may not be fully representative of long-term exposures or exposures during sensitive periods of development. More sophisticated analyses and longitudinal studies may be necessary in order to fully understand this relationship.

Similarly, PCBs have been associated, in some studies, with increased risk of male reproductive tract cancers, but again results were inconsistent. Several small studies observed significant relationships between circulating PCB levels and risk of prostate cancer.[167–169] However, in a large nested case-control study in Japan, there were no significant relationships with plasma organochlorine levels.[170] Similarly, no associations were reported in a case-control study in Ontario.[171] With regards to risk of TGCT, results have also been conflicting.[164,166]

Relationships between male reproductive tract cancers and other exposures have been limited, both in number and in methodology. For metals, associations observed in humans have been inconsistent, but results in animal studies suggest cadmium could lead to testicular and prostate cancers.[172] Effects of other chemicals have yet to be explored.

10.11 Summary and Conclusion

In summary, there is a fairly large body of evidence suggesting that a wide range of chemicals adversely impact the male reproductive tract following occupational or environmental exposure. However, the level of evidence and the consistency of findings within and between studies and between chemical agents has varied, and further research would be beneficial. Most of the studies described here have been cross-sectional in nature. Well-designed longitudinal studies are needed in order to explore the temporal relationships between exposure and outcome, and to account for the common occurrence of wide variability in individual exposure levels over time. In addition, researchers need to begin addressing not just single chemicals or classes of chemicals, but also exposure to mixtures of chemicals that may act additively, synergistically, or antagonistically with one another in relation to men's health endpoints. More research is also needed on genetic, metabolic, demographic, or other characteristics that impart increased individual susceptibility to environmental exposure in relation to these adverse health outcomes, as well as the time points along the life course that are most vulnerable to exposure. Finally, while the overall literature on male reproductive health is useful when considering exposure and aging, there is a clear need for studies focused on older populations, and which examine exposures, endpoints, and important covariates that are most relevant to health concerns later in life.

Abbreviations

DBCP	dibromochloropropane
PCBs	polychlorinated biphenyls
OCs	organochlorine pesticides
DDT	dichlorodiphenyltrichloroethane
MGH	Massachusetts General Hospital
SFF	Study for Future Families
IMPY	2-isoproproxy-4-methyl-pyrimidinol
TCPY	3,5,6-trichloro-2-pyridinol
1N	1-naphthol
3-PBA	3-phenoxybenzoic acid
DBCP	dibromochloropropane
DBP	dibutyl phthalate
MBP	monobutyl phthalate
MEHP	monoethylhexyl phthalate
DEHP	diethylhexyl phthalate
MBzP	monobenzylbutyl phthalate
BBzP	benzylbutyl phthalate
MEP	monoethyl phthalate
DEP	diethyl phthalate
MMP	monomethyl phthalate
DMP	dimethyl phthalate
CASA	computer-aided sperm analysis
MEHHP	mono-2-ethyl-5-hydroxyhexyl phthalate
MEOHP	mono-2-5-oxohexyl phthalate
MECCP	mono-2-ethyl-5-carboxypropyl phthalate
MCPP	mono-3-carboxypropyl phthalate

PBDEs	polybrominated diphenyl ethers
TPP	triphenyl phosphate
PFOA	perfluorooctane octanoate
PFOS	perfluorooctane sulfonate
MP	methy paraben
PP	propyl paraben
BP	butyl paraben
TDCPP	[tris(1,2,-dichloro-2-propyl) phosphate]
DBPs	disinfection by-products
THMs	trihalomethanes
HAAs	haloacetic acids
BMI	body mass index
SHBG	steroid hormone binding globulin
FSH	follicle-stimulating hormone
LH	Luteinizing hormone
DDE	dichlorodiphenyldichloroethylene
HCB	hexachlorobenzene
DAPs	diakyl phosphates
DMP	dimethylphosphate
DEP	diethylphosphate
DETP	diethylthiophosphate
FAI	free androgen index
PVC	polyvinyl chlorine
GnRH	gonadotropin-releasing hormone
T4	thyroixine
T3	triiodothyronine
TSH	thyroid-stimulating hormone
TGCT	testicular germ cell tumors

References

1. J. D. Meeker and R. Hauser, in *Environmental Impacts on Reproductive Health and Fertility*, eds. T. J. Woodruff, S. Janssen, L. Guillette and L. Giudice, Cambridge University Press, Cambridge, 2010, pp. 154–160.
2. S. H. Swan, E. P. Elkin and L. Fenster, *Environ Health Perspect*, 2000, **108**, 961–966.
3. E. Carlsen, A. Giwercman, N. Keiding and N. E. Skakkebaek, *BMJ*, 1992, **305**, 609–613.
4. A. G. Andersen, T. K. Jensen, E. Carlsen, N. Jorgensen, A. M. Andersson, T. Krarup, N. Keiding and N. E. Skakkebaek, *Hum Reprod*, 2000, **15**, 366–372.
5. A. F. Stewart and E. D. Kim, *Urology*, 2011, **78**, 496–499.
6. G. Toft, L. Hagmar, A. Giwercman and J. P. Bonde, *Reprod Toxicol*, 2004, **19**, 5–26.
7. ATSDR (Agency for Toxic Substances and Disease Registry), Atlanta, GA, 2000.

8. ATSDR (Agency for Toxic Substances and Disease Registry), Atlanta, GA, 2002.
9. W. J. Crinnion, *Altern Med Rev*, 2010, **15**, 101–109.
10. B. Bush, A. H. Bennett and J. T. Snow, *Arch Environ Contam Toxicol*, 1986, **15**, 333–341.
11. R. Rozati, P. P. Reddy, P. Reddanna and R. Mujtaba, *Fertil Steril*, 2002, **78**, 1187–1194.
12. J. W. Dallinga, E. J. Moonen, J. C. Dumoulin, J. L. Evers, J. P. Geraedts and J. C. Kleinjans, *Hum Reprod*, 2002, **17**, 1973–1979.
13. J. Richthoff, L. Rylander, B. A. Jonsson, H. Akesson, L. Hagmar, P. Nilsson-Ehle, M. Stridsberg and A. Giwercman, *Environ Health Perspect*, 2003, **111**, 409–413.
14. A. Rignell-Hydbom, L. Rylander, A. Giwercman, B. A. Jonsson, P. Nilsson-Ehle and L. Hagmar, *Hum Reprod*, 2004, **19**, 2066–2075.
15. A. Rignell-Hydbom, L. Rylander, A. Giwercman, B. A. Jonsson, C. Lindh, P. Eleuteri, M. Rescia, G. Leter, E. Cordelli, M. Spano and L. Hagmar, *Environ Health Perspect*, 2005, **113**, 175–179.
16. J. P. Bonde, G. Toft, L. Rylander, A. Rignell-Hydbom, A. Giwercman, M. Spano, G. C. Manicardi, D. Bizzaro, J. K. Ludwicki, V. Zvyezday, E. C. Bonefeld-Jorgensen, H. S. Pedersen, B. A. Jonsson and A. M. Thulstrup, *Environ Health Perspect*, 2008, **116**, 269–277.
17. R. Hauser, Z. Chen, L. Pothier, L. Ryan and L. Altshul, *Environ Health Perspect*, 2003, **111**, 1505–1511.
18. R. Hauser, N. P. Singh, Z. Chen, L. Pothier and L. Altshul, *Hum Reprod*, 2003, **18**, 2525–2533.
19. Y. L. Guo, P. C. Hsu, C. C. Hsu and G. H. Lambert, *Lancet*, 2000, **356**, 1240–1241.
20. P. C. Hsu, W. Huang, W. J. Yao, M. H. Wu, Y. L. Guo and G. H. Lambert, *JAMA*, 2003, **289**, 2943–2944.
21. N. H. Aneck-Hahn, G. W. Schulenburg, M. S. Bornman, P. Farias and C. de Jager, *J Androl*, 2007, **28**, 423–434.
22. K. P. Phillips and N. Tanphaichitr, *J Toxicol Environ Health B Crit Rev*, 2008, **11**, 188–220.
23. M. J. Perry, *Hum Reprod Update*, 2008, **14**, 233–242.
24. M. D. Whorton, T. H. Milby, H. A. Stubbs, B. H. Avashia and E. Q. Hull, *J Toxicol Environ Health*, 1979, **5**, 929–941.
25. A. J. Wyrobek, G. Watchmaker, L. Gordon, K. Wong, D. Moore, 2nd and D. Whorton, *Environ Health Perspect*, 1981, **40**, 255–265.
26. Y. Xia, S. Cheng, Q. Bian, L. Xu, M. D. Collins, H. C. Chang, L. Song, J. Liu, S. Wang and X. Wang, *Toxicol Sci*, 2005, **85**, 615–623.
27. C. Padungtod, D. A. Savitz, J. W. Overstreet, D. C. Christiani, L. M. Ryan and X. Xu, *J Occup Environ Med*, 2000, **42**, 982–992.
28. M. Kamijima, H. Hibi, M. Gotoh, K. Taki, I. Saito, H. Wang, S. Itohara, T. Yamada, G. Ichihara, E. Shibata, T. Nakajima and Y. Takeuchi, *J Occup Health*, 2004, **46**, 109–118.

29. A. Abell, E. Ernst and J. P. Bonde, *Scand J Work Environ Health*, 2000, **26**, 492–500.
30. A. Oliva, A. Spira and L. Multigner, *Hum Reprod*, 2001, **16**, 1768–1776.
31. S. B. Larsen, A. Giwercman, M. Spano and J. P. Bonde, *Reprod Toxicol*, 1998, **12**, 581–589.
32. R. K. Juhler, S. B. Larsen, O. Meyer, N. D. Jensen, M. Spano, A. Giwercman and J. P. Bonde, *Arch Environ Contam Toxicol*, 1999, **37**, 415–423.
33. S. H. Swan, R. L. Kruse, F. Liu, D. B. Barr, E. Z. Drobnis, J. B. Redmon, C. Wang, C. Brazil and J. W. Overstreet, *Environ Health Perspect*, 2003, **111**, 1478–1484.
34. J. D. Meeker, L. Ryan, D. B. Barr, R. F. Herrick, D. H. Bennett, R. Bravo and R. Hauser, *Environ Health Perspect*, 2004, **112**, 1665–1670.
35. J. D. Meeker, N. P. Singh, L. Ryan, S. M. Duty, D. B. Barr, R. F. Herrick, D. H. Bennett and R. Hauser, *Hum Reprod*, 2004, **19**, 2573–2580.
36. J. D. Meeker, D. B. Barr and R. Hauser, *Hum Reprod*, 2008, **23**, 1932–1940.
37. Y. Xia, Y. Han, B. Wu, S. Wang, A. Gu, N. Lu, J. Bo, L. Song, N. Jin and X. Wang, *Fertil Steril*, 2008, **89**, 1743–1750.
38. G. Ji, Y. Xia, A. Gu, X. Shi, Y. Long, L. Song, S. Wang and X. Wang, *Reprod Toxicol*, 2011, **31**, 171–176.
39. H. Toshima, Y. Suzuki, K. Imai, J. Yoshinaga, H. Shiraishi, Y. Mizumoto, S. Hatakeyama, C. Onohara and S. Tokuoka, *Int J Hyg Environ Health*, 2011.
40. S. W. Tsaih, S. Korrick, J. Schwartz, M. L. Lee, C. Amarasiriwardena, A. Aro, D. Sparrow and H. Hu, *Environ Health Perspect*, 2001, **109**, 995–999.
41. S. Benoff, A. Jacob and I. R. Hurley, *Hum Reprod Update*, 2000, **6**, 107–121.
42. I. Hernandez-Ochoa, G. Garcia-Vargas, L. Lopez-Carrillo, M. Rubio-Andrade, J. Moran-Martinez, M. E. Cebrian and B. Quintanilla-Vega, *Reprod Toxicol*, 2005, **20**, 221–228.
43. J. Mendiola, J. M. Moreno, M. Roca, N. Vergara-Juarez, M. J. Martinez-Garcia, A. Garcia-Sanchez, B. Elvira-Rendueles, S. Moreno-Grau, J. J. Lopez-Espin, J. Ten, R. Bernabeu and A. M. Torres-Cantero, *Environ Health*, 2011, **10**, 6.
44. J. D. Meeker, M. G. Rossano, B. Protas, M. P. Diamond, E. Puscheck, D. Daly, N. Paneth and J. J. Wirth, *Environ Health Perspect*, 2008, **116**, 1473–1479.
45. J. Jurasovic, P. Cvitkovic, A. Pizent, B. Colak and S. Telisman, *Biometals*, 2004, **17**, 735–743.
46. S. Telisman, B. Colak, A. Pizent, J. Jurasovic and P. Cvitkovic, *Environ Res*, 2007, **105**, 256–266.
47. C. M. Choy, Q. S. Yeung, C. M. Briton-Jones, C. K. Cheung, C. W. Lam and C. J. Haines, *Fertil Steril*, 2002, **78**, 426–428.

48. J. J. Wirth, M. G. Rossano, D. C. Daly, N. Paneth, E. Puscheck, R. C. Potter and M. P. Diamond, *Epidemiology*, 2007, **18**, 270–273.
49. J. D. Meeker, S. Sathyanarayana and S. H. Swan, *Philos Trans R Soc Lond B Biol Sci*, 2009, **364**, 2097–2113.
50. D. A. Murature, S. Y. Tang, G. Steinhardt and R. C. Dougherty, *Biomed Environ Mass Spectrom*, 1987, **14**, 473–477.
51. S. M. Duty, M. J. Silva, D. B. Barr, J. W. Brock, L. Ryan, Z. Chen, R. F. Herrick, D. C. Christiani and R. Hauser, *Epidemiology*, 2003, **14**, 269–277.
52. R. Hauser, J. D. Meeker, S. Duty, M. J. Silva and A. M. Calafat, *Epidemiology*, 2006, **17**, 682–691.
53. S. M. Duty, A. M. Calafat, M. J. Silva, J. W. Brock, L. Ryan, Z. Chen, J. Overstreet and R. Hauser, *J Androl*, 2004, **25**, 293–302.
54. S. M. Duty, N. P. Singh, M. J. Silva, D. B. Barr, J. W. Brock, L. Ryan, R. F. Herrick, D. C. Christiani and R. Hauser, *Environ Health Perspect*, 2003, **111**, 1164–1169.
55. R. Hauser, J. D. Meeker, N. P. Singh, M. J. Silva, L. Ryan, S. Duty and A. M. Calafat, *Hum Reprod*, 2007, **22**, 688–695.
56. C. Herr, A. zur Nieden, H. M. Koch, H. C. Schuppe, C. Fieber, J. Angerer, T. Eikmann and N. I. Stilianakis, *Int J Hyg Environ Health*, 2009, **212**, 648–653.
57. B. A. Jonsson, J. Richthoff, L. Rylander, A. Giwercman and L. Hagmar, *Epidemiology*, 2005, **16**, 487–493.
58. L. Liu, H. Bao, F. Liu, J. Zhang and H. Shen, *Environ Int*, 2011.
59. N. Pant, A. Pant, M. Shukla, N. Mathur, Y. Gupta and D. Saxena, *Hum Exp Toxicol*, 2011, **30**, 507–514.
60. D. K. Li, Z. Zhou, M. Miao, Y. He, J. Wang, J. Ferber, L. J. Herrinton, E. Gao and W. Yuan, *Fertil Steril*, 2011, **95**, 625–630 e621–624.
61. J. D. Meeker and K. K. Ferguson, *Environ Health Perspect*, 2011, **119**, 1396–1402.
62. J. Mendiola, N. Jorgensen, A. M. Andersson, A. M. Calafat, X. Ye, J. B. Redmon, E. Z. Drobnis, C. Wang, A. Sparks, S. W. Thurston, F. Liu and S. H. Swan, *Environ Health Perspect*, 2010, **118**, 1286–1291.
63. J. D. Meeker, T. Yang, X. Ye, A. M. Calafat and R. Hauser, *Environ Health Perspect*, 2011, **119**, 252–257.
64. K. Akutsu, S. Takatori, S. Nozawa, M. Yoshiike, H. Nakazawa, K. Hayakawa, T. Makino and T. Iwamoto, *Bull Environ Contam Toxicol*, 2008, **80**, 345–350.
65. N. Abdelouahab, Y. Ainmelk and L. Takser, *Reprod Toxicol*, 2011, **31**, 546–550.
66. N. Cherry, F. Labreche, J. Collins and T. Tulandi, *Occup Environ Med*, 2001, **58**, 635–640.
67. I. Figa-Talamanca, M. E. Traina and E. Urbani, *Occup Med (Lond)*, 2001, **51**, 174–188.
68. E. K. Sheiner, E. Sheiner, R. D. Hammel, G. Potashnik and R. Carel, *Ind Health*, 2003, **41**, 55–62.

69. J. H. Raymer, L. C. Michael, W. B. Studabaker, G. W. Olsen, C. S. Sloan, T. Wilcosky and D. K. Walmer, *Reprod Toxicol*, 2011.
70. U. N. Joensen, R. Bossi, H. Leffers, A. A. Jensen, N. E. Skakkebaek and N. Jorgensen, *Environ Health Perspect*, 2009, **117**, 923–927.
71. J. D. Meeker and H. M. Stapleton, *Environ Health Perspect*, 2010, **118**, 318–323.
72. L. Fenster, K. Waller, G. Windham, T. Henneman, M. Anderson, P. Mendola, J. W. Overstreet and S. H. Swan, *Epidemiology*, 2003, **14**, 650–658.
73. T. J. Luben, A. F. Olshan, A. H. Herring, S. Jeffay, L. Strader, R. M. Buus, R. L. Chan, D. A. Savitz, P. C. Singer, H. S. Weinberg and S. D. Perreault, *Environ Health Perspect*, 2007, **115**, 1169–1176.
74. J. Jurewicz, W. Hanke, M. Radwan and J. P. Bonde, *Int J Occup Med Environ Health*, 2009, **22**, 305–329.
75. A. M. Andersson, T. K. Jensen, A. Juul, J. H. Petersen, T. Jorgensen and N. E. Skakkebaek, *J Clin Endocrinol Metab*, 2007, **92**, 4696–4705.
76. T. G. Travison, A. B. Araujo, A. B. O'Donnell, V. Kupelian and J. B. McKinlay, *J Clin Endocrinol Metab*, 2007, **92**, 196–202.
77. J. A. Cauley, S. K. Ewing, B. C. Taylor, H. A. Fink, K. E. Ensrud, D. C. Bauer, E. Barrett-Connor, L. Marshall and E. S. Orwoll, *J Clin Endocrinol Metab*, **95**, 4314–4323.
78. M. Grossmann, *J Clin Endocrinol Metab*, **96**, 2341–2353.
79. D. B. O'Connor, D. M. Lee, G. Corona, G. Forti, A. Tajar, T. W. O'Neill, N. Pendleton, G. Bartfai, S. Boonen, F. F. Casanueva, J. D. Finn, A. Giwercman, T. S. Han, I. T. Huhtaniemi, K. Kula, F. Labrie, M. E. Lean, M. Punab, A. J. Silman, D. Vanderschueren and F. C. Wu, *J Clin Endocrinol Metab*, **96**, E1577–1587.
80. A. M. Traish, M. M. Miner, A. Morgentaler and M. Zitzmann, *Am J Med*, 2011, **124**, 578–587.
81. H. A. Feldman, C. Longcope, C. A. Derby, C. B. Johannes, A. B. Araujo, A. D. Coviello, W. J. Bremner and J. B. McKinlay, *J Clin Endocrinol Metab*, 2002, **87**, 589–598.
82. V. Persky, M. Turyk, H. A. Anderson, L. P. Hanrahan, C. Falk, D. N. Steenport, R. Chatterton, Jr. and S. Freels, *Environ Health Perspect*, 2001, **109**, 1275–1283.
83. M. E. Turyk, H. A. Anderson, S. Freels, R. Chatterton, Jr., L. L. Needham, D. G. Patterson, Jr., D. N. Steenport, L. Knobeloch, P. Imm and V. W. Persky, *Environ Res*, 2006, **102**, 299–307.
84. A. Goncharov, R. Rej, S. Negoita, M. Schymura, A. Santiago-Rivera, G. Morse and D. O. Carpenter, *Environ Health Perspect*, 2009, **117**, 1454–1460.
85. L. Hagmar, J. Bjork, A. Sjodin, A. Bergman and E. M. Erfurth, *Arch Environ Health*, 2001, **56**, 138–143.
86. T. B. Haugen, T. Tefre, G. Malm, B. A. Jonsson, L. Rylander, L. Hagmar, C. Bjorsvik, T. Henrichsen, T. Saether, Y. Figenschau and A. Giwercman, *Reprod Toxicol*, **32**, 261–267.

87. A. H. Giwercman, A. Rignell-Hydbom, G. Toft, L. Rylander, L. Hagmar, C. Lindh, H. S. Pedersen, J. K. Ludwicki, V. Lesovoy, M. Shvets, M. Spano, G. C. Manicardi, D. Bizzaro, E. C. Bonefeld-Jorgensen and J. P. Bonde, *Environ Health Perspect*, 2006, **114**, 1348–1353.
88. W. Dhooge, E. den Hond, G. Koppen, L. Bruckers, V. Nelen, E. van de Mieroop, M. Bilau, K. Croes, W. Baeyens, G. Schoeters and N. van Larebeke, *J Expo Sci Environ Epidemiol*, 2011, **21**, 106–113.
89. R. Recio, G. Ocampo-Gomez, J. Moran-Martinez, V. Borja-Aburto, M. Lopez-Cervante, M. Uribe, L. Torres-Sanchez and M. E. Cebrian, *Environ Health Perspect*, 2005, **113**, 1160–1163.
90. J. Blanco-Munoz, M. M. Morales, M. Lacasana, C. Aguilar-Garduno, S. Bassol and M. E. Cebrian, *Hum Reprod*, 2010, **25**, 1787–1795.
91. G. Toft, A. Flyvbjerg and J. P. Bonde, *Environ Health*, 2006, **5**, 32.
92. J. D. Meeker, S. R. Ravi, D. B. Barr and R. Hauser, *Reprod Toxicol*, 2008, **25**, 184–191.
93. J. D. Meeker, L. Ryan, D. B. Barr and R. Hauser, *Epidemiology*, 2006, **17**, 61–68.
94. Y. Han, Y. Xia, J. Han, J. Zhou, S. Wang, P. Zhu, R. Zhao, N. Jin, L. Song and X. Wang, *Chemosphere*, 2008, **72**, 785–790.
95. J. D. Meeker, D. B. Barr and R. Hauser, *Reprod Toxicol*, 2009, **27**, 155–160.
96. S. Telisman, P. Cvitkovic, J. Jurasovic, A. Pizent, M. Gavella and B. Rocic, *Environ Health Perspect*, 2000, **108**, 45–53.
97. X. Zeng, T. Lin, Y. Zhou and Q. Kong, *J Toxicol Environ Health A*, 2002, **65**, 513–521.
98. X. Zeng, T. Jin, J. P. Buchet, X. Jiang, Q. Kong, T. Ye, A. Bernard and G. F. Nordberg, *Environ Res*, 2004, **96**, 338–344.
99. A. Menke, E. Guallar, M. S. Shiels, S. Rohrmann, S. Basaria, N. Rifai, W. G. Nelson and E. A. Platz, *BMC Public Health*, 2008, **8**, 72.
100. O. Akinloye, A. O. Arowojolu, O. B. Shittu and J. I. Anetor, *Reprod Biol*, 2006, **6**, 17–30.
101. A. Mahmoud, P. Kiss, M. Vanhoorne, D. De Bacquer and F. Comhaire, *Int J Androl*, 2005, **28**, 150–155.
102. A. J. McGregor and H. J. Mason, *Hum Exp Toxicol*, 1991, **10**, 199–203.
103. T. P. Ng, H. H. Goh, Y. L. Ng, H. Y. Ong, C. N. Ong, K. S. Chia, S. E. Chia and J. Jeyaratnam, *Br J Ind Med*, 1991, **48**, 485–491.
104. B. H. Alexander, H. Checkoway, C. van Netten, C. H. Muller, T. G. Ewers, J. D. Kaufman, B. A. Mueller, T. L. Vaughan and E. M. Faustman, *Occup Environ Med*, 1996, **53**, 411–416.
105. E. M. Erfurth, A. Schutz, A. Nilsson, L. Barregard and S. Skerfving, *Br J Ind Med*, 1990, **47**, 639–644.
106. J. P. Bonde, *Br J Ind Med*, 1990, **47**, 508–514.
107. J. P. Bonde and E. Ernst, *Hum Exp Toxicol*, 1992, **11**, 259–263.
108. N. H. Hjollund, J. P. Bonde, T. K. Jensen, E. Ernst, T. B. Henriksen, H. A. Kolstad, A. Giwercman, N. E. Skakkebaek and J. Olsen, *Reprod Toxicol*, 1998, **12**, 91–95.

109. E. A. Kim, H. K. Cheong, K. D. Joo, J. H. Shin, J. S. Lee, S. B. Choi, M. O. Kim, J. Lee and Iu and D. M. Kang, *Neurotoxicology*, 2007, **28**, 263–269.
110. D. G. Ellingsen, E. Haug, P. I. Gaarder, R. Bast-Pettersen and Y. Thomassen, *Scand J Work Environ Health*, 2003, **29**, 230–238.
111. T. Agusa, T. Kunito, H. Iwata, I. Monirith, C. Chamnan, T. S. Tana, A. Subramanian and S. Tanabe, *Chemosphere*, 2007, **68**, 590–596.
112. L. Barregard, G. Lindstedt, A. Schutz and G. Sallsten, *Occup Environ Med*, 1994, **51**, 536–540.
113. F. I. Hsieh, T. S. Hwang, Y. C. Hsieh, H. C. Lo, C. T. Su, H. S. Hsu, H. Y. Chiou and C. J. Chen, *Environ Health Perspect*, 2008, **116**, 532–536.
114. G. Pan, T. Hanaoka, M. Yoshimura, S. Zhang, P. Wang, H. Tsukino, K. Inoue, H. Nakazawa, S. Tsugane and K. Takahashi, *Environ Health Perspect*, 2006, **114**, 1643–1648.
115. J. D. Meeker, A. M. Calafat and R. Hauser, *J Androl*, 2009, **30**, 287–297.
116. J. Mendiola, N. Jorgensen, A. M. Andersson, A. M. Calafat, M. J. Silva, J. B. Redmon, A. Sparks, E. Z. Drobnis, C. Wang, F. Liu and S. H. Swan, *Int J Androl*, 2011, **34**, 369–378.
117. S. Li, J. Dai, L. Zhang, J. Zhang, Z. Zhang and B. Chen, *Biomed Environ Sci*, 2011, **24**, 31–39.
118. C. A. Richter, L. S. Birnbaum, F. Farabollini, R. R. Newbold, B. S. Rubin, C. E. Talsness, J. G. Vandenbergh, D. R. Walser-Kuntz and F. S. vom Saal, *Reprod Toxicol*, 2007, **24**, 199–224.
119. T. Hanaoka, N. Kawamura, K. Hara and S. Tsugane, *Occup Environ Med*, 2002, **59**, 625–628.
120. J. D. Meeker, A. M. Calafat and R. Hauser, *Environ Sci Technol*, 2010, **44**, 1458–1463.
121. T. Takeuchi and O. Tsutsumi, *Biochem Biophys Res Commun*, 2002, **291**, 76–78.
122. T. Galloway, R. Cipelli, J. Guralnik, L. Ferrucci, S. Bandinelli, A. M. Corsi, C. Money, P. McCormack and D. Melzer, *Environ Health Perspect*, 2010, **118**, 1603–1608.
123. M. E. Turyk, V. W. Persky, P. Imm, L. Knobeloch, R. Chatterton and H. A. Anderson, *Environ Health Perspect*, 2008, **116**, 1635–1641.
124. J. D. Meeker, P. I. Johnson, D. Camann and R. Hauser, *Sci Total Environ*, 2009, **407**, 3425–3429.
125. U. N. Joensen, R. Bossi, H. Leffers, A. A. Jensen, N. E. Skakkebaek and N. Jorgensen, *Environ Health Perspect*, 2009, **117**, 923–927.
126. R. T. Zoeller and J. D. Meeker, in *Environmental Impacts on Reproductive Health and Fertility*, eds. T. J. Woodruff, S. Janssen, L. Guillette and L. Giudice, Cambridge University Press, Cambridge, UK, 2010.
127. E. A. Jannini, A. Crescenzi, N. Rucci, E. Screponi, E. Carosa, A. de Matteis, E. Macchia, G. d'Amati and M. D'Armiento, *J Clin Endocrinol Metab*, 2000, **85**, 3453–3457.
128. C. Mendis-Handagama and S. Ariyaratne, *Arch Androl*, 2004, **50**, 347–357.

129. R. R. Maran, *Arch Androl*, 2003, **49**, 375–388.
130. E. M. Velazquez and G. Bellabarba Arata, *Arch Androl*, 1997, **38**, 85–92.
131. J. D. Meeker, N. P. Singh and R. Hauser, *J Androl*, 2008, **29**, 379–388.
132. J. D. Meeker, L. Godfrey-Bailey and R. Hauser, *J Androl*, 2007, **28**, 397–406.
133. J. D. Meeker and M. Boas, in *Encyclopedia of Environmental Health*, ed. J. Nriagu, Elsevier Ltd, Oxford, UK, 2011.
134. E. Salay and D. Garabrant, *Chemosphere*, 2009, **74**, 1413–1419.
135. J. D. Meeker, L. Altshul and R. Hauser, *Environ Res*, 2007, **104**, 296–304.
136. K. Steenland, L. Cedillo, J. Tucker, C. Hines, K. Sorensen, J. Deddens and V. Cruz, *Environ Health Perspect*, 1997, **105**, 1126–1130.
137. S. S. Zaidi, V. K. Bhatnagar, S. J. Gandhi, M. P. Shah, P. K. Kulkarni and H. N. Saiyed, *Hum Exp Toxicol*, 2000, **19**, 497–501.
138. M. Lacasana, I. Lopez-Flores, M. Rodriguez-Barranco, C. Aguilar-Garduno, J. Blanco-Munoz, O. Perez-Mendez, R. Gamboa, S. Bassol and M. E. Cebrian, *Toxicol Appl Pharmacol*, 2010, **243**, 19–26.
139. J. D. Meeker, D. B. Barr and R. Hauser, *Reprod Toxicol*, 2006, **22**, 437–442.
140. B. Dundar, F. Oktem, M. K. Arslan, N. Delibas, B. Baykal, C. Arslan, M. Gultepe and I. E. Ilhan, *Environ Res*, 2006, **101**, 140–145.
141. K. K. Doumouchtsis, S. K. Doumouchtsis, E. K. Doumouchtsis and D. N. Perrea, *J Endocrinol Invest*, 2009, **32**, 175–183.
142. B. Singh, V. Chandran, H. K. Bandhu, B. R. Mittal, A. Bhattacharya, S. K. Jindal and S. Varma, *Biometals*, 2000, **13**, 187–192.
143. M. Bloom, H. Spliethoff, J. Vena, S. Shaver, R. Addink and G. Eadon, *Environ Toxicol Pharmacol*, 2008, **25**, 386–392.
144. A. Julander, M. Karlsson, K. Hagstrom, C. G. Ohlson, M. Engwall, I. L. Bryngelsson, H. Westberg and B. van Bavel, *Int Arch Occup Environ Health*, 2005, **78**, 584–592.
145. J. D. Meeker, A. M. Calafat and R. Hauser, *Environ Health Perspect*, 2007, **115**, 1029–1034.
146. C. G. Roehrborn and L. K. Black, *BJU Int*, 2011, **108**, 806–813.
147. J. S. Townsend, L. C. Richardson and R. R. German, *Am J Mens Health*, 2010, **4**, 353–360.
148. H. O. Adami, R. Bergstrom, M. Mohner, W. Zatonski, H. Storm, A. Ekbom, S. Tretli, L. Teppo, H. Ziegler and M. Rahu, *et al.*, *Int J Cancer*, 1994, **59**, 33–38.
149. R. Bergstrom, H. O. Adami, M. Mohner, W. Zatonski, H. Storm, A. Ekbom, S. Tretli, L. Teppo, O. Akre and T. Hakulinen, *J Natl Cancer Inst*, 1996, **88**, 727–733.
150. E. Huyghe, T. Matsuda and P. Thonneau, *J Urol*, 2003, **170**, 5–11.
151. N. Sincic, T. Kulis, A. Znaor and F. Bray, *Cancer Epidemiol*, 2011.
152. L. E. Fleming, J. A. Bean, M. Rudolph and K. Hamilton, *J Occup Environ Med*, 1999, **41**, 279–288.
153. G. Frost, T. Brown and A. H. Harding, *Occup Med (Lond)*, 2011, **61**, 303–310.

154. L. E. Fleming, O. Gomez-Marin, D. Zheng, F. Ma and D. Lee, *Am J Ind Med*, 2003, **43**, 227–233.
155. E. Kasahara, E. F. Sato, M. Miyoshi, R. Konaka, K. Hiramoto, J. Sasaki, M. Tokuda, Y. Nakano and M. Inoue, *Biochem J*, 2002, **365**, 849–856.
156. M. C. Alavanja, C. Samanic, M. Dosemeci, J. Lubin, R. Tarone, C. F. Lynch, C. Knott, K. Thomas, J. A. Hoppin, J. Barker, J. Coble, D. P. Sandler and A. Blair, *Am J Epidemiol*, 2003, **157**, 800–814.
157. M. C. Alavanja, D. P. Sandler, C. F. Lynch, C. Knott, J. H. Lubin, R. Tarone, K. Thomas, M. Dosemeci, J. Barker, J. A. Hoppin and A. Blair, *Scand J Work Environ Health*, 2005, **31 Suppl 1**, 39–45; discussion 35–37.
158. S. Koutros, M. C. Alavanja, J. H. Lubin, D. P. Sandler, J. A. Hoppin, C. F. Lynch, C. Knott, A. Blair and L. E. Freeman, *J Occup Environ Med*, 2010, **52**, 1098–1105.
159. M. R. Bonner, B. A. Williams, J. A. Rusiecki, A. Blair, L. E. Beane Freeman, J. A. Hoppin, M. Dosemeci, J. Lubin, D. P. Sandler and M. C. Alavanja, *Cancer Causes Control*, 2010, **21**, 871–877.
160. C. H. Christensen, E. A. Platz, G. Andreotti, A. Blair, J. A. Hoppin, S. Koutros, C. F. Lynch, D. P. Sandler and M. C. Alavanja, *Environ Health Perspect*, 2010, **118**, 92–96.
161. W. J. Lee, A. Blair, J. A. Hoppin, J. H. Lubin, J. A. Rusiecki, D. P. Sandler, M. Dosemeci and M. C. Alavanja, *J Natl Cancer Inst*, 2004, **96**, 1781–1789.
162. F. Giannandrea, L. Gandini, D. Paoli, R. Turci and I. Figa-Talamanca, *J Environ Sci Health B*, 2011, **46**, 780–787.
163. K. A. McGlynn, S. M. Quraishi, B. I. Graubard, J. P. Weber, M. V. Rubertone and R. L. Erickson, *J Natl Cancer Inst*, 2008, **100**, 663–671.
164. M. P. Purdue, L. S. Engel, H. Langseth, L. L. Needham, A. Andersen, D. B. Barr, A. Blair, N. Rothman and K. A. McGlynn, *Environ Health Perspect*, 2009, **117**, 1514–1519.
165. M. L. Biggs, M. D. Davis, D. L. Eaton, N. S. Weiss, D. B. Barr, D. R. Doody, S. Fish, L. L. Needham, C. Chen and S. M. Schwartz, *Cancer Epidemiol Biomarkers Prev*, 2008, **17**, 2012–2018.
166. K. A. McGlynn, S. M. Quraishi, B. I. Graubard, J. P. Weber, M. V. Rubertone and R. L. Erickson, *Cancer Res*, 2009, **69**, 1901–1909.
167. L. Hardell, S. O. Andersson, M. Carlberg, L. Bohr, B. van Bavel, G. Lindstrom, H. Bjornfoth and C. Ginman, *J Occup Environ Med*, 2006, **48**, 700–707.
168. J. M. Ritchie, S. L. Vial, L. J. Fuortes, H. Guo, V. E. Reedy and E. M. Smith, *J Occup Environ Med*, 2003, **45**, 692–702.
169. J. M. Ritchie, S. L. Vial, L. J. Fuortes, L. W. Robertson, H. Guo, V. E. Reedy and E. M. Smith, *Environ Res*, 2005, **98**, 104–113.
170. N. Sawada, M. Iwasaki, M. Inoue, H. Itoh, S. Sasazuki, T. Yamaji, T. Shimazu and S. Tsugane, *Environ Health Perspect*, 2010, **118**, 659–665.
171. K. J. Aronson, J. W. Wilson, M. Hamel, W. Diarsvitri, W. Fan, C. Woolcott, J. P. Heaton, J. C. Nickel, A. Macneily and A. Morales, *J Expo Sci Environ Epidemiol*, 2010, **20**, 434–445.
172. R. A. Goyer, J. Liu and M. P. Waalkes, *Biometals*, 2004, **17**, 555–558.

CHAPTER 11

Breast Cancer – Importance of Life Stage with Respect to Environmental Influences

SALLY S. WHITE[a] AND SUZANNE E. FENTON*[b]

[a] Research Fellow, NTP Labs Branch, Division of the National Toxicology Program, NIEHS/NIH, 111 TW Alexander Dr, Bldg 101, MD E1-08, Research Triangle Park, NC 27709, USA; [b] Group Leader, Reproductive Endocrinology, NTP Labs Branch, Division of the National Toxicology Program, NIEHS/NIH, 111 TW Alexander Dr, Bldg 101, MD E1-08, Research Triangle Park, NC 27709, USA
*E-mail: fentonse@niehs.nih.gov

11.1 Introduction

11.1.1 Breast Cancer & Aging Overview

Globally, the incidence of breast cancer increases with age. This is true not just for women, but is also the case for men (see Figure 11.1), as well as for rodents used in research and larger mammals, such as non-human primates, dogs, and cats. In the 2012 American Cancer Society "Breast Cancer Facts and Figures 2011–2012" report,[6] it is documented that between 2004 and 2008, 95% of new breast cancer cases occurred in women aged 40 or older, the median age at diagnosis was 61, and women aged 75–79 exhibited the highest incidence, with a rate of 421.3 cases per 100 000. The 2012 statistics from Susan G. Komen

Issues in Toxicology No. 16
Aging and Vulnerability to Environmental Chemicals: Age-related Disorders and their Origins in Environmental Exposures
Edited by Bernard Weiss

Published by the Royal Society of Chemistry, www.rsc.org

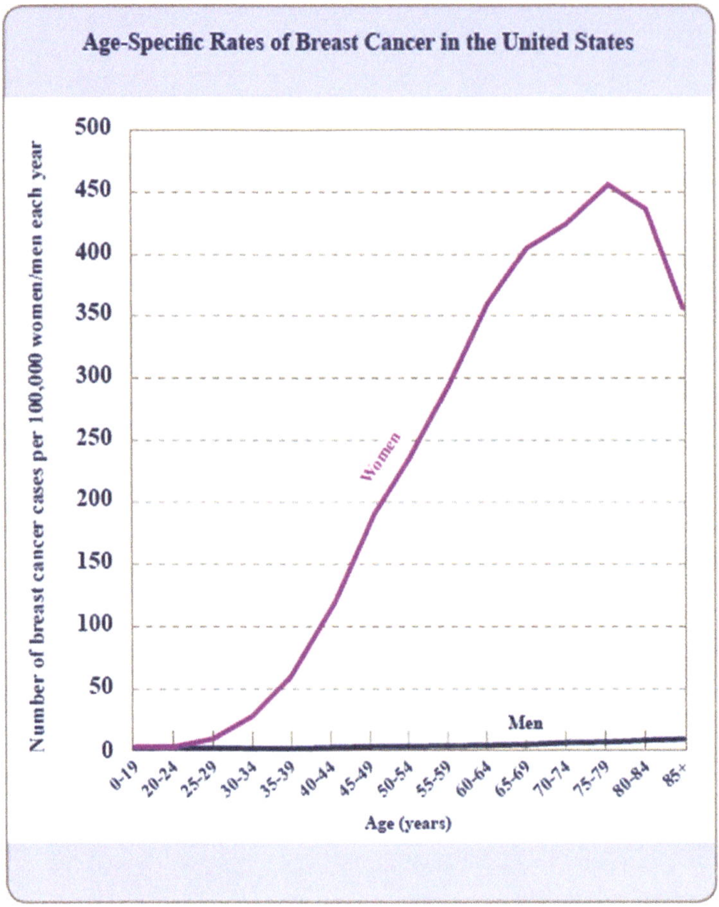

Figure 11.1 Age-specific female and male breast cancer rates in the US. The curve for men (blue) remains relatively flat and depicts the low incidence of diagnosis with breast cancer. The curve for women (pink) depicts increasing incidence of newly diagnosed breast cancer as a function of increasing age. The number of women diagnosed with breast cancer is very low in those younger than age 30 years, but increases steadily in those age 30 to 69 years, and is followed by a decline after age 79, likely due to increased age-related deaths.
Image from Ref. 105.

approximate a slightly higher value of 450 cases per 100 000 women (Figure 11.1).[105]

However, breast cancer is not strictly a disease of aging. While there is a positive correlation between the risk of developing breast cancer and increasing age, breast cancer can and does occur in young women and men. Furthermore, a number of factors beyond age and sex contribute to risk. A Northern European study that evaluated several cancer outcomes in twins (nearly 45 000 sets) determined that only about 27% of cancer risk was attributable to heritable factors (genetic predisposition being only a weak indicator), leaving another 73% of risk modifiable by lifestyle and environmental factors.[1] It has become increasingly clear that biological, social, and environmental factors, and the life stage at which exposures to environmental factors occur, play a substantial role in modifying the risk for developing and dying from breast cancer. Breast cancer is not a single disease process, but rather it is described as a number of different cancer subtypes with varying etiologies,[2,3] their tissue of origin being the common element. Given this complexity, certain forms of breast cancer are thought of more readily as diseases of aging. In fact, differential subtype distribution is exhibited by age,[4] making it less likely that there may be a single cure.

Irrespective of the often late age at diagnosis, breast cancer cannot be thought of simply as a disease of aging, because it may be that critical precursor incidents originate in early life. Normal programming events in the tissue begin in the fetus, continue into adolescence and adulthood, and may be adversely modified at multiple life stages.[5] As such, the timing of these life stage-specific events represent windows of sensitivity during which perturbations of normal processes–*via* chemical, pharmaceutical, or radiological assaults, for example–may alter normal development in a way that increases the vulnerability of the tissue to form tumors, particularly if the tissue receives multiple cumulative assaults. The goals of this chapter are to 1) inform on the critical life stages of the breast shown to exhibit susceptibility to environmental factors, 2) explain the importance of considering breast cancer as a complex, multiple-subtype set of cancers, influenced by environmental factors, and 3) discuss research gaps and promising new approaches to research that will move forward the fields of primary prevention and successful treatment of breast cancer.

11.1.2 Contemporary Breast Issues of Public Concern

The fact that 1 in 8 US women develop breast cancer over a lifetime,[6] and that this trend has not diminished in recent years, has prompted both a 2011 Institute of Medicine report, "Breast Cancer and the Environment: A Life Course Approach",[7] and a 2012 Federal Advisory Committee report, issued by the Interagency Breast Cancer and Environmental Research Coordinating Committee (IBCERCC),[8] calling for primary prevention of this costly disease. The large-scale efforts that have been made by federal agencies, reputable academicians, and nonprofit organizations to communicate the current understanding of and remaining questions surrounding breast cancer have resulted in increased public awareness of breast cancer's prevalence and the potential role of the environment in the disease. Along with breast cancer prevention, a number of other health concerns have gained attention in the field of breast biology, with a focus on adverse changes in the organ, particularly in children and adolescents.

Precocious or early puberty in girls has been an increasing public concern in recent years. While the designation of precocious puberty refers to the appearance of multiple secondary sexual characteristics before age 8, it is the earliest sign of puberty in girls—the appearance of breast buds—that will be addressed here.[9] Thelarche, the onset of breast development, in prepubertal girls is occurring at a younger age than it did two decades ago. An expert panel, convened to address the validity of this trend at the "Role of Environmental Factors on the Timing and Progression of Puberty" workshop, agreed that both thelarche and menarche are trending toward earlier occurrence in American girls from 1940 to 1994 but that the data on boys are insufficient to suggest a trend during this same time period.[10] The panel agreed that the weight of evidence deriving from both human and animal studies supported an association between exposures to endocrine-disrupting chemicals (EDCs) and the amount of body fat, with earlier pubertal end points.[11] Early pubertal landmarks were considered to be "adverse" from a public health perspective by this panel of experts.

In a study published in 1997,[12] premature thelarche was observed in 8% of white girls and 25% of black girls in a study of 17 000 American girls. However, in a study only 10 years later, breast bud development was observed at age 7 and 8, respectively, in 10% and 18% of white girls, and 23% and 43% of black girls (as well as 15% and 31% of Hispanic girls, not assessed in the prior study), suggesting that the incidence of precocious breast development among girls in the US is still increasing with time.[13] A similar decrease in the age of breast development has been noted in school age girls in Copenhagen, Denmark, without a correlated change in the hormones of puberty, suggesting a gonadatropin-independent shift in pubertal timing.[4,15] In fact, they demonstrated that after a 15 year follow-up, breast development was occurring up to 1 year earlier without a significant change in first menses timing. These studies suggest that the rapidly changing environment in which these children are developing may play an important role in this epidemic. There are a number of factors that may contribute to premature thelarche, and we will address these in concert with a discussion on the regulation and dysregulation of breast development. It should also be noted that although timing of breast development has shifted earlier over the last decades, time to first menses has changed very little, if statistically at all, confirming separate regulatory pathways for these pubertal landmarks.[10,14,16] With this large change in breast developmental timing, comes an increase in the time span from initiation of breast development to menarche[17] (see Table 11.1). Whether earlier breast developmental timing or longer time to full breast development is linked to breast cancer risk has not been determined in women.

Another contemporary issue in human breast health is gynecomastia, or the appearance of breast tissue in males. While gynecomastia can be a symptom of multiple disease processes involving hypogonadal or related conditions that interfere with normal testosterone synthesis in adult men, its etiology in boys is infrequently and incompletely understood. While the condition is not unusual in newborn boys, due to the high concentrations of maternal hormones in breast milk, it subsides over the 2–3 week period following birth. Older men, normally affected by decreasing circulating testosterone levels, may develop

Table 11.1 Approximate probability of Tanner Stage B2 (breast bud onset) or menarche in Copenhagen school girls in 1991–1993 and 2006–2008, relative to their chronological age.

Age	*Probability of B2* ***1991–1993 (n = 1100)***	*Probability of B2** ***2006–2008 (n = 995)***	*Probability of Menarche* ***1991–1993 (n = 1100)***	*Probability of Menarche* ***2006–2008 (n = 995)***
6	0	0	0	0
8	0	8%	0	0
10	20%	50%	5%	5%
12	75%	92%	10%	10%
14	100%	100%	60%	70%
16	100%	100%	95%	98%
Median:		**9.74 (95% CI: 9.59–10.01) years**		**13.05 (95% CI: 12.82–13.23) years**

Data estimated from Aksglaede *et al.* 2009, Figure 1. Median ages for puberty endpoints in 2006–2008 were Turnbull estimates.
*Significant acceleration in B2 from the prior measurements.

gynecomastia; it is estimated that 1 in 4 men between the ages of 50 and 80 are affected.[18] Puberty is another time in life when gynecomastia may be common. There exists a clear correlation between obesity and gynecomastia, although to be precise, gynecomastia is not simply an increase in adiposity in the chest, but entails specific growth of the glandular tissue.[19] Furthermore, it is well documented that fat cells produce the enzyme that converts steroid precursors to estrogens, which in turn can drive breast tissue growth in boys/men.[20] As is the case with females, the breast tissue of males is responsive to environmental exposures. One case study describes three prepubertal boys who developed significant breast enlargement following the use of a shampoo containing lavender and tea tree oils, compounds that are known to be without effect in adults, but are suspected to be estrogenic.[21]

In adult males, there is some concern that breast cancer may be misdiagnosed as gynecomastia, as both of these health disorders occur more often with age. Unlike gynecomastia, however, breast cancers are almost always unilateral, making confusion between these diagnoses less probable. Furthermore, breast cancer in men is relatively rare and accounts for only about 1% of all cases.[22] In fact, it is more than 100-fold more common in women. Whether gynecomastia predisposes a man to increased risk of breast cancer is a research area that merits further attention, because it is thought that altered circulating or local breast estrogen production may play a role in the development of both disease endpoints. Controlled estrogenic effects are important in early formation of both male and female breast tissue, a subject that we will turn our attention to here.

11.2 Breast Development

11.2.1 Overview of Unique Developmental Features

A complex and unique tissue, the breast exhibits important characteristics that result in substantial differences in the etiology, as well as our understanding of breast cancer, when compared to cancers of other tissues. Importantly, male and female breast tissue differs in both development and adult morphology, yet breast cancer can arise in both sexes. Also, unlike most organs, the female breast is affected by multiple events of development and differentiation across time, at multiple life stages, not limited to early life and puberty. The breast undergoes continuous change during the menstrual cycle, progressing from a simple gland to a well-budded array of ducts as the ovaries transition through the cycle. Also, in adult life during pregnancy and lactation, the breast exhibits profound tissue remodeling.[23] Around the age of 50, when the brain and ovaries begin to show signs of reproductive senescence, the breast transitions through a peri-menopausal series of structural changes, ending in a simple ductal frame. Furthermore, as a consequence, each event represents a unique opportunity for perturbation of the precise developmental processes that normally occur. That is, each time that the structure and composition of the gland changes during these tightly-regulated physiological events, there exists the potential for environmental factors to interfere with the processes, potentially altering the vulnerability of the glandular cells to develop into cancer.

11.2.2 Human Breast Development Timing and Regulation

Development of the human mammary gland begins during early fetal life. This process first involves the thickening of the milk streak—a band of cells in the ectoderm that will eventually develop into breast tissue—at 4–6 weeks of gestational age, followed by development of discrete mammary buds under the skin around 10–13 weeks of pregnancy. The supporting stroma is formed after this time, during approximately gestational weeks 20–32. Following development of the supporting stroma, and likely due to signals from those surrounding cells, the epithelium begins to branch through the mesenchyme during the second half of gestation, which allows the formation of a lumen within these epithelial structures. Important growth commences and functional receptors (*e.g.*, estrogen receptors) begin to be expressed as branching of these early ducts occurs prior to and up to the time of birth.[23–25]

At birth, the infant breast possesses secretory function and may exhibit fullness, which quickly dissipates along with the maternal source of hormones. The majority of breast development occurs after birth. The early neonatal breast tissue is a simple set of ducts with a few branches embedded in the surrounding stroma, all emptying into the nipple. Prior to puberty, the breast epithelium and supporting tissue grow isometrically, at the same rate as the body. At puberty, breast growth accelerates rapidly, growing allometrically. The breast typically does not reach full size until after menarche and when menstrual cycles become regular. Once this occurs, then the breast epithelium undergoes slight lobular structural changes each month, with the hormonal oscillations of the menstrual cycle. Additional rapid developmental events occur in the tissue during pregnancy. The gland transitions from a relatively restful state to one that very quickly fills the breast fat with differentiated lobulo-alveoli, ready to provide nourishment for the impending child. This process of lactational differentiation is a known protective factor against breast cancer.[26] The younger in life a woman gives birth, and potentially the more times this process of differentiation occurs in a woman's life, affects the amount of protection from breast cancer that is conferred. Although the exact mechanism for this protection is not known, many hypothesize that it is due to involution of the gland at weaning, which is a rapid regression of lobular structures due to extensive apoptosis. Involution-like structural changes occur in the breast again, peri-menopausally, with the accompanying systemic hormonal changes.[23–25]

Rodent mammary glands develop through similar processes as those described in humans, though the absolute amount of time for the various steps varies (see Figure 11.2 for a comparison). However, the relative amount of time spent in the different phases of development, the hormones and growth factors controlling the growth, the types of structures present, and the numerous periods of structural change over a lifetime are consistent across species.[8]

Developmental Event	Human	Rodent
milk streak evident	EW4-6	GD10-11 (mice)
mammary epithelial bud forms	EW10-13	GD12-14 (mice), GD 14-16 (rat)
female nipple and areola form	EW12-16	GD18 (mice)/GD20 (rat)
branching and canalization of epithelium	EW20-32	GD16 to birth (mice), GD 18 to birth (rat)
secretion is possible	EW32-40 (ability lost postnatally)	at birth, with hormonal stimuli
isometric development of ducts	birth to puberty	birth to puberty
TEBs present (peri-pubertal)	8-13 year old girls	23 to 60 days old (rodents)
formation of lobular units	EW32-40, or within 1-2 yr. of first menstrual cycle	puberty and into adulthood

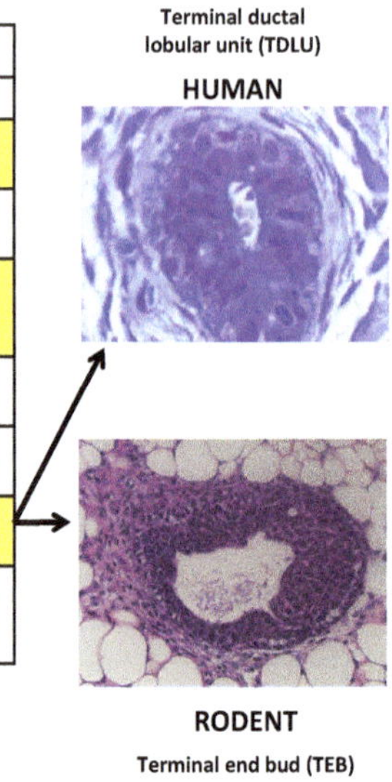

Figure 11.2 Similarity of developmental events in human and rodent mammary tissue over time. Photos depict the terminal end bud (TEB) in the rodent and the morphologically similar structure, terminal ductal lobular unit (TDLU), in the human. They are the most sensitive structures to environmental carcinogens. EW = embryonic week, GD = gestational day. (Table from Ref. 5 photos courtesy of J Russo and MB Macon).

Rodent model studies are the primary means by which an understanding of the developmental and hormone/growth factor-mediated events in humans, and their temporality, has been garnered. Figure 11.3 demonstrates the complex and dramatic changes the rodent mammary gland transitions through over the life course, from prepubertal development until old age. While rodents in general provide important animal models for breast studies, differences in 1) the specific timing of certain events (Figure 11.2), 2) the precise structures present in the gland, and 3) the predominance of specific tumor subtypes and location of metastases exist between species. This topic has been given a careful overview in the recent IBCERCC document.[8]

During the most rapid mammary growth phase—namely puberty—both rodents and humans develop rapidly dividing duct ends that lead the way in epithelial filling of the fat pad. Rodents exhibit end structures that are uniquely referred to as terminal end buds (TEBs). These terminal duct ends, found in both rats and mice, are tear-drop shaped, several cells thick, and are morphologically and functionally analogous to terminal ductal lobular units (TDLUs) in humans (see Figure 11.2 for a visual comparison). In both cases, these terminal sites for the growing ducts comprise clusters of rapidly proliferating cells, which give rise to the eventual adult parenchyma of the tissue. It should be noted that because of the highly proliferative nature of these structures, they are particularly vulnerable to carcinogens.[27] Put simply, in

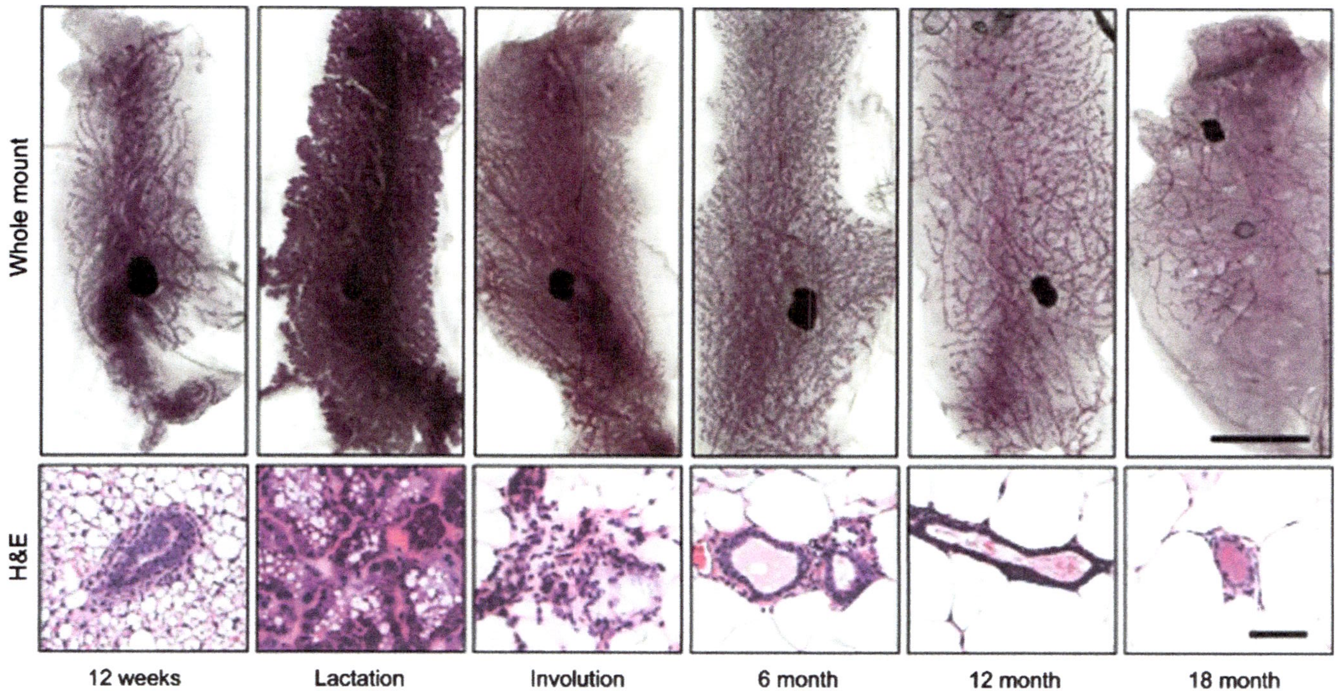

Figure 11.3 Mouse mammary gland morphogenesis. Carmine-stained whole mounts (top row) and hematoxylin- and eosin-stained sections (H&E, bottom row) provide images of fourth inguinal mammary glands. On the far left, 12-week old adult mice have developed a ductal tree that fills the fat pad. Lactating mice show extensive glandular growth and cellular differentiation, and this phenotype is rapidly lost during postlactational involution. Aging mice show gradual degeneration of the mammary gland so that by 18 months, only a spindly ductal structure remains. Scale bar for whole mount, 1 cm; for H&E, 50 μm. Image adapted from Ref. 28.

rapidly dividing cells, mutations, and other exposure-induced "errors" may more likely evade detection by the cellular repair machinery, and be incorporated into new cells and transmitted to future generations. The TDLU and TEBs are present only during the peripubertal period, making the time spent in this phase of development a sensitive window for environmental insults. This represents one example of how the breast may exhibit critical windows of susceptibility, and supports the argument that attempting to identify the assault or causative factors in breast carcinogenesis at the time of diagnosis has been a costly mistake. Is it theorized that girls who start breast development at an early age may be at a heightened susceptibility for breast cancer because they do not complete breast development until several years later, once they attain menses and normal menstrual cycles. Thus they may have TDLU in their breast tissue for longer periods of time than girls who seem to "develop overnight" and may be inadvertently exposing themselves to a variety of environmental insults.

11.3 Altered Breast Development

11.3.1 Altered Development in Humans

While studies of non-cancer endpoints in the human breast are most often logistically limited, certain developmental measures can be addressed in a non-invasive manner. These include the timing of breast appearance, as discussed previously, and lactational ability. Both of these measures can provide information concerning effects of the environment on the developing breast.

The trend for earlier breast development is clear, both in the US and in European cohorts.[15] While epidemiologic data have suggested associations between altered human breast development and exogenous chemical exposures—from both intentionally ingested materials such as packaged foods and personal care products, as well as contact with contaminated environmental materials—the specific causative agents have not been identified in most studies. The role of EDCs in altering breast timing has become apparent by accident, for example: an incident of increased breast enlargement in hundreds of young children in Milan, Italy, likely induced by estrogen-like contamination of their meat supply,[29] and an outbreak of early breast development in four young African-American girls who used shampoos that contained estrogen and placental extract exhibited reversible effects once the shampoo use ceased.[30]

There are very few examples of well-powered epidemiological studies that have demonstrated effects of lifestyle or the environment on breast developmental timing. One reason is the prohibitive costs associated with longitudinal studies of children, another is the complexity of the studies—mixture exposures, invasiveness of blood collection, rapid growth stage—and finally, long-term follow-up is required in order to relate early life exposures to later life health anomalies. One excellent example of an EDC that seems to affect breast developmental timing is dioxin, a pollutant readily formed upon combustion of plastics. The effects were initially identified following an accidental environmental release in Seveso, Italy. Significant delays in breast development have been documented in Seveso adolescents with the highest circulating blood levels of dioxin-like contaminants,[31] and similar delays in breast development have also been observed in Dutch children with the highest prenatal/lactational dioxin levels.[32] Although later life effects associated with higher dioxin exposure are not yet identifiable in the Netherlands cohort, an epidemiological study addressing cancer risk in Seveso, Italy, correlated TCDD exposure with an increased risk of breast cancer.[33] Specifically, the investigators found a breast cancer hazard ratio (HR) of 2.1 [95% confidence interval (CI), 1.0–4.6)] associated with 10-fold increases in serum TCDD levels. At the time that study was undertaken, the female participants with the greatest TCDD exposure were not yet between the ages of 40 and 60. A recent follow-up (conducted in 2008), determined that individual serum TCDD measurements were positively associated with overall cancer incidence among women, but there was a non-significant increase in the breast cancer hazard ratio (HR = 1.44; 95% CI, 0.89–2.33) associated with a 10-fold increase in serum TCDD over the approximately 30-year follow-up period.[34] Because this cohort of women were young when exposed to TCDD (between 0 and 40 years), some of them have still not reached menopause, thus future re-evaluation will help understand the age-related extent of risk of breast cancer associated with early life dioxin exposure.

There are even fewer examples of environmental effects on lactational impairment in women, even though it is clear that environmental chemicals can enter breast tissue, affect the gland, and be excreted into milk.[35,36] Again, there are many reasons that these types of studies have not been conducted. One reason is that the studies must involve large numbers of pregnant women that intend to breastfeed, so that women who want to breastfeed, but cannot, can be identified and studied. However, environmental exposures that prevent effective lactation may have their effects early in life, as already discussed, or during development of the lactating tissue of the breast, during pregnancy. Those effects would need to be teased out, and samples obtained prior to and during pregnancy would be most beneficial for analyses. One example of an EDC that may interfere with lactation time is the metabolite dichlorodiphenyl dichloroethene (DDE). DDE is formed from its parent compound, dichlorodiphenyltrichloroethane or DDT (highly used organochlorine insecticide), and is a highly persistent environmental chemical that is known to have estrogenic effects. Use of this compound has been eliminated in the US and many other countries, but it is still detected worldwide in milk and fat biospecimens. Infants of nearly 860 US mothers with higher levels of milk-borne DDE were breast-fed for shorter times; in fact there was a significant negative association between DDE levels and duration of lactation in all women and in first time lactations.[37]

Chemical tests in government and industry-run 2-year rodent bioassays, as well as specific studies addressing altered mammary gland development in rodent models, have allowed more precise identification of specific agents of concern. These studies have also illuminated the biochemical and histological details of altered development, shedding light on potential mechanisms by which altered development could predispose the tissue to cancer or compromised lactational function.

11.3.2 Altered Development in Rodent Studies

Extensive rodent studies have been performed to date to determine the health effects of only about 1–2% of the chemicals on the US market.[38] However, not all of these tests have included evaluation of the mammary gland. The number of test chemicals assessed for mammary-specific effects is dwarfed by the number assessed for more traditional endpoints of interest, such as hepatotoxicity or mutagenicity. Often, the mammary gland is overlooked during testing if a gross tumor is not visually observed at necropsy.[39] This is unfortunate, as rodents exhibit mammary development that parallels that of humans, and as such offer a unique opportunity to examine the histological origins and mechanisms of environmentally-induced alterations in mammary gland development.

The entire rodent mammary gland can be slide-mounted and stained in order to visualize the parenchymal epithelium within the stroma of the fat pad. This preparation of the sample allows assessments of such developmental measures as the length of ductal outgrowth, number of duct branch points, and the presence and number of structures associated with the developmental stage of the gland, such as TEBs in younger animals, lobules and terminal ducts in mature animals, and lobulo-alveoli in lactating dams. Changes in these endpoints, along with stromal and immune cell changes, among treated animals as compared to concurrent controls, suggest the potential for the agent to alter normal mammary gland development and function.

The agents observed to impact the rodent gland are frequently grouped into classes, including (1) carcinogens, and (2) EDCs, which are further broken down into (a) steroid hormones, both exogenous (pharmaceuticals) and endogenous, (b) phytoestrogens, from dietary exposure to certain plants, (c) environmental metals, and (d) chemicals, used in a variety of products ranging from food packaging and upholstery to pesticides and personal care products. For EDCs, the potential mode of action is almost certainly deemed to be hormonal in nature—as it is with steroid hormones and phytoestrogens—though the specific mechanisms of action may vary substantially between agents. A short list of compounds is now known to alter rodent mammary gland development after early life exposures, including (but not limited to) atrazine, bisphenol A (BPA), dibutylphthalate, diethylstilbestrol (DES), dioxin, methoxychlor, nonylphenol, phytoestrogens, polybrominated diphenyl ethers, and perfluorooctanoic acid (PFOA).[38] While this is a structurally disparate group of chemicals, there is the suggestion that because of their mammary gland-specific outcomes, there may be some common mode(s) of action among them, resulting in a similar phenotypic effect.

Given this, it is important to add to the discussion of environmental factors that their potential contribution to breast cancer risk may not simply be by direct action. Rather, those environmental factors which are known or suspected to alter development may contribute to risk of cancer by predisposing the tissue to secondary assaults from other environmental agents. This is referred to as the two-hit model,[40] wherein the agent affects development in such a way as to increase its basal vulnerability to a secondary event. Examples of these types of effects might include an increase in certain receptor types making the tissue more sensitive to a ligand, an increase in stromal density, altered inflammatory cell populations, or an increase in the number of ductal cells. Secondary events might come in the form of another environmental exposure at a later point in life, or a genetically-driven event such as a mutated tumor suppressor gene that allows precancerous cells to evade detection and elimination. Examples of the numerous effects of EDCs and carcinogens on mammary development, lactation, and breast cancer are shown in Tables 11.2 and 11.3 respectively. These tables and corresponding references were previously presented in the IBCERCC document. This is not an all-inclusive list, but demonstrates some similarity of effects across species.

11.4 Breast Cancer

11.4.1 It's not all about Genetics

As discussed previously, breast cancer is a prevalent cancer in women worldwide, increasing in probability with age. It was once believed that the basis for diseases such as breast cancer was genetics or a single mutagenic event.[41] However, epidemiologic evidence suggests that only a small proportion of breast cancer cases (approximately 5–10%)[6] are determined by gene-based inheritance, such as a single gene mutation like BRCA 1 or 2, and only 10–30% of the breast cancer cases can be attributed to heritable factors of any kind.[1,42] Over the last several years, novel genes that contribute to breast cancer risk in some families have been discovered. One example is the ATM gene, which causes severe disease when both alleles are mutated, but can increase risk of breast cancer in some women when only one allele is mutated.[43] Nonetheless, somewhere between 70–90% of all breast cancer cases are influenced by lifestyle or environment. Currently, a number of environmental factors have been identified as known/accepted risk factors,[6,8,44] and many more remain possible contributors to breast cancer risk.

11.4.2 Known/Accepted, Non-Genetic Risk Factors

As discussed throughout, two risk factors of primary importance in breast cancer are sex—being female—and age. These are clearly risk factors that are not within an individual's control. But, within these overlying risk factors are other modifiable risk factors, or risk factors that can be altered by an individual or a population. Some modifiable risk factors include being overweight, a lack of exercise, and eating a diet low in vegetables, fruits, and whole grains and fiber. Specifically, a body mass index (BMI) of 25 or higher increases the risk for breast cancer after menopause.[45] However, some studies have suggested that a high BMI, a BMI of 31 or higher, may reduce the risk of breast cancer

Table 11.2 Examples of endocrine disrupting chemicals affecting the breast. (Taken from Ref. 8.)

Endocrine Disruptor	*Description*	*Animal*, in vivo, in vitro	*Human epidemiology*
Bisphenol A (BPA)	• A component of polycarbonate plastics and epoxy resins • Large production volume • Widespread human exposure • Leaches into food through food container linings • Found in dental sealants and composites • "Weak" estrogen	• Binds to nuclear ER-α and -β • Activates membrane-bound form of the ER (ncmER), estrogen-related receptor gamma (ERR-γ), GPR30, and aryl hydrocarbon receptor (AhR); possible thyroid hormone and androgen receptor interaction • Induces hyperplastic lesions in mammary tissue of prenatally exposed mice and rats, at doses that approach human exposures • Alters growth of non-human primate mammary gland • Increases susceptibility to carcinogen-induced mammary tumors in rodents	None
Nonylphenol	• Found in the lining of food containers and wraps, cleaning compounds, and spermicides • Known to have estrogenic properties	• Induces dose-dependent increase in mammary cell proliferation, mammary epithelial branching and budding, and hastened differentiation in prenatally exposed female rats • Produces DNA mutations and chromosomal abnormalities, with increased tumor risk	None
Phthalates	• Used to soften plastics for medical tubing and children's toys • Disperses or retains scent in health/beauty products	• Abnormal mammary alveolar branching and hypoplasia in female perinatally-exposed rats • Retained nipples in perinatally-exposed adolescent male rats	• One study showing increased breast cancer risk in Northern Mexico cohort of women at highest phthalate burden

	• Widespread environmental contamination; has been measured in human infants following critical care procedures	• Dilation of mammary alveolar buds and ducts in adult male rats • BBP increased proliferative index of TEBs and altered genomic profile in weanling rats	
Metals	• Naturally occurring, they mimic or perturb normal hormonal milieu • Exposure through water, air, and cigarette smoking	• Cadmium can alter mammary development in mice and rats with low levels of prenatal exposure mimicking estrogen	• Urinary cadmium levels in women associated with a Breast Imaging-Reporting and Data Systems (BI-RADS®) density category of "extremely dense"
Dichlorodiphenyl-trichloroethane (DDT) (MIXTURE)	• Insecticide that controls insect-borne disease • Use peaked in US in 1959 • Banned by US EPA in 1972 • Degrades to *p,p′*-DDE, the most prevalent and persistent metabolite in the environment	• DDT and congeners known to exhibit anti-androgenic and estrogenic activity • Limited evidence for acting as a promoter of mammary tumors in rats	• No associations in pooled and meta-analysis; one study showing early life exposure associated with increased breast cancer risk in women
Dieldrin	• Persistent agricultural pesticide • Used in US from 1950s to 1970s; US ban in 1987	• Causes increased tumor burden in Her2/neu transgenic mice exposed during pregnancy and lactation	• One prospective study showed positive association
Polychlorinated biphenyls (PCBs) (MIXTURE)	• Mixed set of organochlorine isomers • Bioaccumulate in the body • Known exposures from fish, milk • Varying modes of action – some estrogenic, androgenic, or dioxin-like	• Affect pubertal endpoints in girls and rodents • Possible mutant p53 interaction	• Majority of studies null; suggestions from several studies that high PCB levels and CYP1A1 genotypes may interact to increase breast cancer risk • Declared 'possibly carcinogenic' to humans by IARC/EPA

Table 11.2 (*Continued*)

Endocrine Disruptor	*Description*	*Animal*, in vivo, in vitro	*Human epidemiology*
Atrazine	• One of the most heavily used herbicides on food and grain crops in the U.S. • Its use is banned in the European Union. • Unknown mode of action in mammary tissue	• Causes early onset of mammary tumors and an increased incidence of tumors in specific rat strains. • Alters pubertal timing in rodents • Promotes mammary tumor proliferation in rodent models • Deters development of mammary tissue and impacts lactational ability in rats	• Ecologic data for well water and breast cancer risk • One proposed mode of action for atrazine-induced rat mammary tumors, accelerated reproductive senescence, was declared not relevant for breast tumorigenesis in humans by the FIFRA SAP in 2000.
2,3,7,8-tetrachlorodibenzo-p-dioxin (TCDD)	• Industrial incineration and chemical reaction-dependent pollutant • Bioaccumulative, lipophilic contaminant • Binds the aryl hydrocarbon receptor (AhR) • Known carcinogen	• Increased susceptibility of mammary tumor incidence and shorter latency in developmentally exposed female rats exposed to carcinogen • Alters pubertal endpoints in rodents	• Slowed breast development in highest-exposed girls in 2 countries • Suggestive data for breast cancer from industrial accident in Seveso, Italy – not conclusive
Polybrominated Diphenyl Ether (PBDE) (MIXTURE)	• Widely used to retard fire ignition time in textiles, construction materials, and polymers used in electronics • Bioaccumulative and lipophilic compound	• Altered reproductive endpoints in rodents; delayed mammary gland development, and thyroid hormone and behavioral alterations • Effects on breast cancer risk not yet assessed	None
Perfluorooctanoic Acid (PFOA)	• Possesses long half-life in humans (2–4 years) and mice • Used in fire-fighting foams, electronics, and to make products that are grease- and water-proof • Final degradation product of other >8-carbon perfluorinated materials	• Effects on mammary gland of mice include delayed development, altered lactation, decreased weight gain in offspring, and changes in gene expression • Mammary delays at body burdens that overlap with human exposure burden in contaminated parts of the US	• Delayed pubertal timing in girls • Low-powered case-control study of Greenlandic Inuit women demonstrated significant correlation of serum perfluorinated chemicals and breast cancer risk

A large amount of information on pesticides is included in this section because much work has occurred in this area. US EPA has helped to accelerate knowledge of potential health effects of pesticides by requiring testing before they are marketed.

prior to menopause.[46] Obesity—defined as a BMI ≥ 30–further modifies not only incidence, but also survival, and is associated with lower survival, whether diagnosis is pre- or postmenopausal.[47] In addition to measured BMI, weight gain (specifically during adult life) may contribute to postmenopausal cancer risk, but be protective against premenopausal cancer risk. Interestingly, height alone (one component of BMI) has been positively associated with increased risk for both pre- and postmenopausal breast cancer.[45,48]

Alcohol consumption is another known contributor to breast cancer risk, and increasing consumption is correlated with increasing risk. A meta-analysis conducted on data from 53 epidemiological studies, on 58 515 women with invasive breast cancer and 95 067 controls, specifically found that for each additional 10 grams of alcohol consumed per day, relative risk of breast cancer was significantly increased by 7.1% (95% CI, 5.5–8.7%).[49] Furthermore, other studies have replicated this finding, and a recent study from the Nurses' Health Study has shown that even low alcohol intake can be a contributor to breast cancer risk. The risk from low alcohol intake was independent of age, but was associated with ER+/PR+ tumor subtypes.[50] Furthermore, it has also been demonstrated that risk imparted by alcohol consumption is entirely independent of smoking status, and is the same in both smokers and non-smokers.[51]

Increased breast density is considered one of the strongest risk factors for breast cancer, regardless of how it has been measured.[52] Women with the highest measures of breast density have a 4- to 6-fold increased risk of breast cancer *versus* women with non-dense breasts.[53] Breast density is thought to be a "stronger risk factor for breast cancer than any others except age and genetic mutations".[52] Breast density, while not strictly genetic, is not an environmental factor in the same respect as most of those described here. The density of the breast reflects the epithelial and stromal contributions to the breast, and can be measured subjectively or quantitatively. The most common measure of breast density in the clinical setting is the Breast Imaging Reporting and Data Systems (BI-RADS) density method. This is a subjective measure used by radiologists to classify a mammogram as follows: D1: Fatty; D2: Scattered density; D3: Heterogeneously dense; or D4: Extremely dense. Computer-assisted methods are also available to provide quantitative measures of breast density.[54,55] The density of the tissue can be altered by hormonal status, BMI, prior pregnancies, and lactational events, as well as life-stage, such as menopausal status.[56] Those factors which are known to affect density are also independent contributors to breast cancer risk. While the precise mechanism by which density increases risk is unknown, some environmental chemicals, such as PFOA and BPA, have been shown to increase mammary gland density in animal studies following prenatal exposures.[57,58] Similarly, increased risk is imparted by having a personal history of benign breast disease, such as atypical ductal hyperplasia, atypical lobular hyperplasia, and a history of prior biopsies.

A number of known environmental risk factors are linked to hormone status, and the function of the tissue. Specifically, these risk factors are linked to a woman's lifetime exposure to estrogen and progesterone. Having children late in life or not having children at all increases one's risk of developing breast cancer.[59–62] Independent of pregnancy, never breast feeding also contributes to cancer risk.[63] Early age at menarche (first period, not including breast developmental timing) and late age at menopause also contribute to total lifetime exposure to the normal steroid hormones and increase breast cancer risk in both the US and other countries.[64–66] While the precise mechanisms behind these risk factors are not known, it is believed that the increased number of menstrual cycles over the life time causes an elevation in overall breast cell proliferation events, which may increase the risk for mutations to be incorporated into cell populations and give rise to cancer. Direct evidence that hormonal status during specific life stages contributes to risk is now available due to the large number of women that took estrogen and progesterone (combined) hormone therapy, only to have a significantly increased risk of breast cancer.[67] Another example is that women who have recent steroid hormone contraceptive use are at an increased risk for breast cancer *versus* those women that used contraceptives over 10 years prior to diagnosis.[68] Timing of exposure does seem to be a critical element, that keeps recurring as this field rapidly progresses.

Diethylstilbestrol (DES) is a synthetic estrogen that was given to pregnant women between the 1940s and 1970s, ostensibly to reduce the risk of miscarriage. It is now known that DES is a potent reproductive carcinogen to the developing fetus. In a cohort of exposed ($\sim$4800) and unexposed ($\sim$2100) women followed since the 1970s, breast cancer risk among women exposed to DES *in utero* was significantly elevated, and that population exhibited an overall hazard ratio (HR) of 1.82 (95% confidence interval (CI), 1.04–3.18), with the highest risks being exhibited among those with the highest cumulative gestational doses.[69,70] When broken down more carefully by age, women $\geq$ 40 years of age had a hazard ratio of 1.91 (95% CI, 1.09–3.33), and women $\geq$50 years of age exhibited an even higher risk of 3.00 (95% CI, 1.01–.98).[70] In the most recent analysis of data from these women,[69] there was nearly a 2-fold higher chance of breast cancer in DES-exposed daughters than those not exposed (3.9% vs. 2.2%; HR, 1.82; 95% CI, 1.04–3.18). Furthermore, the mothers who were prescribed the drug also exhibited an increased risk of breast cancer, with a relative risk of 1.4 (95% CI, 1.1–1.9).[71]

As DES and early menarche illustrate, exposure to certain chemicals or endogenous hormones during early life, respectively, is known to contribute to breast cancer risk. Additionally, early exposure to ionizing radiation is also a known contributor to risk. Unfortunately, most of these data derive from populations exposed to nuclear weapon detonations at Hiroshima and Nagasaki, where exposure increased the risk of developing breast cancer, especially among those that received the exposure during adolescence.[72–74] Similarly, exposure of the breast area to radiation for diagnostic or treatment purposes increases the risk of developing cancer by more than four-fold, especially if the exposure occurs before age 30 or if the subpopulation exhibits genetic susceptibilities that predispose them to breast cancer.[75] These data are primarily from women who were treated for scoliosis, recurrent infections of the lung, cancer unrelated to the breast, or upper gastrointestinal tract problems in their adolescent or teenage years.

11.4.3 Possible Environmental Risk Factors

In addition to known contributors to risk, there are a number of environmental factors that may not have yet been accepted as risk factors, given limited epidemiologic data. Animal studies however, have provided some opportunity to test the potential for factors to alter breast cancer risk in validated models for human breast cancer, when these factors have not yet been studied in humans. Conversely, some factors have been suspected in human risk, but have not yet been validated in animal studies.

Childhood BMI has been suggested to be positively correlated with breast cancer risk. Obesity in childhood is implicated in early puberty,[76] and both obesity and early puberty may cause increased endogenous estrogen exposure over the lifetime. Both the higher levels of circulating estrogens and the potentially greater duration of time from menarche to menopause could contribute to higher lifetime exposures to estrogens and thus higher risk of developing breast cancer. Studies in mice however, have not found a clear association between high dietary fat intake and mammary gland development, as Balb/c and C57BL/6 exhibit opposing responses—absence of weight gain and stimulation of gland development in the former, as compared to weight gain and inhibition of gland development in the latter.[77] Environmental chemicals can induce both obesity[78] and altered puberty timing (discussed previously). Therefore, it is possible that environmental factors are affecting not only the breast, but also a modifiable component, body fat.

There is some evidence that healthy dietary patterns may protect against breast cancer. It was documented many years ago that when Asian women immigrate to the US, their incidence of breast cancer increases and this increased risk is transferred to subsequent generations, such that they reach the incidence rates of white American women.[79] It is broadly accepted that modifiable exposures related to lifestyle or environment (*i.e.*, dietary components, industrial chemical exposure, health and beauty aids), and not genetics, explain the international differences in breast cancer risk. One meta-analysis found an 11% decrease in breast cancer risk within the group with the healthiest eating habits as compared to those in the least healthy.[80] Studies in both Chinese and the Korean populations found that eating Western diets as opposed to traditional diets contributed to breast cancer risk.[81,82]

Dietary exposures of concern also includes phytoestrogen intake. Phytoestrogens are plant-derived compounds, structurally and pharmacologically similar to mammalian estrogens. The phytoestrogen content of soy is particularly high and thought to impart the proposed health benefits of soy foods. Often, a contemporary "healthy" diet includes reduced intake of animal products, replaced instead with soy products, such as tofu and soy milk. Genistein is the most studied of the phytoestrogens present in soy foods. Its actions on the developing mammary gland have been studied because soy formula use for infants became increasingly popular in the US in the late 1980s and 1990s.[83] Effects of soy on the developing mammary tissue in both rats and mice vary substantially, based on the route and timing of exposure, as well as the dose and rodent strain.[84] For example, postnatal exposures in the rat appeared to accelerate the structural maturation of the gland, and in one study, even increase the multiplicity of mammary tumors,[85] whereas prenatal exposures in the mouse slowed structural maturation of the gland.[86] While these data may appear conflicting, they highlight the significance of timing in determining the outcome in the mammary gland of an event such as a dietary or chemical exposure. Most studies of genistein however, have examined exposures during development and tell little about potential protective effects of adult dietary exposure and breast cancer risk. Decreased soy intake may also be a major component of increased breast cancer risk in immigrant Asian women, as discussed above.

Working at night, also referred to as shift work, is considered a probable risk factor for breast cancer, and the mechanism by which it induces carcinogenesis is likely through the suppression of melatonin that results from altered light–dark timing and subsequently an altered circadian rhythm. Studies in rodent models have confirmed these hypotheses. The contribution of shift work to breast cancer risk specifically has not been definitively identified, though one review found that six of nine epidemiologic studies suggested a moderate increase in breast cancer risk with shift work.[87]

As discussed, in the case of DES, chemical exposures have the capacity to greatly alter breast cancer risk. A number of synthetic chemicals in personal care products or present in the environment as pollutants, have been pinpointed as estrogenic agents that women and girls are likely to come into contact with, which may disrupt normal hormone signaling and ultimate risk factors in breast carcinogenesis. Animal studies have demonstrated the endocrine-disrupting capacity for agents such as BPA and polybrominated diphenyl ethers, and they have been supported with human data for agents such as phthalates, dichlorodiphenyl trichloroethane (DDT), dioxin, polychlorinated biphenyls, and certain heavy metals. These all represent agents that may thus have the capacity to contribute to breast cancer risk, if exposure occurs at the appropriate life-stage. More information of the effects of these chemicals on risk for breast cancer can be found in Table 11.2, and in the appendix of the IBCERCC document.[8]

11.4.4 Effect-Modifying Factors

11.4.4.1 Ethnicity–Subtype Interaction

The genetic makeup, race, and/or ethnicity of populations (not just individuals) are known to be risk factor(s) for breast cancer. Importantly, these underlying factors that cannot be changed by an individual, can impart specific risks when combined with the many risk factors already discussed. It is now clear that women of African–American descent are more apt to be diagnosed with more aggressive, harder to treat tumor subtypes (*i.e.*, ER negative) than are women of European ancestry.[88] African–American girls also appear to be the most affected by changes in puberty timing[13] and childhood obesity,[89] and display more severe Vitamin D deficiency, as well as exhibiting increased gene polymorphisms in the Vitamin D receptor pathway, which may make them more prone to ER negative tumor development.[90] The Carolina Breast Cancer Study has also determined that basal-like tumors (triple-negative) were seen at the highest incidence among premenopausal African–American women.[91] This type of tumor is among the most likely to cause poor prognosis.

11.4.4.2 Smoking

Even though smoking is known as a risk factor for overall cancer, its effect-modifying actions on tissue-specific cancers is not definitive. Cigarettes contain many chemicals identified as carcinogens.[92] Tobacco smoke can induce enzyme reactions known to induce estrogenic and anti-estrogenic effects in specific cells of the body. For many years, the link between smoking and breast cancer risk was seen as weak; some studies detected an association, while others did not. However, that changed when the risk for breast cancer took into consideration gene-by-environment interactions. Specifically, when numerous studies were pooled to form a cohort of more than 5000 cases and 5000 controls, and the data was reanalyzed (a meta-analysis), the results showed that women expressing genetic variants of NAT2 had slowed detoxification of the carcinogenic compounds in tobacco smoke. These women were at increased risk of breast cancer due to smoking.[93] However, another well-powered re-analysis of several cohorts did not find associations between NAT2 gene variants and breast cancer risk.[94] More recently, 8772 women with breast cancer, in a cohort of 111 140 participants (Nurses' Health Study), were studied for effects of smoking. The investigators determined that active smoking was associated with a modest increase in breast cancer risk, especially if that smoking occurred prior to the first birth.[95] Furthermore, the Canadian Expert Panel on Tobacco Smoke and Breast Cancer Risk[96] concluded that "1)... the association between active smoking and both pre- and postmenopausal breast cancer are consistent with causality", and "2) The association between second-hand smoke and breast cancer in younger, primarily premenopausal women who have never smoked is consistent with causality".

Although the specific environmental factors discussed could be thought of as either effect-modifying factors, or in some cases true risk factors, the notion of a "first-hit" in a "two-hit" model is an important line of discussion. That is, an agent that contributes a first hit would initiate or predispose the tissue to an increased susceptibility to a secondary agent, which would then promote the carcinogenesis event. Tables 11.2 and 11.3 give several examples of environmental factors, both potentially one hit (carcinogens) and two-hit (EDC) compounds, that have been shown to have an association with breast cancer in women. Volatile organic chemicals, such as benzene and the dry cleaning agent, trichloroethylene have been hypothesized to have caused an outbreak of breast

Table 11.3 Examples of chemical carcinogens affecting the breast. (Taken from Ref. 8.)

Chemical	*Description*	*Animal*, in vivo, in vitro	*Human epidemiology*
Tobacco Smoke (MIXTURE)	• Cigarettes contain about 3600 chemicals • Affects the metabolism and/or mutagenicity of hormones and/or other carcinogens in breast tissue • Human studies demonstrate that tobacco constituents can reach breast tissue	• Of over 60 known carcinogens in tobacco smoke, several are known to induce mammary tumors in lab animals	• The Canadian Expert Panel on Tobacco Smoke and Breast Cancer Risk declares that both active and passive smoke exposure increase breast cancer risk • The Nurses' Health Study confirms that active smoking, especially prior to first child, increases breast cancer risk
Polycyclic Aromatic Hydrocarbons (PAHs) (MIXTURE)	• Formed from incomplete combustion of hydrocarbons • Pervasive in the environment	• Induce mammary tumors in laboratory rats	• Presence of PAH-DNA adducts is associated with breast cancer risk in Long Island Breast Cancer Project • Associations between PAHs and breast cancer risk could be restricted to subgroups of women with high-risk genotypes
Aryl Aromatic Amines	• Exposure from mainstream and passive tobacco smoke, synthetic fuels, and from metabolic reduction of polycyclic nitroaromatic hydrocarbons (ubiquitous in diesel exhaust and in airborne particulates)	• Some aryl aromatic amines are potentially mutagenic and carcinogenic to human breast cells • Induces mammary tumor formation in rodents	• Pooled and meta-analysis showing increased risk with smoking for women with slow N-acetyltransferase genotypes (detoxifies aromatic amines)

Heterocyclic Amines (HCAs)	• Formed when meat is cooked • Present in tobacco smoke	• Some are powerful mammary carcinogens in rodents	• 2010 Meta-analysis demonstrated a 17% increase in odds of breast cancer, determined by meat intake (31 epidemiological studies represented)
N-*Nitrosamines*	• Exposure through diet, endogenous formation in the stomach, tobacco smoke, occupation, rubber products, and medical therapies • Have been detected in pacifiers and baby bottle nipples • Mutagenic compounds	• Induce rodent mammary tumors that are histologically similar to human cancers and can metastasize • Transform cultured mouse mammary cells • Cause cultured human mammary epithelial cells to undergo unscheduled DNA synthesis	• None

cancer in men and women in a Marine base in NC and other parts of the US.[97,98]

Many examples of these compounds being successful first and second "hits" in rodent models for breast cancer also exist. For example, the high use herbicide, atrazine has been shown to exacerbate tumor development in both mice and rats,[99–101] acting as a second hit to alter the hormonal milieu, creating a permissive environment for tumor development. Secondly, Table 11.2 lists numerous EDCs that demonstrate a first hit, where an increased number of rapidly proliferating target cells (TEBS) are present for an extended period of time following an early life exposure to the EDC. The increased population of TEBs are then at the mercy of another chemical or carcinogen exposure that comes along. Without the "first hit" of the endocrine disrupting chemical during development, the "second-hit" or the carcinogenic agent, might have had too few targets, probabilistically, to plant the seeds of future carcinogenesis.

11.5 Conclusions

11.5.1 Life-Stage Consideration is Crucial

An important modifier, and possibly the most significant outside of sex, is the stage of life at which an individual diagnosed with breast cancer experiences an exposure—radiological, chemical, pharmaceutical—potentially determining lifetime breast cancer risk. The timing or life-stage—neonatal, peripubertal, lactational, pre-menopausal, postmenopausal, *etc.*—at which one of the known or suspected risk factors previously listed is encountered is a critical element in breast cancer risk[5,8,44] (See Figure 11.4). The timing of early life environmental exposures or lifestyle modifications can cause accelerated weight gain as a child, altered pubertal timing, and even delayed conception of the first child, all of which are known to substantially modify breast cancer risk.

A few recent human studies, as well as numerous animal studies, have supported the hypothesis that the life-stage during which specific environmental factors are present plays a key role in the contribution of those environmental factors to breast cancer risk. For at least three decades, the majority of studies examining environmental factors that were associated with breast cancer diagnoses measured factors present around the time of diagnosis. As discussed, epidemiologic evidence from exposure to DES and ionizing radiation offered the first solid proof of the sensitivity of life-stage with respect to the outcome of the exposure, as well as the high latency between exposure and the changes in the gland, which may culminate in breast cancer.

Since the mid-1990s, several nested case-control and case-control studies have been conducted, and most have not observed a significant association between breast cancer risk and serum, or adipose tissue levels of DDT or its degradate, *p,p′*-DDE, the most prevalent and persistent metabolite in the environment. However, a fairly recent study took a novel approach and evaluated the risk of breast cancer in women based not only on how much

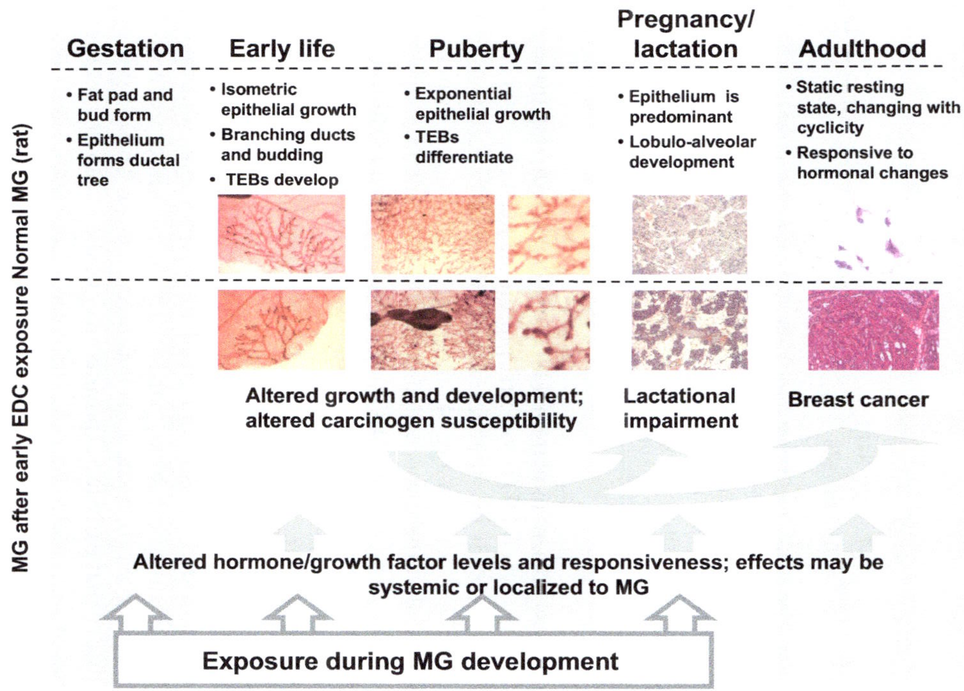

Figure 11.4 Stages of normal rat MG development and effects of environment on subsequent events. Effects of early life EDC exposures can lead to altered developmental programming in the breast and have been reported neonatally, at puberty, and well into adulthood, when effects on lactation or mammary tumorigenesis become evident. The normal morphology and pace of pubertal development are often altered, and these effects can be observed using MG whole-mount preparations. Transient or permanent effects may be due to gene imprinting, altered gene expression, modified endogenous MG signaling, or changes in hormonal milieu. Arrows indicate plausible (black) or more certain (gray) mechanistic pathways. Photomicrographs for early life and puberty were all taken at 16× magnification on a macroscope (adapted from Ref. 104); photomicrographs for pregnancy/lactation and adulthood were taken at 10× magnification on a standard microscope (from SE Fenton). Bars = 2 mm. Adapted from Ref. 38.

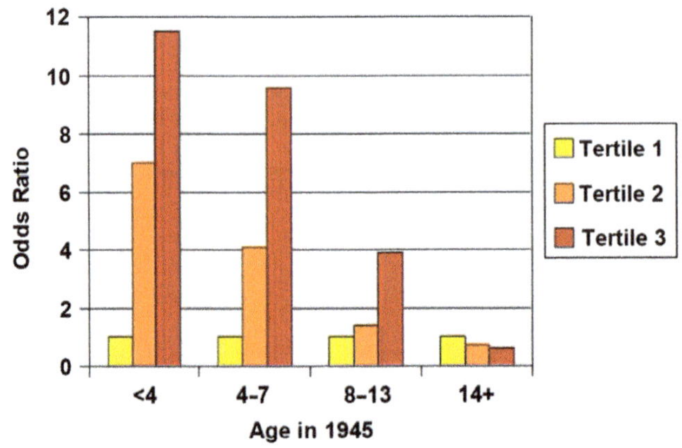

Figure 11.5 Associations of serum *p,p'*-DDT with early breast cancer in mothers in the Child Health and Development Studies, according to their age in 1945, a proxy for age at first exposure to DDT. Tertiles are based on the distribution of the *p,p'*-DDT in the controls. Tertile 1 is the reference category for odds ratios shown. Breast cancer is defined as diagnosis before age 50. See 102 for details.
Adapted from Ref. 103.

measurable compound was present in maternal blood prior to birth, but also on how old the individual was when DDT was first put on the market in 1945.[102] This study reported a significant five-fold rise in risk of breast cancer among women exposed to *p,p'*-DDT prior to age 14, and when broken down into age increments demonstrated that there was a significant effect of potential age of exposure on breast cancer risk (see Figure 11.5 for specifics). In an evaluation of the existing epidemiologic literature on DDT exposure and breast cancer risk, Cohn reports that the studies to date have been limited in their ability to assess exposure during early life, when windows of sensitivity exist for the breast, thus may be failing to link DDT causally to breast cancer.[103] Cohn uses DDT as a case study, and specifically points out that epidemiologic studies are often designed in a manner that focuses on immediate observations, and thus limits their potential to identify causality, particularly with disease processes that entail extended periods of progression, such as breast cancer. These reports further support the theory that early life exposures may be the most relevant for breast cancer etiology.

Epidemiological efforts are unlikely to clearly identify risk factors linked to life-stage without performing longitudinal studies. With such potential risk factors as elevated BMI in childhood, advanced puberty timing, and exposure to mixtures of environmental compounds, longitudinal studies will need to be conducted, ideally with existing cohorts, in order to follow participants with known childhood medical histories through menopause and beyond. This would allow us to gain a realistic picture of the roles of such factors in breast cancer risk, as well as further understanding of the time(s) in an individual's life when they are most sensitive to these factors.

11.5.2 Prevention – a Primary Purpose or an Afterthought?

Transdisciplinary research—that which brings together multiple facets of research, such as animal biologists and clinicians working hand-in-hand on a single question—may be the fastest and most efficient way to determine what environmental factors we must avoid and if and when we are to begin to *prevent* breast cancer. Prevention, in this context, is meant as simply that—we decrease the incidence of breast cancer because we stopped the exposures that caused it. This is the same idea that is conveyed in the "no texting while driving" laws. If you stop texting while driving, the number of drivers killed in accidents will go down to the level prior to the texting explosion. Because this disease takes many, many years from exposures to disease, animal models will be critical tools in gaining further understanding of life-stage sensitivities and the classes of chemicals that contribute to breast cancer risk. Mechanisms to "shelter" sensitive tissues from events that contribute to breast cancer risk, regulations to monitor or eliminate exposures such as early life clinical radiation and inadvertent chemical exposures in our water supply, laws to enable risk assessors to crack down on environmental polluters, federal testing that requires evaluation of mammary gland effects for every new pharmaceutical and chemical that comes onto the market, and training of the next generation of clinicians in environmental health sciences are imperative. That is, we must prevent exposures as much as possible, by reducing exposures cumulatively and especially during these sensitive windows of susceptibility. We must also inform the public, and it will be especially important to include outreach specialists and breast cancer advocates in the transdisciplinary studies outlined previously. There might be intentional efforts to reduce levels of chemicals of concern in products—such as baby bottles or formula for infants, makeup or jewelry targeted toward peri-pubertal girls, and our health and beauty-aid products intended for daily use, like toothpaste and anti-perspirant—which might be used by pregnant and lactating women and their children during these windows of sensitivity.

Further preventative measures might include moving toward green chemistry, as a means of reducing exposure to estrogenic and carcinogenic agents, and promoting healthy living through better diets, greater physical activity, and reduced contact with agents known to contribute to risk. Education will also continue to be a primary element in prevention, with an end goal of minimizing exposure.

11.5.3 Future Research – Age or Stage?

To begin the long road toward prevention of this disease that affects both young and old women and men, we need far greater knowledge of the specific environmental factors that are found in cord blood, infant, child, and adolescent blood or urine, and breast milk so that we can mitigate the exposures in the body during influential developmental stages of the breast. Specifically in the case of men, we have no idea what the risk factors might be for breast cancer. Continued research will be needed in order to further elucidate which breast life-stages are most susceptible to which combination of assaults. Complementary epidemiologic and animal studies will be needed in order to identify human-specific risk to these exposures, and determine the mechanistic underpinnings. The influence of environmental factors on individuals of different ethnicities/race, socio-economic status, and tumor subtype is expected to vary. It is a very complicated matter to resolve, but our future understanding of these matters must include evaluation of tumor subtype, and we should no longer consider breast cancer a single disease.

Study designs should no longer consider adult-only environmental exposures or measurement of exposures around the time of cancer diagnosis as acceptable. Future studies will need to be longitudinal, to understand the history of the gland and potential early risk and modifying factors. One way to enhance the ability to perform these types of studies is through development of nationwide biospecimen banks and databases containing details of collected specimens that other investigators can utilize to develop collaborations across centers and disciplines of research.

Furthermore, our means of testing chemicals, pharmaceuticals, and food additives for health effects in rodents and cells needs to change radically. Beyond the study design issues discussed, current methods are simply too cumbersome, being extremely time- and resource-prohibitive. Additionally, there is little to no regulatory impetus to test for breast-specific effects, and breast tissue is often not evaluated in these tests. Higher-throughput methods of testing chemicals/pharmaceuticals/food additives currently in production and on the market for their potential to affect breast health need to be developed. To do this, the tests must include either relevant cells cultured with the normal cells found in the breast, or include mammary evaluation in rodent models. Breast cancer affects too many women to allow this important tissue to keep being disregarded. Identifying new analytical strategies to clear these many chemicals of any potential for harm to the breast, and establishing regulations that enforce this testing, will be the charge of the future researchers and risk assessors, as our world continues to be polluted with chemicals.

We have now come full circle to the very reason for writing this chapter – breast cancer has long since been regarded a disease of aging, but we know that it is the mixture of risk factor exposures at critical stages of breast development that leads some individuals and populations to be more vulnerable to the disease than others. It may also be the life-stage sensitivity interaction with genes and environment that leads to the development of one subtype of tumor *versus* another. Future studies should focus on the specifics of this complex disease, such as when there was an interaction of genes and environment by subtype, race/ethnicity, known risk factors, *etc.*, and then we may begin to decrease the incidence of this disease.

References

1. P. Lichtenstein, N. V. Holm, P. K. Verkasalo, A. Iliadou, J. Kaprio, M. Koskenvuo, E. Pukkala, A. Skytthe and K. Hemminki, Environmental

and heritable factors in the causation of cancer--analyses of cohorts of twins from Sweden, Denmark, and Finland, *N Engl J Med*, 2000, **343**(2), 78–85.

2. C. Curtis, S. P. Shah, S. F. Chin, G. Turashvili, O. M. Rueda, M. J. Dunning, D. Speed, A. G. Lynch, S. Samarajiwa, Y. Yuan, S. Gräf, G. Ha, G. Haffari, A. Bashashati, R. Russell and S. McKinney; METABRIC Group: A. Langerød, A. Green, E. Provenzano, G. Wishart, S. Pinder, P. Watson, F. Markowetz, L. Murphy, I. Ellis, A. Purushotham, A. L. Børresen-Dale, J. D. Brenton, S. Tavaré, C. Caldas and S. Aparicio, The genomic and transcriptomic architecture of 2,000 breast tumours reveals novel subgroups, *Nature*, 2012, **486**(7403), 346–352.
3. S. P. Shah, A. Roth, R. Goya, A. Oloumi, G. Ha, Y. Zhao, G. Turashvili, J. Ding, K. Tse, G. Haffari, A. Bashashati, L. M. Prentice, J. Khattra, A. Burleigh, D. Yap, V. Bernard, A. McPherson, K. Shumansky, A. Crisan, R. Giuliany, A. Heravi-Moussavi, J. Rosner, D. Lai, I. Birol, R. Varhol, A. Tam, N. Dhalla, T. Zeng, K. Ma, S. K. Chan, M. Griffith, A. Moradian, S. W. Cheng, G. B. Morin, P. Watson, K. Gelmon, S. Chia, S. F. Chin, C. Curtis, O. M. Rueda, P. D. Pharoah, S. Damaraju, J. Mackey, K. Hoon, T. Harkins, V. Tadigotla, M. Sigaroudinia, P. Gascard, T. Tlsty, J. F. Costello, I. M. Meyer, C. J. Eaves, W. W. Wasserman, S. Jones, D. Huntsman, M. Hirst, C. Caldas, M. A. Marra and S. Aparicio, The clonal and mutational evolution spectrum of primary triple-negative breast cancers, *Nature*, 2012, **486**(7403), 395–399.
4. C. K. Anders, C. Fan, J. S. Parker, L. A. Carey, K. L. Blackwell, N. Klauber-DeMore and C. M. Perou, Breast carcinomas arising at a young age: unique biology or a surrogate for aggressive intrinsic subtypes?, *J Clin Oncol*, 2011, **29**(1), e18–20.
5. S. E. Fenton, Endocrine-disrupting compounds and mammary gland development: early exposure and later life consequences, *Endocrinology*, 2006, **147**(Suppl 6), S18–24.
6. American Cancer Society. "Breast Cancer Facts and Figures 2011–2012," Atlanta: American Cancer Society, Inc., 2011. Web. 1 May 2012. <http://www.cancer.org/acs/groups/content/@epidemiologysurveilance/documents/document/acspc-030975.pdf>.
7. Institute of Medicine. "Breast Cancer and the Environment: A Life Course Approach." Institute of Medicine, December 7, 2011. Web. 1 May 2012. <http://www.iom.edu/Reports/2011/Breast-Cancer-and-the-Environment-A-Life-Course-Approach.aspx>.
8. Inter-Agency Breast Cancer and the Environment Research Coordinating Committee (IBCERCC). "Breast Cancer and the Environment: Prioritizing Prevention". 2012. http://www.niehs.nih.gov/about/boards/ibcercc/.
9. W. A. Marshall and J. M. Tanner, Variations in pattern of pubertal changes in girls, *Arch Dis Child*, 1969, **44**(235), 291–303.
10. S. Y. Euling, S. G. Selevan, O. H. Pescovitz and N. E. Skakkebaek, Role of environmental factors in the timing of puberty, *Pediatrics*, 2008, **121**(Suppl 3), S167–171.

11. S. Y. Euling, M. E. Herman-Giddens, P. A. Lee, S. G. Selevan, A. Juul, T. I. Sorensen, L. Dunkel, J. H. Himes, G. Teilmann and S. H. Swan, Examination of US puberty-timing data from 1940 to 1994 for secular trends: panel findings, *Pediatrics*, 2008, **121**(Suppl 3), S172–191.
12. M. E. Herman-Giddens, E. J. Slora, R. C. Wasserman, C. J. Bourdony, M. V. Bhapkar, G. G. Koch and C. M. Hasemeier, Secondary sexual characteristics and menses in young girls seen in office practice: a study from the Pediatric Research in Office Settings network, *Pediatrics*, 1997, **99**(4), 505–512.
13. F. M. Biro, M. P. Galvez, L. C. Greenspan, P. A. Succop, N. Vangeepuram, S. M. Pinney, S. Teitelbaum, G. C. Windham, L. H. Kushi and M. S. Wolff, Pubertal assessment method and baseline characteristics in a mixed longitudinal study of girls, *Pediatrics*, 2010, **126**(3), e583–590.
14. L. Aksglaede, K. Sorensen, J. H. Petersen, N. E. Skakkebaek and A. Juul, Recent decline in age at breast development: the Copenhagen Puberty Study, *Pediatrics*, 2009, **123**(5), e932–939.
15. K. Sørensen, A. Mouritsen, L. Aksglaede, C. P. Hagen, S. S. Mogensen and A. Juul, Recent secular trends in pubertal timing: implications for evaluation and diagnosis of precocious puberty, *Horm Res Paediatr.*, 2012, **77**(3), 137–145.
16. F. M. Biro, B. Huang, S. R. Daniels and A. W. Lucky, Pubarche as well as thelarche may be a marker for the onset of puberty, *J Pediatr Adolesc Gynecol*, 2008, **21**(6), 323–328.
17. A. Mouritsen, L. Aksglaede, K. Sorensen, S. S. Mogensen, H. Leffers, K. M. Main, H. Frederiksen, A. M. Andersson, N. E. Skakkebaek and A. Juul, Hypothesis: exposure to endocrine-disrupting chemicals may interfere with timing of puberty, *Int J Androl*, 2010, **33**(2), 346–359.
18. Mayo Clinic. Gynecomastia. http://www.mayoclinic.com/health/gynecomastia/DS00850 1998–2012 Mayo Foundation for Medical Education and Research.
19. E. Iuanow, M. Kettler and P. J. Slanetz, Spectrum of disease in the male breast, *AJR Am J Roentgenol*, 2011, **196**(3), W247–259.
20. H. Sasano, M. Kimura, S. Shizawa, N. Kimura and H. Nagura, Aromatase and steroid receptors in gynecomastia and male breast carcinoma: an immunohistochemical study, *J Clin Endocrinol Metab*, 1996, **81**(8), 3063–3067.
21. D. V. Henley, N. Lipson, K. S. Korach and C. A. Bloch, Prepubertal gynecomastia linked to lavender and tea tree oils, *N Engl J Med*, 2007, **356**(5), 479–485.
22. J. R. Weiss, K. B. Moysich and H. Swede, Epidemiology of male breast cancer, *Cancer Epidemiol Biomarkers Prev*, 2005, **14**(1), 20–26.
23. J. Russo and I. Russo, Development of the human mammary gland. In: D. C. Neville MC (ed.), *The Mammary Gland: Development, Regulation, and Function*, New York: Plenum Press, 1987, pp. 67–93.

24. C. W. Elston and I. O. Ellis (1998). Normal structure and developmental abnormalities. In: C. W. Elston and I. O. Ellis (ed.), *The breast*, Edinburgh: Churchill Livingstone, 1998, pp. 1–19.
25. B. A. Gusterson and T. Stein, Human breast development., *Semin Cell Dev Biol.*, 2012.
26. H. Ma, L. Bernstein, M. C. Pike and G. Ursin, Reproductive factors and breast cancer risk according to joint estrogen and progesterone receptor status: a meta-analysis of epidemiological studies, *Breast Cancer Res*, 2006, **8**(4), R43.
27. J. Russo, L. K. Tay, D. R. Ciocca and I. H. Russo, Molecular and cellular basis of the mammary gland susceptibility to carcinogenesis, *Environ Health Perspect*, 1983, **49**, 185–199.
28. D. C. Radisky and L. C. Hartmann, Mammary involution and breast cancer risk: transgenic models and clinical studies, *J Mammary Gland Biol Neoplasia*, 2009, **14**(2), 181–191.
29. G. M. Fara, G. Del Corvo, S. Bernuzzi, A. Bigatello, C. Di Pietro, S. Scaglioni and G. Chiumello, Epidemic of breast enlargement in an Italian school, *Lancet*, 1979, **2**(8137), 295–297.
30. C. M. Tiwary, Premature sexual development in children following the use of estrogen- or placenta-containing hair products, *Clin Pediatr (Phila)*, 1998, **37**(12), 733–739.
31. E. Den Hond, H. A. Roels, K. Hoppenbrouwers, T. Nawrot, L. Thijs, C. Vandermeulen, G. Winneke, D. Vanderschueren and J. A. Staessen, Sexual maturation in relation to polychlorinated aromatic hydrocarbons: Sharpe and Skakkebaek's hypothesis revisited, *Environ Health Perspect*, 2002, **110**(8), 771–776.
32. M. M. Leijs, J. G. Koppe, K. Olie, W. M. van Aalderen, P. Voogt, T. Vulsma, M. Westra and G. W. ten Tusscher, Delayed initiation of breast development in girls with higher prenatal dioxin exposure; a longitudinal cohort study, *Chemosphere*, 2008, **73**(6), 999–1004.
33. M. Warner, B. Eskenazi, P. Mocarelli, P. M. Gerthoux, S. Samuels, L. Needham, M. Westra and G. W. ten Tusscher, Serum dioxin concentrations and breast cancer risk in the Seveso Women's Health Study, *Environ Health Perspect*, 2002, **110**(7), 625–628.
34. M. Warner, P. Mocarelli, S. Samuels, L. Needham, P. Brambilla and B. Eskenazi, Dioxin exposure and cancer risk in the Seveso Women's Health Study, *Environ Health Perspect*, 2011, **119**(12), 1700–1705.
35. W. J. Rogan, A. Bagniewska and T. Damstra, Pollutants in breast milk, *N Engl J Med*, 1980, **302**(26), 1450–1453.
36. L. L. Needham, P. Grandjean, B. Heinzow, P. J. Jorgensen, F. Nielsen and D. G. Patterson, *et al.*, Partition of environmental chemicals between maternal and fetal blood and tissues., *Environ Sci Technol.*, 2011, **45**, 1121–1126.
37. W. J. Rogan, B. C. Gladen, J. D. McKinney, N. Carreras, P. Hardy, J. Thullen, J. Tingelstad and M. R. Tully, Polychlorinated biphenyls (PCBs) and dichlorodiphenyl dichloroethene (DDE) in human milk: effects

on growth, morbidity, and duration of lactation, *Am J Public Health*, 1987, **77**(10), 1294–1297.

38. R. A. Rudel, S. E. Fenton, J. M. Ackerman, S. Y. Euling and S. L. Makris, Environmental exposures and mammary gland development: state of the science, public health implications, and research recommendations, *Environ Health Perspect*, 2011, **119**(8), 1053–1061.
39. S. L. Makris, Current assessment of the effects of environmental chemicals on the mammary gland in guideline rodent studies by the US Environmental Protection Agency (US EPA), Organisation for Economic Co-operation and Development (OECD), and National Toxicology Program (NTP)., *Environ Health Perspect*, 2011, **119**(8), 1047–1052.
40. A. G. Knudson, Hereditary cancer: two hits revisited, *J Cancer Res Clin Oncol*, 1996, **122**(3), 135–140.
41. D. Hanahan and R. A. Weinberg, The hallmarks of cancer, *Cell*, 2000, **100**(1), 57–70.
42. National Cancer Institute, National Cancer Institute: Genetics of Breast and Ovarian Cancer (PDQÛ) Retrieved June 1, 2012, from http://www.cancer.gov/cancertopics/pdq/genetics/breast-and-ovarian/HealthProfessional/page2, 2012.
43. L. Shen, Z. H. Yin, Y. Wan, Y. Zhang, K. Li and B. S. Zhou, Association between ATM polymorphisms and cancer risk: a meta-analysis, *Mol Biol Rep*, 2012, **39**(5), 5719–5725.
44. Institute of Medicine. "Breast Cancer and the Environment: A Life Course Approach." Instistute of Medicine, December 7, 2011. Web. 1 May 2012. <http://www.iom.edu/Reports/2011/Breast-Cancer-and-the-Environment-A-Life-Course-Approach.aspx>.
45. P. A. van den Brandt, D. Spiegelman, S. S. Yaun, H. O. Adami, L. Beeson, A. R. Folsom, G. Fraser, R. A. Goldbohm, S. Graham, L. Kushi, J. R. Marshall, A. B. Miller, T. Rohan, S. A. Smith-Warner, F. E. Speizer, W. C. Willett, A. Wolk and D. J. Hunter, Pooled analysis of prospective cohort studies on height, weight, and breast cancer risk., *Am J Epidemiol*, 2000, **152**(6), 514–527.
46. A. Vrieling, K. Buck, R. Kaaks and J. Chang-Claude, Adult weight gain in relation to breast cancer risk by estrogen and progesterone receptor status: a meta-analysis, *Breast Cancer Res Treat*, 2010, **123**(3), 641–649.
47. M. Protani, M. Coory and J. H. Martin, Effect of obesity on survival of women with breast cancer: systematic review and meta-analysis, *Breast Cancer Res Treat*, 2010, **123**(3), 627–635.
48. J. Green, B. J. Cairns, D. Casabonne, F. L. Wright, G. Reeves and V. Beral, Height and cancer incidence in the Million Women Study: prospective cohort, and meta-analysis of prospective studies of height and total cancer risk, *Lancet Oncol*, 2011, **12**(8), 785–794.
49. N. Hamajima, K. Hirose, K. Tajima, T. Rohan, E. E. Calle, C. W. Heath, R. J. Coates, J. M. Liff, R. Talamini, N. Chantarakul, S. Koetsawang, D. Rachawat, A. Morabia, L. Schuman, W. Stewart, M. Szklo, C. Bain, F. Schofield, V. Siskind, P. Band, A. J. Coldman, R. P. Gallagher,

T. G. Hislop, P. Yang, L. M. Kolonel, A. M. Nomura, J. Hu, K. C. Johnson, Y. Mao, S. De Sanjosé, N. Lee, P. Marchbanks, H. W. Ory, H. B. Peterson, H. G. Wilson, P. A. Wingo, K. Ebeling, D. Kunde, P. Nishan, J. L. Hopper, G. Colditz, V. Gajalanski, N. Martin, T. Pardthaisong, S. Silpisornkosol, C. Theetranont, B. Boosiri, S. Chutivongse, P. Jimakorn, P. Virutamasen, C. Wongsrichanalai, M. Ewertz, H. O. Adami, L. Bergkvist, C. Magnusson, I. Persson, J. Chang-Claude, C. Paul, D. C. Skegg, G. F. Spears, P. Boyle, T. Evstifeeva, J. R. Daling, W. B. Hutchinson, K. Malone, E. A. Noonan, J. L. Stanford, D. B. Thomas, N. S. Weiss, E. White, N. Andrieu, A. Brémond, F. Clavel, B. Gairard, J. Lansac, L. Piana, R. Renaud, A. Izquierdo, P. Viladiu, H. R. Cuevas, P. Ontiveros, A. Palet, S. B. Salazar, N. Aristizabel, A. Cuadros, L. Tryggvadottir, H. Tulinius, A. Bachelot, M. G. Lê, J. Peto, S. Franceschi, F. Lubin, B. Modan, E. Ron, Y. Wax, G. D. Friedman, R. A. Hiatt, F. Levi, T. Bishop, K. Kosmelj, M. Primic-Zakelj, B. Ravnihar, J. Stare, W. L. Beeson, G. Fraser, R. D. Bullbrook, J. Cuzick, S. W. Duffy, I. S. Fentiman, J. L. Hayward, D. Y. Wang, A. J. McMichael, K. McPherson, R. L. Hanson, M. C. Leske, M. C. Mahoney, P. C. Nasca, A. O. Varma, A. L. Weinstein, T. R. Moller, H. Olsson, J. Ranstam, R. A. Goldbohm, P. A. van den Brandt, R. A. Apelo, J. Baens, J. R. de la Cruz, B. Javier, L. B. Lacaya, C. A. Ngelangel, C. La Vecchia, E. Negri, E. Marubini, M. Ferraroni, M. Gerber, S. Richardson, C. Segala, D. Gatei, P. Kenya, A. Kungu, J. G. Mati, L. A. Brinton, R. Hoover, C. Schairer, R. Spirtas, H. P. Lee, M. A. Rookus, F. E. van Leeuwen, J. A. Schoenberg, M. McCredie, M. D. Gammon, E. A. Clarke, L. Jones, A. Neil, M. Vessey, D. Yeates, P. Appleby, E. Banks, V. Beral, D. Bull, B. Crossley, A. Goodill, J. Green, C. Hermon, T. Key, N. Langston, C. Lewis, G. Reeves, R. Collins, R. Doll, R. Peto, K. Mabuchi, D. Preston, P. Hannaford, C. Kay, L. Rosero-Bixby, Y. T. Gao, F. Jin, J. M. Yuan, H. Y. Wei, T. Yun, C. Zhiheng, G. Berry, J. Cooper Booth, T. Jelihovsky, R. MacLennan, R. Shearman, Q. S. Wang, C. J. Baines, A. B. Miller, C. Wall, E. Lund, H. Stalsberg, X. O. Shu, W. Zheng, K. Katsouyanni, A. Trichopoulou, D. Trichopoulos, A. Dabancens, L. Martinez, R. Molina, O. Salas, F. E. Alexander, K. Anderson, A. R. Folsom, B. S. Hulka, L. Bernstein, S. Enger, R. W. Haile, A. Paganini-Hill, M. C. Pike, R. K. Ross, G. Ursin, M. C. Yu, M. P. Longnecker, P. Newcomb, L. Bergkvist, A. Kalache, Farley™ and S. Holck, O. Meirik, Collaborative Group on Hormonal Factors in Breast Cancer, Alcohol, tobacco and breast cancer--collaborative reanalysis of individual data from 53 epidemiological studies, including 58,515 women with breast cancer and 95,067 women without the disease, *Br J Cancer*, 2002, **87**(11), 1234–1245.

50. W. Y. Chen, B. Rosner, S. E. Hankinson, G. A. Colditz and W. C. Willett, Moderate alcohol consumption during adult life, drinking patterns, and breast cancer risk, *JAMA*, 2011, **306**(17), 1884–1890.

51. C. Pelucchi, I. Tramacere, P. Boffetta, E. Negri and C. La Vecchia, Alcohol consumption and cancer risk, *Nutr Cancer*, 2011, **63**(7), 983–990.
52. V. A. McCormack and I. dos Santos Silva, Breast density and parenchymal patterns as markers of breast cancer risk: a meta-analysis, *Cancer Epidemiol Biomarkers Prev*, 2006, **15**(6), 1159–1169.
53. N. F. Boyd, G. S. Dite, J. Stone, A. Gunasekara, D. R. English, M. R. McCredie, G. G. Giles, D. Tritchler, A. Chiarelli, M. J. Yaffe and J. L. Hopper, Heritability of mammographic density, a risk factor for breast cancer, *N Engl J Med*, 2002, **347**(12), 886–894.
54. G. Ursin, H. Ma, A. H. Wu, L. Bernstein, M. Salane, Y. R. Parisky, M. Astrahan, C. C. Siozon and M. C. Pike, Mammographic density and breast cancer in three ethnic groups, *Cancer Epidemiol Biomarkers Prev*, 2003, **12**(4), 332–338.
55. J. W. Byng, N. F. Boyd, E. Fishell, R. A. Jong and M. J. Yaffe, The quantitative analysis of mammographic densities, *Phys Med Biol*, 1994, **39**(10), 1629–1638.
56. G. Masala, D. Ambrogetti, M. Assedi, D. Giorgi, M. R. Del Turco and D. Palli, Dietary and lifestyle determinants of mammographic breast density. A longitudinal study in a Mediterranean population, *Int J Cancer*, 2006, **118**(7), 1782–1789.
57. S. S. White, K. Kato, L. T. Jia, B. J. Basden, A. M. Calafat, E. P. Hines, J. P. Stanko, C. J. Wolf, B. D. Abbott and S. E. Fenton, Effects of perfluorooctanoic acid on mouse mammary gland development and differentiation resulting from cross-foster and restricted gestational exposures, *Reprod Toxicol*, 2009, **27**(3–4), 289–298.
58. M. Durando, L. Kass, J. Piva, C. Sonnenschein, A. M. Soto, E. H. Luque and M. Muñoz-de-Toro, Prenatal bisphenol A exposure induces preneoplastic lesions in the mammary gland in Wistar rats, *Environ Health Perspect*, 2007, **115**(1), 80–86.
59. B. MacMahon, P. Cole, T. M. Lin, C. R. Lowe, A. P. Mirra, B. Ravnihar, E. J. Salber, V. G. Valaoras and S. Yuasa, Age at first birth and breast cancer risk, *Bull World Health Organ*, 1970, **43**(2), 209–221.
60. T. J. Key, P. K. Verkasalo and E. Banks, Epidemiology of breast cancer, *Lancet Oncol*, 2001, **2**(3), 133–140.
61. J. Russo, R. Moral, G. A. Balogh, D. Mailo and I. H. Russo, The protective role of pregnancy in breast cancer, *Breast Cancer Res*, 2005, **7**(3), 131–142.
62. S. J. Lord, L. Bernstein, K. A. Johnson, K. E. Malone, J. A. McDonald, P. A. Marchbanks, M. S. Simon, B. L. Strom, M. F. Press, S. G. Folger, R. T. Burkman, D. Deapen, R. Spirtas and G. Ursin, Breast cancer risk and hormone receptor status in older women by parity, age of first birth, and breastfeeding: a case-control study, *Cancer Epidemiol Biomarkers Prev*, 2008, **17**(7), 1723–1730.
63. Collaborative Group on Hormonal Factors in Breast Cancer, Breast cancer and breastfeeding: collaborative reanalysis of individual data from 47 epidemiological studies in 30 countries, including 50302 women with

breast cancer and 96973 women without the disease., *Lancet*, 2002, **360**(9328), 187–195.

64. A. Shin, Y. M. Song, K. Y. Yoo and J. Sung, Menstrual factors and cancer risk among Korean women, *Int J Epidemiol*, 2011, **40**(5), 1261–1268.
65. J. M. Yuan, M. C. Yu, R. K. Ross, Y. T. Gao and B. E. Henderson, Risk factors for breast cancer in Chinese women in Shanghai, *Cancer Res*, 1988, **48**(7), 1949–1953.
66. J. B. Kampert, A. S. Whittemore and R. S. Paffenbarger, Combined effect of childbearing, menstrual events, and body size on age-specific breast cancer risk, *Am J Epidemiol*, 1988, **128**(5), 962–979.
67. G. A. Colditz, S. E. Hankinson, D. J. Hunter, W. C. Willett, J. E. Manson, M. J. Stampfer, C. Hennekens, B. Rosner and F. E. Speizer, The use of estrogens and progestins and the risk of breast cancer in postmenopausal women, *N Engl J Med*, 1995, **332**(24), 1589–1593.
68. P. A. Marchbanks, J. A. McDonald, H. G. Wilson, S. G. Folger, M. G. Mandel, J. R. Daling, L. Bernstein, K. E. Malone, G. Ursin, B. L. Strom, S. A. Norman, P. A. Wingo, R. T. Burkman, J. A. Berlin, M. S. Simon, R. Spirtas and L. K. Weiss, Oral contraceptives and the risk of breast cancer, *N Engl J Med*, 2002, **346**(26), 2025–2032.
69. R. N. Hoover, M. Hyer, R. M. Pfeiffer, E. Adam, B. Bond, A. L. Cheville, T. Colton, P. Hartge, E. E. Hatch, A. L. Herbst, B. Y. Karlan, R. Kaufman, K. L. Noller, J. R. Palmer, S. J. Robboy, R. C. Saal, W. Strohsnitter, L. Titus-Ernstoff and R. Troisi, Adverse health outcomes in women exposed in utero to diethylstilbestrol, *N Engl J Med*, 2011, **365**(14), 1304–1314.
70. J. R. Palmer, L. A. Wise, E. E. Hatch, R. Troisi, L. Titus-Ernstoff, W. Strohsnitter, R. Kaufman, A. L. Herbst, K. L. Noller, M. Hyer and R. N. Hoover, Prenatal diethylstilbestrol exposure and risk of breast cancer, *Cancer Epidemiol Biomarkers Prev*, 2006, **15**(8), 1509–1514.
71. E. R. Greenberg, A. B. Barnes, L. Resseguie, J. A. Barrett, S. Burnside, L. L. Lanza, R. K. Neff, M. Stevens, R. H. Young and T. Colton, Breast cancer in mothers given diethylstilbestrol in pregnancy, *N Engl J Med*, 1984, **311**(22), 1393–1398.
72. C. E. Land, J. D. Boice, R. E. Shore, J. E. Norman and M. Tokunaga, Breast cancer risk from low-dose exposures to ionizing radiation: results of parallel analysis of three exposed populations of women, *J Natl Cancer Inst*, 1980, **65**(2), 353–376.
73. K. Ozasa, Y. Shimizu, A. Suyama, F. Kasagi, M. Soda, E. J. Grant, R. Sakata, H. Sugiyama and K. Kodama, Studies of the mortality of atomic bomb survivors, Report 14, 1950–2003: an overview of cancer and noncancer diseases, *Radiat Res*, 2012, **177**(3), 229–243.
74. M. Tokunaga, J. E. Norman, M. Asano, S. Tokuoka, H. Ezaki, I. Nishimori and Y. Tsuji, Malignant breast tumors among atomic bomb survivors, Hiroshima and Nagasaki, 1950–74, *J Natl Cancer Inst*, 1979, **62**(6), 1347–1359.

75. M. S. Linet, T. L. Slovis, D. L. Miller, R. Kleinerman, C. Lee, P. Rajaraman and A. Berrington de Gonzalez, Cancer risks associated with external radiation from diagnostic imaging procedures., *CA Cancer J Clin.*, 2012, **62**(2), 75–100.
76. P. B. Kaplowitz, Link between body fat and the timing of puberty, *Pediatrics*, 2008, **121**(Suppl 3), S208–217.
77. L. K. Olson, Y. Tan, Y. Zhao, M. D. Aupperlee and S. Z. Haslam, Pubertal exposure to high fat diet causes mouse strain-dependent alterations in mammary gland development and estrogen responsiveness, *Int J Obes (Lond)*, 2010, **34**(9), 1415–1426.
78. A. Janesick and B. Blumberg, Minireview: PPARgamma as the target of obesogens, *J Steroid Biochem Mol Biol*, 2011, **127**(1–2), 4–8.
79. R. G. Ziegler, R. N. Hoover, M. C. Pike, A. Hildesheim, A. M. Nomura, D. W. West, A. H. Wu-Williams, L. N. Kolonel, P. L. Horn-Ross, J. F. Rosenthal and M. B. Hyer, Migration patterns and breast cancer risk in Asian-American women, *J Natl Cancer Inst*, 1993, **85**(22), 1819–1827.
80. S. F. Brennan, M. M. Cantwell, C. R. Cardwell, L. S. Velentzis and J. V. Woodside, Dietary patterns and breast cancer risk: a systematic review and meta-analysis, *Am J Clin Nutr*, 2010, **91**(5), 1294–1302.
81. C. X. Zhang, S. C. Ho, J. H. Fu, S. Z. Cheng, Y. M. Chen and F. Y. Lin, Dietary patterns and breast cancer risk among Chinese women, *Cancer Causes Control*, 2011, **22**(1), 115–124.
82. Y. A. Cho, J. Kim, A. Shin, K. S. Park and J. Ro, Dietary patterns and breast cancer risk in Korean women, *Nutr Cancer*, 2010, **62**(8), 1161–1169.
83. National Toxicology Program, Multigenerational reproductive study of genistein (Cas No. 446-72-0) in Sprague-Dawley rats (feed study), *Natl Toxicol Program Tech Rep Ser*, 2008, **539**, 1–266.
84. A. Warri, N. M. Saarinen, S. Makela and L. Hilakivi-Clarke, The role of early life genistein exposures in modifying breast cancer risk, *Br J Cancer*, 2008, **98**(9), 1485–1493.
85. L. Hilakivi-Clarke, E. Cho, I. Onojafe, M. Raygada and R. Clarke, Maternal exposure to genistein during pregnancy increases carcinogen-induced mammary tumorigenesis in female rat offspring, *Oncol Rep*, 1999, **6**(5), 1089–1095.
86. E. Padilla-Banks, W. N. Jefferson and R. R. Newbold, Neonatal exposure to the phytoestrogen genistein alters mammary gland growth and developmental programming of hormone receptor levels, *Endocrinology*, 2006, **147**(10), 4871–4882.
87. G. Costa, E. Haus and R. Stevens, Shift work and cancer - considerations on rationale, mechanisms, and epidemiology, *Scand J Work Environ Health*, 2010, **36**(2), 163–179.
88. K. Amend, D. Hicks and C. B. Ambrosone, Breast cancer in African-American women: differences in tumor biology from European-American women, *Cancer Res*, 2006, **66**(17), 8327–8330.

89. Centers for Disease Control and Prevention. Overweight and Obesity. http://www.cdc.gov/obesity/data/childhood.html Accessed Sept 24, 2012. last updated Aug 28, 2012.
90. S. Yao, G. Zirpoli, D. H. Bovbjerg, L. Jandorf, C. C. Hong, H. Zhao, L. E. Sucheston, L. Tang, M. Roberts, G. Ciupak, W. Davis, H. Hwang, C. S. Johnson, D. L. Trump, S. E. McCann, F. Ademuyiwa, K. S. Pawlish, E. V. Bandera and C. B. Ambrosone, Variants in the vitamin D pathway, serum levels of vitamin D, and estrogen receptor negative breast cancer among African-American women: a case-control study, *Breast Cancer Res*, 2012, **14**(2), R58.
91. L. A. Carey, C. M. Perou, C. A. Livasy, L. G. Dressler, D. Cowan, K. Conway, G. Karaca, M. A. Troester, C. K. Tse, S. Edmiston, S. L. Deming, J. Geradts, M. C. Cheang, T. O. Nielsen, P. G. Moorman, H. S. Earp and R. C. Millikan, Race, breast cancer subtypes, and survival in the Carolina Breast Cancer Study, *JAMA*, 2006, **295**(21), 2492–2502.
92. National Toxicology Program, Report on Carcinogens, 12th edition, 2011. Retrieved June 1, 2012, from http://ntp.niehs.nih.gov/ntp/roc/twelfth/roc12.pdf.
93. C. B. Ambrosone, S. Kropp, J. Yang, S. Yao, P. G. Shields and J. Chang-Claude, Cigarette smoking, N-acetyltransferase 2 genotypes, and breast cancer risk: pooled analysis and meta-analysis, *Cancer Epidemiol Biomarkers Prev*, 2008, **17**(1), 15–26.
94. D. G. Cox, L. Dostal, D. J. Hunter, L. Le Marchand, R. Hoover, R. G. Ziegler, M. J. Thun and Breast and Prostate Cancer Cohort Consortium, N-acetyltransferase 2 polymorphisms, tobacco smoking, and breast cancer risk in the breast and prostate cancer cohort consortium, *Am J Epidemiol*, 2011, **174**(11), 1316–1322.
95. F. Xue, W. C. Willett, B. A. Rosner, S. E. Hankinson and K. B. Michels, Cigarette smoking and the incidence of breast cancer, *Arch Intern Med*, 2011, **171**(2), 125–133.
96. K. C. Johnson, A. B. Miller, N. E. Collishaw, J. R. Palmer, S. K. Hammond, A. G. Salmon, K. P. Cantor, M. D. Miller, N. F. Boyd, J. Millar and F. Turcotte, Active smoking and secondhand smoke increase breast cancer risk: the report of the Canadian Expert Panel on Tobacco Smoke and Breast Cancer Risk (2009), *Tob Control*, 2011, **20**(1), e2.
97. D. Zucchino, Camp Lejeune residents blame rare cancer cluster on the water. *Los Angeles Times*, August 26, 2009.
98. A. Boudreau and S. Bronstein, CNN Special Investigations Unit (September 24, 2009). Male breast cancer patients blame water at Marine base. Retrieved May 1, 2012, from http://articles.cnn.com/2009-09-24/health/marines.breast.cancer_1_breast-cancer-cancer-spread-drinking-water?_s=PM:HEALTH.
99. K. Fukamachi, B. S. Han, C. K. Kim, N. Takasuka, Y. Matsuoka, E. Matsuda, T. Yamasaki and H. Tsuda, Possible enhancing effects of atrazine and nonylphenol on 7,12-dimethylbenz[a]anthracene-induced

mammary tumor development in human c-Ha-ras proto-oncogene transgenic rats, *Cancer Sci*, 2004, **95**(5), 404–410.
100. M. Ueda, T. Imai, T. Takizawa, H. Onodera, K. Mitsumori, T. Matsui and M. Hirose, Possible enhancing effects of atrazine on growth of 7,12-dimethylbenz(a) anthracene-induced mammary tumors in ovariectomized Sprague-Dawley rats, *Cancer Sci*, 2005, **96**(1), 19–25.
101. L. T. Wetzel, L. G. Luempert, C. B. Breckenridge, M. O. Tisdel, J. T. Stevens, A. K. Thakur, P. J. Extrom and J. C. Eldridge, Chronic effects of atrazine on estrus and mammary tumor formation in female Sprague-Dawley and Fischer 344 rats, *J Toxicol Environ Health*, 1994, **43**(2), 169–182.
102. B. A. Cohn, M. S. Wolff, P. M. Cirillo and R. I. Sholtz, DDT and breast cancer in young women: new data on the significance of age at exposure, *Environ Health Perspect*, 2007, **115**(10), 1406–1414.
103. B. A. Cohn, Developmental and environmental origins of breast cancer: DDT as a case study, *Reprod Toxicol*, 2011, **31**(3), 302–311.
104. R. R. Enoch, J. S. Stanko, S. N. Greiner, G. L. Youngblood, J. L. Rayner and S. E. Fenton, Mammary gland development as a sensitive end-point following acute prenatal exposure to a low dose atrazine metabolite mixture in female Long Evans rats, *Environ Health Perspect*, 2007, **115**(4), 541–547.
105. Susan G. Komen for the Cure. "Understanding Breast Cancer: Risk Factors and Prevention." Susan G. Komen for the Cure. Web. 1 May 2012. <http://ww5.komen.org/BreastCancer/GettingOlder.html>.

CHAPTER 12

Environmental Chemicals and Prostate Cancer Risk

JASPREET S. JONEJA, WEN-YANG HU, RICARDO R. RIOS AND GAIL S. PRINS*

Department of Urology, University of Illinois at Chicago, Chicago, IL, USA 60612
*E-mail: gprins@uic.edu

12.1 Introduction

Male reproductive health is defined by both the proper development of the reproductive system and maintenance of function throughout adult life, including the capacity to reproduce. While female sexual differentiation, considered the default developmental pathway, is largely independent of estrogens and androgens, male sexual differentiation is driven by androgens produced by the fetal testes and is entirely androgen-dependent.[1,2] Many environmental chemicals (ECs) have been shown to directly or indirectly interfere with androgen action or mimic estrogenic action, thus impacting male developmental programming and reproductive tract maturation, as well as initiating direct effect in adults. Several compounds—including endocrine-disrupting chemicals (EDCs), industrial compounds, cigarette smoke, air pollution, radiation, electromagnetic fields, processed foods, alcohol, and pharmaceuticals—have been implicated in various abnormalities of the reproductive tract organs.

The present discussion is organized around the potential involvement of ECs in direct and indirect effects on the prostate gland in adults, as well as early life exposures to these compounds, which may predispose this sensitive developing

Issues in Toxicology No. 16
Aging and Vulnerability to Environmental Chemicals: Age-related Disorders and their Origins in Environmental Exposures
Edited by Bernard Weiss

Published by the Royal Society of Chemistry, www.rsc.org

tissue to prostate cancer upon aging. As a cross-reference, Table 12.1 summarizes the evidence and provides references for individual ECs with regards to prostate cancer (PC).

PC is the most common non-cutaneous cancer and the second leading cause of cancer deaths in North American men.[3] It is known that steroids play a role in the initiation and progression of PC, which is the basis for hormonal treatment strategies that include androgen ablation and androgen receptor (AR) blockade.[4,5] Increasing evidence indicates that in addition to androgens, estrogens play key roles in prostate carcinogenesis and progression, although the mechanisms are not fully understood.[6–9] In men, chronically elevated estrogens have been associated with increased risk of PC,[10] while in rodents, estrogens in combination with androgens induce PC.[11] In addition to the direct effects of steroids, it is currently recognized that age, race, genetics (family history), diet, and environmental factors can impact prostate cancer risk.[12]

Recent advances in stem cell research indicate that stem cells and early stage progenitor cells may be direct carcinogenic targets and, potentially, the cells of origin in cancer initiation and progression. Novel *in vitro* and *in vivo* models using stem and early stage progenitor cells isolated from normal human prostates have been developed and used to initiate hormonal carcinogenesis.[7] These *in vitro* prostasphere and *in vivo* chimeric prostate models with carcinogenic induction serve as suitable models for examining stem cell perturbations and carcinogenic actions of ECs on human prostate cells. Using these models, our laboratory has recently found evidence that human prostate epithelial stem cell exposures to natural and environmental estrogens and other ECs such as dioxin and inorganic arsenic can alter stem cell self-renewal and differentiation and gene expression programs.[13] Thus it is likely that various ECs influence carcinogenic risk in the human prostate gland, in part by permanently reprogramming the stem cell population.

12.2 Evidence and Mechanisms

12.2.1 Farming and Pesticides

Regarding links between prostate cancer and environmental factors in humans (outside of diet), the most compelling data come from the established occupational hazard of farming and increased prostate cancer rates.[14–16] While several variables may contribute to higher PC rates in farmers, chronic or intermittent exposures to pesticides are the most likely explanation.[15,17,18] This is supported by a large epidemiology study (Agricultural Health Study)—a collaborative effort between the National Cancer Institute, the National Institute of Environmental Health Sciences, and the Environmental Protection Agency in the United States—that has examined agricultural lifestyles and health in ~90 000 participants in North Carolina and Iowa since 1993 (www.aghealth.org). Evaluation of >55 000 pesticide applicators revealed a direct link between exposure to methyl bromide, a fungicide with an unknown mode of action, and increased PC rates. Furthermore, 6 out of 45 common

Table 12.1 Summary of evidence for prostate cancer risks in humans and animal model systems as a result of exposure to environmental chemicals.

Environmental Chemicals	*Evidence for cancer risk in humans*	*References*	*Evidence for cancer risk in experimental models*	*References*
Environmental Estrogen				
DES			Elevated prostate cancer risk	[31,32,33]
BPA	Elevated prostate cancer risk	[40,41]	Elevated prostate cancer risk	[41,42]
PCBs	Elevated prostate cancer risk	[44,45,46]	Elevated prostate cancer risk	[47]
Atrazine	Elevated prostate cancer risk	[52,53]	Elevated prostate cancer risk	[51]
	Decreased prostate cancer risk	[54,55]		
Anti-androgens				
Vinclozalin			Decreased prostate cancer risk	[69]
			Elevated prostate cancer risk	[50,71]
DDT/DDE	Elevated prostate cancer risk	[18]		
Heavy metals				
Arsenic	Elevated prostate cancer risk	[59,66]	Elevated prostate cancer risk	[62,65]
Cadmium	Elevated and decreased prostate cancer risk	[56]	Elevated prostate cancer risk	[57,58]
Pesticides				
Methyl bromide	Elevated prostate cancer risk	[15]		
Chlorpyrifos	Elevated prostate cancer risk	[15,19]		
Fonofos	Elevated prostate cancer risk	[15,19]		
Coumaphos	Elevated prostate cancer risk	[15,19]		
Phorate	Elevated prostate cancer risk	[15,19]		
Permethrin	Elevated prostate cancer risk	[15,19]		
Butylate	Elevated prostate cancer risk	[15,19]		
UV filters				
4-methyl-benzylidene camphor (4-MBC)			Elevated prostate cancer risk	[48,49]
3-benzylidene camphor (3-BC)			Elevated prostate cancer risk	[48,49]
Dioxin				
TCDD	Decreased prostate cancer risk	[79]		

agricultural pesticides showed correlation with exposure and increased PC in men with a familial history, suggesting gene–environment interactions. These six agents were chlorpyrifos, fonofos, coumaphos, phorate, permethrin, and butylate.[15,19] The first four of these compounds are thiophosphates and share a common chemical structure. While these agents are regarded as acetylcholine esterase inhibitors and have not been shown to have direct estrogenic or anti-androgenic activities, a literature search revealed that these compounds have significant capacity as p450 enzyme inhibitors. In particular, chlorpyrifos, fonofos, and phorate strongly inhibit CYP1A2 and CYP3A4, which are the major p450s that metabolize estradiol, estrone, and testosterone in the liver.[20,21]

Furthermore, the human prostate constitutively expresses CYP1A2 and CYP3A4 enzymes that are involved in intraprostatic metabolism of steroids, drugs, and dietary compounds.[22–24]

This raises the possibility that exposure to these compounds may interfere with steroid hormone metabolism by the liver as well as the prostate, and in doing so, alter steroid balance and availability, which in turn may contribute to increased PC risk. A similar mechanism of endocrine disruption *in vivo* has been identified for polychlorinated biphenols (PCBs) and polyhalogenated aromatic hydrocarbons [including dioxins, bisphenol A (BPA), and dibenzofurans] through potent inhibition of estrogen sulfotransferase, which effectively elevates bioavailable estrogens in various target organs.[25,26]

12.2.2 Environmental Estrogens

In men, chronically elevated estrogens have been associated with increased risk of PC.[10] In rodents, estrogens, in combination with androgens, induce PC.[27] For the sake of simplicity, we here refer to environmental estrogens as molecules with identified estrogenic activity (estrogen mimics), mostly through activation of estrogen receptors (ERs).

12.2.2.1 Diethylstilbesterol (DES)

DES exposure is considered an important model of endocrine disruption and provides proof of principle for exogenous estrogenic agents as disruptors of multiple endorgans. Maternal exposure to DES during pregnancy was found to result in more extensive prostatic squamous metaplasia in human male offspring than observed with maternal estradiol alone.[28] While prostatic metaplasia eventually resolved following DES withdrawal, ectasia and persistent distortion of ductal architecture remained.[29] This has led to the postulation that men prenatally exposed to DES may be at increased risk for prostatic disease later in life, although this has not been borne out in the limited population studies conducted to date.[30] However, extensive studies with DES in rodent models predict marked abnormalities in the adult prostate, including increased susceptibility to adult-onset carcinogenesis following early DES exposures.[31–33]

12.2.2.2 BPA

BPA is a synthetic polymer used in the production of polycarbonate plastics and expoxy resins and significant levels have been found in the urine of 93% of US population in a recent screen by the Centers for Disease Control and Prevention.[34] The relative binding affinity of BPA for either nuclear ERα and ERβ or capacity for BPA to activate ER-dependent transcription is ~10 000 lower than estradiol or DES.[35,36] While these data might suggest that BPA has minimal estrogenic activity, 1 μM BPA is 50% as efficacious as 1 μM 17β-estradiol in activating an estrogen-responsive luciferase reporter.[37] This indicates that, although BPA may have a significantly lower potency than endogenous estrogens *in vitro*, it is a full agonist for both ERα and ERβ. Furthermore, BPA induces ER through non-genomic pathways with an EC50 equivalent to 17β-estradiol, suggesting that *in vivo* estrogenic activity of BPA may be due to non-genomic activation of ER.[38,39] The effects of BPA with regard to carcinogenic potential, including the prostate gland, have recently been reviewed by an expert panel.[40] In short, there is evidence from rodent models and human prostate cell lines that BPA can influence carcinogenesis, modulate PC cell proliferation, and for some tumors, stimulate progression. The recent reports have provided evidence that early life exposure to BPA may increase susceptibility to hormonal carcinogenesis in the prostate gland, possibly by developmentally reprogramming carcinogenic risk.[41] Studies using a rat model showed that brief neonatal exposure to a low dose of BPA ($10\,\mu g\,kg^{-1}$ BW per day) significantly increased the incidence and grade of prostatic intraepithelial neoplasia following adult estrogen exposure. This model of sensitivity to hormonal carcinogenesis is relevant to humans in that relative estradiol levels increase in the aging male and may contribute to prostate disease risk.[42] Global analysis of the DNA methylome in prostates neonatally exposed to BPA revealed that multiple genes involved in signaling pathways have permanent DNA methylation alterations that directly lead to complex changes in gene transcription programs throughout life.[41,43] Altered expression of DNA methyl transferases (Dmnt 3a and b) and methyl binding proteins (MBDs) by early-life exposures may underpin the DNA methylation modifications.[43] Together, these findings indicate that early-life exposures to ECs may increase susceptibility to prostate carcinogenesis through epigenetic reprogramming.

12.2.2.3 PCBs

Persistent organic pollutants, such as PCBs, are fat soluble chemicals that bioaccumulate in the human body. Many have estrogenic or anti-androgenic activity and as such, may perturb male reproductive activity. A recent analysis of adipose tissue concentrations of PCBs in Swedish men with and without PC revealed a significant association between PCB levels in the higher quandrants and PC odds ratio, with the most marked associations for PCB153 and trans-chlordane.[44] A more extensive epidemiologic study of capacitor manufacturing plant workers highly exposed to PCBs revealed a strong exposure–response relationship for PC mortality.[44] This supports previous findings of correlations between PCB 153 and 180 and PC risk in electric utility workers.[45,46] While estrogenic activity of these compounds is a suspected mode of action, there is also evidence that PCBs inhibit estrogen sulfotransferase activity in the liver and effectively increase bioavailable estrogen in the body.[25] Recently, Aroclor-1254, a mixture of 60 PCB pollutants, was tested on rat prostate cells *in vitro* and shown to disrupt gap junctions and expression of connexin 32 and 43, and increase double-stranded DNA breaks, suggesting that PCBs may be able to transform prostate cells leading to carcinogenesis.[47] Further investigation using animal models is warranted for PCBs and PC risk.

12.2.2.4 Ultraviolet (UV) Filters

There are a few recent reports that UV light filters used to protect against the sun have estrogenic activity.[48] Specifically, 4-methylbenzylidene camphor and 3-benzylidene camphor are ERβ ligands.[49] While little, if any, work has been done with regard to these UV filters and human PC, a few recent reports indicate that developmental exposure to the compounds can alter prostate gland development and estrogen target gene expression in the rat.[48,50] This raises the possibility that the fetal prostate may be affected following maternal use of these compounds.

12.2.2.5 Atrazine

Atrazine at environmentally relevant levels has been shown to result in chronic prostatitis in rats, which is believed to be a predisposing factor to PC.[51] Atrazine exposure was associated with a 4–6 fold increase in PC in men working in an atrazine production facility;[52,53] however, this was refuted in a subsequent case-controlled analysis of these workers.[54] Furthermore, a large epidemiologic study of California agriculture workers exposed to atrazine found no increased risk for PC.[55] Atrazine stimulates aromatase activity, thus resulting in elevated circulating estradiol and reduced testosterone levels, and this shift in the estradiol : testosterone ratio is known to contribute to prostate diseases in several animal model systems. Furthermore, atrazine exposure and its resultant elevation in estradiol have been shown to elevate circulating prolactin levels, which have also been correlated with increased PC risk. Thus indirect effects of atrazine on prostate disease risk are likely attributable to the hormonal perturbations elicited by this chemical.

12.2.2.6 Cadmium

Cadmium is known to bind to ERs and function as an estrogenic mimic. While some large epidemiologic reports have indicated a relationship between cadmium exposure and PC rates, others have refuted these findings.[56] Nonetheless, there are intriguing reports in the literature which show that cadmium has proliferative action with human prostate cells *in vitro*, through an ER-dependent mechanism, and that this exposure is associated with acquisition of androgen independence.[57] Furthermore, prostatic tumors have been shown to be experimentally induced by oral exposure to cadmium.[58] Since cadmium bioaccumulates in the body, further epidemiologic analysis of cadmium and PC risk is warranted, particularly in men with occupational exposures.

12.2.2.7 Arsenic

Arsenic is a semi-metallic element found naturally in soils, ground water and surface water, and is a notable carcinogen at environmentally relevant doses.[59–61]

Exposure to inorganic arsenic (iAs) is widespread for humans with millions exposed to potentially harmful levels worldwide, primarily through drinking water and food, as well as occupational inhalation exposure (http://www.epa.gov/teach/).

The US-EPA standard for arsenic in drinking water is 10 ppb; however, geographic hotspots exist in the southwest US, Bangladesh, Taiwan and elsewhere with excessive drinking water levels, reaching 200 to >500 ppb. In 2009, the International Agency for Research on Cancer classified arsenics as "carcinogenic to humans" based on sufficient evidence in humans for lung, skin, and urinary bladder cancers. Additionally, epidemiology and animal studies show heightened risk for PC with chronic iAs exposure.[62–64] Epidemiologic studies have shown an association between arsenic exposure and PC mortality in Taiwan, a finding that was substantiated by a later study in the United States.[59,65] In this context, there is a recent report that arsenic can induce malignant transformation of prostate epithelial cells *in vitro* and drive them toward an androgen-independent state.[66] Importantly, it has been documented that arsenic may mediate some of these effects through endocrine disruption, specifically through interaction and interference with multiple steroid receptor family members, including ERs, ARs, and retinoid acid receptors/retinoid X receptors, perhaps through common zinc-finger interactions.[66,67] Thus it is possible that endocrine disruption by arsenic can contribute to PC risk.

12.2.3 Anti-Androgens

While there are no known environmental androgens, environmental chemicals can also function through anti-androgenic pathways. Since prostate cancer is an androgen-dependent disease, we will briefly examine the known effects of some of these agents on the prostate gland.

12.2.3.1 Vinclozolin

Vinclozolin is a fungicide that is used as a pesticide on crops. It has known anti-androgenic properties, interfering with AR activity.[68] Since vinclozolin effects are driven through AR antagonism, it is not surprising that there are no reported associations between this compound and PC, an androgen-dependent disease. Exposure of rats to vinclozolin during development results in reduced prostate gland growth and size, which would be expected for an anti-androgen.[69] Of interest, however, are recent studies with maternal (i.e. *in utero*) exposure to vinclozolin in rats which produce transgenerational effects on offspring through epigenetic alterations.[69] These permanent perturbations include adverse consequences on the prostate gland, such as premature acinar atrophy and aging-associated prostatitis for four generations.[70] This may be particularly significant in light of recent evidence that chronic inflammation may play a role in prostate cancer initiation.[71]

12.2.3.2 Dichlorodiphenyltrichloroethane/dichlorodiphenyl-dichloroethylene (DDT/DDE)

DDT and its metabolic derivative *p,p′*-DDE were widely used as pesticides in the United States, and they are still used in other countries worldwide. In addition to AR antagonistic effects,[72] *p,p′*-DDE at high concentrations has been shown to function as an inhibitor of 5α-reductase, the intraprostatic enzyme responsible for converting testosterone to the more potent androgen, dihydrotestosterone.[73] While many reproductive abnormalities, including reduced prostate growth, have been attributed to DDT/DDE exposure, there is limited data for an exposure to DDT/*p,p′*-DDE and PC risk. A recent assessment of pesticide exposures in British Columbia farmers noted a significant association between DDT exposure and PC risk (odds ratio = 1.68) and this deserves follow-up investigations in other populations and cohorts.[18]

12.2.4 Dioxins

Dioxins [polychlorinated dibenzo-*p*-dioxins (PCDDs)] resist degradation and are thus considered persistent organic pollutants. 2,3,7,8-tetrachlorodibenzo-*p*-dioxin (TCDD) is the most toxic dioxin and causes a variety of effects, including immunotoxicity, hepatotoxicity, teratogenicity, and tumor promotion.[74] Changes in gene expression induced by TCDD and related chemicals are initiated by binding to the aryl hydrocarbon receptor (AhR),[75] and crosstalk between AhR and ERα is well established. Activated AhR inhibits ER activity through several mechanisms, whereas ERα has a positive role in AhR signaling.[76] Additionally, an inverse relationship was found between serum TCDD levels and serum testosterone in chemical production workers.[77]

Adult TCDD exposure at general population levels is associated with a decreasing risk of benign prostate hyperplasia (BPH) with higher exposure levels.[78] Further, TCDD increased tumor-free survival in transgenic TRAMP mice that spontaneously develop PC, while AhR activation decreased lymph node metastasis, suggesting that TCDDs may protect against prostate cancer in adulthood. In contrast, *in utero* exposure to TCDD in mice interferes with prostate bud patterning and is associated with hyperplastic lesions in aged animals. Together, these findings suggest that timing of TCDD exposures may dictate their effects on subsequent prostate disease.[79]

12.3 Environmental Chemicals and Prostate Stem/Progenitor Cells

The prostate gland contains a simple columnar epithelium with three differentiated cell types— basal, luminal, and neuroendocrine—that are embedded in a fibro-muscular stroma.[80,81] The major epithelial cell population is luminal secretory cells, which express cytokeratins (CK) 8/18 and AR and are androgen-dependent for growth, survival, and production of secretory proteins such as prostate specific antigen (PSA). Basal epithelial cells are interspersed along the basement membrane and express p63 and CK5 but are largely AR negative and androgen-independent. The scarce population of neuroendocrine cells is scattered within the basal layer and is identified by the expression of chromogranin A and synaptophysin. Strong evidence now exists for the presence of a rare population of adult stem cells within the human prostate gland; these cells are capable of self-renewal, as well as differentiation into early progenitor cells, which give rise to the three differentiated epithelial cell populations.[81–85]

It is widely accepted that adult stem cells are involved in normal tissue replenishment throughout life, while cancer stem cells support cancer growth,[86,87] although the cell(s) of origin for prostate cancer may include luminal, basal, neuroendocrine, progenitor, and stem cells.[81,88] It is increasingly evident that the resultant prostate cancers contain cancer stem cells that continuously seed and maintain tumor growth.[89,90] As the property of self-renewal allows for a long life span of stem cells, undifferentiated stem/progenitor cells are highly susceptible to environmental injuries over time and have the capacity to transmit their "injury memory" to the differentiated progeny.[91] Since the prostate gland is most susceptible to environmental insults during early development, it is reasonable to predict that prostate stem and early stage progenitor cells may be the primary targets of estrogenic exposures throughout life.[7]

Recently, our laboratory reported that that human prostate stem/progenitor cells from normal, disease-free prostates express high levels of estrogen receptors, including ERα, ERβ, and GPR30, and exhibit a proliferative response to 1 nM 17β-estradiol.[13] New studies using side-population fluorescence activated cell sorting (FACS) analysis of primary prostate epithelial cell cultures (Hoechst 33342 exclusion with and without verapamil) show a dose-dependent increase in human prostate stem cell numbers after 4 days of culture in 10–1000 nM E2 (Figure 12.1 A). Together, these results demonstrate that normal human prostate stem and progenitor cells are responsive to estrogens with increased rates of self-renewal, implicating them as direct estrogen targets. Furthermore, treatment of primary prostate epithelial cells with 10 nM BPA

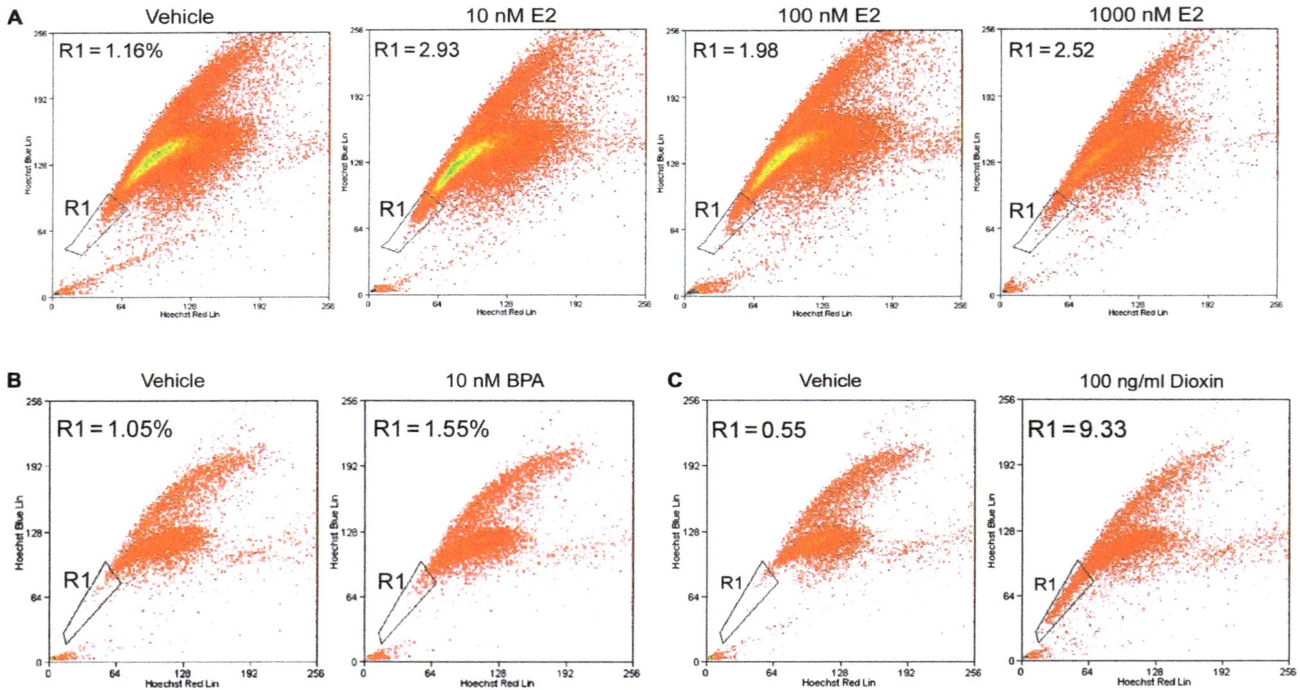

Figure 12.1 Effects of E2, BPA, arsenite and dioxin on prostate stem/progenitor cell proliferation, evaluated by side population analysis and prostasphere assay. (A) E2 (10–1000 nM) treatment increased the percentage of side population cells (R1) at all doses, as measured by Hoechst 33342 dye efflux using flow cytometry analysis. Prostate epithelial cells were stained with 5 μg mL^{-1} of Hoechst 33342 either in the absence (graphs shown) or presence (not shown) of 50 μM of verapamil hydrochloride before analysis. (B) BPA (10 nM) treatment also increased the percentage of side population cells (R1). (C) Dioxin (100 ng mL^{-1}) treatment increased the percentage of side population cells (R1).

increased the percentage of side population of prostate stem/progenitor cells (Figure 12.1 B), similar to the E2 exposures. Dioxin (100 ng mL^{-1}) markedly increased side population numbers in 2-D prostate epithelial cell cultures, indicating a stimulation of stem cell self-renewal (Figure 12.1 C).[13] Together, these findings support the hypothesis that ECs may target the prostate stem and early-stage progenitor cell populations which may contribute to increased prostate cancer risk following exposures.

12.4 Conclusion

There is accumulating and consistent evidence that exposures to ECs over a life time are associated with an increased risk of PC. Published findings for the individual chemicals are summarized in Table 12.1. While the findings for individual compounds and classes of compounds may be somewhat limited and at times contradictory, the evidence must be considered as a whole. Overall, there are clear trends that support a link between early-life EC exposures, as well as accumulation of persistent ECs throughout life, and an increased risk of PC. This is supported with a wealth of research using animal models, as well as *in vitro* systems, that has allowed researchers to dissect potential mechanisms of action. Clearly, continued animal and epidemiologic studies are required over the next several years to accurately determine risks of cancers as a function of accumulating ECs in the environment. These evaluations will be critical for the establishment of proper guidelines and federal regulations regarding use, exposure, and dispersal of these compounds. The development of biomarkers for EC exposures would also be of great future benefit to the medical and regulatory community as we try to link exposures with disease outcomes. In summary, while there has been significant progress in determining human PC risks from ECs, there is much that remains to be done in the decades to come.

References

1. R. Swerdloff and B. C. Robaire, Handbook of Andrology, *The American Society of Andrology*, 2010, p. 2-1.
2. B. R. Zirkin and B. C. Robaire, Handbook of Andrology, *The American Society of Andrology*, 2010, p. 4-1.
3. A. Jemal, R. Siegel, E. Ward, Y. Hao, J. Xu, T. Murray and M. J. Thun, *CA: A Cancer Journal for Clinicians*, 2008, **58**, 71.
4. M. A. Eisenberger, B. A. Blumenstein, E. D. Crawford, G. Miller, D. G. McLeod, P. J. Loehrer, G. Wilding, K. Sears, D. J. Culkin, I. M. Thompson Jr., A. J. Bueschen and B. A. Lowe, *N. Engl. J. Med.*, 1998, **339**, 1036.
5. C. Huggins and C. F. Hodges, *Cancer Res.*, 1941, **1**, 293.
6. S. J. Ellem and G. P. Risbridger, *Nat. Rev*, 2007, **7**, 621.
7. W. Y. Hu, G. B. Shi, H. M. Lam, D. P. Hu, S. M. Ho, I. C. Madueke, A. Kajdacsy-Balla and G. S. Prins, *Endocrinology*, 2011, **152**, 2150.

8. G. S. Prins, L. Birch, W. Y. Yang and S. M. Ho, *Reprod. Toxicol.*, 2007, **23**, 374.
9. G. S. Prins and K. S. Korach, *Steroids*, 2008, **73**, 233.
10. F. Modugno, J. L. Weissfeld, D. L. Trump, J. M. Zmuda, P. Shea, J.A. Cauley and R. E. Ferrell, *Clin. Cancer Res.*, 2001, **7**, 3092.
11. M. C. Bosland and Urol, *Oncol*, 1996, **2**, 103.
12. D. L. LaSalle Jr. and S. H. Reuben, 2008–2009 Annual Report: The President's Cancer Panel, National Institutes of Health, Bethesda, MD, April 2010.
13. W. Y. Hu, G. B. Shi, D. P. Hu and G. S. Prins, *Mol. Cell. Endocrinol.*, 2012, **354**, 63.
14. H. Morrison, D. Savitz, R. Semenciw, B. Hulka, Y. Mao, D. Morison and D. Wigle, *Am. J. Epidemiol.*, 1993, **137**, 270.
15. M. C. Alavanja, C. Samanic, M. Dosemeci, J. Lubin, R. Tarone, C. F. Lynch, C. Knott, K. Thomas, J. A. Hoppin, J. Barker, J. Coble, D. P. Sandler and A. Blair, *Am. J. Epidemiol.*, 2003, **157**, 800.
16. T. E. Meyer, A. L. Coker, M. Sanderson and E. Symanski, *Occup. Environ. Med.*, 2007, **64**, 155.
17. G. Van Maele-Fabry, G. Libotte, J. Willems and D. Lison, *Cancer Causes Control*, 2006, **17**, 353.
18. R. R. Band, Z. A. Abonto, J. Bert, B. Lang, R. Fang, R. P. Gallagher and N. D. Le, *Prostate*, 2011, **71**, 168.
19. R. Mahajan, M. R. Bonner, J. A. Hoppin and M. C. Alavanja, *Environ. Health Perspect.*, 2006, **114**, 1205.
20. K. A. Usmani, R. L. Rose and E. Hodgson, *Drug Metab. Dispos.*, 2003, **31**, 384.
21. K. A. Usmani, T. M. Cho, R. L. Rose and E. Hodgson., *Drug Metab. Dispos.*, 2006, **34**, 1606.
22. N. Finnström, C. Bjelfman, T. Söderström, G. Smith, L. Egevad, B. Norlén, C. R. Wolf and A. Rane, *Eur. J. Clin. Invest.*, 2001, **31**, 880.
23. T. Lawson and C. Kolar, *Cancer Lett.*, 2002, **175**, 141.
24. K. M. Sterling and K. R. Cutrineo, *J. Cell Biol.*, 2004, **91**, 423.
25. M. H. Kester, S. Bulduk, D. Tibboel, W. Meinl, H. Glatt, C. N. Falany, M. W. Coughtrie, A. Bergman, S. H. Safe, G. G. Kuiper, A. G. Schuur, A. Brouwer and T. J. Visser, *Endocrinology*, 2000, **141**, 1897.
26. M. H. Kester, S. Bulduk, H. van Toor, D. Tibboel, W. Meinl, H. Glatt, C. N. Falany, M. W. Coughtrie, A. G. Schuur, A. Brouwer and T.J. Visser, *J Clin. Endocrinol. Metab.*, 2002, **87**, 1142.
27. I. Leav, S. Ho, P. Ofner, F. Merk, P. Kwan and D. Damassa, *J. Natl. Cancer Inst.*, 1988, **80**, 1045.
28. S. G. Driscoll and S. G. Taylor, *Obstet and Gynecol*, 1980, **56**, 537.
29. C. Y. Yonemura, G. R. Cunha, Y. Sugimura and S. L. Mee, *Acta Anat.*, 1995, **153**, 1.
30. R. M. Giusti, K. Iwamoto and E. E. Hatch, *Ann. Intern. Med.*, 1995, **122**, 778.
31. J. Rajfer and D. S. Coffey, *Invest. Urol*, 1978, **16**, 186.

32. Y. Arai, T. Mori, Y. Suzuki and H. A. Bern, *Int. Rev. Cytol.*, 1983, **84**, 235.
33. L. Huang, Y. Pu, S. Alam, L. Birch and G. S. Prins, *J. Androl.*, 2004, **25**, 330.
34. A. M. Calafat, X. Ye, L. Y. Wong, J. A. Reidy and L. L. Needham, *Environ. Health Perspect.*, 2008, **116**, 39.
35. G. G. Kuiper, J. G. Lemmen, B. Carlsson, J. C. Corton, S. H. Safe, P. T. van der Saag, B. van der Burg and J. A. Gustafsson, *Endocrinology*, 1998, **139**, 4252.
36. J. G. Lemmen, R. J. Arends, P. T. van der Saag and B. van der Burg, *Environ. Health Perspect.*, 2004, **112**, 1544.
37. T. Kurosawa, H. Hiroi, O. Tsutsumi, T. Ishikawa, Y. Osuga, T. Fujiwara, S. Inoue, M. Muramatsu, M. Momoeda and Y. Taketani, *Endocr. J.*, 2002, **49**, 465.
38. K. H. Song, K. Lee and H. S Choi, *Endocrinology*, 2002, **143**, 2208.
39. D. E. Walsh, P. Dockery and C. M. Doolan, *Mol. Cell. Endocrinol.*, 2005, **230**, 23.
40. R. Keri, S. M. Ho, P. A. Hunt, K. E. Knudsen, A. M. Soto and G. S. Prins, *Reprod. Toxicol.*, 2007, **24**, 240.
41. S. M. Ho, W. Y. Tang, J. Belmonte and G. S. Prins., *Cancer Res.*, 2006, **66**, 5624.
42. J. M. Kaufman and A. Vermeulen, *Endocr. Rev.*, 2005, **26**, 833.
43. W. Y. Tang, L. M. Morey, Y. Y. Cheung, L. Birch, G. S. Prins and S.M. Ho, *Endocrinology*, 2012, **153**, 42.
44. L. Hardell, S. O. Andersson, M. Carlberg, L. Bohr, B. van Bavel, G. Lindström, H. Björnfoth and C. J. Ginman, *Occup. Environ. Med.*, 2006, **48**, 700.
45. L. E. Charles, D. Loomis, C. M. Shy, B. Newman, R. Millikan, L. A. Nylander-French and D. Couper, *Am. J. Epidemiol.*, 2003, **157**, 683.
46. J. M. Ritchie, S. L. Vial, L. J. Fuortes, H. Guo, V. E. Reedy and E. M. Smith, *J. Occup. Environ. Med.*, 2003, **45**, 692.
47. F. Cillo, M. de Eguileor, F. Gandolfi and T. Brevini, *Endocr.-Relat. Cancer*, 2007, **14**, 257.
48. M. Schlumpf, P. Schmid, S. Durrer, M. Conscience, K. Maerkel, M. Henseler, M. Gruetter, I. Herzog, S. Reolon, R. Ceccatelli, O. Faass, E. Stutz, H. Jarry, W. Wuttke and W. Lichtensteiger, *Toxicology*, 2004b, **205**, 113.
49. M. Schlumpf, H. Jarry, W. Wuttke and W. Lichtensteiger, *Toxicology*, 2004a, **199**, 109.
50. M. D. Anway, A. S. Cupp, M. Uzumcu and M. K. Skinner, *Science*, 2005, **308**, 1466.
51. T. E. Stoker, C. Robinette and R. L. Cooper, *Toxicol. Sci.*, 1999, **52**, 68.
52. P. A. MacLennan, E. Delzell, N. Sathiakumar, S. L. Myers, H. Cheng, W. Grizzle, V. W. Chen and X. C. Xu, *J. Occup. Environ. Med.*, 2002, **44**, 1048.
53. J. Sass, *J. Occup. Environ. Med.*, 2004, **45**, 343.

54. P. A. Hessel, R. Kalmes, T. J. Smith, E. Lau, P. J. Mink and J. Mandel, *J. Occup. Environ. Med.*, 2004, **46**, 379.
55. J. A. Rusiecki, A. De Roos, W. J. Lee, M. Dosemeci, J. H. Lubin, J.A. Hoppin, A. Blair and M. C. Alavanja, *J. Natl. Cancer Inst.*, 2004, **96**, 1375.
56. M. E. Parent and J. Siemiatycki, *Epidemiologic Reviews*, 2001, **23**, 138.
57. L. Benbrahim-Tallaa, J. Liu, M. M. Webber and M. P. Waalkes, *Prostate*, 2007b, **67**, 135.
58. M. P. Waalkes, *J. Inorg. Biochem.*, 2000, **79**, 241.
59. C. J. Chen, T. Kuo and M. Wu, *Lancet*, 1988, **1**, 414.
60. W. H. Watson and J. D. Yager, *Toxicol. Sci.*, 2007, **98**, 1.
61. K. Straif, L. Benbrahim-Tallaa, R. Baan, Y. Grosse, B. Secretan, F. El Ghissassi, V. Bouvard, N. Guha, C. Freeman, L. Galichet and V. Cogliano, *Lancet Oncol.*, 2009, **10**, 453.
62. L. Benbrahim-Tallaa and M. P. Waalkes, *Environ. Health Perspect.*, 2008, **116**, 158.
63. C. Y. Yang, C. C. Chang and H. F. Chiu, *J. Toxicol. Environ. Health, Part A*, 2008, **71**, 1559.
64. E. J. Tokar, L. Benbrahim-Tallaa, J. M. Ward, R. Lunn, R. L. Sams and M. P. Waalkes, *Crit. Rev. Toxicol.*, 2010, **40**, 912.
65. D. R. Lewis, J. W. Southwick, R. Ouellet-Hellstrom, J. Rench and R. Calderon, *Environ. Health Perspect.*, 1999, **107**, 359.
66. J. C. Davey, J. E. Bodwell, J. A. Gosse and J. Hamilton, *Toxicol. Sci.*, 2007, **98**, 75.
67. X. Zhou, X. Sun, K. L. Cooper, F. Wang, K. J. Liu and L. G. Hudson, *J. Biol. Chem.*, 2011, **286**, 22855.
68. R. Kavlok and A. Cummings, *Crit. Rev. Toxicol.*, 2005, **35**, 721.
69. W. Yu, B. Lee, S. Nam, B. Ahn, J Hong, J. Do, Y. Kim, Y. Lee and Y. Yun, *J. Vet. Med. Sci*, 2004, **66**, 847.
70. L. Benbrahim-Tallaa, M. M. Webber and M. P. Waalkes, *Environ. Health Perspect.*, 2007, **115**, 243.
71. W. G. Nelson, T. L. DeWeese and A. M. DeMarzo, *Cancer Metastasis Rev.*, 2002, **21**, 3.
72. L. E. Gray, C. Wolf, C. Lambright, P. Mann, M. Price, R. L. Cooper and J. Ostby, *J. Toxicol. Ind. Health*, 1999, **15**, 94.
73. S. Lo, I. King, A. Alléra and D. Klingmüller, *Toxicol. In Vitro*, 2007, **21**, 502.
74. N. Kuroda, Y. Kinoshita, Y. Sun, M. Wada, N. Kishikawa, K. Nakashima, T. Makino and H. Nakazawa, *J. Pharm. Biol. Anal*, 2003, **30**, 1743.
75. M. Kuroda, K. Oikawa, T. Ohbayashi, K. Yoshida, K. Yamada, J. Mimura, Y. Matsuda, Y. Fujii-Kuriyama and K. Mukai, *FEBS Lett*, 2005, **579**, 167.
76. J. Matthews and J. A. Gustafsson, *Nucl. Recept. Signal*, 2006, **4**, e016.
77. G. M. Egel, M. H. Sweeney, M. A. Fingerhut, K. K. Wille, T.M. Schnorr and W. E. Halperin, *Am. J. Epidemiol.*, 1994, **139**, 272.

78. A. Gupta, N. Ketchum, C. G. Roehrborn, A. Schecter, C. C Aragaki and J. E. Michalek, *Environ. Health Perspect.*, 2006, **114**, 1649.
79. C. M. Vezina, T. M. Lin and R. E. Peterson, *Biochem. Pharmacol.*, 2009, **77**, 566.
80. J. T. Isaacs, E. R. Barrack, W. B. Isaacs and D. S. Coffey in *The Prostatic Cell: Structure and Function-Part A*, (eds) G. P. Murphy, A. A. Sandburg and J. P. Karr, Publisher: Alan R Liss, New York, 1981, p. 1–24.
81. X. Wang, M. Kruithof-de Julio, K. D. Economides, D. Walker, H. Yu, M. V. Halili, Y. P. Hu, S. M. Price, C. Abate-Shen and M. M. Shen, *Nature*, 2009, **461**, 495.
82. P. E. Burger, X. Xiong, S. Coetzee, S. N. Salm, D. Moscatelli, K. Goto and E. L. Wilson, *Proc. Natl. Acad. Sci. U. S. A.*, 2005, **102**, 180.
83. A. De Marzo, W. Nelson, A. Meeker and D. Coffey, *J. Urol.*, 1998, **160**, 2381.
84. K. G Leong, B. E. Wang, L. Johnson and W. Q. Gao, *Nature*, 2008, **456**, 804.
85. J. Miki and J. Rhim, *Prostate Cancer Prostatic Dis.*, 2008, **11**, 32.
86. S. C. Presnell, B. Petersen and M. Heidaran, *Semin. Cell Dev. Biol.*, 2002, **13**, 369.
87. S. Smith, W. Neaves and S. Teitelbaum, *Science*, 2007, **316**, 5830.
88. S. Kasper, *Stem Cell Rev.*, 2008, **4**, 193.
89. G. Gu, J. Yuan, M. Wills and S. Kasper, *Cancer Res.*, 2007, **67**, 4708.
90. S. Kasper, *Urol. Oncol.*, 2009, **27**, 301.
91. A. S. Cheng, A. C. Culhane, M. W. Chan, C. R. Venkataramu, M. Ehrich, A. Nasir, B. A. Rodriguez, J. Liu, P. S. Yan, J. Quackenbush, K. P. Nephew, T. J. Yeatman and T. H. Huang, *Cancer Res.*, 2008, **68**, 1786.

CHAPTER 13

The Aging Kidney and Exposure to the Nephrotoxic Metals Cadmium and Mercury

CHRISTY C. BRIDGES* AND RUDOLFS K. ZALUPS

Mercer University School of Medicine, Division of Basic Medical Sciences, Macon, Georgia 31207, USA
*E-mail: Bridges_cc@mercer.edu

13.1 Introduction

Aging is an inevitable fact of life. Owing to advances in modern medicine over the past century, the life-expectancy of humans in developed and developing countries has lengthened significantly. According to the World Health Organization, the global life expectancy has risen from 64 years in 1990 to 68 years in 2011.[1] In developed countries such as the United States, the average life expectancy has increased from 47.3 years in 1900 to 77.9 years in 2007.[2] Similar trends exist for other developed and developing countries, such as the United Kingdom, Japan, Chile and Sri Lanka. Increases in life expectancy have led to an increase in the aged and elderly population. World-wide, it is currently estimated that approximately 650 million individuals are over the age of 60. Because of lengthening life expectancies, this figure is expected to increase to 2 billion by 2050.[1] In the United States alone, the percentage of individuals over the age of 65 has increased approximately tenfold in the past century. In 1900,

Issues in Toxicology No. 16
Aging and Vulnerability to Environmental Chemicals: Age-related Disorders and their Origins in Environmental Exposures
Edited by Bernard Weiss

Published by the Royal Society of Chemistry, www.rsc.org

approximately 3.1 million individuals, or 4.1% of the population, were over the age of 65. This number increased to approximately 35 million (12.4% of the population) in 2000.[3] A thorough understanding of the impact of aging on organ systems, such as the kidney, will be critical when managing the healthcare of elderly and aged individuals. Furthermore, aging may enhance individual susceptibility to disease as well as increase one's risk of being negatively affected by exposure to environmental and/or occupational toxicants. Because of increased life expectancy and increased pollution in the environment, it is likely that elderly and aged individuals will be exposed more often and possibly to higher levels of toxic pollutants than individuals were decades ago. Given this trend, it is important that we understand not only the normal aging process, but also the effects of exposure of aging individuals to potential nephrotoxicants, such as the toxic metals cadmium (Cd) and mercury (Hg).

13.2 Aging and the Normal Kidneys

Aging results in many deleterious structural and physiological changes in the kidneys. These changes may be related entirely to renal cell senescence or, alternatively, they may be consequences of multiple factors, such as age-related hemodynamic changes, renal or non-renal disease, and/or life-long exposure to environmental and/or occupational toxicants. The aging kidneys are capable of maintaining normal renal function and systemic homeostasis in healthy individuals, despite the fact that the normal aging process has been shown to have significant deleterious structural and physiological consequences. These changes are thought to significantly affect the functional reserve of the kidneys in that the kidneys have a reduced capacity to respond to challenges such as changes in hemodynamics and exposure to toxicants. Because of this reduction in functional reserve, the kidneys, and possibly other organs, may be more susceptible to physiologic, pathologic, and toxicologic challenges.

13.2.1 Structural Changes within the Glomerulus

One of the primary targets of the aging process is the renal glomerulus. Significant ultrastructural changes occur within numerous glomeruli as a result of the normal aging process. Indeed it has been reported that approximately 30%–40% of all glomeruli become sclerotic by the eighth decade of life.[4–7] Structural characteristics of a typical sclerotic glomerulus include a thickened glomerular basement membrane (GBM), expanded mesangial matrix, and shrinkage and occlusion of the glomerular capillaries (Figure 13.1).[6,8–10]

Although the pathogenesis of this process is not completely understood, it is thought that age-related glomerulosclerosis and the resulting drop in glomerular filtration rate (GFR) are the results of multiple factors, including increased susceptibility to inflammatory cytokines, alterations in blood flow, and damage to the glomerular filtration barrier (Figure 13.2).[11–13] A reduction in the total number of functioning nephrons appears to be an additional

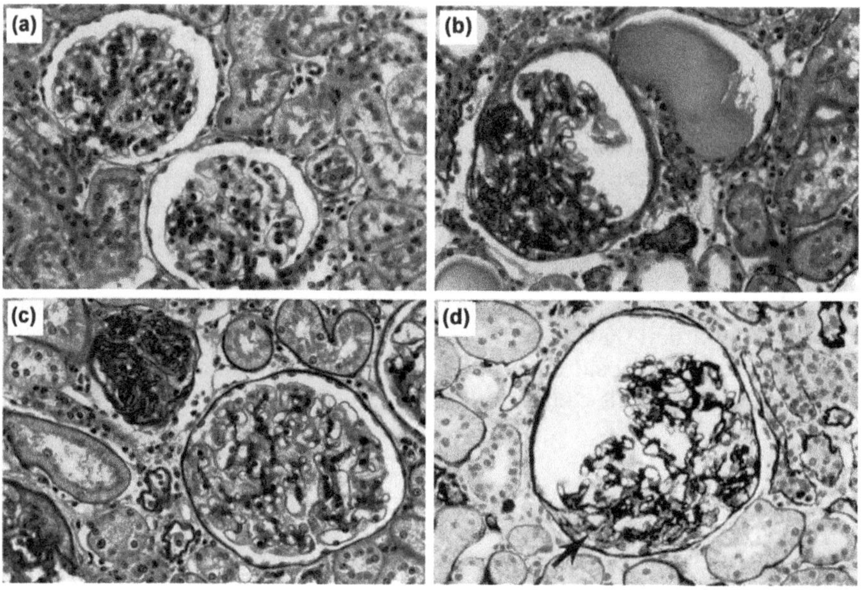

Figure 13.1 Glomeruli of young rats display normal glomerular morphology (a) [periodic-acid Schiff (PAS) stain]; At 24 months of age rat kidneys contained glomeruli that were characteristic of both focal segmental glomerulosclerosis (b) and global glomerulosclerosis (c). Adhesions (arrow) between Bowman's capsule and the glomerular tuft were also observed in some glomeruli (d) [Silver stain]. (400×).
Reprinted with permission from Ref. 14.

contributing factor in the development of glomerulosclerosis. As nephrons are lost, vascular and glomerular changes occur in remaining functional nephrons in an attempt to compensate for the reduction in GFR.[11,15] These changes lead to glomerular hypertrophy, hyperperfusion, and hyperfiltration, which increase the single nephron GFR (SNGFR) and thus predispose affected glomeruli to sclerotic changes.[11,16–18]

Indeed a positive correlation between glomerular hypertrophy and the development of glomerulosclerosis has been demonstrated in aging mice.[19] In addition, proliferation of mesangial cells and expansion of mesangial matrix, both of which are often associated with glomerular hypertrophy, appear to precede and contribute to the development of glomerulosclerosis.[20] Alternatively, age-related glomerulosclerosis may occur *via* immunologic mechanisms whereby formation of circulating or *in situ* immune complexes leads to glomerulonephritis.[13]

Interestingly, glomeruli in the outer cortex appear to be affected earlier and more severely by sclerotic changes than those in the juxtamedullary region.[6,21,22] As cortical glomeruli degenerate, glomerular capillaries atrophy, which leads to sclerosis. Interestingly, in juxtamedullary glomeruli, a direct channel is formed between the afferent and efferent arterioles, resulting in

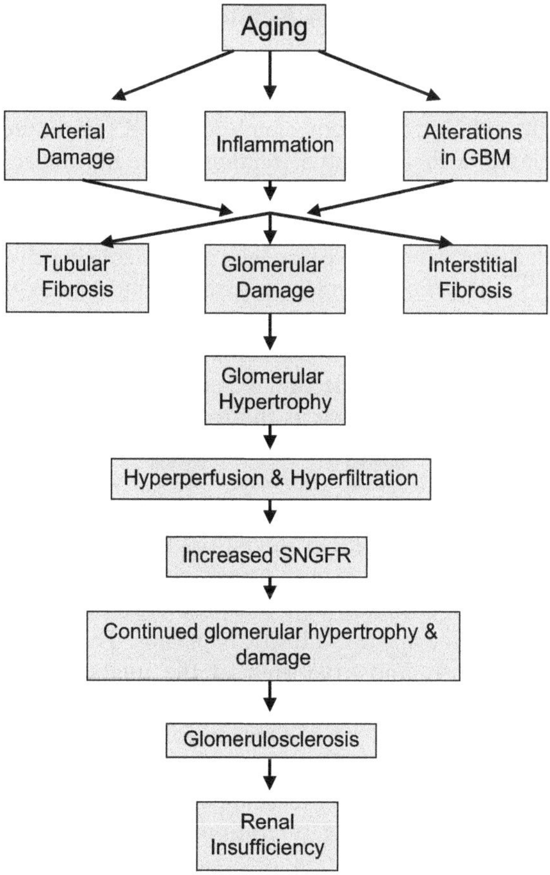

Figure 13.2 Possible pathogenesis of age-related glomerulosclerosis. Many factors have been proposed to contribute to age-related glomerulosclerosis; these include hemodynamic and structural alterations at the site of the glomerulus. These changes may lead to glomerular hypertrophy followed by hyperperfusion and hyperfiltration of affected glomeruli. Owing to these hypertrophic changes, single nephron glomerular filtration rate increases and may lead to glomerular injury, and ultimately glomerulosclerosis and renal insufficiency.

arterioles that do not communicate hemodynamically with a glomerulus.[11] In general, these aberrant glomeruli tend to be larger than other cortical glomeruli; therefore, a significant reduction in the functionality of this population of glomeruli likely leads to significant reductions in whole-body GFR. An important marker of glomerular damage is proteinuria, which results from a disruption of the glomerular filtration barrier. Indeed recent studies have suggested that injury to and dysfunction of podocytes, which are key components of the glomerular filtration barrier, may play a role in the pathogenesis of age-related glomerulosclerosis.[23–25]

13.2.2 Structural Changes in Renal Tubules and Interstitium

Age-related changes have also been observed within renal tubules. These changes include atrophy and degeneration, formation of diverticula, irregular thickening of the tubular basement membrane, and tubulointerstitial fibrosis, which is associated with interstitial inflammation, fibroblast activation, and increased deposition of collagen.[10,26–28] Ding and colleagues[26] examined senescent tubular epithelial cells and found increased expression of transforming growth factor β-1 (TGF-β1), which plays a role in cell cycle regulation, and $p21^{WAF1/CIP1}$, a cyclin-dependent kinase inhibitor thought to be involved in regulating cell growth. Although the reason for the upregulation of TGF-β1 and $p21^{WAF1/CIP1}$ is unclear, it is possible that this increased expression leads to a dysregulation of the cell cycle and consequently, cell growth. Similarly, increased expression of genes such as the hypoxia-inducible factor 1 (HIF-1), which mediates cell and tissue responses to hypoxia,[29] appears to play a role in the development of interstitial fibrosis.[30] In addition, accumulations of macrophages and myofibroblasts, which are involved in collagen deposition, have been shown to be present in interstitial areas of fibrosis.[31] Given the presence of myofibroblasts, it is not surprising that increased deposition of collagens (types I and III),[31] as well as noncollagenous proteins,[27] has been detected in the interstitial space of fibrotic nephrons. This deposition is thought to contribute to fibrosis and expansion of the interstitium. An increase in apoptosis of tubular and interstitial cells has also been observed in areas of fibrosis.[10] This apoptosis may be one reason for the documented decreases in volume, length, and number of tubular segments from fibrotic nephrons.[13,28,32] As a consequence of these structural changes, alterations in tubular function are also likely to occur. These alterations include a reduced ability to concentrate/dilute urine,[33] maintain acid/base balance,[34] and filter solutes, especially sodium.[28,35]

13.2.3 Physiologic Changes in the Kidney

Since the aging kidney is subjected to considerable changes in structure, it is not surprising to find that GFR also changes significantly as the kidney ages.[6,9,22,28,36,37] Estimates indicate that beginning at an age of 30–40 years, total GFR decreases by approximately 10% per decade of life.[9,13,17,37,38] The rate of decline has been shown to increase after the age of 65.[35,37,39] The Baltimore Longitudinal Study of Aging, which collected data from patients aged 17 to 96, over a 23-year period, found that creatinine clearance (*i.e.*, GFR) declined by 0.75 mL min^{-1} per year.[40,41] This decrease is most likely a consequence of multiple factors, including damage to and inadequate regeneration of podocytes, glomerulosclerosis, and an eventual reduction in the total number of functioning nephrons.[25,42,43] Interestingly, the findings from the Baltimore Longitudinal Study suggested that GFR may not decrease in every patient. Although the overall findings of this study suggested that GFR is reduced steadily over time, of the 254 patients evaluated, 92 (36%) showed no significant reduction in GFR.[40] Since the publication of this study, weakness in the design and analysis of data have been noted by others.[44] Interestingly, several recent studies have proposed a link between one's genetic background and the tendency to develop age-related glomerular changes that lead to reductions in GFR.[45–48] Thus individual genetic differences may account for the lack of change in GFR observed in some patients. Despite the mixed findings of the Baltimore Longitudinal Study, there is overwhelming evidence to suggest that a decline in GFR is a normal consequence of aging.[5,13,37,44]

In addition to changes in GFR, aging also appears to affect renal blood flow (RBF) to the kidney.[5,9,22] Maximum RBF is reached around the third decade, following which RBF has been shown to decrease by approximately 10% per decade of life.[6] This decrease appears to be related to changes in the vascular resistance in afferent and efferent arterioles rather than to changes in cardiac output[49] or renal perfusion.[50] Because the decrease in total GFR is generally less than the decrease in RBF, filtration fraction (FF) increases in most patients.[5,13,22,38] It should be pointed out that although overall RBF decreases, variable changes in blood flow occur at the level of the individual nephron. Within a single, hypertrophied nephron, RBF increases as a result of the hypertrophic changes that occur within that nephron.[51,52] Increases in RBF may lead to increased intraglomerular pressure, which may then lead to glomerular injury.

Renal functional reserve may also be altered in elderly and aged individuals. Renal functional reserve is the ability of the kidney to increase its basal RBF and GFR by 20% or more after a stimulus, such as a protein load.[36,53] Studies of renal functional reserve in elderly individuals have yielded mixed results. While some studies found that the functional reserve of the kidneys is preserved to some extent in healthy elderly individuals,[54,55] a separate study reported that renal functional reserve is reduced or depleted in the elderly and aged, in order to accommodate for the age-related decline in renal function and as an attempt to preserve normal renal function.[56] Another study found that the renal functional reserve of the elderly remained intact, but its magnitude was lower in older individuals than in younger individuals.[57] Similarly, *in vivo* studies using aged Sprague-Dawley rats provided evidence for an age-related decline in renal functional reserve.[58] Moreover, it has been shown that functional reserve of the kidneys is decreased or absent in patients with diseases such as diabetes and hypertension.[59–62]

Aging and cell senescence also leads to changes at the cellular level. Under normal conditions, the mitotic index for renal epithelial cells is low, with proliferation occurring in approximately 1% of renal tubular cells. This percentage declines with age and may impair the ability of renal tubules to repair themselves.[63] Similarly, studies in mouse kidneys have shown that the normal burst of proliferation observed following an acute insult to renal tubules is reduced in aged kidneys.[64] These data are supported by the findings of Shurin and colleagues, who assessed plasma levels of various cytokines in individuals ranging from 45 to 78 years old[65] and found that levels of insulin-like growth factor-1 (IGF-1) were lower in aged individuals.[65] Others have reported decreases in epidermal growth factor (EGF).[52] Furthermore, results from cDNA microarray profiling of genes from human kidneys indicate that many genes are down-regulated in aged kidneys. Most of these genes appear to be related to energy metabolism, as well as nucleotide, amino acid, and protein turnover. An increase in gene expression was noted in a selected set of genes responsible for immune and inflammatory responses.[47] Indeed, in separate studies, increases in the expression of tumor necrosis factor (TNF)-α and interleukin (IL)-6, which are both involved in inflammatory processes, were found to be associated with aging.[66–68] In addition to changes in cytokines responsible for growth and inflammation, it appears that aging also negatively affects the regulatory control of apoptosis, leading to an increase in the basal levels of apoptosis in the kidney.[69]

13.3 Aging and Kidney Disease

There is a clear association between aging and the development of kidney disease. One can speculate that as the kidneys age, they lose their capacity to cope with certain challenges. Therefore, when an aged kidney is challenged, physiologically, pathologically, or toxicologically, renal function will likely be affected. Indeed an epidemiological study analyzing 437 cases of acute renal failure in Spain demonstrated that acute renal failure was 3.5 times more prevalent in adults over the age of 70 than in younger adults.[70] Similarly, an analysis of data obtained from the Third National Health and Nutrition Examination Study (NHANES) in the United States identified an association between age and the incidence of chronic renal failure.[71] It was noted that, even in the absence of other diseases such as hypertension and diabetes, approximately 11% of individuals over the age of 65 have been diagnosed with moderate to severe renal failure.[71] The progression of renal failure also appeared to occur more rapidly in aged patients than in younger patients.[71] Another study of elderly patients with acute or chronic renal failure suggested that older individuals are at greater risk of morbidity associated with their disease.[72]

Comorbidities such as hypertension and diabetes are common in the elderly population and are likely to increase the susceptibility of individuals to renal disease.[73,74] In the United States, approximately 30% of the adult population is affected by hypertension,[75] the incidence of which has been shown to increase with age. Approximately 70% of adults over the age of 65 have been diagnosed with the disease.[75] A similar trend exists for diabetes, which affects approximately 8% of the population in the United States.[76] Of individuals aged 65 and older, nearly 27% have been diagnosed with diabetes.[76] The presence of diseases such as hypertension and/or diabetes in aging patients likely enhances the normal age-related decline in renal function compared with healthy individuals.[77] Therefore, it is reasonable to suggest that aged and elderly patients with superimposed diseases are more susceptible to the development of acute or chronic renal failure.

It is also important to consider the increase in prescription drug use in the elderly and aged population. Aging not only leads to a reduction in renal function, but can also lead to a reduced ability to metabolize drugs and eliminate drug metabolites.[78] For example, non-steroidal anti-inflammatory drugs (NSAIDs) such as salicylate may be used frequently by aged and elderly individuals. In fact, the use of these drugs by the aged and elderly population is estimated to be three times that of the younger population.[78] In addition, time required to eliminate drugs such as salicylate has been shown to be greater in the elderly population than in younger individuals.[79] This reduction may be due, in part, to age-related loss of renal function. Considering the increased use and reduced elimination of certain drugs in the elderly and aged population, it is possible that the use of these drugs may predispose individuals to kidney diseases, such as analgesic nephropathy (which often leads to renal insufficiency or failure).

13.4 Aging and Exposure to Toxic Metals

Owing to naturally occurring and chemically manufactured toxicants in the environment, individuals are exposed frequently over their lifetime to toxicants that have the capacity to negatively affect various organ systems. Just as aging in the presence of diseases can have a negative impact on renal function and may enhance the development of renal disease, exposure of elderly and aged individuals to nephrotoxicants may promote or enhance the progression of renal disease. Since not all relevant nephrotoxicants can be addressed here, we will focus on two prevalent environmental metal toxicants, cadmium and mercury. Because of their abundance in the environment and in numerous occupational settings, exposure of humans to each of these metal toxicants is nearly unavoidable. The toxic effects of cadmium and mercury have been characterized extensively and a great deal is known about the mechanisms by which they gain access to target cells. Based on that knowledge and the frequency of human exposure, we have chosen to use cadmium and mercury as example nephrotoxicants in our discussion of aging and exposure to toxic metals.

As discussed in previous sections, the major age-related change within the nephron is glomerulosclerosis. As the sclerotic process progresses and glomeruli become non-functional, this decrease in functional renal mass leads to hypertrophy of remaining functional glomeruli. Glomerular and tubular hypertrophy is associated with hyperperfusion and an increase in SNGFR.[80] Consequently, the luminal and basolateral surfaces of renal tubular epithelial cells are potentially exposed to higher levels of xenobiotics, metabolic wastes, and nephrotoxicants. In addition, these substances may be taken up more readily by hypertrophied tubular cells because of increases in the expression of certain cellular transport mechanisms. The increased exposure to, and probable uptake of, available xenobiotics, metabolic wastes, and nephrotoxicants likely enhances the risk of hypertrophied tubular cells being affected adversely by these substances.[11] These adverse effects could conceivably lead to additional cell death and glomerulosclerosis, which would further reduce the functional renal mass of the patient.

13.4.1 Cadmium

Cadmium (Cd) is a prevalent environmental pollutant and nephrotoxicant. Industrial uses of cadmium include manufacture of batteries, pigments, coatings, and plastics.[81] Current regulations regarding cadmium emissions and disposal have reduced occupational exposure to cadmium, yet the environments and surrounding areas where cadmium is/was used industrially remain heavily contaminated. Additionally, the use of this metal in phosphate fertilizers can leave soil and water heavily contaminated with cadmium residue. Cadmium concentrates in soils and subsequently accumulates in plants, particularly root vegetables, as well as grains and tobacco.[82] Cadmium is also present in high concentrations in aquatic animals such as seals and mollusks, and in crustaceans such as oysters and crabs.[82]

Diet is the primary means by which the general, non-smoking population is exposed to cadmium.[82] In contrast, individuals who smoke are exposed to this metal primarily *via* the inhalation of cigarette smoke due to the high concentration of cadmium in tobacco.[82] Each cigarette contains approximately 1–2 μg of cadmium.[83] About 10% of the cadmium contained in a cigarette is inhaled,[84] with approximately 50% of that being absorbed in the lungs.[85] Therefore, it is estimated that individuals who smoke one pack of 20 cigarettes each day will absorb approximately 1–2 μg of cadmium daily.[86] Cadmium is also present in air and drinking water in various regions of the world, although the concentration of cadmium in air is relatively low and drinking water is generally not a major source of exposure for the general population.[82,86,87]

In a recent assessment by the US Centers for Disease Control and Prevention, as part of the NHANES, blood and urine content of cadmium was analyzed in over 5000 individuals. In individuals over the age of 20, the average blood level was $0.376\,\mu g\,L^{-1}$ while the average urinary concentration of cadmium was $0.232\,\mu g\,L^{-1}$.[88] Both urinary and blood levels of cadmium have remained fairly steady over the past decade. These data suggest that individuals continue to be exposed chronically to cadmium. Thus, a thorough understanding of the effects of exposure to cadmium on an organ system is important to overall human health.

13.4.1.1 Renal Handling of Cadmium

Cadmium appears to gain access to renal epithelial cells by several different mechanisms. When bound to the metal-binding protein, metallothionein (MT), it is thought to be taken up *via* receptor-mediated endocytosis. Cadmium is also a strong electrophilic cation, which enables it to compete for and interact with membrane transporters that are involved in the uptake of nutritive metals, such as calcium, iron, and zinc. Alternatively, cadmium(II) ions may form linear complexes with select sulfhydryl (thiol)-containing biomolecules, such as glutathione (GSH), cysteine (Cys), or homocysteine (Hcy).[89,90] These cadmium-thiol complexes may gain access to cells at the site of membrane transporters normally involved in the transport of endogenous amino acids, oligopeptides, organic anions, or organic cations.[91,92]

Following exposure and absorption, a significant amount of cadmium is transported to the liver, where it becomes associated with MT to form CdMT.[93,94] It is believed by numerous investigators that when cadmium induces hepatocellular necrosis, CdMT is released into sinusoidal blood. This is especially true following acute exposure to nephrotoxic doses. CdMT is filtered freely at the glomerulus and is then thought to be taken up at the luminal plasma membrane of proximal tubular epithelial cells *via* receptor-mediated endocytosis.[92,95–102] This route of uptake appears to be a major route of proximal tubular entry for cadmium.[103] Indeed, the cells of the proximal convoluted tubule are the primary sites adversely affected by CdMT.[93,97,99,104–108] Following uptake by proximal tubular cells, CdMT is delivered to endosomes and lysosomes, where Cd^{2+} is dissociated from MT and transported into the cytoplasm *via* the divalent metal transporter 1 (DMT1).[96,109] DMT1 is also localized in the luminal plasma membrane of the epithelial cells lining the ascending thick limb of the loop of Henle, the distal convoluted tubule, and the principal cells of the cortical collecting duct,[110] where it may play a role in the uptake of cadmium ions and lead to adverse effects within these cells.

Cadmium ions may also be taken up from the proximal tubular lumen by a mechanism involving ligand exchange. Cadmium may dissociate from MT or other ligands under certain conditions,[111] and the process of ligand exchange may allow the cadmium ion to exchange from a protein or non-protein thiol to the binding site of a cation transporter. Certain zinc transporters appear to be capable of utilizing cadmium ions as substrates. ZIP8 (SLC39A8) and ZIP14 (SLC39A14) have both been identified in the kidney and have been shown *in vitro* to mediate the uptake of cadmium ions into cultured renal epithelial cells stably transfected with either of these carriers.[112–115] Cadmium ions and complexes appear to utilize additional mechanisms to gain access to renal epithelial cells; however, those mechanisms and processes remain unclear at present.

13.4.1.2 Renal Effects of Cadmium Exposure

Exposure to cadmium can be assessed by measuring cadmium concentrations in urine or blood. Urinary excretion of cadmium is considered to be a reliable indicator of renal and body burden and typically represents chronic levels of exposure.[86,116,117] In contrast, plasma levels of cadmium usually reflect a more recent exposure, such as one occurring within the previous month.[86,116,118] Cadmium has a long half-life within the body, partly due to its incorporation into bone.[81] Therefore, following exposure, decades may be required for complete elimination of this toxic metal.[86]

Following chronic exposure to cadmium, approximately 50% of the total body stores accumulate in the kidney.[119,120] Thus, it is not surprising to find that this organ is a primary target of cadmium toxicity, which leads to reductions in GFR and generalized tubular dysfunction (*i.e.*, Fanconi's syndrome).[116,120,121] One of the earliest signs of renal damage is the presence of urinary biomarkers, such as β_2-microglobulin, *N*-acetyl-β-D-glucosamidase (NAG), and kidney injury molecule-1 (Kim-1).[116] β_2-microglobulin is a low molecular weight protein that is filtered freely at the glomerulus and is normally absorbed by proximal tubules.[122] Following tubular damage, a small fraction of β_2-microglobulin escapes absorption and is excreted in urine. Alternatively, NAG is derived from mitochondria within proximal tubular epithelial cells and thus, following cellular damage, this enzyme is released into tubular fluid for eventual elimination in urine.[123] More recently, Kim-1, which is a transmembrane protein not normally detectable in urine, has been shown to be a useful marker of renal tubular cell injury and/or death.[124]

Recently, studies have shown that chronic exposure to even low levels of cadmium can result in early signs of renal toxicity.[121,125–129] The earliest sign of cadmium-induced renal damage is microproteinuria, which is usually identified by the presence of β_2-microglobulin in urine.[82,86] After exposure to greater doses of cadmium, tubular damage is evidenced by the presence of a Fanconi's syndrome, which is typically characterized by glucosuria, aminoaciduria, hyperphosphaturia, and hypercalciuria.[82] In addition, the glomerulus is injured and consequently, GFR declines. This decline results in increased detectable levels of urinary protein.[82,86,130] The incidence of kidney stones also increases in individuals exposed chronically to (or to larger doses of) cadmium, possibly due to the increased concentration of calcium in tubular fluid and urine.[131] Owing to the fact that the active form of vitamin D (1,25 dihydroxy-cholecalciferol) is formed in the kidneys, it is possible that renal damage would impede the conversion of the inactive form of this vitamin to the active form. Indeed, studies from cadmium-polluted areas report an association between cadmium-induced renal damage and lowered plasma levels of active vitamin D.[132,133] Interestingly, the renal changes that are observed following chronic exposure to a low dose of cadmium are similar to those observed with normal aging of the kidneys.[86]

13.4.1.3 Aging and the Effects of Cadmium Exposure on the Kidneys

Epidemiological studies have demonstrated a positive correlation between age and the renal accumulation of cadmium in individuals exposed chronically to this metal.[128,134] Since the normal filtration capacity of the kidney appears to decline with aging, exposure of elderly individuals to cadmium appears to potentiate the negative effects of age-related renal dysfunction. Consequently, it is reasonable to postulate that exposure of elderly and aged individuals to cadmium may be especially detrimental to target organs. In aged kidneys, the threshold at which nephrotoxic effects are observed may be lower than in the kidneys of a younger individual. Indeed, it has been suggested that long-term exposure to cadmium exacerbates the age-related decline in GFR.[135,136] Moreover, exposure to cadmium or other nephrotoxicants may further reduce or completely eliminate the renal functional reserve and the ability of the remaining functional renal mass to maintain normal homeostasis when challenged.[137–139] Sprague-Dawley rats exposed chronically to oral cadmium have been shown to have less renal functional reserve than unexposed rats.[58] Similarly, in an epidemiological study assessing renal function in cadmium/zinc smelter workers with detectable amounts of cadmium in their urine, it was found that age-related reduction in renal functional reserve was enhanced following exposures to cadmium that resulted in microproteinuria.[140] Collectively, these studies suggest that exposure to cadmium, and perhaps other nephrotoxicants, can abolish renal functional reserve, which may increase the susceptibility of these individuals to renal failure resulting from other risk factors, such as hypertension and diabetes.

Given that smoking is a common route of exposure to cadmium, it is not surprising to find that urinary and blood levels of cadmium increase with age in current smokers.[128,141,142] Individuals who smoke may have blood cadmium levels as high as 4–5 times greater than that of non-smokers.[86] This increased exposure to cadmium may lead to an increased susceptibility of smokers to the nephrotoxic effects of cadmium. Furthermore, increased exposure to cadmium may eventually play a role in the development of chronic kidney disease.

Aging kidneys are often characterized by areas of glomerular and tubular hypertrophy, hyperfiltration, and glomerulosclerosis. This pathological scenario is somewhat similar to the experimental model created by a uninephrectomy. In uninephrectomized animals, the contralateral kidney undergoes significant compensatory hypertrophy in order to maintain normal fluid and solute homeostasis.[52,143] As part of the compensatory mechanism, the transcription and translation of numerous proteins, including membrane transporters and metal-binding proteins (MT1 and MT2), are upregulated significantly.[52,143,144] An increase in the number and/or activity of transport proteins involved in the proximal tubular uptake of cadmium may enhance the nephropathy induced by this metal. When uninephrectomized and sham Sprague-Dawley rats were exposed to cadmium, the renal burden of cadmium was greater in the contralateral kidney of uninephrectomized rats than in the corresponding kidney of sham rats.[108] In addition, urinary excretion of NAG and cadmium was greater in uninephrectomized rats than in sham rats. Furthermore, when a toxic dose of cadmium was administered to each group of rats, it was found that uninephrectomized rats were more susceptible to the toxic effects of cadmium than corresponding sham rats.[108] Considering these data, it is logical to suggest that exposure to cadmium following a reduction in functional renal mass may lead to more severe nephropathy.[108]

Diseases that affect renal health, such as hypertension and diabetes, are common in elderly and aged individuals. Therefore, it is important to understand the relationship between aging, cadmium exposure, and superimposed diseases. A link between aging and body levels of cadmium following chronic exposure has been clearly established. Similarly, numerous epidemiological and animal studies have provided evidence suggesting an association between exposure to cadmium and the occurrence and severity of diabetes.[145,146] While diabetes alone may lead to decreased GFR, albuminuria, and morphological alterations along the nephron.[147] chronic exposure to cadmium may enhance the onset of these negative renal effects.[145] Indeed studies in which normal Sprague-Dawley rats were injected intraperitoneally with cadmium showed that administration of cadmium induced hyperglycemia.[148,149] This hyperglycemia may be the result of increases in levels of the gluconeogenic enzymes, glucose-6-phosphatase, fructose-1,6-diphosphatase, phosphoenol pyruvate carboxykinase, and pyruvate carboxylase.[149] Exposure of rats to cadmium chloride also appears to decrease the gene expression and release of insulin.[150–152] Taken together, these studies suggest that exposure to cadmium may increase one's susceptibility of developing diabetes. Exposure to cadmium may also promote the development of signs and symptoms in a diabetic patient. Diabetes-induced renal pathology may be observed earlier in patients that are exposed chronically to low levels of cadmium compared with un-exposed patients. This theory is supported by studies comparing streptozotocin-induced diabetic Wistar rats and non-diabetic Wistar rats.[153] The findings from these studies showed that urinary levels of protein, NAG, and γ-glutamyltransferase were greater in diabetic rats than in controls, suggesting that renal damage was more extensive in diabetic rats.[153] In addition, diabetic rats were found to excrete less cadmium in urine and consequently had a greater renal burden of cadmium than that of non-diabetic rats, suggesting the presence of glomerular damage.[153] In a similar study it was found that exposure of diabetic Sprague-Dawley rats to cadmium significantly increased the urinary excretion of albumin, transferring, and IgG.[154] In a separate study, varying concentrations of CdMT were injected into normal or obese hyperglycemic (ob/ob) mice.[155] Pathological signs of nephron damage (proteinuria and calciuria) were observed at lower concentrations of cadmium in the ob/ob mice than in normal mice, suggesting that the hyperglycemic state increases susceptibility to cadmium-induced nephropathy.[155]

The results of multiple epidemiological studies correlate well with the aforementioned animal studies and provide additional support for the notion that exposure to cadmium enhances the renal pathology associated with diabetes. In a cross-sectional study carried out in the Torres Strait Islands, located between Australia and New Guinea, investigators identified a strong positive correlation between urinary markers of cadmium exposure and diabetic nephropathy.[156] Similarly, a cross-sectional study of 1699 Belgian subjects suggested that diabetic patients may be more susceptible to the nephrotoxic effects of cadmium.[157] Moreover, Åkesson and colleagues assessed the effect of cadmium exposure on diabetes-induced renal dysfunction in 10 766 subjects and reported that the nephrotoxic effects of cadmium exposure could be observed at lower levels in diabetic patients compared with non-diabetic patients.[121]

Interestingly, cadmium levels in men and women appear to differ significantly. The body burden of cadmium in women tends to be significantly greater than that in men. In a study of healthy Thai men and women, it was found that the average urinary excretion of cadmium in non-smoking women was similar to that of men who smoked cigarettes.[158] In a study of 57 non-smoking women, it was found that urinary and blood levels of cadmium correlated with age and body iron stores.[159] Women with lower serum ferritin were found to have higher levels of cadmium.[159,160] In general, women have lower iron stores than men; when iron stores are low, the divalent metal transporter 1 (DMT1) in the intestine is upregulated to facilitate increased intestinal uptake of ferrous iron (Fe^{2+}).[161] DMT1 has also been shown to mediate the intestinal uptake of cadmium;[161,162] therefore, upregulation of this carrier could potentially increase the absorption of dietary cadmium ions from the lumen of the intestine. Indeed, it has been proposed that an increase in DMT1 expression and consequent increase in cadmium absorption is the primary reason for the greater levels of cadmium detected in women.[158–160]

13.4.2 Mercury

Mercury is a toxic metal found in many environmental and occupational settings. It exists in elemental (metallic), inorganic, and/or organic forms. Elemental mercury (Hg^0) is unique in that it exists as a liquid at room temperature. Inorganic mercury may be found as mercurous (Hg^{1+}) or mercuric (Hg^{2+}) ions, which are usually bonded with anionic species of chlorine, sulfur, or oxygen to form mercurous or mercuric salts. In the environment, inorganic mercury is usually found in the mercuric form. Organic forms of mercury include phenylmercury, dimethylmercury, and monomethylmercury. Of these forms, methylmercury (CH_3Hg^+) is the most frequently encountered in the environment. It is formed primarily when inorganic mercuric ions are methylated by microorganisms present in soil and water.[163–166]

Humans may be exposed to mercury in occupational and environmental settings, as well as through dental amalgams, and medicinal and dietary sources.[163,164,166,167] The majority of human exposure, however, results from the ingestion of food and water contaminated with CH_3Hg^+. Much of the dietary intake of this metal is *via* ingestion of large predatory fish, such as northern pike, salmon, swordfish, and shark, which may contain high levels of CH_3Hg^+. Upon ingestion, CH_3Hg^+ is absorbed readily by the gastrointestinal tract of humans and other mammals.[163] Mercuric ions can then enter systemic circulation where they can be delivered to target organs.

13.4.2.1 Renal Handling of Mercury

Inorganic and organic forms of mercury accumulate readily in the kidney. While the kidney is the primary site of accumulation of and intoxication by inorganic forms of mercury, organic forms of mercury, which primarily affect the central nervous system, also have serious toxicological effects in the kidney.[168–171] Within this organ, the primary site of uptake and accumulation of mercuric species is the proximal tubule.[166] It should be noted that following exposure to CH_3Hg^+, a fraction of absorbed CH_3Hg^+ will be oxidized within tissues and cells to form Hg^{2+}.[172–175] It is also important to note that within biological systems, mercurous, mercuric, or methylmercuric ions do not exist as inorganic salts, or in an unbound, "free" ionic state.[176] Rather, mercuric ions are found bonded to one or more thiol-containing biomolecules, such as GSH, Cys, Hcy, *N*-acetylcysteine (NAC), and albumin. For Hg^{2+}, this bonding occurs in a linear II, coordinate covalent manner while thiol-conjugates of CH_3Hg^+ form linear I, coordinate covalent complexes.[179,180]

Renal accumulation of as much as 50% of a nontoxic dose of Hg^{2+} occurs rapidly in the kidneys within a few hours of exposure.[177] The vast majority of this Hg^{2+} accumulates in the epithelial cells of the proximal tubule.[166] A preponderance of data collected in the past decade indicates that mercuric ions gain access to proximal tubular cells *via* mechanisms present on both the luminal and basolateral plasma membranes.[178–182] Early studies utilizing isolated perfused proximal tubules indicate that the primary transportable, biological form of mercury across the luminal membrane of the proximal tubule is a Cys *S*-conjugate (Cys-*S*-Hg-*S*-Cys).[183–185] Additional studies in isolated perfused tubules indicate that amino acid transporters located in the luminal plasma membrane are likely involved in the uptake of mercuric conjugates from the tubular lumen.[178,179] It has been hypothesized that since Cys-*S*-Hg-*S*-Cys is similar in size and shape to the amino acid cystine, this mercuric conjugate may be a substrate of a cystine transporter. Studies using Madin-Darby Canine Kidney (MDCK) cells stably transfected with the sodium-independent cystine transporter, system $b^{0,+}$, provide strong evidence implicating this carrier in the uptake of Cys-*S*-Hg-*S*-Cys from the lumen into the proximal tubular cell.[186] Similar studies have also identified the Hcy *S*-conjugate of Hg (Hcy-*S*-Hg-*S*-Hcy) as a substrate for system $b^{0,+}$.[187] To our knowledge, a sodium-dependent mechanism for the luminal uptake of Cys-*S*-Hg-*S*-Cys and Hcy-*S*-Hg-*S*-Hcy by proximal tubular cells has not yet been identified. In contrast, experimental evidence from *Xenopus laevis* oocytes indicates that Cys- and Hcy-*S*-conjugates of CH_3Hg^+ (Cys-*S*-CH_3Hg^+ and Hcy-*S*-CH_3Hg^+ respectively) are substrates of the sodium-dependent amino acid carrier, system $B^{0,+}$.[188] Currently, there are no experimental data supporting a role for system $B^{0,+}$ in the uptake of Cys-*S*-Hg-*S*-Cys or Hcy-*S*-Hg-*S*-Hcy.[188]

Approximately 40–60% of the mercury that accumulates in proximal tubular cells is taken up at the basolateral plasma membrane.[180,182,185,189–192] Numerous *in vitro* studies using cultured MDCK cells stably transfected with the organic anion transporter (OAT)-1 provide strong evidence indicating that mercuric conjugates of Cys, Hcy, and NAC (NAC-*S*-Hg-*S*-NAC) are taken up by this carrier.[193–203] Cys-*S*-Hg-*S*-Cys has also been shown to be a transportable substrate of another isoform of OAT, namely OAT3.[204] Both, OAT1 and OAT3 are localized in the basolateral plasma membrane of proximal tubular epithelial cells.[195,196] Based on published reports, it appears that OAT1 is the primary mechanism involved in the basolateral transport of

Cys-*S*-Hg-*S*-Cys, NAC-*S*-Hg-*S*-NAC, and Hcy-*S*-Hg-*S*-Hcy into proximal tubular cells.[180,181,185,189–192,204–206] In addition to conjugates of inorganic mercury, Cys-, NAC-, and Hcy-*S*-conjugates of CH_3Hg^+ have also been identified as substrates for OAT1.[201–203] Collectively, these data provide strong support for a role of OAT1 and OAT3 in the basolateral uptake of certain mercuric complexes.

Once mercuric ions gain access to the intracellular compartment of cells, they form strong bonds with protein and non-protein thiol-containing biomolecules. Intracellular mercuric ions also induce, and bind to, MT and/or GSH.[207,208] Bonding to these biomolecules often prevents or reduces greatly the export of mercuric ions from the cell. However, it is well-documented that mercuric ions can be extracted from renal tubular cells following treatment with a metal complexing agent, such as 2,3-bis(sulfanyl)propane-1-sulfonic acid (formally known as 2,3-dimercaptopropane-1-sulfonic acid, DMPS)[209] or 2,3-dimercaptosuccinic acid (DMSA).[209–214] It is thought that DMPS and DMSA gain access to proximal tubular cells at the basolateral membrane *via* OAT1, OAT3 and/or the sodium-dependent dicarboxylate transporter (NaC2).[215–218] It is hypothesized that once internalized, DMPS and DMSA form complexes with intracellular Hg^{2+} and these complexes are then exported across the luminal membrane *via* the multidrug resistance-associated protein 2 (MRP2). In a recent study, TR^- rats, which lack Mrp2, were exposed to a non-nephrotoxic dose of $HgCl_2$ and treated subsequently with DMPS or DMSA. The results of this study provided strong evidence for a role of Mrp2 in the DMPS- and DMSA-mediated extraction of mercuric ions from proximal tubular cells.[219,220] In addition, *in vitro* studies utilizing inside-out, brush-border membrane vesicles prepared from *Sf9* cells transfected with human MRP2 provided direct evidence indicating that DMPS- and DMSA-*S*-conjugates of Hg^{2+} are transportable substrates of MRP2.[219,220] Mrp2 also appears to play a role in the NAC-mediated extraction of mercuric ions following exposure to CH_3Hg^+.[221] *In vivo* studies in TR^- rats suggest that Mrp2 plays a role in the transport of CH_3Hg-*S*-NAC from within proximal tubular cells into the tubular lumen.[222] The ability of Mrp2 to utilize CH_3Hg-*S*-NAC as a substrate was also shown directly *via* studies using inside-out, brush-border membrane vesicles prepared from the kidneys of TR^- rats.[222] Similarly, Mrp2 has been implicated in the DMPS- and DMSA-mediated elimination of CH_3Hg^+ from proximal tubular cells using TR^- rats and inside-out, brush-border membrane vesicles from MRP2-expressing *Sf9* cells as experimental models.[223] Collectively, these data provide strong support for the hypothesis that MRP2 plays an important role in the renal elimination of mercuric ions following exposure to forms of Hg^{+2} or CH_3Hg^+.

13.4.2.2 Renal Effects of Mercury Exposure

Exposure to all forms of mercury can have nephrotoxic effects;[168–171] however, exposure to conjugates of inorganic mercury induces the most severe acute nephropathy. Following exposure to a low dose of $HgCl_2$, cellular damage can be observed in the *pars recta* of the proximal tubule, suggesting that this region of the nephron is the most sensitive to the toxic effects of mercury.[166] Exposure to higher doses of $HgCl_2$ not only results in more rapid induction of cellular necrosis, but also leads to necrosis in the *pars convoluta* and distal segments of the nephron.[224,225] Following exposure to a nephrotoxic dose of mercury, injury can be detected at the cellular level in *pars recta* segments in as little as three hours.[226] Changes in mitochondrial structure are evident and pyknotic nuclei can be identified. After six hours, cells begin to lose microvilli, mitochondrial swelling worsens, and dilation of the endoplasmic reticulum can be detected.[224] Reductions in enzymatic activity in the *pars recta* have also been reported.[225] Twelve hours after exposure to $HgCl_2$, electron microscopic analyses of cells reveal rupture of the plasma membrane, loss of microvilli, decreased contact with the basement membrane, and loss of cell shape.[227] After 24 hours, cellular fragments can be identified in the tubular lumen, junctional complexes between cells are absent, and nuclear structure is compromised.[225–227] When tubular epithelial cells are injured and die, numerous brush-border and intracellular enzymes, such as alkaline phosphatase, γ-glutamyltransferase, lactate dehydrogenase, aspartate aminotransferase (AST), and alanine aminotransferase (ALT) can be detected in urine.[213,228–232] As the extent of mercury-induced renal injury progresses, there is also a simultaneous increase in the urinary excretion of mercuric ions.[233–235]

Exposure to $HgCl_2$ can also have detrimental effects on glomeruli. Hall and colleagues[236] exposed rats to a non-nephrotoxic dose of $HgCl_2$ for 21 weeks. At the end of the exposure period there were no significant differences in the parameters of renal function (*i.e.*, plasma urea nitrogen, plasma creatinine, protein excretion); yet significant histological changes were noted in the kidneys. Tubular, interstitial and glomerular lesions were found to be significantly worse in rats exposed to $HgCl_2$ than in control animals.[236] Similarly, in rats exposed to methylmercury over a two-year period, fibrotic changes were identified in a fraction of glomeruli.[237] In addition, deposits of IgG, IgM, and C3 were detected along the glomerular basement membrane,[237] suggestive of the development of membranous glomerulonephritis.[166,238–240] Glomerular changes such as fibrosis and glomerulonephritis often lead to reductions in GFR. Therefore, it is not surprising that following exposure to mercury, reductions in GFR have been observed.[224,241]

Based on these studies, it is clear that acute and chronic exposure to mercuric compounds has numerous, deleterious effects in the kidneys. Considering that aged and elderly individuals have reduced functional renal mass (due to glomerulosclerosis, tubular atrophy, and interstitial fibrosis), it is possible that exposure of these individuals to mercuric compounds may be even more detrimental to renal health.

13.4.2.3 *Aging and the Effects of Mercury Exposure on the Kidney*

Although the aged and elderly make up a significant percentage of the population, and exposure to mercury and mercuric compounds appears to be increasing, little is known about the relationship between aging kidneys and the renal effects of mercury exposure. Several *in vitro* studies suggest that accumulation of mercuric ions is greater in aged animals than younger animals. Hirayama and Yasutake[242] exposed C57BL/6N mice, ages two weeks to 45 weeks, to a single dose of methylmercury and found that accumulation of mercuric ions was greater in older mice than in younger mice. This study also found that urinary excretion of mercury was lower in older mice, suggesting that more mercury was retained within the kidneys and other organs.[242] Interestingly, increases in the expression of MT and GSH, which have been shown to occur with aging, may lead to increased binding and retention of mercuric ions within target cells.[243]

As the kidneys age, the total number of functioning nephrons decreases significantly. This decline in functional renal mass is somewhat similar to an experimental model in which animals are uninephrectomized. Although the uninephrectomized rat model does not mimic exactly the changes that occur in an aging kidney, similarities exist between the two systems. In each, a significant number of nephrons are lost and remaining nephrons must go through a compensatory, hypertrophic phase in order to maintain normal fluid and electrolyte homeostasis.[51,52,143] It has been suggested by a number of investigators that hyperfiltration and hyperperfusion occurring in hypertrophied nephrons may result in these nephrons being exposed to higher levels of potential nephrotoxicants such as mercury. This increased exposure may increase the susceptibility of these nephrons to the deleterious effects of mercury or other nephrotoxicants.[231,244–250]

Several studies in uninephrectomized rats support the idea that hypertrophied nephrons are more sensitive to the toxic effects of mercury. Ramos-Frendo and colleagues[246] exposed uninephrectomized and sham rats to a nephrotoxic dose of $HgCl_2$ and found that the development of acute renal failure was more pronounced in uninephrectomized animals than in sham animals. Similarly, Houser and Berndt[244] exposed uninephrectomized and sham Sprague-Dawley rats to a nephrotoxic dose of $HgCl_2$, following which they assessed renal susceptibility to mercuric ions. Exposure to $HgCl_2$ included glomerular and tubular dysfunction, which appeared to be more severe in uninephrectomized rats than in sham rats.[244] In a separate, more detailed study using uninephrectomized and sham Sprague-Dawley rats exposed to a nephrotoxic dose of $HgCl_2$, it was discovered that mercuric ions were redistributed within the kidney following uninephrectomy. The concentration of mercuric ions was greater in the renal cortex and outer stripe of the outer medulla in uninephrectomized rats than in sham animals.[245] Not surprisingly, the urinary excretion of mercury (per kidney) was greater in uninephrectomized rats than in shams.[244,245] A similar study was carried out in uninephrectomized and sham Long Evans hooded rats, which were exposed to nephrotoxic doses of $HgCl_2$.[231] It was found that mercury-induced proximal tubular necrosis was more extensive in uninephrectomized animals than in sham animals. In addition, the urinary excretion of cellular enzymes and plasma proteins, including lactate dehydrogenase, γ-glutamyltransferase and albumin, was greater in uninephrectomized animals than in sham animals.[231,251] Collectively, the results of these studies indicate that kidneys of animals with reduced renal mass are more susceptible to the toxic effects of mercury. Similarly, elderly and aged individuals who have reduced renal function, due to normal aging processes and/or superimposed disease processes may be more susceptible to renal injury following exposure to a nephrotoxicant such as mercury.

Chronic kidney disease, which may lead to end-stage renal failure, frequently affects the elderly and aged population. This disease, which is often caused by uncontrolled diabetes and hypertension, is characterized by a progressive and permanent loss of functioning nephrons. In the United States, which has one of the highest rates of chronic kidney disease in the world,[252] nearly 50% of patients with this disease are over the age of 65.[253] Because many patients in the early stages of chronic kidney disease are asymptomatic, a diagnosis is often not made until renal function has been compromised significantly and GFR is well below the normal range. During this period, patients may continue to be exposed to nephrotoxicants such as mercury. Such exposure may enhance morbidity and mortality as these patients may be more sensitive to the toxic effects of mercury. In rat models of chronic kidney disease (*i.e.*, 75% nephrectomy), the disposition of mercuric ions differs significantly from that in sham or uninephrectomized animals.[254] The renal accumulation of mercuric ions has been shown to be significantly lower in 75% nephrectomized rats compared with uninephrectomized rats. This finding is likely related to the fact that GFR is reduced more in 75% nephrectomized rats than in uninephrectomized rats. Based on these data, it has been suggested that the uptake of a large fraction of the mercuric ions that accumulate within the kidney is dependent upon filtration of these ions at the glomerulus.[251,254] A reduction in GFR would be expected to decrease the amount of mercury filtered at the glomerulus and presented to the tubular epithelial cells. This theory is consistent with the finding that the concentration of mercuric ions in blood is significantly greater in 75% nephrectomized rats than uninephrectomized or sham rats. Interestingly, the hepatic accumulation and fecal excretion of mercury have been shown to be significantly greater in 75% nephrectomized rats than in sham or uninephrectomized rats. The increased concentration of mercuric ions could enhance the injurious effects of mercury in hepatocytes, which may lead to a decline in overall health.[251,254]

13.5 Summary

The aging process in the kidneys has been studied and characterized extensively. It is well known that glomerulosclerosis leads to decreases in GFR and RBF. However, there is little information regarding the response of aged kidneys to environmental toxicants such as cadmium or mercury. Because of the prevalence of these metals in the environment, human exposure is nearly unavoidable. Furthermore, it is well-known that acute and chronic exposures to each of these toxic metals can be detrimental to the kidneys of normal adults, thus it can be postulated that exposure of the elderly and aged to these metals may lead to additional reductions in renal function. Individuals with compromised renal function, either from aging, disease, or a combination of aging and disease, are especially susceptible to nephrotoxicants. The few studies available have demonstrated an association between exposure to mercury or cadmium and an increase in the incidence and severity of renal disease. It is important to note that early signs of renal dysfunction often go unnoticed, thus individuals with reduced renal function are often unaware that they are at risk during the early stages of disease. Exposure to nephrotoxicants may occur during this early period, and this exposure may be especially detrimental to these individuals. Therefore, a thorough and complete understanding of the way in which nephrotoxicants are handled by aging kidneys is of utmost importance. Because of the paucity of data available on this topic, additional studies are clearly necessary.

References

1. World Health Organization, World Health Statistics, Geneva, *Switzerland*, 2011, **1**, 45–53, Available at: www.who.int/shoisi/whostat/2011/en/index.html.
2. Centers for Disease Control and Prevention, Health, US, with a special feature on death and dying. National Center for Health Statistics, Hyattsville, MD, 2010, **10**, 10, Available at www.cdc.gov/nchs/data/hus/hus10.pdf.
3. F. S. Hobbs, United States Census Bureau, 2002, 58–59, Available at: www.census.gov/prod/2002pubs/censr-4.pdf.
4. C. Kaplan, B. Pasternack, H. Shah and G. Gallo, *Am. J. Pathol.*, 1975, **80**, 227.
5. M. Epstein, *J. Am. Soc. Nephrol.*, 1996, **7**, 1106.
6. D. Rodriguez-Puyol, *Kidney Int.*, 1998, **54**, 2247.
7. B. Kappel and S. Olsen, *Virchows Arch. A: Pathol. Anat. Histol*, 1980, **387**, 271.
8. X. J. Zhou, Z. G. Laszik, F. G. Silva, in *The Aging Kidney in Health and Disease*, eds. J. F. M. Núñez, J. S. Cameron and D.G. Oreopoulos, Springer, New York, 2008, p. 39.
9. E. V. Lerma, *Clin. Geriatr. Med.*, 2009, **25**, 325.
10. S. E. Thomas, S. Anderson, K. L. Gordon, T. T. Oyama, S. J. Shankland and R. J. Johnson, *J. Am. Soc. Nephrol.*, 1998, **9**, 231.
11. J. M. Lopez-Novoa, in *The Aging Kidney in Health and Disease*, eds. J. F. M. Núñez, J. S. Cameron, and D. G. Oreopoulos, Springer, New York, 2008, p. 113.
12. J. E. Wiggins, S. R. Patel, K. A. Shedden, M. Goyal, B. L. Wharram, S. Martini, M. Kretzler and R. C. Wiggins, *J. Am. Soc. Nephrol.*, 2010, **21**, 587.
13. F. G. Silva, *Int. Urol. Nephrol.*, 2005, **37**, 185.
14. Thomas *et al.*, *J. Am. Soc. Nephrol.*, 1998, **9**, 231–242.
15. R. Zatz and C. K. Fujihara, *Kidney Int. Suppl.*, 1994, **45**, S27.

16. A. B. Fogo, *Kidney Int. Suppl.*, 2000, **75**, S15.
17. J. R. Weinstein and S. Anderson, *Adv. Chronic Kidney Dis.*, 2010, **17**, 302.
18. S. Anderson and B. M. Brenner, *Am. J. Med.*, 1986, **80**, 435.
19. L. Ferder, F. Inserra, L. Romano, L. Ercole and V. Pszenny, *J. Am. Soc. Nephrol.*, 1994, **5**, 1147.
20. J. Floege, R. J. Johnson and W. G. Couser, *Clin. Investig*, 1992, **70**, 857.
21. A. Ljungqvist and C. Lagergren, *J. Anat.*, 1962, **96**, 285.
22. D. Choudhury, D. S. C. Raj, M. Levi, in *The Kidney*, eds. B. M. Brenner and F. C. Rector, Elsevier, Philadelphia, 2004, vol. 2 , p. 2305.
23. J. Wiggins, *Semin. Nephrol.*, 2009, **29**, 587.
24. M. Camici, A. Carpi, G. Cini, F. Galetta and N. Abraham, *Front. Biosci. (Schol Ed)*, 2011, **3** , 995.
25. B. L. Wharram, M. Goyal, J. E. Wiggins, S. K. Sanden, S. Hussain, W. E. Filipiak, T. L. Saunders, R. C. Dysko, K. Kohno, L. B. Holzman and R. C. Wiggins, *J. Am. Soc. Nephrol.*, 2005, **16**, 2941.
26. G. Ding, N. Franki, A. A. Kapasi, K. Reddy, N. Gibbons and P. C. Singhal, *Exp. Mol. Pathol.*, 2001, **70**, 43.
27. C. K. Abrass, M. J. Adcox and G. J. Raugi, *Am. J. Pathol.*, 1995, **146**, 742.
28. X. J. Zhou, D. Rakheja, X. Yu, R. Saxena, N. D. Vaziri and F. G. Silva, *Kidney Int.*, 2008, **74**, 710.
29. Q. Ke and M. Costa, *Mol. Pharmacol.*, 2006, **70**, 1469.
30. K. Kimura, M. Iwano, D. F. Higgins, Y. Yamaguchi, K. Nakatani, K. Harada, A. Kubo, Y. Akai, E. B. Rankin, E. G. Neilson, V. H. Haase and Y. Saito, *Am. J. Physiol. Renal Physiol*, 2008, **295**, F1023.
31. S. Nakatsuji, J. Yamate and S. Sakuma, *Vet. Pathol.*, 1998, **35**, 352.
32. R. D. Lindeman and R. Goldman, *Exp. Gerontol.*, 1986, **21**, 379.
33. J. W. Rowe, N. W. Shock and R. A. DeFronzo, *Nephron*, 1976, **17**, 270.
34. S. Adler, R. D. Lindeman, M. J. Yiengst, E. Beard and N. W. Shock, *J. Lab. Clin. Med.*, 1968, **72**, 278.
35. J. F. Macías-Núñez, J. M. Lopez-Novoa, in *The Aging Kidney in Health and Disease*, eds. J. F. Macias Nunez, J. S. Cameron and D. G. Oreopoulos, Springer, New York, 2008, p. 93.
36. C. G. Musso and D. G. Oreopoulos, *Nephron Physiol Suppl 1.*, 2011, **119**, 1.
37. D. F. Davies and N. W. Shock, *J. Clin. Invest.*, 1950, **29**, 496.
38. C. Baylis and R. Schmidt, *Semin. Nephrol.*, 1996, **16**, 265.
39. N. W. Shock, *Geriatrics*, 1946, **1**, 232.
40. R. D. Lindeman, J. Tobin and N. W. Shock, *J. Am. Geriatr. Soc.*, 1985, **33**, 278.
41. N. W. Shock, R. C. Greulick, R. Andres, D. Arenberg, P. T. Costa, E. G. Lakatta and J. D. Tobin, *Public Health Service, United States Department of Health and Human Services Publication No. 84-2450*, 1984, 175, Available at: www.grc.nia.nih.gov.blsahistory/blsa-1984/index.html.

42. A. D. Rule, L. D. Cornell and E. D. Poggio, *Nephron Physiol.*, 2011, **119**(Suppl 1), p. 6.
43. S. Hoshi, Y. Shu, F. Yoshida, T. Inagaki, J. Sonoda, T. Watanabe, K. Nomoto and M. Nagata, *Lab. Invest*, 2002, **82**, 25.
44. R. J. Glassock and C. Winearls, *Trans. Am. Clin. Climatol. Assoc.*, 2009, **120**, 419.
45. F. Zheng, A. R. Plati, A. Banerjee, S. Elliot, L. J. Striker and G. E. Striker, *Sci. Aging Knowledge Environ*, 2003, **2003**, PE20.
46. A. Melk, B. M. Schmidt, O. Takeuchi, B. Sawitzki, D. C. Rayner and P. F. Halloran, *Kidney Int.*, 2004, **65**, 510.
47. A. Melk, E. S. Mansfield, S. C. Hsieh, T. Hernandez-Boussard, P. Grimm, D. C. Rayner, P. F. Halloran and M. M. Sarwal, *Kidney Int.*, 2005, **68**, 2667.
48. Y. Zha, T. Taguchi, A. Nazneen, I. Shimokawa, Y. Higami and M. S. Razzaque, *Am. J. Nephrol.*, 2008, **28**, 755.
49. R. Naeije, A. Fiasse, E. Carlier, M. Opsomer and M. Leeman, *Eur. J. Clin. Pharmacol.*, 1993, **44**, 35.
50. N. K. Hollenberg, D. F. Adams, H. S. Solomon, A. Rashid, H. L. Abrams and J. P. Merrill, *Circ. Res.*, 1974, **34**, 309.
51. N. J. Fine LG, D. A. Kujubu and A. Knecht, in *The Kidney: Physiology and Pathophysiology*, eds. D.W. Seldin and G. Giebisch, Raven Press, New York, 2nd edn, 1992, p. 3113.
52. J. P. Hayslett, *Physiol. Rev.*, 1979, **59**, 137.
53. J. P. Bosch, S. Lew, S. Glabman and A. Lauer, *Am. J. Med.*, 1986, **81**, 809.
54. J. Bohler, D. Gloer, P. Reetze-Bonorden, E. Keller and P. J. Schollmeyer, *Clin. Nephrol.*, 1993, **39**, 145.
55. D. Fliser, M. Zeier, R. Nowack and E. Ritz, *J. Am. Soc. Nephrol.*, 1993, **3**, 1371.
56. C. Esposito, A. Plati, T. Mazzullo, G. Fasoli, A. De Mauri, F. Grosjean, F. Mangione, F. Castoldi, N. Serpieri, F. Cornacchia and A. Dal Canton, *J. Nephrol*, 2007, **20**, 617.
57. C. G. Musso, J. Reynaldi, B. Martinez, A. Pierangelo, M. Vilas and L. Algranati, *Int. Urol. Nephrol.*, 2011, **43**, 253.
58. K. Uriu, K. Kaizu, Y. L. Qie, A. Ito, I. Takagi, K. Suzuka, Y. Inada, O. Hashimoto and S. Eto, *Toxicol. Appl. Pharmacol.*, 2000, **169**, 151.
59. A. Raes, R. Donckerwolcke, M. Craen, M. C. Hussein and J. Vande Walle, *Pediatr. Nephrol.*, 2007, **22**, 1903.
60. J. Zaletel, D. Cerne, K. Lenart, S. Zitta, G. Jurgens, W. Estelberger and A. Kocijancic, *Wien. Klin. Wochenschr.*, 2004, **116**, 246.
61. F. B. Gabbai, *Semin. Nephrol.*, 1995, **15**, 482.
62. I. M. Pecly, V. Genelhu and E. A. Francischetti, *Int. J. Clin. Pract.*, 2006, **60**, 1198.
63. R. Schmitt and L. G. Cantley, *Am. J. Physiol. Renal Physiol*, 2008, **294**, F1265.
64. R. Schmitt, X. Zhu and L. G. Cantley, *J. Am. Soc. Nephrol.*, 2006, **17**, 530A.

65. G. V. Shurin, Z. R. Yurkovetsky, G. S. Chatta, I. L. Tourkova, M. R. Shurin and A. E. Lokshin, *Cytokine*, 2007, **39**, 123.
66. H. Bruunsgaard, M. Pedersen and B. K. Pedersen, *Curr. Opin. Hematol.*, 2001, **8**, 131.
67. R. Gerli, D. Monti, O. Bistoni, A. M. Mazzone, G. Peri, A. Cossarizza, M. Di Gioacchino, M. E. Cesarotti, A. Doni, A. Mantovani, C. Franceschi and R. Paganelli, *Mech. Ageing Dev.*, 2000, **121**, 37.
68. J. Mysliwska, E. Bryl, J. Foerster and A. Mysliwski, *Mech. Ageing. Dev.*, 1999, **107**, 1.
69. A. M. Joaquin and S. Gollapudi, *J. Am. Geriatr. Soc.*, 2001, **49**, 1234.
70. J. Pascual, L. Orofino, F. Liano, R. Marcen, M. T. Naya, L. Orte and J. Ortuno, *J. Am. Geriatr. Soc.*, 1990, **38**, 25.
71. J. Coresh, B. C. Astor, T. Greene, G. Eknoyan and A. S. Levey, *Am. J. Kidney Dis.*, 2003, **41**, 1.
72. T. Ali, I. Khan, W. Simpson, G. Prescott, J. Townend, W. Smith and A. Macleod, *J. Am. Soc. Nephrol.*, 2007, **18**, 1292.
73. A. H. Abdelhafiz, S. H. Brown, A. Bello and M. El Nahas, *Nephron Clin. Pract.*, 2010, **116**, c19.
74. F. G. Silva, *Int. Urol. Nephro.l*, 2005, **37**, 419.
75. Centers for Disease Control and Prevention, Prevalence of hypertension and controlled hypertension - United States, 2005–2008, *Morbidity and Mortality Weekly Report*, Atlanta, GA, 2011, **1**, 94–97, Available at: www.cdc.gov/mmwr/preview/mmwrhtml/su6001a21.htm.
76. Centers for Disease Control and Prevention, *National Diabetes Fact Sheet: National Estimates and General Information on Diabetes and Prediabetes in the United States*, Atlanta, GA, 2011, **1**, 1–12, Available at: www.cdc.gov/diabetes/pubs/pdf/ndfs_2011.pdf.
77. K. Abdel-Kader and P. M. Palevsky, *Clin. Geriatr. Med.*, 2009, **25**, 331.
78. M. Jerkic, S. Vojvodic and J. M. Lopez-Novoa, *Int. Urol. Nephrol.*, 2001, **32**, 539.
79. G. Cuny, R. J. Royer, J. M. Mur, J. M. Serot, G. Faure, P. Netter, A. Maillard and F. Penin, *Gerontology*, 1979, **25**, 49.
80. N. S. Bricker and L. G. Fine, in *The Kidney*, eds. B. M. Brenner BM and F. C. Rector, Saunders, Philadelphia, 2nd edn, 1981, **1**, p. 1056.
81. Agency for Toxic Substance and Drug Registry, *Cadmium*, 2008, **1**, 1–512, Available at: www.atsdr.cdc.gov/ToxProfiles/tp5.pdr.
82. World Health Organization, *Cadmium - Environmental Health Criteria 134*, Geneva, Switzerland, 1992, Available at: www.inchem.org/documents/ehc/ehc/ehc134.htm.
83. L. Friberg, M. Piscator, G. Nordberg, T. Kjellstrom, *Cadmium in the Environmnent*, CRC Press, Cleveland, 2nd edn,1974.
84. C. G. Elinder, T. Kjellstrom, B. Lind, L. Linnman, M. Piscator and K. Sundstedt, *Environ. Res.*, 1983, **32**, 220.
85. C. G. Elinder, B. Lind, T. Kjellstrom, L. Linnman and L. Friberg, *Arch. Environ. Health.*, 1976, **31**, 292.

86. L. Jarup, M. Berglund, C. G. Elinder, G. Nordberg and M. Vahter, *Scand. J. Work. Environ. Health.*, 1998, **24**(Suppl 1), 1.
87. I. M. Olsson, I. Bensryd, T. Lundh, H. Ottosson, S. Skerfving and A. Oskarsson, *Environ. Health. Perspect.*, 2002, **110**, 1185.
88. Centers for Disease Control and Prevention, *Fourth National Report on Human Exposure to Environmental Chemicals*, Atlanta, 2009.
89. D. L. Rabenstein, A. A. Isab, W. Kadima and P. Mohanakrishnan, *Biochim. Biophys. Acta*, 1983, **762**, 531.
90. D. L. Rabenstein, in *Glutathione: Chemical, Biochemical and Medical Aspects, Coenzymes and Cofactors*, eds. D. Dolphin, O. Auromovibic and R. Poulson, Wiley, New York, 1989, vol. 3, p. 147.
91. Y. Wang, R. K. Zalups and D. W. Barfuss, *Toxicol. Lett.*, 2010, **193**, 61.
92. R. K. Zalups and S. Ahmad, *Toxicol. Appl. Pharmacol,.*, 2003, **186**, 163.
93. E. Felley-Bosco and J. Diezi, *Toxicol. Appl. Pharmacol.*, 1989, **98**, 243.
94. O. Barbier, G. Jacquillet, M. Tauc, P. Poujeol and M. Cougnon, *Am. J. Physiol. Renal Physiol*, 2004, **287**, F1067.
95. R. E. Dudley, L. M. Gammal and C. D. Klaassen, *Toxicol. Appl. Pharmacol*, 1985, **77**, 414.
96. C. Erfurt, E. Roussa and F. Thevenod, *Am. J. Physiol. Cell Physiol*, 2003, **285**, C1367.
97. M. Murakami, K. Sano and M. Webb, *Arch. Toxicol.*, 1987, **60**, 365.
98. C. Dorian, V. H. Gattone and C. D. Klaassen, *Toxicol. Appl. Pharmacol.*, 1992, **117**, 242.
99. C. Dorian, V. H. Gattone and C. D. Klaasen, *Toxicol. Appl. Pharmacol.*, 1992, **114**, 173.
100. E. C. Foulkes, *Toxicol. Appl. Pharmacol.*, 1978, **45**, 505.
101. M. Nordberg, T. Jin and G. F. Nordberg, *IARC Sci. Publ*, 1992, 293.
102. M. Webb, in *Cadmium*, eds. E. C. Foulkes, Springer-Verlag, Berlin/New York, 1986.
103. F. Thevenod, *Nephron Physiol.*, 2003, **93**, 87.
104. G. F. Nordberg, R. Goyer and M. Nordberg, *Arch. Pathol*, 1975, **99**, 192.
105. M. G. Cherian and M. Nordberg, *Toxicology*, 1983, **28**, 1.
106. E. Felley-Bosco and J. Diezi, *Toxicol. Appl. Pharmacol.*, 1987, **91**, 204.
107. M. Murakami, K. Cain and M. Webb, *J. Appl. Toxicol.*, 1983, **3**, 237.
108. R. K. Zalups, R. M. Gelein and M. G. Cherian, *J. Pharmacol. Exp. Ther.*, 1992, **262**, 1256.
109. M. Abouhamed, N. A. Wolff, W. K. Lee, C. P. Smith and F. Thevenod, *Am. J. Physiol. Renal Physiol*, 2007, **293**, F705.
110. C. J. Ferguson, M. Wareing, D. T. Ward, R. Green, C. P. Smith and D. Riccardi, *Am. J. Physiol. Renal Physiol*, 2001, **280**, F803.
111. A. M. Scheuhammer and M. G. Cherian, *Toxicol. Appl. Pharmacol.*, 1986, **82**, 417.
112. B. Wang, S. N. Schneider, N. Dragin, K. Girijashanker, T. P. Dalton, L. He, M. L. Miller, K. F. Stringer, M. Soleimani, D. D. Richardson and D. W. Nebert, *Am. J. Physiol. Cell Physiol*, 2007, **292**, C1523.

113. K. Girijashanker, L. He, M. Soleimani, J. M. Reed, H. Li, Z. Liu, B. Wang, T. P. Dalton and D. W. Nebert, *Mol. Pharmacol.*, 2008, **73**, 1413.
114. H. Fujishiro, S. Okugaki, K. Kubota, T. Fujiyama, H. Miyataka and S. Himeno, *J. Appl. Toxicol.*, 2009, **29**, 367.
115. F. Thevenod, *Biometals*, **23**, 857.
116. W. C. Prozialeck and J. R. Edwards, *Biometals*, 2010, **23**, 793.
117. C. G. Elinder, L. Gerhardsson and G. Oberdorster, in *Biological Monitoring of Toxic Metals*, eds. T. W. Clarkson, L. Friberg, G. F. Nordberg and P. R. Sager, Plenum Press, London, 1988, p. 1.
118. G. F. Nordberg, K. Nogawa, M. Nordberg and J. M. Friedmann, in *Handbook on the Toxicology of Metals*, eds. G. F. Nordberg, B. A. Fowler, M. Nordbergand L. Friberg, Elsevier, Amsterdam, 2007, p. 445.
119. G. F. Nordberg and M. Nordberg, in *Biological Monitoring of Toxic Metals*, eds. T. W. Clarkson, L. Friberg, G. F. Nordberg and P. R. Sager, Plenum Press, New York, 2001, p. 151.
120. N. Johri, G. Jacquillet and R. Unwin, *Biometals*, 2010, **23**, 783.
121. A. Akesson, T. Lundh, M. Vahter, P. Bjellerup, J. Lidfeldt, C. Nerbrand, G. Samsioe, U. Stromberg and S. Skerfving, *Environ. Health Perspect.*, 2005, **113**, 1627.
122. K. Tsuchiya, S. Iwao, M. Sugita and H. Sakurai, *Environ. Health Perspect.*, 1979, **28**, 147.
123. T. Jin, G. Nordberg, X. Wu, T. Ye, Q. Kong, Z. Wang, F. Zhuang and S. Cai, *Environ. Res.*, 1999, **81**, 167.
124. W. C. Prozialeck, V. S. Vaidya, J. Liu, M. P. Waalkes, J. R. Edwards, P. C. Lamar, A. M. Bernard, X. Dumont and J. V. Bonventre, *Kidney Int.*, 2007, **72**, 985.
125. L. Jarup and T. Alfven, *Biometals*, 2004, **17**, 505.
126. L. Jarup, L. Hellstrom, T. Alfven, M. D. Carlsson, A. Grubb, B. Persson, C. Pettersson, G. Spang, A. Schutz and C. G. Elinder, *Occup. Environ. Med.*, 2000, **57**, 668.
127. C. W. Noonan, S. M. Sarasua, D. Campagna, S. J. Kathman, J. A. Lybarger and P. W. Mueller, *Environ. Health. Perspect.*, 2002, **110**, 151.
128. M. E. Mortensen, L. Y. Wong and J. D. Osterloh, *Int. J. Hyg. Environ. Health*, **214**, 305.
129. M. Huang, S. J. Choi, D. W. Kim, N. Y. Kim, C. H. Park, S. D. Yu, D. S. Kim, K. S. Park, J. S. Song, H. Kim, B. S. Choi, I. J. Yu and J. D. Park, *J. Toxicol. Environ. Health. A*, 2009, **72**, 1493.
130. L. Jarup, B. Persson and C. G. Elinder, *Occup. Environ. Med*, 1995, **52**, 818.
131. L. Jarup and C. G. Elinder, *Br. J. Ind. Med.*, 1993, **50**, 598.
132. K. Aoshima and M. Kasuya, *Toxicol. Lett*, 1991, **57**, 91.
133. I. Tsuritani, R. Honda, M. Ishizaki, Y. Yamada, T. Kido and K. Nogawa, *J. Toxicol. Environ. Health*, 1992, **37**, 519.

134. M. Huang, S. J. Choi, D. W. Kim, N. Y. Kim, H. S. Bae, S. D. Yu, D. S. Kim, H. Kim, B. S. Choi, I. J. Yu and J. D. Park, *Environ. Toxicol.*, 2011, Available at: http://onlinelibrary.wiley.com/doi/10.1002/tox20750/pdf.
135. H. C. Gonick, *Indian J. Med. Res.*, 2008, **128**, 335.
136. R. Lauwerys, A. Bernard and A. Cardenas, *Toxicol. Lett.*, 1992, 33.
137. G. A. Porter, *Toxicol. Lett.*, 1989, **46**, 269.
138. H. A. Roels, P. Hoet and D. Lison, *Ren. Fail*, 1999, **21**, 251.
139. P. W. Mueller, R. G. Price and W. F. Finn, *Environ. Health Perspect.*, 1998, **106**, 227.
140. H. A. Roels, R. R. Lauwerys, A. M. Bernard, J. P. Buchet, A. Vos and M. Oversteyns, *Br. J. Ind. Med.*, 1991, **48**, 365.
141. T. Watanabe, A. Koizumi, H. Fujita, H. Fujimoto, A. Ishimori and M. Ikeda, *Tohoku J. Exp. Med*, 1982, **138**, 443.
142. M. Baecklund, N. L. Pedersen, L. Bjorkman and M. Vahter, *Environ. Res*, 1999, **80**, 222.
143. L. G. Fine and J. Norman, *Annu. Rev. Physiol.*, 1989, **51**, 19.
144. R. K. Zalups, J. Fraser and J. Koropatnick, *Am. J. Physiol*, 1995, **268**, F643.
145. J. R. Edwards and W. C. Prozialeck, *Toxicol. Appl. Pharmacol.*, 2009, **238**, 289.
146. G. F. Nordberg, T. Jin, X. Wu, J. Lu, L. Chen, L. Lei, F. Hong and M. Nordberg, *Biochimie*, 2009, **91**, 1282.
147. B. F. Schrijvers, A. S. De Vriese and A. Flyvbjerg, *Endocr. Rev.*, 2004, **25**, 971.
148. R. R. Bell, J. L. Early, V. K. Nonavinakere and Z. Mallory, *Toxicol. Lett.*, 1990, **54**, 199.
149. K. D. Chapatwala, M. Boykin, A. Butts and B. Rajanna, *Drug Chem. Toxicol.*, 1982, **5**, 305.
150. L. J. Lei, T. Y. Jin and Y. F. Zhou, *Biomed. Environ. Sci.*, 2007, **20**, 295.
151. Z. Merali and R. L. Singhal, *Br. J. Pharmacol.*, 1980, **69**, 151.
152. L. J. Lei, T. Y. Jin and Y. F. Zhou, *Wei Sheng Yan Jiu*, 2005, **34**, 394.
153. T. Jin, G. Nordberg, J. Sehlin, H. Wallin and S. Sandberg, *Toxicology*, 1999, **142**, 69.
154. A. Bernard, C. Schadeck, A. Cardenas, J. P. Buchet and R. Lauwerys, *Toxicol. Lett*, 1991, **58**, 51.
155. T. Jin, G. F. Nordberg, J. Sehlin, P. Leffler and J. Wu, *Toxicology*, 1994, **89**, 81.
156. M. Haswell-Elkins, S. Satarug, P. O'Rourke, M. Moore, J. Ng, V. McGrath and M. Walmby, *Environ. Res.*, 2008, **106**, 379.
157. J. P. Buchet, R. Lauwerys, H. Roels, A. Bernard, P. Bruaux, F. Claeys, G. Ducoffre, P. de Plaen, J. Staessen, A. Amery, P. Lijnen, L. Thijs, D. Rondia, F. Sartor, A. Saint Remy and L. Nick, *Lancet*, 1990, **336**, 699.
158. S. Satarug, P. Ujjin, Y. Vanavanitkun, J. R. Baker and M. R. Moore, *Toxicol. Lett.*, 2004, **148**, 177.
159. M. Berglund, A. Akesson, B. Nermell and M. Vahter, *Environ. Health Perspect.*, 1994, **102**, 1058.

160. A. Åkesson, M. Berglund, A. Schutz, P. Bjellerup, K. Bremme and M. Vahter, *Am. J. Public Health*, 2002, **92**, 284.
161. D. W. Kim, K. Y. Kim, B. S. Choi, P. Youn, D. Y. Ryu, C. D. Klaassen and J. D. Park, *Arch. Toxicol.*, 2007, **81**, 327.
162. D. A. Vesey, *Toxicol. Lett.*, 2010, **198**, 13.
163. Agency for Toxic Substances and Drug Registry, *Mercury,* Public Health Service, United States Department of Health and Human Services, Centers for Disease Control, Atlanta, 2008.
164. T. W. Clarkson and L. Magos, *Crit. Rev. Toxicol.*, 2006, **36**, 609.
165. J. P. Rooney, *Toxicology*, 2007, **234**, 145.
166. R. K. Zalups, *Pharmacol. Rev.*, 2000, **52**, 113.
167. J. F. Risher and C. T. De Rosa, *J. Environ. Health*, 2007, **70**, 9.
168. M. J. Murphy, E. J. Culliford and V. Parsons, *Resuscitation*, 1979, **7**, 35.
169. B. Rowens, D. Guerrero-Betancourt, C. A. Gottlieb, R. J. Boyes and M. S. Eichenhorn, *Chest*, 1991, **99**, 185.
170. E. R. Samuels, H. M. Heick, P. N. McLaine and J. P. Farant, *J. Anal. Toxicol.*, 1982, **6**, 120.
171. A. Yasutake, K. Hirayama and M. Inoue, *Arch. Toxicol.*, 1989, **63**, 479.
172. J. C. Gage, *Br. J. Ind. Med*, 1964, **21**, 197.
173. T. Norseth and T. W. Clarkson, *Arch. Environ. Health.*, 1970, **21**, 717.
174. T. Norseth and T. W. Clarkson, *Biochem. Pharmacol.*, 1970, **19**, 2775.
175. S. Omata, M. Sato, K. Sakimura and H. Sugano, *Arch. Toxicol.*, 1980, **44**, 231.
176. W. L. Hughes, *Ann. N. Y. Acad. Sci*, 1957, **65**, 454.
177. R. K. Zalups, *Toxicology*, 1993, **79**, 215.
178. V. T. Cannon, D. W. Barfuss and R. K. Zalups, *J. Am. Soc. Nephrol.*, 2000, **11**, 394.
179. V. T. Cannon, R. K. Zalups and D. W. Barfuss, *Pharmacol. Exp. Ther.*, 2001, **298**, 780.
180. R. K. Zalups, *Toxicol. Appl. Pharmacol.*, 1998, **151**, 192.
181. R. K. Zalups and L. H. Lash, *Biochem. Pharmacol.*, 1997, **53**, 1889.
182. R. K. Zalups and K. H. Minor, *J. Toxicol. Environ. Health*, 1995, **46**, 73.
183. R. K. Zalups and D. W. Barfuss, *J. Toxicol. Environ. Health*, 1995, **44**, 385.
184. R. K. Zalups and D. W. Barfuss, *Toxicology*, 1996, **109**, 15.
185. R. K. Zalups and D. W. Barfuss, *J. Am. Soc. Nephrol.*, 1998, **9**, 551.
186. C. C. Bridges, C. Bauch, F. Verrey and R. K. Zalups, *J. Am. Soc. Nephrol*, 2004, **15**, 663.
187. C. C. Bridges and R. K. Zalups, *Am. J. Pathol.*, 2004, **165**, 1385.
188. C. C. Bridges and R. K. Zalups, *J. Pharmacol. Exp. Ther.*, 2006, **319**, 948.
189. R. K. Zalups and D. W. Barfuss, *Toxicology*, 1995, **103**, 23.
190. R. K. Zalups and D. W. Barfuss, *Toxicol. Appl. Pharmacol.*, 1998, **148**, 183.
191. R. K. Zalups, *Toxicol. Appl. Pharmacol.*, 1995, **132**, 289.
192. R. K. Zalups, *J. Toxicol. Environ. Health A*, 1998, **55**, 13.

193. B. Ferrier, M. Martin and F. Roch-Ramel, *J. Pharmacol. Exp. Ther*, 1983, **224**, 451.
194. A. S. Koh, T. A. Simmons-Willis, J. B. Pritchard, S. M. Grassl and N. Ballatori, *Mol. Pharmacol.*, 2002, **62**, 921.
195. R. Kojima, T. Sekine, M. Kawachi, S. H. Cha, Y. Suzuki and H. Endou, *J. Am. Soc. Nephrol.*, 2002, **13**, 848.
196. H. Motohashi, Y. Sakurai, H. Saito, S. Masuda, Y. Urakami, M. Goto, A. Fukatsu, O. Ogawa and K. Inui, *J. Am. Soc. Nephrol.*, 2002, **13**, 866.
197. J. B. Pritchard, *Am. J. Physiol.*, 1988, **255**, F597.
198. A. Shimomura, A. M. Chonko and J. J. Grantham, *Am. J. Physiol.*, 1981, **240**, F430.
199. T. Tanaka, A. Naganuma, N. Miura and N. Imura, *Toxicol. Appl. Pharmacol*, 1992, **112**, 58.
200. K. J. Ullrich, G. Rumrich, G. Fritzsch and S. Kloss, *Pflugers Arch*, 1987, **408**, 38.
201. R. K. Zalups and S. Ahmad, *Kidney Int.*, 2005, **68**, 1684.
202. R. K. Zalups and S. Ahmad, *J. Pharmacol. Exp. Ther.*, 2005, **315**, 896.
203. R. K. Zalups and S. Ahmad, *J. Pharmacol. Exp. Ther.*, 2005, **314**, 1158.
204. A. G. Aslamkhan, Y. H. Han, X. P. Yang, R. K. Zalups and J. B. Pritchard, *Mol. Pharmacol.*, 2003, **63**, 590.
205. R. K. Zalups and S. Ahmad, *J. Am. Soc. Nephrol.*, 2004, **15**, 2023.
206. R. K. Zalups, A. G. Aslamkhan and S. Ahmad, *Kidney Int.*, 2004, **66**, 251.
207. M. G. Cherian and T. W. Clarkson, *Chem. Biol. Interact.*, 1976, **12**, 109.
208. R. K. Zalups and J. Koropatnick, *J. Pharmacol. Exp. Ther.*, 2000, **295**, 74.
209. J. Ruprecht, *Scientific Monograph for Dimaval.* Houston, TX, 2008, Available at: heyl-berlin.de.
210. H. V. Aposhian, *Annu. Rev. Pharmacol. Toxicol.*, 1983, **23**, 193.
211. H. V. Aposhian, R. M. Maiorino, D. Gonzalez-Ramirez, M. Zuniga-Charles, Z. Xu, K. M. Hurlbut, P. Junco-Munoz, R. C. Dart and M. M. Aposhian, *Toxicology*, 1995, **97**, 23.
212. H. V. Aposhian, R. M. Maiorino, M. Rivera, D. C. Bruce, R. C. Dart, K. M. Hurlbut, D. J. Levine, W. Zheng, Q. Fernando, D. Carter, *et al.*, *J. Toxicol. Clin. Toxicol.*, 1992, **30**, 505.
213. F. Planas-Bohne, *Toxicology*, 1981, **19**, 275.
214. R. K. Zalups, *J. Pharmacol. Exp. Ther.*, 1993, **267**, 791.
215. M. Rodiger, X. Zhang, B. Ugele, N. Gersdorff, S. H. Wright, G. Burckhardt and A. Bahn, *Can. J. Physiol. Pharmacol.*, 2010, **88**, 141.
216. A. Bahn, M. Knabe, Y. Hagos, M. Rodiger, S. Godehardt, D. S. Graber-Neufeld, K. K. Evans, G. Burckhardt and S. H. Wright, *Mol. Pharmacol.*, 2002, **62**, 1128.
217. B. C. Burckhardt, B. Drinkuth, C. Menzel, A. Konig, J. Steffgen, S. H. Wright and G. Burckhardt, *J. Am. Soc. Nephrol.*, 2002, **13**, 2628.
218. F. Islinger, M. Gekle and S. H. Wright, *J. Pharmacol. Exp. Ther*, 2001, **299**, 741.

219. C. C. Bridges, L. Joshee and R. K. Zalups, *Toxicol. Sci.*, 2008, **105**, 211.
220. C. C. Bridges, L. Joshee and R. K. Zalups, *J. Pharmacol. Exp. Ther.*, 2008, **324**, 383.
221. D. A. Aremu, M. S. Madejczyk and N. Ballatori, *Environ. Health Perspect.*, 2008, **116**, 26.
222. M. S. Madejczyk, D. A. Aremu, T. A. Simmons-Willis, T. W. Clarkson and N. Ballatori, *J. Pharmacol. Exp. Ther.*, 2007, **322**, 378.
223. R. K. Zalups and C. C. Bridges, *Toxicol. Appl. Pharmacol*, 2009, **235**, 10.
224. E. M. McDowell, R. B. Nagle, R. C. Zalme, J. S. McNeil, W. Flamenbaum and B. F. Trump, *Virchows Arch. B. Cell. Pathol.*, 1976, **22**, 173.
225. R. C. Zalme, E. M. McDowell, R. B. Nagle, J. S. McNeil, W. Flamenbaum and B. F. Trump, *Virchows Arch. B. Cell. Pathol*, 1976, **22**, 197.
226. A. E. Rodin and C. N. Crowson, *Am. J. Pathol*, 1962, **41**, 485.
227. T. L. Gritzka and B. F. Trump, *Am. J. Pathol.*, 1968, **52**, 1225.
228. R. K. Zalups, *Toxicol. Appl. Pharmacol.*, 2000, **164**, 15.
229. C. A. Gotelli, E. Astolfi, C. Cox, E. Cernichiari and T. W. Clarkson, *Science*, 1985, **227**, 638.
230. R. G. Price, *Toxicology*, 1982, **23**, 99.
231. R. K. Zalups and G. L. Diamond, *Virchows Arch. B. Cell. Pathol. Incl. Mol. Pathol.*, 1987, **53**, 336.
232. R. K. Zalups, C. Cox and G. L. Diamond, Histological and urinalysis assessment of nephrotoxicity induced by mercuric chloride in normal and uninephrectomized rats, in *Biological Monitoring of Toxic Metals*, eds. T. W. Clarkson, L. Friberg, G. F. Nordberg and P. R. Sager, First Edition, Plenum Publishing Corporation, New York, 1988, 531.
233. T. W. Clarkson and L. Magos, *Br. J. Pharmacol. Chemother*, 1967, **31**, 560.
234. L. Magos and T. Stoytchev, *Br. J. Pharmacol*, 1969, **35**, 121.
235. B. Trojanowska, J. K. Piotrowski and S. Szendzikowski, *Toxicol. Appl. Pharmacol.*, 1971, **18**, 374.
236. R. L. Hall, W. L. Wilke and M. J. Fettman, *Vet. Hum. Toxicol.*, 1986, **28**, 305.
237. K. Eto, A. Yasutake, K. Miyamoto, H. Tokunaga and Y. Otsuka, *Tohoku. J. Exp. Med.*, 1997, **182**, 197.
238. P. Druet, E. Druet, F. Potdevin and C. Sapin, *Ann. Immunol. (Paris)*, 1978, **129 C**, 777.
239. P. E. Bigazzi, *Clin. Immunol. Immunopathol.*, 1992, **65**, 81.
240. P. E. Bigazzi, *J. Toxicol. Clin. Toxicol.*, 1988, **26**, 125.
241. R. C. Vanholder, M. M. Praet, P. A. Pattyn, I. R. Leusen and N. H. Lameire, *Kidney Int*, 1982, **22**, 162.
242. K. Hirayama and A. Yasutake, *J. Toxicol. Environ. Health*, 1986, **18**, 49.
243. W. R. Swindell, *Ageing Res. Rev*, 2011, **10**, 132.
244. M. T. Houser and W. O. Berndt, *Toxicol. Appl. Pharmacol.*, 1986, **83**, 506.
245. M. T. Houser and W. O. Berndt, *Toxicol. Appl. Pharmacol*, 1988, **93**, 187.

246. B. Ramos-Frendo, R. Perez-Garcia, J. M. Lopez-Novoa and L. Hernando-Avendano, *Biomedicine*, 1979, **31**, 167.
247. R. K. Zalups, *Exp. Mol. Pathol.*, 1991, **54**, 10.
248. R. K. Zalups, *J. Toxicol. Environ. Health*, 1997, **50**, 173.
249. R. K. Zalups, D. W. Barfuss and P. J. Kostyniak, *Toxicol. Appl. Pharmacol.*, 1992, **115**, 174.
250. R. K. Zalups, J. M. Klotzbach and G. L. Diamond, *Toxicol. Appl. Pharmacol.*, 1987, **89**, 226.
251. R. K. Zalups, *Toxicol. Appl. Pharmacol.*, 1997, **143**, 366.
252. B. Stengel and C. Couchoud, *J. Am. Soc. Nephrol.*, 2006, **17**, 2094.
253. Centers for Disease Prevention and Control, Chronic Kidney Disease Fact Sheet, Department of Health and Human Services, CDC, Atlanta, 2010, pp. 1.
254. R. K. Zalups, *Toxicol. Appl. Pharmacol.*, 1995, **130**, 121.

CHAPTER 14

Age Related Effects of Cadmium and Possible Roles in Aging Processes

BRUCE A FOWLER

ICF International, Fairfax, VA 22031, USA
E-mail: drtox@earthlink.net

14.1 Introduction

14.1.1 Cadmium Exposures

The element cadmium (Cd) is atomic number 48 in the Periodic Table of Elements and is used in a wide variety of industrial applications, including batteries, solar cells, and various alloys.[1] It is also found as a contaminant in super phosphate fertilizers and municipal sewage sludge,[2] where it may be taken up by certain food crops such as rice, leafy green vegetables, and tobacco plants.[1,2] In addition, filter feeding shellfish, such as oysters, have been found to accumulate Cd from seawater.[3,4] Organ meats from the liver and kidneys of livestock[1] also accumulate cadmium, depending on dietary feed stocks. Statistical associations between dietary intakes of cereals, leafy green vegetables, organ meats, yams, and tofu with urinary Cd were reported in a study of 191 premenopausal women.[5] Interestingly, consumption of tofu showed the strongest association in this study.

Issues in Toxicology No. 16
Aging and Vulnerability to Environmental Chemicals: Age-related Disorders and their Origins in Environmental Exposures
Edited by Bernard Weiss

Published by the Royal Society of Chemistry, www.rsc.org

14.1.2 Cadmium from Diet and Tobacco

The main sources of human exposure to Cd are from consumption of food items containing Cd and from use of tobacco products such as cigarettes. The latter can greatly increase body burden.[5,6] The absorption of Cd from dietary exposures is of the order of 5–10%, while inhalation absorption from sources such as tobacco smoke is estimated to be of the order of 50%.[1] The reduction in smoking rates in the US has recently been shown[7] to reduce urinary Cd excretion patterns. Several factors have been reported to be associated with differences in Cd uptake. Low iron status has been shown to exert a marked increase in uptake of Cd from the gastrointestinal tract.[8–12] Race and ethnic differences among women of child bearing age have also been reported,[13] with higher Cd uptake levels among Hispanics and African Americans. These factors may have important health consequences for these sub-populations at later life stages. A recent study,[14] which modeled the National Health and Nutrition Examination Study (NHANES) dataset for urinary Cd in a representative sample of the general US population from ages 2–70 years, showed that dietary uptakes varied as a function of age and gender, with females showing approximately 2-fold greater uptake than males. Even though Cd uptake among females was higher, both genders showed marked increases in urinary Cd concentrations in the 6–11 year old age range, followed by a monotonic increase throughout later years. These increased uptakes in early life are potentially of great importance since Cd has an estimated half-life in the human body of the order of decades. Thus early life exposures may have health impacts in later years and may impact a number of diseases associated with old age, as well as the aging process itself.

This chapter will review a number of human health studies which have evaluated human exposures to Cd, accumulation of this element in various organ systems, and known health outcomes associated with Cd in the elderly. These results will be compared with those from experimental animal studies which examined accumulation of toxic effects of Cd as a function of age, to assess similarities and differences. Studies focused on the mechanisms of Cd-induced toxicity/carcinogenicity will be evaluated in order to understand the organ system effects of this element at the target cell level of biological organization. Finally, the chapter will include a discussion of how available data from these studies may suggest roles for Cd in contributing to the aging process itself[15] through the production of oxidative stress[16] in target cell populations of major organ systems such as the kidney, lungs, skeleton, endocrine/reproductive, and visual and cardiovascular systems.

14.2 Cadmium Accumulation and Effects in Humans

14.2.1 Kidney and Skeletal Effects

14.2.1.1 Role of Gender

Early occupational studies in Japan of Cd-exposed workers[1,17] and multiparous elderly women consuming Cd-contaminated rice demonstrated age-related accumulation of Cd in kidneys; this was associated with tubular proteinuria, calciuria, and an osteomalacia, known in Japan as Itai-itai disease.[1] Similar losses of bone mineral density have been reported among older females with environmental exposures to Cd in Thailand[18] and Korea,[19] but not Poland.[20] Other studies from the US using data from the NHANES III[21] showed that long-term exposure to environmental cadmium levels was associated with increased bone mineral loss, increased serum levels of follicle stimulating hormone (FSH), and urinary cadmium concentrations in women in the 42–60 year old age group, suggesting that a complex set of factors may be involved in the degree of bone mineral loss in females. It is generally agreed that the skeletal effects of Cd are primarily related to renal toxicity of Cd and depletion of calcium body stores since osteomalacia has also been observed in battery workers who were occupationally exposed to Cd,[1] but Cd-induced hormonal disruptive effects may also play a role at the level of bone cells.

As noted,[14] age and gender comparisons from the NHANES studies, which are representative of the general US population, demonstrated that females had much higher urinary cadmium concentrations than males. The data show a marked increase in urinary concentrations of Cd in the 6–11 year old age group, with females approximately twice as high as males, followed by a monotonic rise into the 8th decade of life. It is worth noting that since Cd has a half-life in humans of the order of decades, the early accumulation pattern may well have health consequences in later life. More recent studies from Japan[22] showed similar age-related increases in both blood and urinary Cd as function of age in women from the general population. Urinary Cd more closely correlated with proteinuria biomarkers than blood Cd. Other studies[15] also reported gender related findings using scalp hair as the biomonitoring matrix for Cd, with females showing higher concentrations than males. The authors also suggested an age-dependent hair accumulation of Cd and suggested that it, along with other toxic elements such as arsenic and mercury, may play a role in aging and even increase the rate of aging. Other Japanese studies[23] which measured urinary markers of oxidative stress, such as 8-OH deoxyguanosine (8-OHDG), found that these markers were positively associated with urinary Cd and negatively associated with selenium. The probable role of Cd-induced oxidative stress in mediating the target organ system effects of Cd and the more global associations of Cd with age-related disease processes will be discussed in greater detail in following sections. As noted, the effects of Cd on target organ systems in humans, such as the kidneys, lungs and skeleton, have been appreciated for many years, but Cd is a broad-spectrum toxic agent that is increasingly being recognized to produce toxicity in a number of other organ systems, as discussed in the following sections.

14.2.2 Effects on the Blood Vasculature

More recent studies have also demonstrated effects on cells of the blood vasculature[24–27] and the retina.[28–31] In agreement with these laboratory findings, several large scale epidemiological studies[32–34] have reported associations of increased risks of hypertension, stroke, and peripheral vascular disease and environmental exposures to Cd in adult populations from the US and Thailand. Reported data also suggest an increase in risk of breast cancer.[35] The breast cancer effects could be related to the known endocrine disrupting effects of Cd[36] and to the increased presence of the cadmium-binding protein, metallothionein, in breast cancer cells.[37] A similar increase from Cd may be present in the risk of human prostate cancer[38] as shown from cadmium studies in animals, discussed later. Taken together, these data indicate that Cd exerts a broad spectrum of health effects that most commonly present themselves in the elderly, with a generally greater manifestation of effects in females.

The putative roles of Cd in mediating the morbidity and mortality of these major diseases are of potentially great public health importance and cost to society. The following sections, which provide a brief overview of data from *in vivo* animal studies and *in vitro* tests systems, provide further experimental support for hypotheses suggesting an important role for this toxic element both in mediating common diseases which typically manifest themselves in the later decades of life, and in the aging process itself.

14.3 Cadmium Accumulation and Effects in Experimental Animal Studies

14.3.1 Rodent Studies

14.3.1.1 Effects of Age and Gender

Wada and colleagues[39] studied the accumulation of Cd in various organs of hamsters aged 3–27 months in relation to Cd binding to the metallothionein fraction following a short-term injection protocol. They reported increased accumulation of Cd in the liver as a function of age, but that the kidney accumulation of Cd was elevated in younger animals but attenuated in older animals. These accumulation patterns followed Cd binding to MT, which was suggested to be responsible for observed Cd accumulation patterns. These studies suggested both organ- and age-related differences in the accumulation of Cd. Rho and Kim[40] reported that anti-oxidant dietary grape formulations exerted marked attenuation of age-relatedand Cd-induced oxidative damage and enhancing effects on anti-oxidant enzyme systems in rats of 16, 18, and 20 months of age. Other studies by Ninomiya, *et al.*[41] in 10 and 40 week old female rats given SC injections of 0, 0.3, 0.9, or 2.7 mg kg^{-1} showed dose-related increases in liver accumulation in the 10 week old animals but attenuated Cd accumulation of Cd in livers of the 40 week old animals, which was associated with increased renal accumulation of Cd at the high Cd dose level in this age group. The results of these studies indicate a marked age difference in response to Cd treatment.

There have been a number of *in vivo* experimental studies in rodents over the last three decades indicating that older animals are more susceptible to cadmium-induced target organ toxicity than younger animals.[42–44] Renal damage has been related to mitochondrial gene deletion in rats[45] and found to accelerate age-related changes in mitochondrial DNA in kidney epithelial cells.[46,47] Other studies[48] on renal metabolism of calciotropic hormones in aged female rats indicated marked decreases in serum 25OH vitamin D and 1,25 di-OH vitamin D and in 1,25 di-OH vitamin D in the renal mitochondrial fraction. These changes were associated with increases in calcitonin and parathyroid hormone. These data were correlated with decreases in renal GFR and altered bone mineralization and suggest that long-term low dose exposure to Cd may produce the known bone demineralization secondary to renal damage *via* this physiological mechanism.

Studies by Yang *et al.*[49] have also noted cadmium-induced death in mesangial cells *via* an apoptotic pathway involving Ca^{2+} release from the ER and cellular autophagy. Other studies[50] have reported that Cd exposure produces altered insulin metabolism *via* pancreatic toxicity, possibly leading to renal vascular damage secondary to development of some forms of diabetes.

Organs, such as the testes[51] are also sensitive to Cd toxicity, and Cd may hence play a role in declining sperm counts observed in modern male populations in developed countries. Ototoxicity from Cd exposure[52] is another important effect that clearly has implications for elderly populations.

14.3.2 Effects of *In Utero* Exposures

Studies in rats concerning the effects of *in utero* exposure to Cd have reported decreased body size.[53] Other studies[54] have reported delayed effects in renal function of offspring of female rats treated with Cd *via* the oral route throughout gestation. The changes were not observed until postnatal day 45 and renal failure, characterized by decreased GFR and altered excretion of electrolytes, was observed at postnatal day 60. The importance of these data rests with the growing appreciation that *in utero* exposures to toxic agents, such as Cd, may produce deleterious delayed health consequences at later life stages.

Cadmium exposure has also been demonstrated to produce cancer in experimental animals and IARC has designated Cd a human carcinogen[55] based on combined lines of evidence. The results of these investigations are also consistent with the observations from analogous studies in humans and provide further impetus for examining the effects of Cd at later stages in life and considering the elderly as a subpopulation at special risk for Cd toxicity. In addition, the observed low-dose effects of Cd exposure in exacerbating the effects of the aging process on important organ systems, such as the kidneys, blood vasculature, lungs and skeleton, suggest an important set of interrelationships from the perspective of public health. The relevance of cadmium in development of cancer is an obvious concern in elderly populations. Further research concerning the roles of Cd as a factor in mediating aging processes of target organ systems disease is clearly warranted. As discussed in the following section, Cd-induced production of reactive oxygen species (ROS) in target cell populations appears to play a major role in the mechanisms of Cd toxicity. The attenuating effects of cellular antioxidant systems, metallothionein, and the stress protein response must also be considered in developing mode of action risk assessment strategies. This observation is of particular importance for elderly organisms in which such protective cellular systems may be diminished as a result of the aging process itself combined with marginal nutritional status.

Based on the information from the human and animal studies discussed it is clear that there are a number of analogous organ system effects that are produced by environmental or low-level exposures to Cd. Furthermore, these effects seem to exacerbate similar effects produced by the aging process, such that organisms at later life stages may be rendered as sensitive subpopulations. This observation has important implications for risk assessment strategies to protect the public health.

14.4 Molecular Mechanisms of Cadmium Toxicity

14.4.1 Roles of Cd-Induced Oxidative Stress and Anti-Oxidant Systems

In order to make a clear linkage between Cd exposures and observed target organ toxicities, it is essential to have an understanding of the underlying mechanisms of action and factors, such as age, that may modulate the shape of the dose–response curve for a given toxicological endpoint. Cd is a broad-spectrum toxic agent which may affect a number of intracellular systems. Cd-induced production of ROS, leading to oxidative stress, appears to play a central role in mediating a number of these effects, which include induction of cellular anti-oxidant systems such as glutathione (GSH), superoxide dismutase (SOD), and the metal-binding protein metallothionein (MT). Attenuated control of ROS leads to alterations of cell signaling pathways which regulate cellular replication and cell death by induction of apoptosis. The health consequences of these events may hence include cancer and physiological decrements in target organ function commonly associated with old age. It must be noted that all of these cellular processes are inter-related and the timing and degree to which these important processes become engaged appear to be largely regulated by production of ROS and the ability of cells to sequester Cd^{2+} ions and regulate the production and activity of ROS.

14.4.1.1 Insulin Signaling Pathway Effects

There are a number of papers describing relationships between genes regulating longevity in the worm *C. elegans* and Cd exposure *in vitro*. Studies by Barsyte *et al.*[56] described the interaction of the insulin-like receptor protein DAF-2, AGE-1 and DAF-16 in mediating resistance to a number of cellular insults which produce oxidative stress. In particular, they found that mutations in daf-2 and age-1, but not daf-16, increased resistance to Cd ion toxicity in a 24-hour assay. They also found that induction of MT1 and MT2 was markedly higher in daf-2 mutant worms. They concluded that the insulin signaling pathway determines lifespan in this species by modulating stress-related proteins such as MT. Regulation of MT hence also influences susceptibility to Cd toxicity in this species. Subsequent studies by Wang *et al.*[57] studied the combined effects of Ca and Cd on the lifespan of *C. elegans* and found that the combination of these elements increased oxidative damage and resulted in the induction of hsp-16. They observed that a mutation in daf-16 increased the toxicity of Ca/Cd on lifespan while mutation of daf-2 attenuated the combined effects of Ca/Cd mixtures on life span. Other studies by Tvermoes *et al.*,[58] who examined the metal-inducible genes numr-1 and numr-2, also demonstrated their role in mediating Cd resistance and increasing *C. elegans*' lifespan. These findings are of interest in that these genes also act through interactive effects on the insulin signaling pathway in this species with daf-16 and skn-1.

Studies using mammalian cells from long-lived mouse systems[59] have also reported increased resistance to oxidative stress produced by agents such as Cd and that these systems also produce reduction of the insulin/GF-1FOXO pathway, which is connected to several other cell signaling pathways. The linkage with the insulin signaling pathways in relation to longevity in both *C.elegans* and long-lived mice is intriguing and seems to suggest an inter-connection with formation of ROS generated by agents such as Cd at a basic molecular level. Studies by other investigators[60,61] using cells from long-lived mice have also demonstrated resistance to Cd-induced oxidative stress, but the results highlighted the complexity of this resistance at several levels of biological organization and the involvement with cell signaling pathways, including the induction of immediate early genes in response to Cd exposure. These investigators[62] also noted the important protective roles played by cellular anti-oxidant systems in mediating oxidative stress and consequently the aging process.

Studies in mammalian systems have shown similar effects in relation to regulation of the anti-oxidant response element (ARE) by the transcriptional factor nrf2 in long-lived Snell dwarf mice.[63] The anti-oxidant systems of these mice (*e.g.*, glutathione) are elevated, and treatment of cells from control mice with an inducer of oxidative stress (arsenite) also increases resistance to other oxidative stress inducers such as Cd. The authors suggest that the enhanced activity of genes regulated by the Nrf2/ARE may confer stress resistance in cells from the Snell dwarf mice and hence increase longevity.

14.4.2 Oxidative Stress, Protein Turnover and Chromosomal Effects

Other recent studies[64] on mouse embryo fibroblasts have demonstrated, using system-based gene expression systems, the confirmation of ROS formation in response to *in vitro* Cd exposure, which was associated with alterations in cell-cycle regulation and disruption of the ubiquitin–proteosome system in these cells. The importance of these data rests with a more complete understanding of the mechanisms and consequences of Cd cellular toxicity to essential cellular machinery that is also intimately involved in the aging process, systemic chronic diseases, and cancer.

Studies using cultured lymphocytes from young (18–30 years) and old (80–93 years) persons[65] exposed to Cd demonstrated that those from the older group had increased decondensation in both facultive and constitutive regions of the heterochromatin relative to that observed in lymphocytes from younger persons. These data suggest that heterochromatin remodeling processes are altered as a function of age and that consequently the effects of metals, such as Cd, on these processes will be changed.

It is important to note that Cd exposure may also alter epigenetic mechanisms of cell injury and cancer. Doi *et al.*[66] recently reported down-regulation of the DNA methyl transferase gene (DNMT3A/3B) in chick embryos incubated with Cd for 60 hours and harvested at a 4 hour time point relative to saline controls. They also reported decreased immunoreactivity of 5′-methyl cytidine (5′MeC) at this time point. The 4 hour time point is an important time period in body wall formation in the chick, and these epigenetic effects may underlie Cd-induced formation of ventral body wall defects in chick embryos. Other recent reports[67] have noted the importance of Cd-induced formation of ROS in mediating the carcinogenic effects of Cd, which results in a panoply of effects on signal transduction pathways, DNA damage, and the roles of antioxidant systems, stress proteins, and molecular regulatory factors in mediating these effects. Again, age-related attenuation of these protective systems may facilitate the development of Cd-induced cancer in elderly individuals.[68]

14.5 Potential Roles of Cadmium in Aging Processes

It is clear from the previous discussion that Cd could play a role in the aging process/longevity *via* formation of ROS and that older organisms, including man, have a more limited capacity to deal with Cd-induced cell injury following lifetime exposures to this element. This limited ability appears to be largely a function of attenuation of cellular antioxidant systems, such as GSH and SOD, but also includes limitations in the stress protein response including synthesis of MT. The net result of this interaction between Cd exposures and the aging process is that older organisms are more susceptible to the toxic effects of Cd on target organ systems, such as the lungs, kidneys, blood vasculature, and skeleton. Hence future risk assessments for Cd should take the elderly into account as a sensitive subpopulation. In addition, based on the previous discussion, the female gender seems to be at elevated risk for Cd toxicity, and further research is needed to understand the mechanisms underlying these gender-specific effects.

14.6 Summary and Conclusions

Based on the evidence, it is clear that Cd is a broad-spectrum toxic agent that accumulates in people over the course of a lifetime and affects a number of organ systems. These effects usually manifest themselves in the later stages of life. Females appear to be a subpopulation at particular risk. From experimental animal and cellular studies, Cd-induced production of oxidative stress in target cell populations is a major underlying cause of toxicity, which seems to occur largely by the process of apoptosis. The toxic effects of Cd are modulated by cellular anti-oxidant systems and binding to MT. It appears that the capacity of these protective molecular systems attenuates with age, and these systems may play a role in the manifestations of toxicity which occurs in the elderly from life-tem exposures to this element. In addition, it has been hypothesized that Cd, which is present in all living organisms, may actually play a role in the aging process itself by persistent production of oxidative stress in target tissues until the capacity of anti-oxidant systems becomes depleted.

References

1. G. F. Nordberg, K. Nogawa, M. Nordberg and L. T. Friberg in *Handbook of the Toxicology of Metals*, eds. G. F. Nordberg, B. A. Fowler, M. Nordberg and L. T. Friberg, Elsevier, Amsterdam, 3rd edn, 2007, pp. 446–479.
2. Ministry of Agriculture and Forestry, *Cadmium in Fertilizers: Risks to Human Health and the Environment*, 2000, pp. 1–120.
3. D. W. Engel, W. Sunda and B. A. Fowler in *Biological Monitoring of Marine Pollutants,* eds. F. J. Vernberg, A. Calabrese, F. P. Thurberg and W. B. Vernberg, Academic Press, New York, 1981, pp. 127–144.
4. R. Copes, N. A. Clark, K. Rideout, J. Palaty and K. Tesche, *Environ. Res.*, 2008, **107**, 160–169.
5. S. V. Adams, P. A. Newcomb, M. M. Shafer, C. Atkinson, E. J. Bowles, K. M. Newton and J. W. Lampe, *Sci. Total Environ.*, 2011, **409**, 1632–1637.
6. P. A. Richter, E. E. Bishop, J. Wang and M. H. Swahn, *J. Environ. Res. Public Health*, 2009, **6**, 1930–1946.
7. M. Tellez-Plaza, A. Navas-Acien, K. L. Caldwell, A. Menke, P. Muntner and E. Guallar, *Environ. Health Perspect.*, 2012, **120**, 204–209.
8. R. Apinan, S. Satarug, R. Ruengweeravut, W. Mahavorasirkul and K. Na-Bangchang, *Environ. Geochem. Health*, 2010, **32**, 237–242.
9. H. M. Meltzer, A. L. Brantsaeter, B. Borch-Ionsen, D. G. Ellingsen, J. Alexander, Y. Thomassen, H. Stigum and T. A. Ydersbond, *Environ. Res.*, 2010, **110**, 497–504.
10. C. M. Gallagher, J.J. Chen and J.S. Kovach, *Environ. Res.*, 2011, **111**, 702–707.
11. B. Julin, M. Vahter, B. Amzal, A. Wolk, M. Berglund and A. Akesson, *Environ. Health*, 2011, **10**, 105–111.
12. M. Berglund, A. L. Lindberg, M. Rahman, M. Yunus, M. Grander, B. Lonnerdal and M. Vahter, *Environ. Res.*, 2011, **111**, 1271–1279.
13. R. S. Mijal and C. B. Holzman, *Environ. Res.*, 2010, **110**, 505–512.
14. P. Ruiz, M. Mumtaz, J. Osterloh, J. Fisher and B. A. Fowler, *Toxicol. Lett.*, 2010, **198**, 44–48.
15. H. Yasuda, K. Yoshida, Y. Yasuda and T. Tsutsui, *Curr. Aging Sci.*, 2012, **5**, 105–111.

16. R. C. Patra, A. K. Rautray and D. Swarup, *Veterinary Medicine International, 2011*, Article ID 457327, 9 pages, 2011. doi:10.4061/2011/457327. (www. hindawi.com/journals/vmi/2011/457327/cta, accessed 01/25/2012).
17. G. Kazantsis, *Biometals*, 2004, **17**, 493–498.
18. P. Limpatanachote, W. Swaddiwudhipong, M. Nishijo, R. Honda, P. Mahasakpan, K. Nambunmee and W. Ruangyuttikarn, *J. Med. Assoc. Thai.*, 2010, **93**, 1451–1457.
19. M. Shin, D. Paek and C. Yoon, *Environ. Res.*, 2011, **111**, 101–109.
20. M. Trzcinka-Ochocka, M. Jakubowski, W. Szymczak, B. Janasik and R. Brodzka, *Environ. Res.*, 2010, **110**, 286–293.
21. C. M. Gallagher, B. S. Moonga and J. S. Kovach, *Environ. Res.*, 2010, **110**, 106–111.
22. M. Ikeda, F. Ohashi, Y. Fukui, S. Sakuragi and J. Moriquchi, *Int. Arch. Occup. Environ. Health*, 2011, **84**, 121–129.
23. B. A. Muzembo, D. Narongpon, N. R. Ngatu, M. Eitoku, R. Hirota and N. Suganuma, *Geriatr. Gerontol. Int.*, 2011 Dec 28. doi: 10.1111/j. 1447-0594.2011.00793.x. (Epub ahead of print).
24. W. C. Prozialeck, J. R. Edwards and J. M. Woods, *Life Sci.*, 2006, **79**, 1493–1506.
25. W. C. Prozialeck, J. R. Edwards, D. W. Nebert, J. M. Woods, A. Barchowsky and W. D. Atchison, *Toxicol. Sci.*, 2008, **102**, 207–218.
26. B. Messner, M. Knoflach, A. Seubert, A. Ritsch, K. Pfaller, B. Henderson, Y. H. Shen, I. Zeller, J. Willeit, G. Laufer, G. Wick, S. Kiechl and D. Bernhard, *Arterioscler., Thromb., Vasc. Biol.*, 2009, **29**, 1392–1398.
27. E. M. Alissa and G. A. Ferns, *J. Toxicol.*, 2011, doi: 10.1155/ 2011/870125,21 pages. (www.hindawi.com accessed 01/25/2012).
28. N. K. Wills, V. M. Ramanujam, J. Chang, N. Kalariya, J .R. Lewis, T. X. Weng and F. J. van Kujik, *Exp. Eye Res.*, 2008, **86**, 41–51.
29. N. M. Kalariya, N. K. Wills, K. V. Ramana, S. K. Srivastava and F. J. van Kujik, *Exp. Eye Res.*, 2009, **89**, 494–502.
30. N. M. Kalariya, B. Nair, D. K. Kalariya, N. K. Wills and F. J. vanKujik, *Toxicol. Lett.*, 2010, **198**, 56–62.
31. A. B. Lansdown, *Met. Ions Life Sci.*, 2011, **8**, 187–246.
32. J. L. Peters, T. S. Perlstein, M. J. Perry, E. McNeely and J. Weuve, *Environ. Res.*, 2010, **110**, 199–206.
33. M. Tellez-Plaza, A. Navas-Acen, C. M. Crainiceanu, A. R. Sharret and E. Guallar, *Am. J. Epidemiol.*, 2010, **172**, 671–681.
34. W. Swaddwudhipong, P. Mahasakpan, P. Limpatanachote and S. Krintratun, *Environ. Res.*, 2010, **110**, 612–616.
35. C. M. Gallagher, J. J. Chen and J. S. Kovach, *Aging*, 2010, **2**, 804–814.
36. C. Byrne, S. D. Divekar, G. B. Storchan, D. A. Parodi and M. B. Martin, *Toxicol. Appl. Pharmacol.*, 2009, **238**, 266–271.
37. L. Gallicchio, J. A. Flaws, B. A. Fowler and O. B. Loffe, *Cancer Detect. Prev.*, 2005.
38. G. S. Prins, *Endocr.-Relat. Cancer*, 2008, **15**, 649–656.

39. O. Wada, M. Ouchi, S. Manabe, H. Iwai, H. Suzuki, H. Matsui and T. Ono, *J. Toxicol. Sci.*, 1981, **6**, 115–22.
40. K. A. Rho and M. K. Kim, *J. Nutr. Sci. Vitaminol.*, 2006, **52**, 33–46.
41. R. Ninomiya, N. Koizumi and D. Fujita, *Environ. Health Prev. Med.*, 1997, **1**, 178–83.
42. T. Yamano, M. Shimizu and T. Noda, *Toxicol. Sci.*, 1998, **46**, 393–402.
43. T. Yamano, S. D. Kosanke and L. E. Rikana, *Toxicol. Appl. Pharmacol.*, 1999, **161**, 225–230.
44. K. Uriu, K. Kaizu, Y. L. Qie, A. Ito, I. Takagi, K. Suzuka, Y. Inada, O. Hashimoto and S. Eto, *Toxicol. Appl. Pharmacol.*, 2000, **169**, 151–158.
45. S. Takebayashi, S. Jimi, M. Segawa and A. Takai, *Clin. Exp. Nephrol.*, 2003, **1**, 18–26.
46. A. Takaki, S. Jimi, M. Segawa and H. Iwasaki, *Ann. N. Y. Acad. Sci.*, 2004, **1011**, 3332–3338.
47. A. Takaki, S. Jimi, M. Segawa, S. Hisano, S. Takebayashi and H. Iwasaki, *Toxicology*, 2004, **203**, 145–154.
48. M. M. Brzoska and J. Moniuszko-Jakoniuk, *Arch. Toxicol.*, 2005, **79**, 636–646.
49. L. Yang, K. Wu, W. Chiu, S. Wang and C. Shih, *Autophagy*, 2009, **5**, 571–572.
50. J. Edwards and W.C. Proziakeck, *Toxicol. Appl. Pharmacol.*, 2009, **3**, 289–293.
51. E. R. Siu, D. D. Mruk, C. S. Porto and C. Y. Cheng, *Toxicol. Appl. Pharmacol.*, 2009, **238**, 240–249.
52. S. Kim, H. Jeong, N. Myung, M. Kim, J. Lee, H. So, R. Park, H. Kim, J. Um and S. Hong, *Environ. Health Perspect.*, 2008, **116**, 854–862.
53. R. Couto-Moraes, L. F. Felicio and M. M. Bernardi, *J. Appl. Toxicol.*, 2010, **3**, 233–241.
54. G. Jacquillet, O. Barbier, I. Rubera, M. Tauc, A. Borderie, M. C. Namorado, D. Martin, G. Sierra, J. L. Reyes, P. Poujeol and M. Cougnon, *Am. J. Physiol: Renal*, 2007, **293**, 1450–1460.
55. International Agency for Research against Cancer (IARC), *Beryllium, Cadmium, Mercury, and Exposures in the Glass Manufacturing Industry*, Vol. 58, 1997.
56. D. Barsyte, D. A. Lovejoy and G. J. Lithgow, *FASEB J.*, 1002, **15**, 627–634.
57. S. Wang, M. Tang, B. Pei, X. Xiao, J. Wang, H. Hang and L. Wu, *Toxicol. Sci.*, 2008, **102**, 345–351.
58. B. E. Tvermoes, W. A. Boyd and J. H. Freedman, *J. Cell Sci.*, 2010, **123**, 2124–2134.
59. S. Murakami, *Exp. Gerontol.*, 2006, **10**, 2014–2019.
60. A. B. Salmon, S. Murakami, A. Bartke, J. Kopchick, K. Yasumura and R. A. Miller, *Am. J. Physiol.: Endocrinol. Metab.*, 2005, **289**, E23–E29.
61. A. B. Salmon, A. A. S. Akha, R. Buffenstein and R. A. Miller, *J. Gerontol. A. Biol. Sci. Med. Sci.*, 2008, **63**, 232–241.
62. A. B. Salmon, A. Richardson and V. I. Perez, *Free Radic. Biol. Med.*, 2010, **48**, 642–673.

63. S. F. Leiser and R. A. Miller, *Mol. Cell. Biol.*, 2010, **30**, 871–874.
64. T. Lezhava, J. Monaselidze, T. Jokhadze, M. Gorgoshidze, M. Kiladze, M. Gaiozishvili, *Age*, 2011, **33**, 433–438.
65. X. Yu, J. F. Robinson, J. S. Sidhu, S. Hong and E. M. Faustman, *Toxicol. Sci.*, 2010, **114**, 356–377.
66. T. Doi, P. Puri, A. McCann, J. Bannigan and J. Thompson, *Toxicol. Sci.*, 2011, **120**, 475–480.
67. P. Koedrith and Y. R. Seo, *Int. J. Mol. Sci.*, 2011, **12**, 9576–9595.
68. E. J. Tokar, L. Benbrahim-Tallaa and M. P. Waalkes, *Met. Ions Life Sci.*, 2011, **8**, 375–401.

CHAPTER 15

Lead Exposure and Osteoporosis: Mechanisms and Clinical Manifestations

J. EDWARD PUZAS,* CATHERINE A. MUZYTCHUK AND JONATHAN D. HOLZ

Department of Orthopaedics, University of Rochester School of Medicine and Dentistry, Rochester, NY 14642, USA
*E-mail: edward_puzas@urmc.rochester.edu

15.1 Introduction

Lead exposure and osteoporosis represent two of the most widespread health concerns facing the people of the United States and the world. These two entities are inextricably linked by virtue of the fact that almost all of the lead in humans resides in their skeleton. Yet the toxic effects of lead on the musculoskeletal system have been an under-investigated topic. As we better understand the interrelationship between environmental toxins and the skeleton, it should improve our ability to diagnose and treat bone diseases such as osteoporosis.

Osteoporosis is a disease characterized by an increased risk of skeletal fracture. The underlying causes for the increased risk are numerous; however, the two most important contributing factors are a decrease in bone mass and bone quality. Bone mass is measured with techniques that can assess the mineral density at susceptible skeletal sites. The lower the bone mineral density,

Issues in Toxicology No. 16
Aging and Vulnerability to Environmental Chemicals: Age-related Disorders and their Origins in Environmental Exposures
Edited by Bernard Weiss

Published by the Royal Society of Chemistry, www.rsc.org

the higher the risk of fracture. Bone quality is an encompassing term that relates to the micro architecture of bone, the organic composition of the tissue, the degree of mineralization and the ability to repair micro damaged areas. More recent data has begun to show that environmental agents such as lead can contribute to decreases in both the mass and quality of the skeleton.

Lead, in its ionic form, affects the functioning of both bone forming cells (osteoblasts) as well as bone resorbing cells (osteoclasts). However, it appears that the effects of this heavy metal are more deleterious on the action of osteoblasts and as such, the normal remodeling process in humans can be compromised. That is, lead decreases the rate of new bone formation relative to the rate of bone resorption and the skeleton loses mass and quality over a lifetime. Interestingly, since lead is stored in the osseous compartment, it is possible to observe harmful effects on bone, even at blood levels that could be considered normal.

In this treatise we will explore the issues of lead in our environment, its route of exposure and accumulation in the skeleton. We will also discuss how this toxin affects the cells of bone to predispose exposed individuals to an increased risk of osteoporosis.

15.2 Lead in the Environment

The widespread use of lead in manufacturing, gasoline, paints and plumbing has led to its dispersal throughout the environment.[1,2] Lead persists in the environment as it binds to soil and cannot be broken down.[3] No safe lower limit of lead exposure has been found and in fact, recently, the Center for Disease Control in the United States has issued a statement acknowledging this. Lead can affect virtually all organs and systems, causing adverse effects in the reproductive system and kidneys, and exerting a wide variety of neurological and cognitive effects, as well as being a potential carcinogen. We believe that we have identified another target of low level lead exposure that may be affecting the morbidity of a large part of the population, *i.e.* the structural skeleton responsible for mechanical support.

15.2.1 Is Lead a Physiologically Important Environmental Toxicant?

The answer is a definitive *yes*. And it may pose serious health issues in bone at levels well below any adopted safety threshold in blood. That is, bone cells are exposed to lead from two different sources, the extracellular fluid and the mineralized compartment of bone. This is due to their proximity to and metabolism of mineralized tissues, where greater than 90% of the body burden of lead resides. In fact, it has been shown that bone cells (both osteoclasts and osteoblasts), when cultured on bone wafers containing lead, show a depressed function in the absence of any detectable lead in the media. If this phenomenon exists *in vivo* then it is likely that we are grossly underestimating the effect of this heavy metal on skeletal metabolism.

Lead toxicity has become a controversial topic. Some organizations suggest that the levels of lead in the environment and in humans are not dangerous. It is true that the average blood lead level has been decreasing since the late 1960's and 1970's and that the childhood lead levels are the lowest in decades, averaging around 6 $\mu g\,dL^{-1}$. These data have been used by organizations such as the Small Property Owners Association (http://www.spoa.com/pages/lead-paint.html) to make the case that lead is no longer a safety issue in our country. They claim that de-leading houses and raising concerns for new sources of lead is an antiquated idea worthy of abandoning. They also state that the risk of lead poisoning in inner-city homes can be brought to zero with minimal measures such as wiping one's feet upon entering the house. Although some of these points are based on research data, many claims have been taken out of context. The overwhelming evidence in the literature supports the fact that lead remains an environmental problem. In fact, as our ability to perform careful clinical and basic science research becomes more refined, it is apparent that 10 $\mu g\,dL^{-1}$ in blood is no longer a safe threshold. A recent case in point shows that there is a decrease in IQ in children with each 1.0 $\mu g\,dL^{-1}$ increase in blood lead levels and that the effect is largest at levels below 10 $\mu g\,dL^{-1}$.[4] This toxin, previously thought to be harmless below 10 $\mu g\,dL^{-1}$, is not.

We now have definitive data demonstrating that a stunting of skeletal growth in children, a predisposition to osteoporosis later in life and a compromised ability to heal osteoporotic fractures are all manifestations of lead-exposed individuals. The fact that women currently entering the menopause had the greatest exposure to lead in their formative years (in the 1960's and early 1970's) suggests that we may on the verge of experiencing a significant increase in lead-related osteoporotic fractures.

15.2.2 Routes of Exposure

Elemental lead has two primary routes of absorption into the body, oral ingestion and inhalation. Lead may also be absorbed through cuts in the skin, however an intact integument represents a barrier to absorption. One third to one half of inhaled lead is absorbed into the bloodstream. Aside from behavior that increases lead exposure, physiological differences contribute to elevated lead exposure in children. The intestinal track of young children absorbs 30–40% of ingested lead, while adults absorb only 5–10%. In spite of reduced absorption in adults, lead bioaccumulates over time due to its slow release from the body. Once ingested, the skeleton acts to sequester lead, effectively removing it from the bioavailable extracellular fluid pool, and documented findings have confirmed that the skeleton is the major reservoir of lead in the body (harboring nearly 95% of the total lead burden). Once stored in the skeleton, the half-life of lead has been estimated to be from 20 to 30 years.[5–7] Lead localized to the bone continues to contribute to toxicity by exposing bone cells to high concentrations, even though circulating and soft tissue levels are low. Additionally in times of excessive skeletal remodeling, such as menopause, paraplegic immobilization, endocrine diseases such as thyrotoxicosis, and after a fracture, the re-release of lead from bone back into circulation[8–11] can elevate blood levels by 2–5 $\mu g\,dL^{-1}$.

15.2.3 Bioaccumulation of Lead

Lead is an insidiously unique toxicant in that no safe level of lead exposure has been found. In general, animals bioaccumulate lead due to its long half-life in the body and persistence in nature, providing continued exposure; however, biomagnification up the food chain does not generally occur. Additionally, increases in environmental lead have given rise to increased body burden, with preindustrial skeletons of native Americans containing 1000 fold lower lead levels than modern counterparts. As lead affects numerous organs and systems, its compartmentalization and deposition throughout the body is of great interest. Of US preschoolers, 10–15%, have blood lead levels above the former Center for Disease Control (CDC) acceptable range.

15.2.4 Blood Levels, Intracellular Concentrations, Mitochondrial Storage

Blood levels are a poor surrogate for assessing long-term lead exposure as the half life for the metal in blood is 30 days[12] and in serum is between 100 and 200 days. However, for assessing short-term exposure where 99% of lead is bound to erythrocytes, blood lead levels can be a sensitive metric. While in the blood, lead is capable of passing through the blood brain barrier and placenta. Furthermore, blood lead levels reflect the interaction of environmental levels with humans as the mean blood lead level of persons between the ages of 1 and 74 has gone from 12.8 $\mu g\,dL^{-1}$ in 1976 to 2.8 $\mu g\,dL^{-1}$ in 1991.

Cellular uptake of lead can vary dramatically between cell types, with dorsal root ganglia allowing no entry[13] and cultured CHO cells taking up lead to achieve a concentration of 97 μM.[14] It seems that cells of the skeleton, such as osteoblasts and chondrocytes, have intracellular lead levels hovering around 120–180 nM.

Mitochondria serve as an intracellular calcium storage site and contain a calcium transporter on the inner membrane to sequester calcium from the cytosol into the mitochondrial matrix. This transporter also moves lead into the mitochondrial matrix and exhibits an even greater affinity for the heavy metal.[15] This lead sequestration could result in higher levels of lead in the mitochondrial compartment and is known to interfere with mitochondrial calcium uptake.[16]

15.2.5 Lead in the Skeleton and Teeth

As a divalent cation, lead exhibits a strong affinity for calcified tissues of the skeleton and dentition, with >90% of the total body burden residing in bone.[17] It has been shown that levels of lead in pre- and post-natally formed dentine and enamel correlate with blood lead levels at the time of their formation,[18] and tooth lead levels have been used as an indicator of exposure in adults as well.[19] Experiments using lead isotopes show that in humans, 40–70% of blood lead originates from re-release of skeletal repositories.[20] Bone and tooth lead levels are more indicative of long-term lead exposure levels, relative to blood, as the half-life of lead in bone is estimated to be over 20 years. Due to a slower relative turnover rate, cortical bone may have a longer half-life of lead retention than trabecular bone. To measure bone lead levels, k-shell X-ray fluorescence spectrometry (k-XRF) can be used. The latest generation of instruments employed utilizes a ^{109}Cd source to excite the lead K shell electrons to produce gamma rays (*i.e.*, X-ray fluorescence) and a four detector array, each with its own multi-channel analyzer. This system is more precise than earlier generations and can accurately detect lead levels in the range of 2–4 $\mu g\,g^{-1}$ bone.

15.3 Skeletal Effects of Lead

15.3.1 Suppression of 1,25-Dihydroxycholecalciferol

Until relatively recently, it was held that skeletally sequestered lead was inert with regard to the body's soft tissues; however, a growing body of evidence shows that lead can exert its toxic effects upon the skeletal system directly and indirectly. One of the most important and far-reaching of these effects is reducing vitamin D levels. The effect of lead on vitamin D was proposed as an explanation for the observed correlation between elevated lead levels and osteoporosis.[21] This correlation was corroborated by associative findings linking lead exposure to reductions in active vitamin D levels[22,23] and the ability of ethylenediaminetetraacetic acid (EDTA) chelation to restore the levels. The mechanism behind the suppression of vitamin D is most likely due to several non-mutually exclusive factors. It is well established that oral lead exposure can lead to appetite suppression and vomiting.[24] Reduction in overall food intake could contribute to reduced vitamin D intake. The ability of EDTA to restore 1,25 $(OH)_2$ vitamin levels without altering levels of 25 (OH) vitamin D points to lead impairment of renal biosynthesis of the active form of the vitamin, and this renal impairment has been shown to be a secondary effect of lead toxicity resulting from a reduction in the heme body pool.[25] Lead-induced musculo-skeletal pathologies result from direct effects of lead on the cells of this system; however, the possible contribution of vitamin D suppression to these skeletal pathologies is an important factor.

15.3.2 Developmental Effects

The spatial distribution of lead in the proximity of the growth plate is evidenced radiographically by lead lines.[26,27] Exposure to lead *in utero* as well as post-natally can disrupt normal skeletal development. It compromises chondrocyte function, leads to skeletal malformations, reduces bone formation rates and prevents children from achieving a normal stature. Ronis *et al.* found that mice exposed to lead from gestational day 4 to day 55 had significantly "reduced somatic growth, longitudinal bone growth, and bone strength" compared to controls.[28] Maternal lead exposure prior to and throughout pregnancy was likewise shown to reduce early post-natal growth as measured by tail length and tail vertebral bone growth.[29] Moreover, data from NHANES II in humans showed that blood lead levels of 20–30 $\mu g\, dL^{-1}$ were associated with decreased height in children aged 1–7.[30,31] The data showed a 1.57 cm decrease in stature and 0.52 cm decrease in head circumference for every 10 $\mu g\, dL^{-1}$ increase in blood lead concentration.[32] Even *in utero* lead may be exerting skeletal effects, as prenatal lead exposure has been linked to shorter birth lengths.[33,34] Interestingly, lead suppression of skeletal growth continues well after the cessation of exposure, a finding that implicates the skeletal release of lead in extending the duration of its effect. Chelation, however, was found to ameliorate suppression of skeletal development by lead.[35]

Lead has been shown to delay growth plate chondrocyte maturation,[36,37] but the most probable mechanism by which lead toxicity on skeletal maturation occurs is through inducing a defect in osteoblast function. Historically, there have been a number of reports describing the effect of lead on osteoblasts.[38–41] These studies have been performed in transformed cell lines, freshly isolated normal cells and in *in vivo* experiments. Uniformly, it has been observed that lead is deleterious to the functioning of these cells. The metal ion has been shown to inhibit secretion of osteonectin, alkaline phosphatase activity and type I collagen synthesis.[42,43] Lead also adversely affects osteoblast cell proliferation and the effect of regulatory growth factors.[44,45]

In animal experiments directly analogous to what occurs in humans, it has been shown that osteoblast activity is suppressed and stem cell frequency is decreased with lead exposure. In dogs, lead exposure resulted in a suppression of osteoblastic activity that continued after cessation of exposure.[46] In mice that were exposed to lead in their drinking water for 6–12 weeks,[47] osteogenic precursor cells isolated from bone marrow demonstrated a decreased number of mineralized nodules, a measure of osteogenic precursor cell frequency. Even a brief exposure of the animals to lead led to an approximately 50% decrease in colony forming ability. This occurred at a dose of 55 ppm lead in the water. This concentration achieved a blood lead level in the mice similar to that observed in exposed humans (*i.e.* approximately 20 $\mu g\, dL^{-1}$).

One of the key paracrine factors that regulates the progression of cells from mesenchymal stem cells into osteoprogenitor cells is TGF-β. The current thinking is that the TGF-β pathway stimulates the expansion of osteoblast numbers and maintains a pool of cells that can be primed for new bone formation.[48] Inhibition of the pathway would then favor a depletion of osteoprogenitor cell number. Recent data support this observation and suggest that the mechanism by which lead has its effects on bone formation may involve a decrease in the pool of phosphorylated TGF-β intermediates in exposed cells.

15.3.3 Delayed Tooth Development and Increased Incidence of Dental Caries

Lead also affects another of its mineralized repositories, delaying tooth development and increasing the incidence of dental caries. Eruption rate and enamel formation are both susceptible to lead.[49] In rats, intraperitoneal injection of lead acetate was responsible for delaying tooth eruption rate and decreasing mineralization.[50] These findings implicate enamel development as a target of lead toxicity. A potential mechanism by which lead might be exerting these effects is disruption of specific enzyme cascades, a mechanism common to other lead pathologies. Enamel mineralization occurs on a protein scaffold (*i.e.* amelogenin), which is then removed by matrix metalloproteinases;[51] lead, however, disrupts the activity of these enzymes.[52]

A number of epidemiological studies have found an association between high lead levels and the presence of dental caries. Analysis of the third NHANES study showed an association between elevated blood lead levels and dental caries in both deciduous and permanent teeth.[53] In a survey of children aged 6–10 years, a positive correlation between lead levels and dental caries was again found, with a stronger association observed in primary teeth than permanent teeth, as well as higher incidence of caries on occlusal, lingual and buccal tooth surfaces.[54] Furthermore, the ability of lead to exert effects beyond initial exposure was again demonstrated when it was found that infants (aged 18–37 months) exposed to lead were more likely to have developed caries on the lingual surface of their primary teeth than later in life.[55]

15.3.4 Fracture Healing and Incidence of Non-Union

Paralleling the inhibitory effect of pre- and perinatal lead exposure on skeletal development, lead exposure in older animals has also been shown to delay fracture healing and increase the incidence of fibrous non-unions.[56] These investigations utilized a closed tibial model of fracture on mice that had been treated with lead for 6 weeks and found that bridging cartilage formation and overall amount of cartilage types II and X were suppressed and delayed, as was maturation and calcification of osseous tissue. No effects on osteoclasts were observed, therefore the observed effects were attributed to disruption of chondrocyte function, resulting in inhibition of endochondral ossification. Lead was shown to exert effects on chondrocyte populations through the modulation of TGF-β and BMP signaling. Taken in concert, these findings on chondrocytes offer a mechanistic explanation of shorter birth lengths. Lead causes an initial increase in chondrogenesis, resulting in increased growth plate activity but with premature closure and overall reduction in bone mineralization and density, while in the fracture callus, this process is paralleled and ossification is delayed and reduced. Not only are these findings important for observing lead effects on fracture healing, but in the larger scope of skeletal pathology, they show that lead can affect chondrocytes through disruption of TGF-β signaling.

15.4 Osteoporosis and the Mechanism of Lead Toxicity in Bone Cells

15.4.1 Osteoporosis

While the developing skeleton may be susceptible to lead toxicity at lower doses or shorter exposure times, the adult skeleton also is a vulnerable target.[57] Along with increased tooth degeneration and disruption of fracture healing, numerous studies have identified a reduction in bone density as an effect of lead exposure. Examination of NHANES II data revealed a positive correlation between blood lead levels and osteoporosis in post-menopausal women.[58] A case study presented by Berlin *et al.* similarly found evidence of elevated skeletal turnover and osteoporotic fracture in a lead poisoned individual.[59] Animal studies have further elucidated lead effects on bone density. After 7 months of low-level lead exposure, adult beagles experienced reductions in bone formation rates.[60] In adult rats exposed to lead, during which they maintained a biologically relevant blood level of $21\ \mu g\ dL^{-1}$ for one year, a significant decrease in bone density was observed.[61] The cellular mechanisms for this effect included a number of bone related processes, as reviewed by Holz *et al.*[62] In lead-exposed adults, Ronis *et al.* found decreased bone density and less formation of new endosteal bone.[63] Lead-induced disruption of bone density resulted from inhibition of osteoblastogenesis,[64] as well as increased osteoclast number, potent inhibition of downstream effects of vitamin D and (it was speculated) inhibition of collagen or collagen precursor synthesis.[65]

15.4.2 Mechanisms of Action for Lead Toxicity

15.4.2.1 Enzyme and Kinase Inhibition

Heavy metals such as lead are transported across cell membranes and can interfere with a number of cellular processes. In particular, kinase activities can be markedly affected. This would include the kinases associated with Smad phosphorylations in the TGF-β and BMP pathways. Since these are key pathways for the control of mesenchymal stem cell expansion and differentiation, they represent a sensitive target for agents such as lead.

15.4.2.2 Generation of Reactive Oxygen Species

Reactive oxygen species (ROS) are oxygen containing molecules with highly reactive unpaired valence electrons. These molecules are produced as normal byproducts of cellular respiration but can exert a number of toxic effects, such as damaging DNA and forming adducts with cellular molecules.[66] One possible source of the ROS that have been associated with musculoskeletal disease is lead. As stated, lead accumulation at concentrations greater than that seen in bone and blood occurs in the articular cartilage, synovial fluid and mineralized cartilage matrix. Furthermore, heavy metals have been shown to induce ROS production through the widely known Fenton reaction, involving iron.[67] Interestingly, Huang *et al.* found that lead induced ROS in *S. alfredii* roots[68] and, more importantly, has been shown to induce oxidative stress in mice.[69] High levels of lead and cadmium have been associated with elevated levels of ROS in humans.[70] Mechanistically, lead depletes cellular defenses against oxidative stress, such as glutathione and protein-bound sulfhydryl groups, and exerts pro-oxidant activity through Fenton-like reactions, phagocytic cell recruitment and redox cycling quinines. These combined effects result in an increasingly oxidized cellular state.[71] DNA damage, formation of other adducts and alterations in ROS sensitive signaling pathways are some of the mechanisms by which ROS play a well-documented role in pathological etiologies, and their role in heavy metal toxicity further illustrates this. Stohs *et al.* reasoned that the cell damage caused by heavy metals was due at least in part to ROS generation, and Ercal *et al.*, reviewing a more recent and broader literature base, go further and state that most heavy metal pathology is exerted through ROS and disruption of oxidative state.[72] Ahamed *et al.* concluded that hypertension, kidney disease, neurodegenerative disease and cognitive impairment could be caused by ROS generated by high-level lead exposure and that increasing evidence for low-level lead exposure similarly affecting these diseases was accruing.[73] Furthermore, lead disrupts the expression of growth factor receptors through ROS intermediates,[74] and lead generated ROS is also known to induce apoptosis.

15.4.3 Bone Mass and Osteoporosis

Osteoporosis is a disease of epidemic proportions in the United States, with an estimated 25 million affected individuals.[75,76] The health care costs associated with treatment of osteoporotic hip and spine fractures and associated morbidity may exceed $15 billion per year. During childhood and adolescence, bone mass accretion occurs through both the activities of the chondrocytes in the growth plates and the bone forming activity of osteoblasts. Thus bone mass and bone mineral density (BMD) gradually increase during growth. Bone mass is a reflection of the relative rates of bone formation and bone resorption, and continues to increase into early adulthood after growth plate closure, until peak bone mass is reached at age 25–30. After peak bone mass is reached, bone resorption rates exceed formation rates, and there is a gradual loss of bone with further aging in both men and women. At menopause, the loss of estrogen results in an acceleration of the rate of bone loss, which occurs over approximately a 10 year period, subsequently slowing to a rate resembling pre-menopausal bone loss. Systemic stimuli of bone resorption, such as cortico-steroids, thyroid or parathyroid disease, can further enhance the rate of bone loss. BMD correlates directly with bone strength and inversely with fracture risk. As bone is lost, an individual can cross a theoretical "fracture threshold," where the BMD and associated bone strength are insufficient to resist non-traumatic forces on the bone and can lead to fractures. Men achieve greater peak bone mass levels and are not subject to the accelerated decline associated with menopause, so bone density levels are less likely to cross the fracture threshold, explaining the 5–6-fold higher incidence of osteoporosis in women as compared to men. Also, there are other genetic determinants of bone mass, such as race. Black men and women have been shown to have higher peak bone mass compared with White and Hispanic individuals, thus accounting for the decreased incidence of osteoporosis among Blacks. Antiresorptive treatments such as estrogen, estrogen analogs and bisphosphonates at menopause have been shown to prevent accelerated bone loss and reduce fracture risk in perimenopausal women.[77–82] The inhibitory effects of lead on chondrocytes and osteoblasts could result in attainment of a lower peak bone mass, predisposing lead-exposed individuals to osteoporosis later in life. Furthermore, lead released from bone matrix during increased resorption, such as at menopause, could increase local concentrations at bone surfaces, worsening the inhibition of osteoblastic bone formation and therefore accelerating the loss of bone by further disturbing the balance of bone formation and resorption. Osteoporosis associated with lead intoxication has been previously reported,[83] consistent with our own findings and those of others who have shown lead toxicity causing osteopenia in animal models.

15.4.3.1 Bone Quality vs. *Bone Density*

Bone densitometry with dual energy X-ray absorptiometry (DXA) has been an extremely valuable tool for the identification of patients with low bone mass. In fact, the operational definition for osteoporosis has been defined as a t-score ≤ -2.5 as measured by DXA. At this time, and probably for a reasonable period into the future, DXA will remain the gold standard for the diagnosis of patients with osteoporosis and a tool to measure the effect of medications.[84] However, as has become more apparent over the past five years, there are a number of measurements of bone strength that cannot be explained solely on changes measured by DXA. This is due to the inherent limitations of the DXA measurements.[85] DXA cannot distinguish i) specific attributes of 3D geometry, ii) cortical *vs.* cancellous density, iii) trabecular architecture and iv) intrinsic material properties of bone matrix. Because of this, the correlation of DXA data with bone strength varies considerably and ranges from $r^2 = 0.5$ to 0.7 at different sites in the body (*i.e.*, radius, vertebrae and proximal femur). Furthermore, the ability of DXA to predict changes in fracture risk after treatment with medications is also low.

When these data are analyzed with logistic regression models, they show that the ability of DXA to predict fracture risk reduction is poor. The percentage change in bone mineral density with various treatments accounts for only a small percentage of the observed reduction in fracture risk.[86–92] The implications of these findings are that changes other than bone density have occurred that account for the increase in strength. That is, osteoclast and osteoblast activity has been able to create a skeletal structure that resists mechanical forces with only a small change in the total amount of bone.

The work by Hochberg *et al.*[93] analyzed the change in BMD as a function of antiresorptive therapy and found a regression line that showed a change in bone strength that was only partially dependent on BMD. In this work, the author plotted the percent change in BMD *vs.* the relative risk of fracture. If BMD could explain entirely the change in fracture risk, then at a "0" percent change in BMD the relative risk of fracture should be 1.0. What they found was an approximate 30% reduction in fracture risk with a 0% change in BMD. This suggested that the medications were altering another parameter of bone strength that was independent of the quantity of bone. This parameter is likely to be the micro architecture of the tissue.

A more careful analysis of skeletal structure has documented at least eight parameters of architecture that can be involved in altering the mechanical strength of the bone. These micro architectural parameters can be measured with micro computed tomography and magnetic resonance imaging. Using three of these analytic measures, Dufresne *et al.* [94] showed that within 1–2 years after the menopause, bone mineral density can decrease by a little more than 3%, but deterioration of the micro architecture and true 3D bone density can occur to levels of 13–20%. These findings highlight the need to evaluate parameters of bone quality other than simple density with DXA. Additionally, the picture appears more complex as age, prior fracture and skeletal turnover also appear to contribute independently to the risk of fracture.[95–98]

15.4.4 Lead and Osteoporosis

Our hypothesis, along with preliminary data in both *in vitro* and *in vivo* animal and human models, suggests that a significant proportion of people with osteoporosis may have the disease due to lead exposure and that lead in the skeleton will prevent normal healing of fractures.

It appears that environmental lead exposure prevents a person from attaining a high peak bone density during skeletal development. This is accomplished mechanistically by interfering with endochondral bone formation and bone remodeling. Additionally, compromising osteoclast and osteoblast function would cause an individual to cross over a "fracture threshold" at an earlier age and predispose them to a decrease in bone strength and osteoporotic fractures.

15.4.4.1 Lead and the DXA Measurement Artifact

The skeletal data on rats with lead exposure is somewhat controversial. Gruber *et al.*[99] demonstrated that lead caused a decrease in bone mass by DXA, histomorphometry, and mineral analysis. In a subsequent study, the effect of lead exposure was ameliorated by calcium supplementation.[100] Lead-exposed rats have also been shown to have decreased femoral weights and L5 vertebral body heights, as well as histomorphometric evidence of osteopenia.[101]

However, the bone density in these studies, as measured by DXA, was higher in the lead treated animals. This is consistent with data in our laboratory which indicates that bone samples doped with increasing quantities of lead have spuriously high BMD with a direct dose–response effect when measured by DXA, an artifact which may be related to interactions of the low energy photons of the DXA with lead atoms. The magnitude of the effect far outweighs the calculated effect of lead on mineral density, which would theoretically be too small to be measurable. If this artifact occurs in measurements of BMD by DXA in humans, there may be serious implications in the interpretation of clinical data, which may necessitate knowing an individual's bone lead content to correct for this problem. Preliminary clinical data indicate a significant ($p<0.05$) inverse relationship between blood lead and the ratio of two densitometric measurements (BMD measured by ultrasound divided by the BMD measured by DXA), in a pilot study of 13 subjects, which supports our contention that DXA of lead-containing bone overestimates its density. This finding may also explain the discrepancy, reported by Escribano *et al.*,[102] between the histomorphometric data, which indicated osteoporosis in lead-treated rats, and DXA densitometric data, which showed higher BMD in the same animals.

15.4.5 Measurement of Bone Lead

The method of K shell X-ray fluorescence has been employed to measure bone lead in occupationally lead-exposed and unexposed individuals.[103] *In vivo* bone lead measurements were first developed by Ahlgren and Mattsson at Lund in Sweden. They used X-rays from a ^{57}Co source to excite lead K-shell electrons. The measurement was made in a finger bone and this system has been in operation since 1972.[104] Subsequently, an improved system was developed by Chettle, Scott, Laird and Somervaille in Birmingham, England. This system used X-rays from a ^{108}Cd source to excite the lead K-shell electrons to produce gamma rays (*i.e.*, X-ray fluorescence), and proved to have three particular advantages over the original approach: measurements were more precise, bone lead content could be directly related to bone mineral and measurements could usefully be made of any superficial bone.[105] The first human measurements were made in 1983 and, initially, the tibia lead concentration was studied. Since then, both the tibia and calcaneus have frequently been selected as representative of cortical and trabecular bone sites respectively. The patella has also been used in this way, and measurements have also been reported of radius, sternum and skull. This measurement approach has been adopted by a number of laboratories around the world. In 1991, Chettle and Webber of McMaster University developed a new system with improved precision, based on the same principles.[106]

Two particular features of the relationship between bone lead and lead exposure have consistently emerged from studies in which K X-ray fluorescence technology has been employed. First, bone lead concentration reflects cumulative lead exposure. Cumulative exposure can be represented by the time-weighted integral of blood lead, monitored regularly in lead-exposed workers. Second, release of lead from bone contributes to circulating lead in blood, thus constituting an endogenous exposure. This relationship is particularly clear when industrial exposure has ceased. For such people, endogenous exposure can often be the dominant contributor to current blood lead.

15.4.6 Skeletal Effects of Lead Exposure – *in vitro* and Animal Studies

Lead has been associated with both low birth weight and short stature, although there is controversy as to whether this results from specific skeletal effects or is related to systemic and nutritional factors.[107–109] Substantial preliminary data demonstrate potent specific effects of low levels of lead on chondrocytes, osteoblasts, osteoclasts, and mesenchymal stem cells. *In vitro* studies have shown that lead has specific effects on growth plate chondrocytes that alter cell phenotype and function.[110] Also, potent inhibitory effects on osteoblast and osteoclast phenotype and function have been demonstrated.[111–113] suggesting that lead may have effects on bone development and remodeling. Importantly, lead toxicity at environmentally relevant levels has been shown to decrease BMD in rats and produce osteoporosis in other animal models.[114–116] Thus while systemic effects of lead on other organ systems may influence the skeleton, there appears to be direct effects of low levels of lead on the cells involved in bone development, remodeling and repair. Examination of the histomorphometry of lead intoxicated rats shows abnormalities of the growth plates, including defective remodeling and altered growth plate thickness, with loss of proliferating cells and disorganization of the growth plate architecture.[117]

15.4.7 Skeletal Effects of Lead Exposure – Clinical Studies

Despite the extensive laboratory research on the effects of lead exposure on bone metabolism, human studies on this association are limited. Laraque *et al.* found that lead-exposed African-American children had a higher mean mineral content than age-matched, white norms.[118] At age 36–47 months, the mean bone mineral content of the radius of the lead-exposed subjects and norms were $0.268\,gm\,cm^{-2}$ *vs.* $0.215\,gm\,cm^{-2}$ respectively ($p<0.005$). The authors attributed the findings to racial differences in bone density. In further analyses, Laraque plotted age against bone density among children with low *vs.* high lead exposure (*i.e.*, blood lead level $\leq 29\,\mu g\,dL^{-1}$ *vs.* $\geq 30\,\mu g\,dL^{-1}$); the difference in bone density was not significant ($p=0.63$). Laraque concluded that lead exposure is not associated with changes in bone mass. However, since the comparison group was made up of children with moderate-level lead exposure (*i.e.*, blood lead level 12–29 $\mu g\,dL^{-1}$), such an analysis cannot exclude the possibility that lead exposure has a threshold effect on bone density at lower blood lead levels.

Although recent studies report a dramatic decrease in the prevalence of lead exposure in the US,[119,120] this does not imply that adults have not had exposure in the past. As recently as the late 1970s, 78% of the entire US population—children and adults—had blood lead levels $\geq 10\,\mu g\,dL^{-1}$,[121] the threshold of concern defined by the Centers for Disease Control (CDC, 1991) at that time. This means that the majority of adults in the US had, at some time in the past, an elevated blood lead level, and therefore currently have elevated bone lead levels, given the extremely long half life of lead in bone ($t_{1/2} = 20$ years).[122] With this large number of adults who have elevated bone lead levels, and the morbidity associated with osteoporosis, it is important to investigate whether an association exists between lead exposure and the disease, osteoporosis. This research, however, should not be limited to adults. Although osteoporosis is an affliction of the elderly, its roots may be established during childhood. An individual who does not achieve peak bone mass during childhood may be at risk for osteoporosis in later life.[123] Since 90% or more of bone mass is achieved by age 17–20 years,[124,125] the association between lead exposure and bone density should be examined among children and skeletally mature adolescents.

15.5 Summary

In summary, lead toxicity in the skeleton is emerging as an important risk factor in diseases of bone, especially in older adults and women. These would include such conditions as growth plate defects, impairment in remodeling, fracture healing and osteoporosis. It appears that an exposure to lead, even at an early age, can predispose individuals to any of these conditions, with the possibility of more serious manifestations later in life. Osteoporosis is the most widespread of these afflictions and consumes the greatest number of health care dollars. When considering the effects of lead exposure on osteoporosis, it is important to note that the effects of lead may begin prior to development of a peak bone density. Considering that the half-life of lead is of the order of decades, even an early exposure can be a life-long hazard to one's skeletal health. This is diagrammatically depicted in Figure 15.1.

Early exposure will prevent attaining a peak bone mass that can protect an individual later in life. Lead exposure also accelerates the rate of bone loss after the menopause, driving a number of individuals, mainly females, across a fracture threshold at younger age. Along with these effects of lead in bone, the heavy metal tends to mask the diagnosis of low bone mass by DXA and prevents the body from normally healing fractures. All things considered, significant lead exposure in humans, though decreasing in incidence, continue to represent a real health hazard to the skeleton.

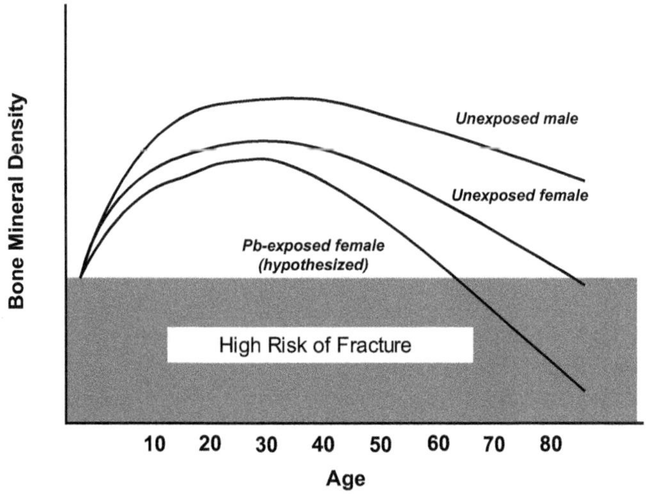

Figure 15.1 The general trends for bone mineral density (*i.e.*, skeletal mass) in males and females is depicted in this stylized diagram. Both males and females achieve a peak bone density between the ages of 20 and 30. Skeletal mass then plateaus for approximately 20 to 30 years, at which time all individuals begin to lose bone. Healthy males that are not exposed to high levels of lead infrequently cross the "fracture threshold" during a normal lifespan. However, females, by virtue of the fact that they never attain the same peak density as males and lose bone more rapidly after the menopause, enter a region of high fracture risk more often than males. All laboratory and clinical evidence points to the observation that lead-exposed females do not reach the same density as unexposed females and lose bone at an even faster rate than their healthy counterparts. This would hypothetically lead to crossing into the high fracture risk region at an earlier age.

References

1. B. L. Gulson, K. J. Mizon, J. D. Davis, J. M. Palmer and G. Vimpani, *Environmental Health Perspectives*, 2004, **112**(1), 52–60.
2. P. Glorennec, C. Peyr, J. Poupon, Y. Oulhote and B. Le Bot, *Journal of Occupational and Environmental Hygiene*, 2010, **7**(5), 253–260.
3. B. Wilson and F. B. Pyatt, *Ecotoxicology and Environmental Safety*, 2007, **66**(2), 224–231.
4. R. Lanphear, J. Hornung, K. Khoury, P. Yolton, D. C. Baghurst, R. L. Bellinger, K. N. Canfield, R. Dietrich, T. Bornschein, S. J. Greene, H. L. Rothenberg, L. Needleman, G. Schnaas, Wasserman and J. Graziano, *Environ Health Perspect*, 2005, **113**, 894–899.
5. N. Khalil, L. A. Morrow, H. Needleman, E. O. Talbott, J. W. Wilson and J. A. Cauley, *Neuropsychology*, 2009, **23**(1), 10–19.
6. E. W. Grimsley and L. Adams-Mount, *South Med J*, 1994, **87**(7), 689–691.

7. J. O. Christoffersson, L. Ahlgren, A. Schütz, S. Skerfving and S. Mattsson, *Arch Environ Health*, 1986, **41**(5), 312–318.
8. E. K. Silbergeld, J. Schwartz and K. Mahaffey, *Environ Res*, 1988, **47**(1), 79–94.
9. M. Shannon, H. Lindy, C. Anast and J. Graef, *Vet Hum Toxicol*, 1988, **30**(6), 586–588.
10. R. H. Goldman, R. White, S. N. Kales and H. Hu, *Am J Ind Med*, 1994, **25**(3), 417–424.
11. E. Symanski and I. Hertz-Picciotto, *Am J Epidemiol*, 1995, **141**(11), 1047–1058.
12. M. B. Rabinowitz, *Environ Health Perspect*, 1991, **91**, 33–37.
13. R. Domann, L. Wunder and D. Busselberg, *Cell Mol Neurobiol*, 1997, **17**(3), 305–314.
14. J. P. Wise, D. M. Stearns, K. E. Wetterhahn and S. R. Patierno, *Carcinogenesis*, 1994, **15**(10), 2249–2254.
15. J. G. Pounds, R. Wright and R. L. Kodell, *Toxicol Appl Pharmacol*, 1982, **66**(1), 88–101.
16. J. G. Pounds, G. J. Long and J. F. Rosen, *Environ Health Perspect*, 1991, **91**, 17–32.
17. F. Barbosa, Jr., J. E. Tanus-Santos, R. F. Gerlach and P. J. Parsons, *Environmental Health Perspectives*, 2005, **113**(12), 1669–1674.
18. M. Arora, B. J. Kennedy, S. Elhlou, N. J. Pearson, D. M. Walker, P. Bayl and S. W. Chan, *Sci Total Environ*, 2006, **371**(1–3), 55–62.
19. J. Pusapukdepob, P. Sawangwong, C. Pulket, D. Satraphat, S. Saowakontha and P. S. Source, *Southeast Asian J Trop Med Public Health*, 2007, **38**(1), 168–177.
20. D. R. Smith, J. D. Osterloh and A. R. Flegal, *Environ Health Perspect*, 1996, **104**(1), 60–66.
21. E. K. Silbergeld, J. Schwartz and K. Mahaffey, *Environ Res*, 1988, **47**(1), 79–94.
22. K. R. Mahaffey, J. F. Rosen, R. W. Chesney, J. T. Peeler, C. M. Smith and H. F. DeLuca, *Am J Clin Nutr*, 1982, **35**(6), 1327–1331.
23. J. F. Rosen, R. W. Chesney, A. Hamstra, H. F. DeLuca and K. R. Mahaffey, *N Engl J Med*, 1980, **302**(20), 1128–1131.
24. A. Pagliuca and G. J. Mufti, *BMJ*, 1990, **300**(6728), 830.
25. L. Patrick, *Altern Med Rev*, 2006, **11**(1), 2–22.
26. A. J. Leone, *Am J Roentgenol Radium Ther Nucl Med*, 1968, **103**(1), 165–167.
27. M. Pearl and L. M. Boxt, *Radiology*, 1980, **136**(1), 83–84.
28. E. I. Chopin and B. J. Alloway, *The Science of the Total Environment*, 2007, **373**(2–3), 488–500.
29. J. D. Hamilton and E. J. O'Flaherty, *Fundam Appl Toxicol*, 1994, **22**(4), 594–604.
30. C. R. Angle and D. R. Kuntzelman, *Journal of Toxicology and Environmental Health*, 1989, **26**(2), 149–156.
31. J. Schwartz, C. Angle and H. Pitcher, *Pediatrics*, 1986, **77**(3), 281–288.

32. C. Ballew, L. K. Khan, R. Kaufmann, A. Mokdad, D. T. Miller and E. W. Gunter, *J Pediatr*, 1999, **134**(5), 623–630.
33. M. Hernandez-Avila, K. E. Peterson, T. Gonzalez-Cossio, L. H. Sanin, A. Aro, L. Schnaas and H. Hu, *Arch Environ Health*, 2002, **57**(5), 482–488.
34. R. Shukla, R. L. Bornschein, K. N. Dietrich, C. R. Buncher, O. G. Berger, P. B. Hammond and P. A. Succop, *Pediatrics*, 1989, **84**(4), 604–612.
35. M. Pearl and L. M. Boxt, *Radiology*, 1980, **136**(1), 83–84.
36. A. Zhitnikov and P. M. Mazhuga, *Tsitol Genet*, 1987, **21**(4), 248–252.
37. A. Zhitnikov and P. M. Mazhuga, *Tsitol Genet*, 1988, **22**(2), 3–7.
38. J. J. Sauk, T. Smith, E. K. Silbergeld, B. A. Fowler and M. J. Somerman, *Toxicol Appl Pharmacol*, 1992, **116**(2), 240–247.
39. R. F. Klein and K. M. Wiren, *Endocrinology*, 1993, **132**(6), 2531–2537.
40. C. R. Angle, D. J. Thomas and S. A. Swanson, *Toxicol Appl Pharmacol*, 1990, **103**(2), 281–287.
41. G. J. Long, J. G. Pounds and J. F. Rosen, *Calcif Tissue Int*, 1992, **50**(5), 451–458.
42. Y. Ma, D. Fu and Z. Liu, *Toxicol Ind Health*, 2012 Mar, **28**(2), 136–146.
43. R. F. Klein and K. M. Wiren, *Endocrinology*, 1993, **132**(6), 2531–257.
44. C. R. Angle, D. J. Thomas and S. A. Swanson, *Toxicol Appl Pharmacol*, 1990, **103**(2), 281–287.
45. F. A. Schanne, R. K. Gupta and J. F. Rosen, *Biochim Biophys Acta*, 1992, **1180**(2), 187–194.
46. C. Anderson and K. D. Danylchuk, *J Environ Pathol Toxicol*, 1980, **3**(5–6), 413–422.
47. A. M. Sharifi, R. Ghazanfari, N. Tekiyehmaroof and M. A. Sharifi, *Toxicol Mech Methods*, 2011, **21**(3), 225–230.
48. K. Janssens, P. ten Dijke, S. Janssens and W. Van Hul, *Endocr Rev*, 2005, **26**(6), 743–774.
49. M. Pearl and N. M. Roland, *ASDC J Dent Child*, 1980, **47**(4), 269–271.
50. R. F. Gerlach, D. B. Toledo, P. D. Novaes, J. Merzel and S. R. Line, *Arch Oral Biol*, 2000, **45**(11), 951–955.
51. M. Matsuzawa, T. J. Sheu, Y. J. Lee, M. Chen, T. F. Li, C. T. Huang, J. D. Holz and J. E. Puzas, *J Periodontal Res*, 2009, **44**(3), 289–296.
52. R. F. Gerlach, A. P. de Souza, J. A. Cury and S. R. Line, *Eur J Oral Sci*, 2000, **108**(4), 327–334.
53. M. E. Moss, B. P. Lanphear and P. Auinger, *JAMA*, 1999, **281**(24), 2294–2298.
54. A. Gemmel, M. Tavares, S. Alperin, J. Soncini, D. Daniel, J. Dunn, S. Crawford, N. Braveman, T. W. Clarkson, S. McKinlay and D. C. Bellinger, *Environ Health Perspect*, 2002, **110**(10), A625–A630.
55. J. R. Campbell, M. E. Moss and R. F. Raubertas, *Environ Health Perspect*, 2000, **108**(11), 1099–1102.
56. J. J. Carmouche, J. E. Puzas, X. Zhang, P. Tiyapatanaputi, D. A. Cory-Slechta, R. Gelein, M. Zuscik, R. N. Rosier, B. F. Boyce,

R. J. O'Keefe and E. M. Schwarz, *Environ Health Perspect*, 2005, **113**(6), 749–755.

57. J. G. Pounds, G. J. Long and J. F. Rosen, *Environ Health Perspect*, 1991, **91**, 17–32.
58. E. K. Silbergeld, J. Schwartz and K. Mahaffey, *Environ Res*, 1988, **47**(1), 79–94.
59. K. Berlin, L. Gerhardsson, J. Börjesson, E. Lindh, N. Lundström, A. Schütz, S. Skerfving and C. Edling, *Scand J Work Environ Health*, 1995, **21**(4), 296–300.
60. C. Anderson and K. D. Danylchuk, *Lab Invest*, 1977, **37**(5), 466–469.
61. H. E. Gruber, H. C. Gonick, F. Khalil-Manesh, T. V. Sanchez, S. Motsinger, M. Meyer and C. F. Sharp, *Miner Electrolyte Metab*, 1997, **23**(2), 65–73.
62. J. D. Holz, T. J. Sheu, H. Drissi, M. Matsuzawa, M. J. Zuscik and J. E. Puzas, *Birth Defects Research Part C*, 2007, **81**(1), 41–50.
63. M. J. Ronis, J. Aronson, G. G. Gao, W. Hogue, R. A. Skinner, T. M. Badger and C. K. Lumpkin, Jr., *Toxicol Sci*, 2001, **62**(2), 321–329.
64. J. R. Campbell and P. Auinger, *Environ Health Perspect*, 2007, **115**(7), 1018–1022.
65. G. M. Hass, W. Landerholm and A. Hemmens, *Am J Pathol*, 1967, **50**(5), 815–847.
66. D. F. Stowe and A. K. Camara, *Antioxid Redox Signal*, 2009, **11**(6), 1373–1414.
67. S. K. Bopp, H. K. Abicht and K. Knauer, *Aquat Toxicol*, 2008, **86**(2), 197–204.
68. H. Huang, T. Li, S. Tian, D. K. Gupta, X. Zhang and X. E. Yang, *Bioresour Technol*, 2008, **99**(14), 6088–6096.
69. J. Xu, L. J. Lian, C. Wu, X. F. Wang, W. Y. Fu and L. H. Xu, *Food Chem Toxicol*, 2008, **46**(5), 1488–1494.
70. A. R. Kiziler, B. Aydemir, I. Onaran, B. Alici, H. Ozkara, T. Gulyasar and M. C. Akyolcu, *Biol Trace Elem Res*, 2007, **120**(1–3), 82–91.
71. S. J. Stohs and D. Bagchi, *Free Radic Biol Med*, 1995, **18**(2), 321–336.
72. N. Ercal, H. Gurer-Orhan and N. Aykin-Burns, *Curr Top Med Chem*, 2001, **1**(6), 529–539.
73. M. Ahamed and M. K. Siddiqui, *Clin Chim Acta*, 2007, **383**(1–2), 57–64.
74. S. J. Flora, M. Mittal and A. Mehta, *Indian J Med Res*, 2008, **128**(4), 501–523.
75. National Institute of Health. Osteoporosis prevention, diagnosis and therapy. *NIH Consensus Statement*, 2000, March 27–29, **17**(1), 1–45.
76. R. N. Rosier, *Clinical Orthopaedics & Related Research*, 2001, **385**, 57–67.
77. S. Adami, M. Passeri, S. Ortolani, M. Broggini, L. Carratelli, I. Caruso, G. Gandolini, L. Gnessi, M. Laurenzi and A. Lombardi, *Bone*, 1995, **17**, 383–390.
78. D. M. Black, S. R. Cummings, D. B. Karpf, J. A. Cauley, D. E. Thompson, M. C. Nevitt, D. C. Bauer, H. K. Genant, W. L. Haskell,

R. Marcus, S. M. Ott, J. C. Torner, S. A. Quandt, T. F. Reiss and K. E. Ensrud, *Fracture Intervention Trial Research Group. Lancet*, 1996, **348**, 1535–1541.
79. H. G. Bone, R. W. Downs, J. R. Tucci, S. T. Harris, R. S. Weinstein, A. A. Licata, M. R. McClung, D. B. Kimmel, B. J. Gertz, E. Hale and W. J. Polvino, *J Clin Endo Metabol*, 1997, **82**, 265–274.
80. C. H. Chesnut, M. R. McClung, K. E. Ensrud, N. H. Bell, H. K. Genant, S. T. Harris, F. R. Singer, J. L. Stock, R. A. Yood and P. D. Delmas, *Am J Med*, 1995, **99**, 144–152.
81. B. Ettinger, D. M. Black, B. H. Mitlak, R. K. Knickerbocker, T. Nickelsen, H. K. Genant, C. Christiansen, P. D. Delmas, J. R. Zanchetta, J. Stakkestad, C. C. Gluer, K. Krueger, F. J. Cohen, S. Eckert, K. E. Ensrud, L. V. Avioli, P. Lips and S. R. Cummings, *JAMA*, 1999, **282**, 637–645.
82. D. B. Karpf, D. R. Shapiro, E. Seeman, K. Ensrud, C. C. Johnson, S. Adami, S. T. Harris, A. C. Santora 2nd, L. J. Hirsch, L. Oppenheimer and D. Thompson, *JAMA*, 1997, **277**, 1159–1164.
83. K. Berlin, L. Gerhardsson, J. Borjesson, E. Lindh, N. Lundstrom, A. Schutz, S. Skerfving and C. Edling, *Scan J Work, Environment, Health*, 1995, **21**, 296–300.
84. D. Marshall, O. Johnell and H. Wedel, *BMJ*, 1996, **312**, 697–711.
85. M. L. Bouxsein, B. S. Coan and S. C. Lee, *Bone*, 1999, **25**, 49–54.
86. C. H. Chesnut, S. Silverman, K. Andriano, H. Genant, A. Gimona, S. Harris, D. Kiel, M. LeBoff, M. Maricic, P. Miller, C. Moniz, M. Peacock, P. Richardson, N. Watts and D. A. Baylink, *Am J Med*, Sep, 2000, **109**(4), 267–276.
87. B. Ettinger, D. M. Black, B. H. Mitlak, R. K. Knickerbocker, T. Nickelsen, H. K. Genant, C. Christiansen, P. D. Delmas, J. R. Zanchetta, J. Stakkestad, C. C. Gluer, K. Krueger, F. J. Cohen, S. Eckert, K. E. Ensrud, L. V. Avioli, P. Lips and S. R. Cummings, *JAMA*, 1999 Aug 18, **282**(7), 637–645.
88. S. Sarkar, B. H. Mitlak, M. Wong, J. L. Stock, D. M. Black and K. D. Harper, *J Bone Miner Res.*, 2002 Jan, **17**(1), 1–10.
89. S. T. Harris, N. B. Watts, H. K. Genant, C. D. McKeever, T. Hangartner, M. Keller, C. H. Chesnut, 3rd, J. Brown, E. F. Eriksen, M. S. Hoseyni, D. W. Axelrod and P. D. Miller, *JAMA*, 1999 Oct 13, **282**(14), 1344–1352.
90. Z. Li, M. P. Meredith and M. S. Hoseyni, *Stat Med Nov 15*, 2001, **20**(21), 3175–3188.
91. D. M. Black, S. R. Cummings, D. B. Karpf, J. A. Cauley, D. E. Thompson, M. C. Nevitt, D. C. Bauer, H. K. Genant, W. L. Haskell, R. Marcus, S. M. Ott, J. C. Torner, S. A. Quandt, K. E. Ensrud. *Lancet*. 1996 Dec 7, **348**(9041), 1535–1541.
92. S. R. Cummings, D. B. Karpf, F. Harris, H. K. Genant, K. Ensrud, A. Z. LaCroix and D. M. Black, *Am J Med Mar*, 2002, **112**(4), 281–289.

93. M. C. Hochberg, S. Greenspan, R. D. Wasnich, P. Miller, D. E. Thompson and P. D. Ross, *J Clinical Endocrinology & Metabolism*, 2002, **87**(4), 1586.
94. T. E. Dufresne, P. A. Chmielewski, M. D. Manhart, T. D. Johnson and B. Borah, *Calcif Tiss Int*, 2003, **73**(5), 423–432.
95. J. A. Kanis, D. Black, C. Cooper, P. Dargent, B. Dawson-Hughes, C. De Laet, P. Delmas, J. Eisman, O. Johnell, B. Jonsson, L. Melton, A. Oden, S. Papapoulos, H. Pols, R. Rizzoli, A. Silman and A. Tenenhouse, *Osteoporosis Int*, 2002, **13**, 527–636.
96. P. D. Ross, H. K. Genant, J. W. Davis, P. D. Miller and R. D. Wasnich, *Osteoporos Int*, 1993, **3**, 120–126.
97. R. Eastell, I. Barton, R. A. Hannon, A. Chines, P. Garnero and P. D. Delmas, *J Bone Miner Res*, 2003, **18**, 1051–1056.
98. P. Garnero, E. Hausherr, M. C. Chapuy, C. Marcelli, H. Grandjean, C. Muller, C. Cormier, G. Bréart, P. J. Meunier and P. D. Delmas, *J Bone Miner Res*, Oct 1996, **11**(10), 1531–1538.
99. H. E. Gruber, H. C. Gonick, F. Khalil-Manesh, T. V. Sanchez, S. Motsinger, M. Meyer and C. F. Sharp, *Mineral & Electrolyte Metabolism*, 1997, **23**(2), 65–673.
100. H. E. Gruber, Y. Ding, A. A. Stasky, M. Meyer, M. R. Pandian, D. Pandian, N. D. Vaziri, J. Grigsby and H. C. Gonick, *Mineral Electrolyte Metabolism*, 1999, **25**, 143–146.
101. A. Escribano, M. Revilla, E. R. Hernandez, C. Seco, J. Gonzalez-Riola, L. F. Villa and H. Rico, *Calcified Tissue International*, 1997, **60**(2), 200–203.
102. A. Escribano, M. Revilla, E. R. Hernandez, C. Seco, J. Gonzalez-Riola, L. F. Villa and H. Rico, *Calcified Tissue International*, 1997, **60**(2), 200–203.
103. A. Aro, C. Amarasiriwardena, M. L. Lee, R. Kim and H. Hu, *Medical Physics*, 2000, **27**, 119–123.
104. L. Ahlgren and S. Mattsson, *Physics in Medicine & Biology*, 1979, **24**(1), 136–145.
105. L. J. Somervaille, D. R. Chettle, M. C. Scott, D. R. Tennant, M. J. McKiernan, A. Skilbeck and W. N. Trethowan, *Br J Ind Med*, 1988, **45**, 174–181.
106. C. L. Gordon, D. R. Chettle and C. E. Webber, *Basic Life Sciences*, 1993, **60**, 285–288.
107. J. G. Pounds, G. J. Long and J. F. Rosen, *Env. Health Perspectives*, 1991, **91**, 17–32.
108. D. G. Hicks, R. J. O'Keefe, K. J. Reynolds, D. A. Cory-Slechta, J. E. Puzas, A. Judkins and R. N. Rosier, *Toxicol Appl Pharmacol*, 1996, **140**, 164–172.
109. P. B. Hammond, S. D. Chernausek, P. A. Succop, R. Shukla and R. L. Bornschein, *Toxicol. Appl. Pharmacol*, 1989, **99**, 474–486.
110. D. G. Hicks, R. J. O'Keefe, K. J. Reynolds, D. A. Cory-Slechta, J. E. Puzas, A. Judkins and R. N. Rosier, *Toxicol Appl Pharmacol*, 1996, **140**, 164–172.

111. J. E. Puzas, M. J. Sickel and M. E. Felter, *Neurotoxicol*, 1992, **13**, 800–806.
112. E. Bonucci, *Clin Orth Rel Res*, 1981, **158**, 252–269.
113. R. F. Klein and K. M. Wiren, *Endocrinol*, 1993, **132**, 264–268.
114. A. Escribano, M. Revilla, E. R. Hernandez, C. Seco, J. Gonzalez-Riola, L. F. Villa and H. Rico, *Calcified Tissue International*, 1997, **60**(2), 200–203.
115. H. E. Gruber, H. C. Gonick, F. Khalil-Manesh, T. V. Sanchez, S. Motsinger, M. Meyer and C. F. Sharp, *Mineral & Electrolyte Metabolism*, 1997, **23**(2), 65–73.
116. F. G. Clegg and J. M. Rylands, *J. Comparative Pathol*, 1966, **76**, 15–22.
117. J. D. Hamilton and E. J. O'Flaherty, *Fundamental Appl Toxicol*, 1994, **22**, 594–604.
118. D. Laraque, L. Arena, J. Karp and D. Gruskay, *Pediatr Radiol*, 1990, **20**, 461–463.
119. D. J. Brody, J. L. Pirkle, R. A. Kramer, K. M. Flegal, T. D. Matte, E. W. Gunther and D. C. Paschal, *JAMA*, 1994, **272**, 277–283.
120. J. L. Pirkle, R. B. Kaufmann, D. J. Brody, T. Hickman, E. W. Gunter and D. C. Paschal, *Environ Health Perspect*, 1998, **106**, 745–750.
121. K. R. Mahaffey, J. L. Annest, J. Roberts, R. S. Murphy, *N Engl J Med.* 1982, **307**, 573–579.
122. R. P. Wedeen, *Neurotox*, 1992, **13**, 843–852.
123. National Institute of Health. Osteoporosis prevention, diagnosis and therapy, NIH Consensus Statement, 2000, March 27–29, **17**(1), 1–45.
124. A. M. Magarey, T. J. Boulton, B. E. Chatterton, C. Schultz, B. E. Nordin and R. A. Cockington, *Acta Paediatrica*, 1999, **88**, 139–146.
125. T. Lloyd, V. M. Chinchilli, D. F. Eggli, N. Rollings and H. E. Kulin, *Arch Pediat Adolesc Med*, 1998, **152**, 998–1002.

CHAPTER 16

Liver Disease

MATT CAVE,* MOHAMMAD K. MOHAMMAD, GAVIN ARTEEL, KEITH CAMERON FALKNER AND CRAIG J. MCCLAIN

Department of Medicine, Division of Gastroenterology, Hepatology, and Nutrition, Department of Pharmacology and Toxicology, University of Louisville, CTR Building Room 503, 505 S. Hancock St., Louisville, KY 40202, USA
*E-mail: matt.cave@louisville.edu

16.1 Introduction

The liver is the largest organ in the body, weighing approximately 1.5 kg in adults, and it is possibly the most complex organ in terms of metabolism. It has a unique dual blood supply, being perfused by both the portal vein and hepatic artery, and comprises multiple cell types having differing functions. Hepatocytes make up over 80% of total liver mass and play a critical role in the metabolism of amino acids and ammonia, biochemical oxidation reactions, and detoxification of a variety of drugs, vitamins, hormones, and environmental toxicants. Kupffer cells represent the largest reservoir of fixed macrophages in the body. They play a protective role against gut-derived toxins that have escaped into the portal circulation, and they are a major producer of cytokines, which can influence the toxicity of environmental toxicants. Hepatic stellate cells are the major storehouse for vitamin A in the body and play an important role in collagen formation during liver injury. Other specific cell types also have unique functions (*e.g.*, bile duct epithelium in bile flow, sinusoidal endothelial cells in adhesion molecule expression and endocytosis). The liver plays a vital

Issues in Toxicology No. 16
Aging and Vulnerability to Environmental Chemicals: Age-related Disorders and their Origins in Environmental Exposures
Edited by Bernard Weiss

Published by the Royal Society of Chemistry, www.rsc.org

role in protein, carbohydrate, and fat metabolism, as well as micronutrient metabolism. It synthesizes plasma proteins, nonessential amino acids, urea (for ammonia excretion), glycogen, and critical hormones such as the anabolic molecule, insulin-like growth factor-1. The liver is a major site for fatty acid metabolism, and bile from the liver is needed for fat absorption from the intestine. The liver plays a critical role in protecting against gut-derived toxins and converting environmental toxicants/xenobiotics into non-toxic agents. While the liver is generally considered somewhat resistant to the effects of aging, important changes do occur. This chapter reviews the effects of aging on the liver and its response to environmental toxicants.

16.2 Aging Associated Changes in Liver Structure and Function

Aging is associated with changes in hepatic morphology, physiology, biochemistry, immune function, and regeneration, which could increase susceptibility to toxicants, resulting in liver disease (Table 16.1). These changes are subsequently discussed.

16.2.1 Morphologic Changes

Aging is associated with a 20% reduction in liver weight. Macroscopically, the liver undergoes 'brown atrophy' with old age, secondary to accumulation of pigmented waste products within the hepatocytes. The major pigment is lipofuscin. Lipofuscin is composed of insoluble, cytoplasmic, highly oxidized proteins related to chronic oxidative stress and end products of lipid peroxidation in lysosomes.

In addition to a reduced number of hepatocytes, several microscopic changes occur with hepatocyte aging, including increased binuclear index, and nuclear polyploidy. Nuclear vacuoles become larger in size and more irregularly shaped with aging. These "terminal hepatocytes" are incapable of cell division. Mitochondrial volume (but not number) increases, and there is a decrease in the

Table 16.1 Age-related hepatic changes conferring increased susceptibility to toxicant exposures.

Category	*Change*
Morphologic	↓ Hepatic mass
Physiologic	Sinusoidal pseudocapillarization
	↓ Bile salt formation and bile flow
	Mitochondrial dysfunction
Biochemical	↓ Phase I activity (cytochrome P450)
	Altered III activity (↓ xenobiotic transporters)
Antioxidant Defenses	↓ Glutathione
Immune Function	↑ Kupffer cells and pro-inflammatory cytokines
Regeneration	↓ Regeneration (shortened telomeres)

smooth endoplasmic reticulum.[1,2] The liver sinusoidal endothelial cells (LSECs) lose fenestrations and became 50% thicker with sub-endothelial collagen deposition (*Pseudocapillarization*).[3,4] The presence of complete basement membrane in liver sinusoids is a sign of age-related degeneration. Unlike "capillarization" seen in other liver pathology, aging is not associated with bridging fibrosis and nodular regeneration.[5] Therefore, pseudocapillarization leads to relative hypoxia of hepatocytes and may be reflected by lower ATP/ADP ratios in older *versus* younger subjects. This process could be important for drug therapy in old age, because the clearance of drugs undergoing oxidative metabolism, such as theophylline and propranolol, has been shown to be impaired.[6] Kupffer cell (resident macrophage) morphology remains unchanged, but both numbers and phagocytic activity increase with aging.[3,7]

16.2.2 Physiologic Changes

The most striking age-related change in liver physiology is the approximately 40% reduction in blood flow primarily due to sinuosoidal pseudocapillarization.[2,4] Declines in hepatic volume and blood flow may strongly contribute to age-related diminished oxygen-dependent hepatocyte functions, including xenobiotic metabolism and drug clearance and the liver's overall functional capacity.[3,8] Also, bile flow and bile salt formation are decreased by about 50%, resulting in reduced hepatic clearance of certain drugs, *e.g.* cardiac glycosides, with biliary elimination.[2,3] Additionally, recent studies have demonstrated a marked age-related increase in the cholesterol content of rat liver microsomes, leading to increased rigidity of the membrane lipid domain, thus impeding the ability of cytochrome P450 isoforms (CYPs) to interact efficiently with other mono-oxygenase components.[3]

16.2.3 Biochemical Changes

There are several biochemical mechanisms that underlie the primary aging process and probably contribute to age-related changes in adaptive responses and functions (*e.g.*, toxicant clearance), thereby increasing susceptibility to environmental or endogenous stresses.[2,9] These mechanisms include: altered xenobiotic metabolism, reduced antioxidant capacity, immune dysfunction, and impaired regeneration.

16.2.3.1 Xenobiotic Metabolism

Foreign compound and drug metabolism occurs generally in three phases. The first phase involves activation of the foreign chemical by oxidative enzymes, predominantly the cytochrome P450 family. Following activation, the metabolite is frequently conjugated with sulfate, glutathione or sugar (glucuronide), which simultaneously reduces the ability of the metabolite to react with either protein or DNA and facilitates excretion of the metabolite. The final phase involves elimination of the conjugate by specialized transporters. The liver is the major organ in the body responsible for drug and foreign compound metabolism, and the levels of these enzyme systems are greatest in this organ.

In general, there is an age-related decline in phase I drug metabolism of the order of 30–50%, which appears to be isozyme specific.[2,10–12] Phase II metabolism appears to be well maintained;[12] however, glutathione levels do decline with advancing age,[13,14] and more importantly, the ability to recover after an event that depletes glutathione is impaired.[15] The effects of aging on Phase III metabolism, which involves transporters on either the basolateral or apical surfaces of hepatocytes, are not well characterized; however, some age-related declines have been observed.

16.2.3.1.1 Phase I Metabolism. Foreign chemicals and drugs are metabolized by relatively few of the cytochromes P450 expressed in the body. The major enzymes include the CYP1A1, CYP1A2, CYP2C8, CYP2C9, CYP2C19, CYP2D6, CYP2E1, and CYP3A4.[12,16,17] The most notable age-related declines occur in the expression of CYP1A2, CYP2C9/10, and CYP2C18/19. Some studies have implicated declines in other isoenzymes, including CYP2A, CYP2E1, and CYP3A4. However, these are inconclusive, in part because these are frequently inducible enzymes, and expression levels may vary widely between individuals as a function of environmental exposure to foreign compounds. Likewise, other isoenzymes, such as CYP1A1, have very low basal levels of expression in the absence of an inducer.

The genes controlling induction of the cytochromes P450 include the Aryl hydrocarbon receptor (AhR), whose ligands include planar aromatic compounds, such as benzo[α]pyrene, and chlorinated compounds, such as 2,3,7,8-tetrachlorodibenzodioxin (TCDD).[18] The cytochromes P450 expressed in liver and which are are induced by this mechanism are CYP1A1 and CYP1A2. Induction of enzymes by this mechanism does not appear to be affected by aging.

A second important system for induction of drug metabolism is the induction of drug metabolism by the N1I class of nuclear receptors, which, in the liver, includes the constitutive androstane receptor (CAR) and the pregnane and xenobiotic receptor (PXR). Increasing interest is being focused on these receptors in liver disease, as CAR activation is thought to reduce obesity in animals fed a high fat diet, while PXR activation is thought to promote obesity in animals fed a high fat diet.[19] As obesity is the major contributor to the development of non-alcoholic fatty liver disease, the intersection of drug and foreign compound metabolism is a current novel area for research. From an aging perspective, these receptors appear to be close homologues of the *Caenorhabditis elegans* receptor, DAF-12.[20] DAF-12 is a critical determinant of lifespan in *C. elegans* and is critical for the larvae to enter the non-feeding, stress-resistant dauer diapause state under unfavorable conditions. This diapause state can greatly increase lifespan in *C. elegans* from 2 weeks to 3–6 months, with the larvae returning to normal development and the reproductive state once conditions are favorable. DAF-12 lies at an intersection of signaling pathways that includes the insulin-like growth factor-1 (IGF-1), transforming growth factor-β, target of rapamycin (TOR), and G-protein-mediated pathways, all of which contain genes that alter the lifespan of *C. elegans* and are implicated in the development of liver disease in humans. *C. elegans* cannot synthesize cholesterol, and the ligand for DAF-12 is thought to be the cholesterol metabolite, dafachronic acid (a potential metabolite of the cytochrome P450, DAF-9, and a Rieske-like oxygenase, DAF 36).[21] Thus, in the absence of a source of cholesterol from the environment, *C. elegans* enters diapause. In mammalian systems, mutations in the IGF-1 signaling pathway are thought to affect lifespan; however, the roles of CAR and PXR are yet to be fully elucidated.

An important consideration of these pathways is, however, the ability of both CAR and PXR to interact with the forkhead family of transcription factors, FoxO1 and FoxA2,[22] mammalian homologs of the *C. elegans* gene DAF-*12*. The forkhead transcription factors are part of the insulin and insulin-like signaling pathway(s) and are important regulators of both gluconeogenesis and lipid metabolism. Both CAR and PXR inhibit Forkhead box protein O1 (FoxO1), which is an important transcription factor for the expression of phosphoenolpyruvate carboxykinase (PEPCK), a critical step in early gluconeogenesis. Thus, activation of CAR or PXR by environmental chemicals tends to reduce gluconeogenesis and decrease circulating glucose levels. PXR can also interact with FoxA2, inhibiting its activity on target genes such as the carnitine palmitoyl transfease 1 (CPT1) gene and the hydroxymethylglutarate-CoA synthetase gene, which are rate-limiting steps in mitochondrial β-oxidation and ketone body synthesis respectively. Both of these processes are critical in lipid catabolism and may partially explain the obeseogenic effects of PXR ligands in animals fed a high fat diet and are likely to augment nonalcoholic fatty liver disease associated with a high fat diet. This suggests that the ability to respond to environmental change is a critical determinant of both lifespan and the development of fatty liver diseases. It also implies that the pathways connected to both processes are somewhat conserved in nematodes and mammals, although the outcomes are subtly different.

A final xenobiotic sensor of relevance in the expression of phase I metabolism and liver disease is the peroxisome proliferator activated receptor α (PPARα), which is activated by phthalates and clofibric acid derivatives. PPARα is intimately involved in the catabolism of fatty acids and is an important transcription regulator of β oxidation, both mitochondrial and peroxisomal, where it induces the CYP4A. In addition, it is an important regulator of CPT1 and 2, fatty acyl CoA oxidase (FACO), and many other genes involved with β- oxidation.[23]

16.2.3.1.2 Phase II Metabolism. Phase II detoxification involves the conjugation of reactive compounds with hydrophilic compounds such as glutathione, sugars (glucuronidation) or sulfate, which reduces the reactively of the parent compound and makes it more easily excreted (as conjugation makes the molecules more hydrophilic and targets them for export by

Phase III transporters). Most studies indicate that phase II enzymes, such as glutathione *S*-transferases, UDP-glucuronoslytranferases, and sulfotranferases, are not altered by aging.[12,24] However, some pharmacokinetic studies do indicate that Phase II metabolism is impaired. This is consistent with the observation that Phase II metabolism is impaired in aged Fisher 344 rats.[25]

16.2.3.1.3 Phase III Metabolism. This group includes protein transporters that function to remove xenobiotics either into the blood or bile depending on the location (on either the apical or basolateral surfaces of the hepatocyte). Studies on the effects of aging on the expression of Phase III systems in humans are limited. Animal studies show that aging is associated with a decline in the expression of organic anion-transporting polypeptides (Oatps), including Oatp 1A1,1B2, and Oatp2b1.[16] Likewise, expression of members of the multidrug resistance protein family (2,3, and 6) are reduced in aging.[16] In contrast, hepatic P-glycoprotein expression has been demonstrated to increase in old age Fisher 344 rats.[26]

16.2.3.2 Antioxidant Defense

The antioxidant capacity of hepatocytes appears to be reduced with age.[2] Mitochondria are both producers and targets of oxidative stress, which is the basis for the mitochondrial theory of aging. Oxidative stress is a cellular state in which the generation of harmful molecules such as reactive oxygen species (ROS), peroxidized lipids, reactive quinones, and electrophiles is greater than the ability of the cell to remove these destructive agents.[27] Both increased ROS production, due to mitochondrial respiratory chain defects,[9] and decreased ROS scavenger levels (*e.g.*, glutathione or GSH) are observed with aging, thus establishing a "vicious cycle" of oxidative stress.[4,9]

Antioxidant defenses in the cell are regulated in part by three redox sensitive transcription factors, Nrf-2, activator protein 1 (AP-1) family members, and nuclear factor kappa b (NF-κB). Nrf-2, or nuclear factor erythroid 2-related factor-2, is a transcription factor that mediates the synthesis of glutathione, which is the most abundant antioxidant in the liver and controls the redox potential of the hepatocyte.[28,29] Nrf-2 is a member of the basic region leucine zipper (bZIP) family of transcription factors and Cap 'n' Collar subfamily, and preferentially forms heterodimers with members of the musculoaponeurotic fibrosarcoma proteins (Mafs). In the absence of environmental stress, Nrf-2 is usually sequestered in the cytosol by Kelch-like ECH-associated protein-1 (Keap-1). This association targets Nrf-2 for ubiquitination and subsequent degradation. Thus, the half-life of Nrf-2 in an unstressed animal is relatively short (15 min). Keap-1 contains several reactive thiol groups which, if modified by agents such as xenobioitic electrophiles, release Nrf-2, allowing it to translocate to the nucleus, heterodimerize with a Maf, and upregulate a wide variety of genes involved with antioxidant stress. This includes those involved with glutathione synthesis, thioredoxin, peroxiredoxin, sulfredoxin, ferritin, metallothionein, and heme oxygenase-1.[30] In addition, Nrf-2 is involved in the expression of molecular chaperones, sub-units of both the 26S and 20S proteosome, and thus increases the cells' ability to degrade unfolded or ubiquitinated proteins. Nrf-2 can also interact with other transcription factors and is thought to antagonize NF-κB signaling and inhibit TNFα production, reducing the inflammatory response.[31] Activators of Nrf-2 tend to be relatively hydrophobic electrophiles rather than pure oxidative stress factors.[32] Stressors like hydrogen peroxide are relatively weak inducers of Nrf-2 signaling, while compounds such as sulforaphane, the isothiocyanate metabolite found in broccoli, are excellent Nrf-2 inducers. Thus, diet and malnutrition in the elderly are likely to have a significant impact on Nrf-2 signaling. Nrf-2 levels decline during aging, as manifested by a reduced response to a stressor.[33] In mice, acetaminophen treatment rapidly depletes glutathione. In young mice, GSH levels soon rebound due to Nrf-2 activation; however, in older mice, the recovery is much slower.[15] This phenomenon is, in part, due to reduced Nrf-2 levels, but changes in the heterodimerization pattern of Nrf-2 are also present.[34] In younger animals, Nrf-2 heterodimerizes with Maf family members to activate genes such as the γ-glutamyl cysteine ligase; however, in older animals, an increase in heterodimerization with c-fos is observed, and this subtly changes the response element binding profile and decreases transactivation potential, leading to a reduced induction of glutathione synthesis. Likewise, age-related declines in Nrf-2 signaling are also likely to affect the inflammatory response, with greater production of pro-inflammatory cytokines.

16.2.3.3 Immune Function

Inflammation is a critical component in the development of liver diseases and marks the progression of steatosis to steatohepatitis in both alcoholic and non-alcoholic liver diseases. During aging there is a phenotypic change in the expression of immune cells of the liver, which include resident populations of macrophages (Kupffer cells) and lymphocytes (including pit cells). Both cell populations change with aging.[35] Kupffer cell numbers increase with aging,[36] as does the basal level of expression of pro-inflammatory cytokines such as TNFα and IL-6. Many liver diseases involve a combination of enhanced immunological responses and the sensitization of hepatocytes, potentially by xenobiotic insults that result in normally resistant hepatocytes becoming susceptible to TNFα-dependent cell death.

Changes in the lymphocyte population of the liver with aging are more complex. The liver contains resident lymphocytes, including NK cells and NKT cells. The origins of these cells are complex and include cells derived from both the thymus and from c-kit$^+$ pluripotent hematopoitic stem cells found in the liver. Mice cells of thymic origin tend to decrease with aging, while the extrathymic-derived cells increase. Likely reflecting this change in phenotype, aging is associated with decreased serum levels of IL2 and increased expression of the pro-inflammatory cytokines, TNFα and IL-6. The levels of these cytokines also reflect a change in the T-cell pool, with an age-related increase and accumulation of more differentiated memory cells and a decline in naïve

T-cells. Some of these cells have the capacity to produce large amounts of pro-inflammatory cytokines. Consistent with this view is an increased expression of pro-inflammatory cytokine genes in the liver with aging. In addition, the number of lymphocytes in the liver increases with age, and, in aged mice, the number of lymphocytes is approximately 3-fold higher. Lymphocytes and Kupffer cells interact *via* a feed-forward mechanism to increase this response and therefore, with aging, the liver's response to an inflammatory stimulus such as endotoxemia, will have a more pro-inflammatory profile, with increases TNFα-secretion and TNFα-dependent hepatocyte death.

16.2.4 Regeneration

The liver has tremendous regenerative capacity. This capacity distinguishes it from other vital organs (*e.g.*, the brain, heart and lungs) that are far less able to replace functional tissue once it has been destroyed. As the main detoxifying organ in the body, the liver has a high likelihood of toxic injury. However, due to its regenerative properties, the liver is able to restore itself to full size and ensure survival of the organism. The liver can fully regenerate within 7–10 days in experimental models (*e.g.*, mice).[37] Although hepatocytes rarely proliferate in the healthy adult liver, virtually all surviving hepatocytes replicate at least once after 70% partial hepatectomy. Residual hepatocytes upregulate both proliferative and liver-specific gene expression in order to preserve tissue-specific function. In addition to hepatocyte proliferation, there is a tightly coordinated response to complement the regenerative process (*e.g.*, angiogenesis, extracellular matrix metabolism), so that the entire organ can be reconstituted within days. During liver regeneration, a complex network of cytokines, growth factors, kinases, and transcription factors drives hepatocytes out of the G_0 phase to enter and progress through replication.[38]

The complex and synchronized regenerative response in the liver can be perturbed and therefore can impact recovery of normal tissue from injury or damage. Indeed, it is now clear that impaired regeneration and/or restitution is critical to the chronicity of numerous hepatic diseases. Although aging does not dramatically affect hepatic histology and architecture, the response to injury can be severely impaired. In animal models, aging has been shown to impair hepatic regeneration.[39] In humans, the risk of liver failure in response to acute injury or hepatic resection increases dramatically in the older patient.[40,41] Aging has also been associated with poor outcome in chronic liver diseases. For example, age at the time of infection is major risk factor for severe liver disease in chronic hepatitis C, and livers from older patients progress through the fibrosis phases more rapidly than those from younger patients.[42,43] It is hypothesized that impaired regeneration contributes, at least in part, to the increased susceptibility of the aged liver to acute and chronic injury.[1]

A major mechanism proposed to contribute to replication senescence in the aged liver is telomere shortening. Telomeres are repeated hexonucleotide sequences at the end of the chromosome. Telomeres function to protect the chromosomes against fusion, non-reciprocal translocations, and deterioration.

During normal cell division, telomere length shortens with each round of division. Thus, the number of telomere repeats normally decreases with age. The rate of telomere shortening is accelerated in organs during chronic inflammation,[44] including in liver.[45] The shortening of telomeres with successive divisions impairs their ability to protect against chromosomal instability. As a result, the cell normally undergoes replicative senescence to prevent clonal expansion of potentially damaged chromosomes. Indeed, loss of this regulation is a key step in carcinogenesis.[46] It is hypothesized that this replicative senescence enhances the rate of remodeling (*i.e.*, fibrosis) during chronic liver injury. In support of that hypothesis, Rudolph, *et al.* demonstrated that livers from telomerase deficient mice progressed to fibrosis and cirrhosis more rapidly during experimental liver disease.[47] In comparison to other organs, hepatic regeneration is robust; but impaired liver regeneration with aging could contribute to age-related susceptibility to hepatotoxicants.

16.3 Occupational and Environmental Hepatotoxicants

As of May 2011, over 60 million unique chemicals were registered with the Chemical Abstracts Service (CAS). Notably, only two years had passed since the registration of the 40 millionth chemical. Due to rapid commercialization, it is impossible to fully understand the potential impact of these new chemicals on liver disease. However, the problem could be significant because 33% of the 677 most common workplace chemicals reported in the National Institute of Occupational Safety and Health (NIOSH) Pocket Guide are associated with hepatotoxicity.[48] Occupational and environmental liver diseases may present with a wide clinical spectrum, ranging from asymptomatic liver enzyme elevation to acute liver failure, cirrhosis, and cancer. In addition to age, an individual's susceptibility to chemical-induced liver disease is determined by polymorphisms in the genes of xenobiotic metabolism, concomitant use of alcohol or prescription medications, nutritional factors, and obesity (as many organic chemicals are lipid soluble).[49,50] Recently, it was demonstrated that hypertriglyceridemia is a risk factor for greater absorption of inhaled organic chemicals because it changes the blood/air partition coefficient to increase solubility of these molecules within the bloodstream.[51] High-level vinyl chloride (VC)[52] and solvent exposures[53] have historically been associated with occupational liver disease, and classical mediators of environmental liver disease include aflatoxins[54] and analines (Epping Jaundice[55,56] and Toxic Oil Syndrome[57]). However, recent population-based studies suggest an emerging role for polychlorinated biphenyls (PCBs), organochlorine insecticides, volatile organic compounds (VOCs), and metals[58–60] in environmental liver disease. These and other historically important chemical hepatotoxicants were recently reviewed.[61]

Toxicant exposure patterns, distribution, metabolism, and elimination may all increase susceptibility to liver injury. Hepatotoxicant exposures vary with age. While occupational exposures occur in adults, children may inadvertently ingest toxic chemicals (*e.g.*, yellow phosphorus from fireworks[62]) or inadvertently be exposed to them through medical care (*e.g.*, Di(2-ethylhexyl) phthalate in IV tubing[63]). Several persistent organic pollutants (POPs) associated with adult liver disease are present in breast milk,[64] but the effects of these chemicals, if any, on pediatric liver disease are uncertain. Likewise, POPs (including PCBs) associated with liver disease bio-accumulate with age, meaning older subjects are more likely to have higher liver and adipose tissue levels. Subsequently, in this chapter, histopathologic subtypes of chemical liver disease as well as selected hepatotoxicants (VC, aflatoxin, and arsenic) are presented with an emphasis on aging.

16.3.1 Pathologic Forms of Liver Injury Attributed to Industrial Chemicals

Chemical liver injury typically results in non-specific hepatitis, although unusual lesions such as hemangiosarcoma may occur. Most industrial chemicals, including solvents, exhibit dose-dependent hepatocyte cytotoxicity and typically result in hepatocellular necrosis.[61] However, both cholestasis[65,66] and acute hepatitis accompanied by rash and eosinophilia resembling an immunologic drug reaction have been reported.[53] Examples of histopathologic liver lesions associated with industrial chemicals are given in Table 16.2.

Recently, our group coined the term, toxicant-associated steatohepatitis (TASH) to describe steatohepatitis in highly exposed chemical workers and associated with increased pro-inflammatory cytokines, insulin resistance, and antioxidant depletion.[52,67] Liver biopsies resembled alcoholic or non-alcoholic steatohepatitis (NASH), but affected workers were non-drinkers and were not obese. Hepatocyte lipid accumulation has historically been considered a benign toxicologic finding and has been described in many forms of chemical hepatitis.[52,61] However, given the increase in cirrhosis and hepatocellular carcinoma associated with the current NASH epidemic, the significance of steatohepatitis due to industrial chemicals must be re-evaluated. Indeed, emerging evidence suggests that steatohepatitis, often with normal serum aminotransferases, may be one of the most common forms of chemical-induced hepatitis.[52,53,67,68] Serum cytokeratin 18 (non-caspase cleaved), a biomarker of necrotic hepatocyte death, is more reliably elevated in these workers.[52,69] Recently, POPs which bio-accumulate with age (including PCBs) have been associated with suspected TASH in epidemiologic studies.[59] Nutritional status, co-exposures, and diseases associated with aging—including diabetes and obesity—appear to confer increased susceptibility to TASH, but more clinical data are needed.[49,52,70]

16.3.2 Vinyl Chloride

Vinyl chloride monomer (VC, C_2H_3Cl, CAS 75-01-4) is a colorless gas and classically described mediator of occupational liver disease.[71] Hepatotoxicity has also been documented in other structurally related haloalkanes (*e.g.*,

Table 16.2 Pathology of Chemical Liver Disease in Humans or Animal Models.

Category	*Selected Examples*
Steatohepatitis	Vinyl chloride, aflatoxin, trichloroethylene, tetrachloroethylene, trichloroethane, carbon tetrachloride, petrochemical mixtures, atrazine, paraquat, chlordecone, polychlorinated biphenyls, nitrobenzene, nitrotoluene, arsenic, methylmercury, thallium, yellow phosphorus, aflatoxin
Necrosis	Carbon tetrachloride and other halogenated aliphatic hydrocarbons, haloaromatic compounds, nitroaromatic compounds, arsenic, yellow phosphorus
Cholestasis	Beryllium, copper, di(2-ethylhexyl) phthalate, methylenedianiline, paraquat, toxic rapeseed oil
Cirrhosis	Arsenic, carbon tetrachloride, polychlorinated biphenyls, trichloroethane, trichloroethylene, trinitrotoluene, vinyl chloride
Peliosis hepatitis	Thorotrast, urethane, vinyl chloride
Granulomas	Beryllium, copper
Pigment deposition	Anthracite, thorotrast, titanium
Cholangiocarcinoma	Thorotrast, polychlorinated biphenyls
Hepatocellular Carcinoma	Arsenic, carbon tetrachloride, polychlorinated biphenyls, tetrachloroethylene, thorotrast, trichloroethylene, trinitrotoluene, vinyl chloride, aflatoxin
Hemangiosarcoma	Vinyl chloride, butoxyethanol, chloronitrobenzene, polyhexamethylene biguanine, urethane, tetrafluoroethylene

Adapted from M. Cave, K. C. Falkner and C. J. McClain in *Zakim and Boyer's Hepatology: A Textbook of Liver Disease*, 6th edn, Elsevier Saunders, Philadelphia, 2011.

carbon tetrachloride) and haloalkenes (*e.g.*, trichloroethylene, TCE).[65,72,73] However, the identification of three cases of vinyl chloride-related hemangiosarcoma at a single B.F. Goodrich chemical plant in Louisville, KY in the 1970's is perhaps the most important sentinel event in occupational hepatology.[71] Subsequent studies have documented associations between VC exposures and a variety of other liver diseases, including hepatocellular carcinoma (HCC),[49] TASH,[52] cirrhosis,[49] peliosis hepatitis, focal hepatocytic hyperplasia (FHH), and focal mixed hyperplasia (FMH).[74] VC exposure, metabolism, hemangiosarcoma, and TASH are subsequently discussed, with emphasis on the effects of aging on VC toxicity.

VC is a high production volume chemical, and worldwide production capacity exceeds 35 million lbs. VC is used for polymer production, most notably, polyvinyl chloride (PVC), and for the synthesis of chlorinated solvents. To date, more than 80,000 American chemical workers have been exposed to VC.[75] At production facilities such as those at Louisville, prior to 1975, high level exposures estimated to exceed 1,000 ppm occurred in "poly cleaners", who entered and manually cleaned PVC batch reactor vessels. VC exposures were subsequently limited by the Occupational Safety and Health Administration's Vinyl Chloride Standard (29 CFR 1910.1017) to less than

1 ppm averaged over an 8 hour work day. In addition to chemical workers, high level occupational exposures occurred in hair dressers, as VC was used as an aerosol propellant in hair spray from approximately 1962 to 1974.[76] VC has been identified as a solvent degradation product, and it is present in landfill leachate, where it potentially places surrounding populations at risk. VC may also leach from PVC pipes which are used to carry drinking water, or may form as a disinfection byproduct.

VC is metabolized in a strikingly similar fashion to ethanol, producing reactive VC metabolites. At concentrations up to approximately 220 ppm, VC is metabolized by CYP2E1, forming the highly reactive genotoxic epoxide, chloroethylene oxide.[77] CYP2E1 polymorphisms were associated with fibrosis, liver injury, and chromosomal damage in Asian VC workers, and possibly hemangiosarcoma at the Louisville plant.[50,78–80] Chloroethylene oxide is either spontaneously or enzymatically converted to chloroacetaldehyde (CAA).[81] CAA may be metabolized by aldehyde dehydrogenase 2 or scavenged by sulfhydryl groups/glutathione. VC exposure may be associated with increased systemic pro-inflammatory cytokines and reduced antioxidant defenses;[52] indeed, GST polymorphisms have been associated with increased biomarkers of genotoxicity and liver disease in VC workers.[79,80] Likewise, we recently showed, *in vitro*, that CAA treatments induced mitochondrial dysfunction, a hallmark of aging.[82] Therefore, VC metabolism, like aging, may be associated with inflammation, oxidative stress, and mitochondrial dysfunction; and genetic variation may confer increased susceptibility.

Hepatic hemangiosarcoma (Figures 16.1, 16.2) is a vascular tumor believed to originate from sinusoidal endothelial cells. Although hemangiosarcoma may occur spontaneously with some frequency in other mammalian species, it is exceptionally rare in humans.[83] However, 26 highly-exposed B.F. Goodrich workers from the Louisville plant have developed hepatic hemangiosarcoma,

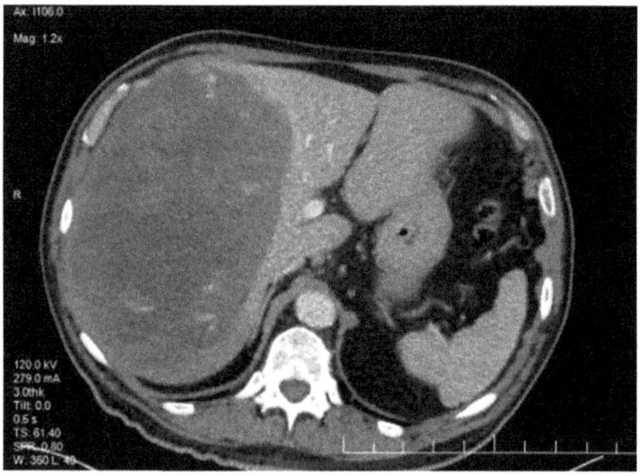

Figure 16.1 Computed tomography scan from a VC worker with a 20 cm hypodense liver mass which was subsequently confirmed to be hemangiosarcoma on biopsy.

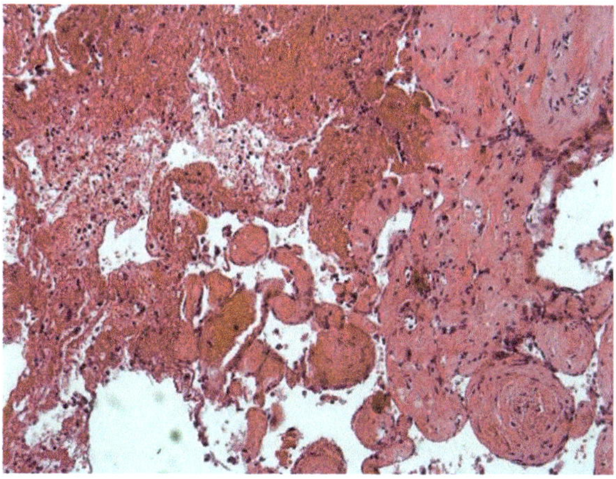

Figure 16.2 Photomicrograph (100×, H&E stain) of a liver biopsy from a second VC worker with hemangiosarcoma.

and this is likely the largest single-site cluster worldwide.[84] This association has been confirmed in large epidemiologic studies of more than 10,000 North American and more than 12,000 European VC workers.[85,86] Consistent with the Louisville data, duration of exposure, cumulative exposure, and employment as an autoclave cleaner were risk factors for hemangiosarcoma in these studies. At cumulative exposures below 1,500 ppm per year, mortality from hemangiosarcoma approached that of the entire cohort, again demonstrating the dose-dependence of this cancer.[86] Peculiarly, even though VC is genotoxic, in Louisville workers, hemangiosarcoma presented with aging, following a long latency period. Hemangiosarcoma presented at a mean age of 57.9 ± 12.2 and at a mean of 32.2 ± 11.9 years after initial occupational VC exposure. Given this prolonged latency period, cases continue to present, even decades after the last VC exposure. Some studies have implicated p53 and polymorphisms in DNA repair genes in VC-related hepatocarcinogenesis.[87–89] However, more work is required to better understand why VC exposures may result in cancer with aging following a prolonged latency period.

As early as 1975, it was recognized that "fatty changes" similar to those observed in alcoholic liver disease were present in about half of biopsied chemical workers with high cumulative exposures.[90] In fact, in his final paper addressing focal hepatocytic hyperplasia (FHH) and focal hepatocytic hyperplasia (FMH,) Hans Popper noted that FHH and FMH were often obscured by "fatty infiltration and/or chronic disease (hepatitis/granuloma)".[74] Our group became interested in this topic following the publication of reports documenting NASH in lean Brazilian petrochemical workers exposed to chemical mixtures including vinyl chloride,[68]and ultrasound studies observing hepatomegaly, steatosis, and fibrosis in VC workers.[91,92] Subsequently, 25 liver biopsies from highly exposed VC workers at the Louisville plant were re-analyzed, yielding an 80% steatohepatitis prevalence (Figure 16.3).[52] Fibrosis

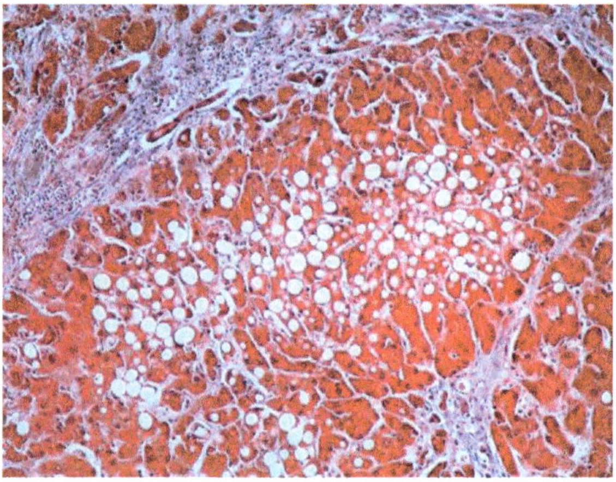

Figure 16.3 Photomicrograph of a liver biopsy (100×, H&E stain) of a VC worker with TASH and cirrhosis.

was present in 55% of TASH cases. Remarkably, serum transaminases were normal in most cases. TASH was associated with insulin resistance, reduced serum adiponectin levels, marked elevation of pro-inflammatory cytokines, and reduced serum antioxidants. TASH was associated with primarily necrotic, rather than apoptotic, hepatocellular death. Similar biochemical findings were present in elastomer/polymer workers with suspected TASH and who were exposed to mixtures of acrylonitrile, 1,3-butadiene, and styrene.[67] Because these modes of action have been associated with aging, interactions between aging and TASH could be anticipated, but have not been studied.

16.3.3 Aflatoxin

While VC is historically associated with occupational liver disease, aflatoxins are classically described, and still relevant, environmental hepatoxicants. Aflatoxins are unavoidable food contaminants, produced by *Aspergillus* species, including *A. flavus*.[54] These mycotoxins are produced by fungal action during the production harvest, storage, and processing of peanuts, corn, and grains, particularly under warm and moist conditions. Aflatoxins were initially identified 50 years ago as the cause of "turkey X disease", but they were subsequently found to produce human disease as well.[54] In developed countries, aflatoxin levels in both food for human consumption and livestock feed are regulated. Two well-defined clinical syndromes have been described in humans: acute aflatoxicosis and hepatocellular carcinoma; although some evidence suggests that aflatoxins may also cause hepatomegaly,[93] cirrhosis,[94] and growth restriction[95] in children, who appear to have increased susceptibility.[96]

Acute aflatoxicosis results from high-dose exposures and occurs periodically in mini-epidemics in developing countries. Aflatoxicosis results in vomiting, hepatic steatosis, bile duct proliferation, hemorrhagic necrosis, pulmonary edema, and hepatic encephalopathy.[54] The largest reported outbreak occurred in Kenya in 2004–2005 following ingestion of contaminated maize and resulted in 317 cases and 125 deaths.[97] Experimental studies have confirmed microvesicular steatosis with glutathione depletion following acute exposure, with aspartate aminotransferase (AST) > alanine aminotransferase (ALT) elevation and impaired mitochondrial respiration similar to Reye's syndrome.[98–100] Thus, acute aflatoxicosis could be considered to represent "fulminant TASH".

In contrast to acute aflatoxicosis, hepatocellular carcinoma is increasingly prevelent, and occurs as a consequence of low-level chronic exposures. Experimental studies have confirmed carcinogenesis with chronic aflatoxin B_1 (AFB1) exposure across multiple species.[54] However, human epidemiological studies have typically focused on aflatoxin (urinary aflatoxin-N^7-guanine) and hepatitis B virus (serum HBV surface antigen) co-exposures in Asia. Notably, in the People's Republic of China, the incidence of HCC is 700,000 cases per year. The first major cohort study, comprising more than 18,000 men in Shanghai, determined HCC relative risks of 3.4, 7, and 59 for aflatoxin, HBV, and combined aflatoxin/HBV exposures. These synergistic results have been confirmed in other studies, and in high risk areas in China, the onset of liver cancer also begins early in life, starting at age 20.[54]

Aflatoxin hepatocarcinogensis has been attributed to the genotoxicity of metabolites of AFB_1 and AFG_1. AFB_1 is oxidized by CYP1A2 and CYP3A4 to metabolites including the epoxide, AFB_1-8,9-oxide, which may form DNA adducts (most notably aflatoxin-N^7-guanine), or be conjugated with glutathione to eventually form aflatoxin-*N*-acetylcysteine (AFB-NAC). Indeed GST polymorphisms have been associated with increased incidence of HCC due to aflatoxin exposures.[54] Ongoing chemoprevention studies focus on the ability of Nrf2 activators, such as oltipraz or broccoli sprouts tea, to enhance detoxification, as measured by increased urinary AFB-NAC and decreased aflatoxin adducts.[54]

16.3.4 Arsenic

Inorganic arsenic is a ubiquitous element and a natural drinking water contaminant. Owing to its toxic potential to humans, it is a high priority hazardous substance in the United States. Chronic exposure to arsenic has been linked with a myriad of possible health effects, including skin lesions, hypertension, cardiovascular disease, respiratory disease, and malignancies of the skin and internal organs.[101] The liver is a well-known target organ of arsenic exposure. Hepatic abnormalities caused by arsenic exposure include hepatomegaly, non-cirrhotic portal fibrosis, and portal hypertension.[102–104] Furthermore, arsenic exposure has been linked to hepatic malignancies, namely hepatic hemangiosarcoma and hepatocellular carcinoma in both humans and in animal models.[105,106] Straub *et al.* demonstrated that mouse liver is also sensitive to more subtle hepatic changes (*e.g.*, hepatic endothelial cell capillarization and vessel remodeling) at lower arsenic exposure levels

(250 ppb) without any gross pathologic effects.[105] It is nevertheless unclear at this time if environmental arsenic exposure at the levels observed in the US causes liver disease.

Another major health concern for the US population is obesity, the prevalence of which is increasing at an alarming rate. Among the myriad of health complications associated with obesity (*e.g.*, diabetes, cardiovascular risk, *etc.*) is non-alcoholic fatty liver disease (NAFLD). Risk factors for primary NAFLD (*i.e.*, not secondary to other proximate causes) are analogous to those of metabolic syndrome (*e.g.*, obesity, type II diabetes, and dyslipidemia). It is also clear however, that there are likely other unidentified risk factors that contribute to the development of disease. A striking feature of arsenic exposure and non-alcoholic fatty liver disease is that there is significant overlap between areas of risk in the US.[107,108] For example, states with clusters of municipal wells with high levels of arsenic (*e.g.*, Michigan, Texas, West Virginia, and Oklahoma) also have high incidences of obesity and diabetes.[109,110] Furthermore, high arsenic in the drinking water is generally localized to private artesian water supplies (not regulated by the EPA) in rural communities, where the incidence of obesity tends to be even higher than in most areas of the country. It is therefore possible that arsenic exposure is an unidentified environmental risk factor in the development of NAFLD. In support of this hypothesis, it was recently demonstrated that liver injury during experimental NAFLD is enhanced by concomitant arsenic exposure in mice.[111] As described subsequently, the course of NAFLD is worsened with aging.

16.4 Aging and Clinical Liver Disease

There are no liver diseases specific to advanced age. However, the clinical course and management of the elderly with liver diseases differs in several aspects from that of young individuals. Reduction in protective enzymes, decline in response to growth factors, and increased pathogen load from the gut all put the aged liver at increased risk for disease.[9,112] In this section, alcoholic liver disease, NAFLD, viral hepatitis, and drug-induced liver injury (DILI) will be discussed with regard to aging and susceptibility.

16.4.1 Alcoholic Liver Disease

Alcohol consumption is common in old age, and approximately 62% of individuals over 60 years old are heavy alcohol drinkers.[113] The majority (90–100%) of individuals with chronic alcohol consumption develop alcoholic fatty liver (AFL). About 30% of AFL individuals develop alcoholic steatohepatitis (ASH), and approximately 10–20% develop alcoholic cirrhosis.[114]

The liver is the main organ for ethanol metabolism. Ethanol is primarily metabolized to acetaldehyde ($\sim$80%) by alcohol dehydrogenase (ADH), and by cytochrome P450 2E1 (CYP2E1) and catalase. ADH transfers electrons from ethanol to the reducing equivalent $NADP^+$; the cytochrome P450 system transfers the electrons to molecular oxygen (O_2), and catalase reduces hydrogen peroxide (H_2O_2) to water. Age associated diminished activity of these enzymes makes the liver vulnerable to the toxicity of alcohol.[115,116] Additionally, the shift in hepatic redox state that occurs with oxidation of ethanol inhibits mitochondrial β-oxidation of fatty acids and increases fatty acid synthesis and esterification,[117] thereby contributing to the development of alcoholic fatty liver (AFL). In the aging population, AFL can lead directly to cirrhosis *via* enhanced fibrogenesis.

More than 28% of alcoholic liver disease (ALD) diagnoses are in patients aged 60 or over.[116] Half of the elderly patients who develop cirrhosis die within a year of its diagnosis.[113] The most common presentation in patients over 70 years is dizziness and non-specific symptoms such as malaise, anorexia, abdominal pain.[112] Because aged individuals often have other diseases, elderly patients who have ALD may have more severe symptoms and a higher frequency of complications.[116] One study identified that 100% of men aged over 70 presenting with ALD had a more severe clinical presentation (jaundice, ascites, portal hypertension, gynecomastia) and cirrhosis on biopsy, compared to 55% of men aged 20–59 years.[112] In patients with severe ASH or cirrhosis, a variety of prognostic criteria exist: edema, esophageal variceal bleeding, and hepatic encephalopathy, all of which increase mortality significantly.[116] The Glasgow score for alcoholic hepatitis considers that age >50 is a significant factor for a worse prognosis.[112] In a British study, mortality from cirrhosis in alcoholic liver disease at years 1 and 3 of follow-up was 34% and 54% respectively in patients over 60, compared with 5% and 24% respectively in patients under 60.[118] Also, age over 55 is associated with an increased incidence of central nervous system damage in patients with ALD when compared to younger individuals.[114] Thus, the severity and prognosis of ALD is worse with aging, and ethanol can increase susceptibility to injury from specific xenobiotics metabolized by CYP2E1.

16.4.2 Nonalcoholic Fatty Liver Disease

NAFLD is composed of a spectrum of liver pathology ranging from steatosis to inflammation, often with fibrosis (non-alcoholic steatohepatitis), to cirrhosis. NAFLD is regarded as the hepatic manifestation of the metabolic syndrome, and its prevalence has risen in parallel with the obesity epidemic. A recent study showed that NAFLD accounted for 75% of chronic liver disease in the United States (NHANES 2005–2008), increasing from 47% in the previous decade (NHANES 1988–1994).[119] Fatty liver was detected by magnetic resonance spectroscopy in 33.6% of the 2,349 adult (age 18–65) participants in the Dallas Heart Study.[120] The prevalence of NAFLD increases with age and ranges from 1–3% in children, 5% in teenagers, 18% in adults aged 20–40, 39% in adults aged 40–50, to over 40% in adults over 70 years of age.[121] Not only is NAFLD more common with aging, it also appears to be more severe. Age (especially >50) was associated with increased fibrosis using multivariate analysis in multiple cross-sectional studies.[121] In the only liver biopsy study of NAFLD in patients over 70, exceptionally high prevalences of fibrosis (40%) and cirrhosis (14%) were observed.[122] In addition to age, insulin resistance is an important determinant of fibrosis progression. However, the interaction between NAFLD and insulin resistance is complex, as NAFLD is also associated with the subsequent development of overt diabetes, metabolic syndrome, and cardiovascular disease.[121] The presence of NAFLD is associated with increased mortality, and ischemic heart disease, cancer, and cirrhosis are the leading causes of death in NAFLD.[121]

Several mechanisms have been proposed to explain increased susceptibility to NAFLD with aging.[121] Foremost among these are age-related loss of lean body mass and an increased prevalence of metabolic syndrome. These conditions are associated with fat redistribution from subcutaneous adipose tissue (SAT) to visceral adipose tissue (VAT). This shift increases the flux of free fatty acids to the liver and eventually overwhelms the oxidative (age-related decrease in mitochondrial function) and antioxidant capacities of the liver, resulting in increased hepatic lipid accumulation, oxidative stress, and inflammation. NAFLD has also been associated with abnormal xenobiotic metabolism, independent of aging. Thus, NAFLD may increase susceptibility to liver injury from xenobiotic compounds. The weight of evidence indicates that NAFLD is associated with down-regulation of CYP1A2 and cellular glutathione (GSH).[123] CYP2E1 is upregulated in the majority of human and rat, but not mouse, studies. Limited human data suggest that specific hepatic uptake transporters may also be downregulated,[124] while ATP-binding cassette (efflux) transporters may be upregulated (albeit with abnormal cellular localization in some cases)[125] with increasing severity of NAFLD. Not only does NAFLD potentially increase susceptibility to xenobiotic toxicity, some toxicants have clearly been associated with the development of NAFLD/TASH (Table 16.2).

16.4.3 Viral Hepatitis

Worldwide, HBV accounts for an estimated 370 million chronic infections.[126] Older age at the time of acute HBV infection is associated with increased rates of progression to chronic HBV.[127] However, spontaneous annual seroclearance rates of hepatitis B surface antigen are higher in older subjects with chronic HBV.[127] While progression to cirrhosis is best correlated with higher HBV DNA levels, older age and male sex are also important risk factors.[128] Older age also increases the risk for development of hepatocellular carcinoma.[129]

Approximately 3% (~170 million) of the world's population has been infected with Hepatitis C (HCV), and adults aged 40–49 have the highest seroprevalence.[127] However, subjects older than 65 are more likely to present with decompensated cirrhosis and HCC.[130] A liver biopsy study in patients over the age of 65 showed that 60% had cirrhosis, 30% had HCC, and 10% had chronic active hepatitis.[112] The probability of fibrosis progression is accelerated with aging; and men aged 61–70 years with HCV had 300 times greater fibrosis progression per year than men aged 21–40 years.[131] Likewise, the median time to development of cirrhosis was 33 years in those infected during the third decade of life, compared to 16 years in those infected at age 40 or older.[132] Older age is also associated with decreased rates of sustained virologic response with HCV pharmacotherapy, and this lack of response has been attributed, in part, to increased drop-outs due to medication side effects. HCV is the leading indication for liver transplantation in the US, but older donor age is associated with increased graft loss due to more aggressive recurrence of HCV infection.[133]

The more rapid course of HCV observed with aging has been proposed to be related to a reduction in hepatic blood flow, reduced mitochondrial function, and cumulative exposures to environmental hepatotoxicants.[118,127] Mixed exposures to 1,2-ethylene dichloride and vinyl chloride have a synergistic effect with hepatitis B virus infection for liver injury (elevated serum aminotransferases) in exposed workers.[134] Likewise chronic HBV was a risk factor for the development of hepatocellular carcinoma in vinyl chloride workers.[134,135] Moreover, aflatoxin co-exposures may synergistically increase the risk for hepatocellular carcinoma in subjects with chronic HBV or HCV infection.[136] Exposure to acrolein, an environmental aldehyde, has been associated with decreased responsiveness *in vitro* to interferon alpha, which is used to treat chronic viral hepatitis.[137]

16.4.4 Drug Induced Liver Injury

Older age is traditionally considered to be a susceptibility factor for drug induced liver injury (DILI).[138] It is estimated that over 1100 drugs and herbals are associated with DILI, and DILI remains the leading cause of acute liver failure (ALF).[139] Furthermore, older age negatively impacted survival of ALF in some, but not all, studies.[140] In the Acute Liver Failure Study Group, acetaminophen (APAP) accounted for 46% of ALF, while non-APAP DILI accounted for 12% of ALF.[141] Older age is a traditional risk factor for both APAP and idiosyncratic DILI (*e.g.*, diclofenac, isoniazid, flucloxacillin, amoxicillin/clavulanic acid, erythromycin, nitrofurantoin, and methotrexate).[138,139] In Spain, 45% of DILI cases during 1994–2004 occurred in patients aged > 60.[142] More recent data from DILI registries challenge the notion that age alone is risk factor for ALF from DILI.[139] However, age continues to be associated with increased susceptibility to cholestatic DILI.[139] In addition to age-related changes in drug absorption, distribution, metabolism, and elimination, age and frailty may be associated with additional risk factors for DILI, including concomitant ethanol use, polypharmacy, malnutrition, NAFLD, and cognitive impairment affecting adherence.[138] From a mechanistic standpoint, mitochondrial toxicity appears to be an early event in idiosyncratic DILI, and age-related mitochondrial damage could confound this problem.[138] Aging related risk factors appear to increase susceptibility to DILI, and mitochondrial dysfunction and malnutrition remain important associated mechanisms. However, more data are needed to better understand this important topic.

16.5 Conclusions

The liver is the largest and most biochemically complex organ in the body. Normal aging is associated with morphologic, physiologic, biochemical, immunologic, and regenerative changes, which may increase susceptibility to hepatotoxic chemicals. Industrial chemicals and food contaminants such as aflatoxin have been associated with a myriad of pathologic liver injuries, ranging from acute hepatitis to chronic hepatitis, cirrhosis, and liver cancer. The hepatic response to toxic chemicals may be even more complex in older individuals with underlying liver diseases, including alcoholic liver disease, nonalcoholic fatty liver disease, and viral hepatitis.

Abbreviations

AFB_1	aflatoxin B1
ADH	alcohol dehydrogenase
ALD	alcoholic liver disease
AFL	alcoholic fatty liver
ALF	acute liver failure
ALT	alanine aminotransferase
ASH	alcoholic steatohepatitis
AST	aspartate aminotransferase
AP-1	activator protein 1
ARE	antioxidant response element
AhR	aryl hydrocarbon receptor
bZIP	basic region leucine zipper
CAA	chloroacetaldehyde
CAR	constitutive androstane receptor
CAS	chemical abstracts service
CYP	cytochrome P450
DILI	drug-induced liver injury
FHH	focal hepatocytic hyperplasia
FMH	focal mixed hyperplasia
GCL	glutamate cysteine ligase
GSH	reduced glutathione
GST	glutathione *S*-transferases
HBV	hepatitis B virus
HCV	hepatitis C Virus
HCC	hepatocellular carcinoma
IGF-1	insulin-like growth factor
Keap1	kelch-like-ECH-associated protein 1
LSECs	liver sinusoidal endothelial cells
NASH	nonalcoholic steatohepatitis
NF-κB	nuclear factor kappa B
NIOSH	National Institute of Occupational Safety and Health
Nrf2	nuclear factor (erythroid-derived 2)-like 2

PCBs	polychlorinated biphenyls
POPs	persistent organic pollutants
PPARα	peroxisome proliferator activated receptor α
PXR	pregnane and xenobiotic receptor
ROS	reactive oxygen species
SAT	subcutaneous adipose tissue
TCDD	2,3,7,8-tetrachlorodibenzodioxin
Fox01	Forkhead box protein 01
PEPCK	Phosphoenolpyruvate carboxykinase
CPT1	carnitine palmitoyl transfersase 1
FACO	fatty acyl CoA oxidase
Otap	organic anion transporting peptide
NFkB	nuclear factor kappa B
Mafs	musculoaponeurotic fibrosarcoma proteins
TASH	toxicant-associated steatohepatitis
TOR	target of rapamycin
VAT	visceral adipose tissue

References

1. M. Hoare, T. Das and G. Alexander, *J. Hepatol.*, 2010, **53**, 950–961.
2. D. G. Le Couteur and A. J. McLean, *Clin. Pharmacokinetics*, 1998, **34**, 359–373.
3. D. L. Schmucker, *Drugs Aging*, 2001.
4. S. J. Mitchell, A. E. Kane and S. N. Hilmer, *Curr. Gerontol. Geriatr. Res.*, 2011, **2011**, 624156.
5. D. G. Le Couteur, A. Warren, V. C. Cogger, B. Smedsrod, K. K. Sorensen, R. De Cabo, R. Fraser and R. S. McCuskey, *Anat. Rec.*, 2008, **291**, 672–683.
6. O. Junaidi and A. M. Di Bisceglie, *Clinics in Geriatric Medicine*, 2007, **23**, 889–903, viii.
7. S. J. Mitchell and S. N. Hilmer, *Ther. Adv. Drug Safety*, 2010, **1**, 65–77.
8. P. L. Jansen, *Best Practice & Research. Clinical Gastroenterology*, 2002, **16**, 149–158.
9. A. J. McLean and D. G. Le Couteur, *Pharmacol. Rev.*, 2004, **56**, 163–184.
10. H. A. Wynne, L. H. Cope, O. F. James, M. D. Rawlins and K. W. Woodhouse, *Age Ageing*, 1989, **18**, 415–418.
11. E. A. Sotaniemi, A. J. Arranto, O. Pelkonen and M. Pasanen, *Clinical Pharmacology and Therapeutics*, 1997, **61**, 331–339.
12. U. Klotz, *Drug Metab. Rev.*, 2009, **41**, 67–76.
13. G. A. Hazelton and C. A. Lang, *The Biochemical Journal*, 1980, **188**, 25–30.
14. C. A. Lang, S. Naryshkin, D. L. Schneider, B. J. Mills and R. D. Lindeman, *The J. Lab. Clin. Med.*, 1992, **120**, 720–725.
15. T. S. Chen, J. P. Richie, Jr. and C. A. Lang, *Drug Metabolism and Disposition: the Biological Fate of Chemicals*, 1990, **18**, 882–887.

16. Y. K. Zhang, K. W. Saupe and C. D. Klaassen, *Drug Metabolism and Disposition: the Biological Fate of Chemicals*, 2010, **38**, 1122–1131.
17. A. Parkinson, D. R. Mudra, C. Johnson, A. Dwyer and K. M. Carroll, *Toxicol. Appl. Pharmacol.*, 2004, **199**, 193–209.
18. M. S. Denison and J. P. Whitlock, Jr., *The Journal of Biological Chemistry*, 1995, **270**, 18175–18178.
19. T. Wada, J. Gao and W. Xie, *Trends Endorinol. Metab.*, 2009, **20**, 273–279.
20. S. P. Mooijaart, B. W. Brandt, E. A. Baldal, J. Pijpe, M. Kuningas, M. Beekman, B. J. Zwaan, P. E. Slagboom, R. G. Westendorp and D. van Heemst, *Ageing Research Reviews*, 2005, **4**, 351–371.
21. B. Gerisch, V. Rottiers, D. Li, D. L. Motola, C. L. Cummins, H. Lehrach, D. J. Mangelsdorf and A. Antebi, *Proc.Natl. Acad. Sci. U.S.A.*, 2007, **104**, 5014–5019.
22. Y. Konno, M. Negishi and S. Kodama, *Drug Metab. Pharmacokinet.*, 2008, **23**, 8–13.
23. E. R. Kallwitz, A. McLachlan and S. J. Cotler, *World J. Gastroenterol.*, 2008, **14**, 22–28.
24. J. B. Schwartz, *Clin. Pharm. Ther.*, 2007, **82**, 87–96.
25. J. S. Lee, W. O. Ward, J. Liu, H. Ren, B. Vallanat, D. Delker and J. C. Corton, *PloS One*, 2011, **6**, e24381.
26. J. S. Warrington, D. J. Greenblatt and L. L. von Moltke, *J. Pharmacol. Exp. Ther.*, 2004, **309**, 730–736.
27. R. N. Hardwick, C. D. Fisher, M. J. Canet, A. D. Lake and N. J. Cherrington, *Drug Metabolism and Disposition: the Biological Fate of Chemicals*, 2010, **38**, 2293–2301.
28. P. D. Ray, B. W. Huang and Y. Tsuji, *Cell. Signalling*, 2012, **24**, 981–990.
29. K. N. Lewis, J. Mele, J. D. Hayes and R. Buffenstein, *Integr. Comp. Biol.*, 2010, **50**, 829–843.
30. H. Y. Cho, S. P. Reddy, A. Debiase, M. Yamamoto and S. R. Kleeberger, *Free Radic. Biol. Med.*, 2005, **38**, 325–343.
31. X. L. Chen, G. Dodd, S. Thomas, X. Zhang, M. A. Wasserman, B. H. Rovin and C. Kunsch, *American Journal of Physiology. Heart and Circulatory Physiology*, 2006, **290**, H1862–1870.
32. T. Nguyen, T. H. Rushmore and C. B. Pickett, *The Journal of Biological Chemistry*, 1994, **269**, 13656–13662.
33. J. H. Suh, S. V. Shenvi, B. M. Dixon, H. Liu, A. K. Jaiswal, R. M. Liu and T. M. Hagen, *Proc.Natl. Acad. Sci. U.S.A.*, 2004, **101**, 3381–3386.
34. S. V. Shenvi, E. Smith and T. M. Hagen, *Aging Cell*, 2012, **11**, 297–304.
35. A. Tsukahara, S. Seki, T. Iiai, T. Moroda, H. Watanabe, S. Suzuki, T. Tada, H. Hiraide, K. Hatakeyama and T. Abo, *Hepatology*, 1997, **26**, 301–309.
36. S. N. Hilmer, V. C. Cogger and D. G. Le Couteur, *The Journals of Gerontology. Series A, Biological Sciences and Medical Sciences*, 2007, **62**, 973–978.
37. R. Taub, *Nat. Rev. Mol. Cell Biol.*, 2004, **5**, 836–847.

38. R. F. Schwabe, E. Seki and D. A. Brenner, *Gastroenterology*, 2006, **130**, 1886–1900.
39. P. Iakova, S. S. Awad and N. A. Timchenko, *Cell*, 2003, **113**, 495–506.
40. A. Regev and E. R. Schiff, *Gastroenterol. Clin. North. Am.*, 2001, **30**, 547–563, x–xi.
41. J. S. Hammond, I. N. Guha, I. J. Beckingham and D. N. Lobo, *Br. J. Surg.*, 2011, **98**, 1188–1200.
42. T. Poynard, P. Bedossa and P. Opolon, *Lancet*, 1997, **349**, 825–832.
43. S. B. Missiha, M. Ostrowski and E. J. Heathcote, *Gastroenterology*, 2008, **134**, 1699–1714.
44. M. W. Djojosubroto, Y. S. Choi, H. W. Lee and K. L. Rudolph, *Mol. Cells*, 2003, **15**, 164–175.
45. H. Aikata, H. Takaishi, Y. Kawakami, S. Takahashi, M. Kitamoto, T. Nakanishi, Y. Nakamura, F. Shimamoto, G. Kajiyama and T. Ide, *Exp. Cell Res.*, 2000, **256**, 578–582.
46. Y. Deng, S. S. Chan and S. Chang, *Nat. Rev. Cancer*, 2008, **8**, 450–458.
47. K. L. Rudolph, S. Chang, M. Millard, N. Schreiber-Agus and R. A. DePinho, *Science*, 2000, **287**, 1253–1258.
48. K. G. Tolman and R. Sirrine, *Clin. Liver Dis.*, 1998, **2**.
49. G. Mastrangelo, U. Fedeli, E. Fadda, F. Valentini, R. Agnesi, G. Magarotto, T. Marchi, A. Buda, M. Pinzani and D. Martines, *Environ. Health Perspect.*, 2004, **112**, 1188–1192.
50. H. I. Hsieh, P. C. Chen, R. H. Wong, J. D. Wang, P. M. Yang and T. J. Cheng, *Toxicology*, 2007, **239**, 34–44.
51. Y. S. Lin, T. J. Smith, D. Wypij, K. T. Kelsey and F. M. Sacks, *Environ. Health Perspect.*, 2002, **110**, 165–168.
52. M. Cave, K. C. Falkner, M. Ray, S. Joshi-Barve, G. Brock, R. Khan, M. Bon Homme and C. J. McClain, *Hepatology*, 2010, **51**, 474–481.
53. N. Brautbar and J. Williams, 2nd, *Int. J. Hyg. Environ. Health*, 2002, **205**, 479–491.
54. T. W. Kensler, B. D. Roebuck, G. N. Wogan and J. D. Groopman, *Toxicol. Sci.*, 2011, **120**(Suppl 1), S28–48.
55. H. Kopelman, P. Scheurer and R. Williams, *Quart. J. Med.*, 1966, **35**, 533–564.
56. L. Nichols, *Int. Arch. Occup. Environ. Health*, 2004, **77**, 592–594.
57. E. Gelpi, M. P. de la Paz, B. Terracini, I. Abaitua, A. G. de la Camara, E. M. Kilbourne, C. Lahoz, B. Nemery, R. M. Philen, L. Soldevilla and S. Tarkowski, *Environ. Health Perspect.*, 2002, **110**, 457–464.
58. M. Patel, K. C. Falkner, C. J. McClain, G. Brock, S. Appana and M. Cave, *Gastroenterology*, 2009, **136**, 289.
59. M. Cave, S. Appana, M. Patel, K. C. Falkner, C. J. McClain and G. Brock, *Environ. Health Perspect.*, 2010, **118**, 1735–1742.
60. J. Liu, W. Drane, X. Liu and T. Wu, *Environ. Res.*, 2009, **109**, 193–199.
61. M.Cave, K. C.Falkner and C. J.McClain, in *Zakim and Boyer's Hepatology: A Textbook of Liver Disease*, eds. T. Boyer, M. Manns and A. Sanyal, Elsevier Saunders, Philadelphia, 6th edn., 2011, pp. 476–492.

62. M. Ates, A. Dirican, D. Ozgor, C. Aydin, B. Isik, C. Ara, M. Yilmaz, M. Ayse Selimoglu, C. Kayaalp and S. Yilmaz, *Liver Transpl.*, 2011, **17**, 1286–1291.
63. H. von Rettberg, T. Hannman, U. Subotic, J. Brade, T. Schaible, K. L. Waag and S. Loff, *Pediatrics*, 2009, **124**, 710–716.
64. H. L. Tsang, S. Wu, C. K. Leung, S. Tao and M. H. Wong, *Environ. Int.*, 2011, **37**, 142–151.
65. H. Zimmerman, *Hepatotoxicity: The Adverse Effects Of Drugs And Other Chemicals On The Liver*, Lippincott Williams & Wilkins, Philadelphia, 2 edn, 1999.
66. G.Farrell, *Drug-Induced Liver Disease*, Churchill Livingstone, New York, 1994.
67. M. Cave, K. C. Falkner, L. Henry, B. Costello, B. Gregory and C. J. McClain, *J Occup. Environ. Med.*, 2011, **53**, 1128–1133.
68. H. P. Cotrim, L. A. De Freitas, C. Freitas, L. Braga, R. Sousa, F. Carvalho, R. Parana, R. Santos-Jesus and Z. Andrade, *Liver Int.*, 2004, **24**, 131–135.
69. M. Cave, K. C. Falkner, B. Costello, B. Gregory, L. D. Henry and C. J. McClain, *The Toxicologist CD Supplement to Toxicological Sciences — An Official Journal of the Society of Toxicology*, 2011, **120**(Suppl 2).
70. M. Cave, I. Deaciuc, C. Mendez, Z. Song, S. Joshi-Barve, S. Barve and C. McClain, *The Journal of Nutritional Biochemistry*, 2007, **18**, 184–195.
71. J. L. Creech, Jr. and M. N. Johnson, *J. Occup Med.*, 1974, **16**, 150–151.
72. R. J. Bull, *Environ. Health Perspect.*, 2000, **108**(Suppl 2), 241–259.
73. L. H. Lash and J. C. Parker, *Pharmacol. Rev.*, 2001, **53**, 177–208.
74. C. H. Tamburro, L. Makk and H. Popper, *Hepatology*, 1984, **4**, 413–418.
75. J. Kielhorn, C. Melber, U. Wahnschaffe, A. Aitio and I. Mangelsdorf, *Environ. Health Perspect.*, 2000, **108**, 579–588.
76. P. F. Infante, S. E. Petty, D. H. Groth, G. Markowitz and D. Rosner, *Int. J. Occup. Environ. Health*, 2009, **15**, 36–42.
77. R. E. Hefner, Jr., P. G. Watanabe and P. J. Gehring, *Environ. Health Perspect.*, 1975, **11**, 85–95.
78. D. Antonino-Green, M. W. Linder, P. Fortwengler, S. Looney, T. E. Geoghegan and R. J. Valdes, *Proc. Am. Assoc. Cancer Res.*, 2000, **41**.
79. F. Ji, Y. J. Zheng, Q. Wang, W. Wang, Y. L. Qiu, F. Wu, S. J. Chai, J. Li and Z. L. Xia, *Zhonghua Lao Dong Wei Sheng Zhi Ye Bing Za Zhi*, 2011, **29**, 583–588.
80. C. Y. Huang, K. L. Huang, T. J. Cheng, J. D. Wang and L. L. Hsieh, *Arch. Toxicol.*, 1997, **71**, 482–488.
81. H. M. Bolt, *Criti. Rev. Toxicol.*, 2005, **35**, 307–323.
82. K. C. Falkner, B. G. Hill, B. Sansbury, C. J. McClain and M. Cave, *Hepatology*, 2010, **52**, 266A.
83. S. M. Cohen, R. D. Storer, K. A. Criswell, N. G. Doerrer, V. L. Dellarco, D. G. Pegg, Z. W. Wojcinski, D. E. Malarkey, A. C. Jacobs,

J. E. Klaunig, J. A. Swenberg and J. C. Cook, *Toxicol. Sci.*, 2009, **111**, 4–18.
84. M. Cave, R. Groce, A. Mahalingashetty, S. Joshi-Barve, L. Reynolds and C. J. McClain, *Hepatology*, 2007, **46**.
85. K. A. Mundt, L. D. Dell, R. P. Austin, R. S. Luippold, R. Noess and C. Bigelow, *Occup. Environ. Med.*, 2000, **57**, 774–781.
86. E. Ward, P. Boffetta, A. Andersen, D. Colin, P. Comba, J. A. Deddens, M. De Santis, G. Engholm, L. Hagmar, S. Langard, I. Lundberg, D. McElvenny, R. Pirastu, D. Sali and L. Simonato, *Epidemiology*, 2001, **12**, 710–718.
87. Y. L. Qiu, P. Sun, W. Wang, T. Wang and Z. L. Xia, *J. Occup. Environ. Med.*, 2011, **53**, 1442–1446.
88. Y. L. Qiu, W. Wang, T. Wang, P. Sun, F. Wu, S. M. Zhu, J. Qian, L. Jin, W. Au and Z. L. Xia, *Int. J. Hyg. Environ. Health*, 2011, **214**, 225–230.
89. G. E. Trivers, H. L. Cawley, V. M. DeBenedetti, M. Hollstein, M. J. Marion, W. P. Bennett, M. L. Hoover, C. C. Prives, C. C. Tamburro and C. C. Harris, *J. Natl Cancer Inst.*, 1995, **87**, 1400–1407.
90. P. Gedigk, R. Muller and H. Bechtelsheimer, *Ann. N. Y. Acad. Sci.*, 1975, **246**, 278–285.
91. T. J. Hsiao, J. D. Wang, P. M. Yang, P. C. Yang and T. J. Cheng, *J. Occup. Environ. Med.*, 2004, **46**, 962–966.
92. M. Maroni, F. Mocci, S. Visentin, G. Preti and A. C. Fanetti, *Occup. Environ. Med.*, 2003, **60**, 60–65.
93. Y. Y. Gong, S. Wilson, J. K. Mwatha, M. N. Routledge, J. M. Castelino, B. Zhao, G. Kimani, H. C. Kariuki, B. J. Vennervald, D. W. Dunne and C. P. Wild, *Environ. Health Perspect.*, 2012.
94. I. Amla, C. S. Kamala, G. S. Gopalakrishna, A. P. Jayaraj, V. Sreenivasamurthy and H. A. Parpia, *Am. J. Clin. Nutr.*, 1971, **24**, 609–614.
95. P. Khlangwiset, G. S. Shephard and F. Wu, *Crit. Rev. Toxicol.*, 2011, **41**, 740–755.
96. J. H. Williams, T. D. Phillips, P. E. Jolly, J. K. Stiles, C. M. Jolly and D. Aggarwal, *Am. J. Clin. Nutr.*, 2004, **80**, 1106–1122.
97. L. Lewis, M. Onsongo, H. Njapau, H. Schurz-Rogers, G. Luber, S. Kieszak, J. Nyamongo, L. Backer, A. M. Dahiye, A. Misore, K. DeCock and C. Rubin, *Environ. Health Perspect.*, 2005, **113**, 1763–1767.
98. L. Zhang, Y. Ye, Y. An, Y. Tian, Y. Wang and H. Tang, *J. Proteome. Res.*, 2011, **10**, 614–623.
99. A. G. Valdivia, A. Martinez, F. J. Damian, T. Quezada, R. Ortiz, C. Martinez, J. Llamas, M. L. Rodriguez, L. Yamamoto, F. Jaramillo, M. G. Loarca-Pina and J. L. Reyes, *Poult. Sci.*, 2001, **80**, 727–734.
100. M. P. Sajan, J. G. Satav and R. K. Bhattacharya, *Indian J. Exp. Biol.*, 1997, **35**, 1187–1190.

101. M. P. Waalkes, J. Liu, H. Chen, Y. Xie, W. E. Achanzar, Y. S. Zhou, M. L. Cheng and B. A. Diwan, *J. Natl. Cancer Inst.*, 2004, **96**, 466–474.
102. D. N. Mazumder, *Toxicol. Appl. Pharmacol.*, 2005, **206**, 169–175.
103. A. Santra, J. Das Gupta, B. K. De, B. Roy and D. N. Guha Mazumder, *Indian J. Gastroenterol.*, 1999, **18**, 152–155.
104. A. Santra, A. Maiti, S. Das, S. Lahiri, S. K. Charkaborty and D. N. Mazumder, *J. Toxicol. Clin. Toxicol*, 2000, **38**, 395–405.
105. A. C. Straub, D. B. Stolz, M. A. Ross, A. Hernandez-Zavala, N. V. Soucy, L. R. Klei and A. Barchowsky, *Hepatology*, 2007, **45**, 205–212.
106. M. P. Waalkes, J. Liu, J. M. Ward and B. A. Diwan, *Toxicol. Appl. Pharmacol.*, 2006, **215**, 295–305.
107. A. H. Mokdad, E. S. Ford, B. A. Bowman, W. H. Dietz, F. Vinicor, V. S. Bales and J. S. Marks, *JAMA*, 2003, **289**, 76–79.
108. A. H. Welch, S. A. Watkins, D. R. Helsel and M. J. Focazio, *U. S. Geological Survey Fact Sheet FS-063-00*, 2000.
109. U. S. G. Survey, 2007.
110. C. f. D. C. a. Prevention, 2007.
111. M. Tan, R. H. Schmidt, J. I. Beier, W. H. Watson, H. Zhong, J. C. States and G. E. Arteel, *Toxicol. Appl. Pharmacol.*, 2011, **257**, 356–364.
112. J. Frith, D. Jones and J. L. Newton, *Age Ageing*, 2009, **38**, 11–18.
113. A. Floreani, *Dig Dis*, 2007, **25**, 138–143.
114. P. Meier and H. K. Seitz, *Curr. Opin. Clin. Nutr. Metab. Care*, 2008, **11**, 21–26.
115. D. L. Schmucker and R. K. Wang, *Exp. Gerontol.*, 1980, **15**, 423–431.
116. H. K. Seitz and F. Stickel, *Clinics in Geriatric Medicine*, 2007, **23**, 905–921, viii.
117. C. S. Lieber, *Annu.Rev. Nutr.*, 2000, **20**, 395–430.
118. O. Falade-Nwulia and C. L. Thio, *Sexual health*, 2011, **8**, 512–520.
119. Z. M. Younossi, M. Stepanova, M. Afendy, Y. Fang, Y. Younossi, H. Mir and M. Srishord, *Clin. Gastroenterol. Hepatol.*, 2011, **9**, 524–530 e521; quiz e560.
120. L. S. Szczepaniak, P. Nurenberg, D. Leonard, J. D. Browning, J. S. Reingold, S. Grundy, H. H. Hobbs and R. L. Dobbins, *Am. J. Physiol. Endocrinol. Metab.*, 2005, **288**, E462–468.
121. L. Gan, S. Chitturi and G. C. Farrell, *Curr. Gerontol. Geriatr. Res.*, 2011, **2011**, 831536.
122. J. Frith, C. P. Day, E. Henderson, A. D. Burt and J. L. Newton, *Gerontology*, 2009, **55**, 607–613.
123. M. D. Merrell and N. J. Cherrington, *Drug. Metab. Rev.*, 2011, **43**, 317–334.
124. A. D. Lake, P. Novak, C. D. Fisher, J. P. Jackson, R. N. Hardwick, D. D. Billheimer, W. T. Klimecki and N. J. Cherrington, *Drug Metabolism and Disposition: the Biological Fate of Chemicals*, 2011, **39**, 1954–1960.
125. R. N. Hardwick, C. D. Fisher, M. J. Canet, G. L. Scheffer and N. J. Cherrington, *Drug Metabolism and Disposition: the Biological Fate of Chemicals*, 2011, **39**, 2395–2402.

126. M. K. Mohommad, Z. Zhou, M. Cave, A. Barve and C. J. McClain, *Nutrition in Clinical Practice: Official Publication of the American Society for Parenteral and Enteral Nutrition*, 2012, **27**, 8–20.
127. A. F. Carrion and P. Martin, *Am. J. Gastroenterol.*, 2012, **107**, 691–697.
128. U. H. Iloeje, H. I. Yang, J. Su, C. L. Jen, S. L. You and C. J. Chen, *Gastroenterology*, 2006, **130**, 678–686.
129. A. S. Lok and B. J. McMahon, *Hepatology*, 2009, **50**, 661–662.
130. D. Thabut, S. Le Calvez, V. Thibault, J. Massard, M. Munteanu, V. Di Martino, V. Ratziu and T. Poynard, *Am. J. Gastroenterol.*, 2006, **101**, 1260–1267.
131. T. Poynard, V. Ratziu, F. Charlotte, Z. Goodman, J. McHutchison and J. Albrecht, *J. Hepatol.*, 2001, **34**, 730–739.
132. E. Minola, D. Prati, F. Suter, F. Maggiolo, F. Caprioli, A. Sonzogni, M. Fraquelli, S. Paggi and D. Conte, *Blood*, 2002, **99**, 4588–4591.
133. J. R. Lake, J. S. Shorr, B. J. Steffen, A. H. Chu, R. D. Gordon and R. H. Wiesner, *Am. J. Transplant.*, 2005, **5**, 549–557.
134. H. I. Hsieh, J. D. Wang, P. C. Chen and T. J. Cheng, *Occup. Environ. Med.*, 2003, **60**, 774–778.
135. C. L. Du and J. D. Wang, *Occup. Environ. Med.*, 1998, **55**, 528–532.
136. C. P. Wild and R. Montesano, *Cancer Lett.*, 2009, **286**, 22–28.
137. S. Joshi-Barve, K. Amancherla, M. Patil, A. Bhatnagar, S. Mathews, L. Gobejishvili, M. Cave, C. McClain and S. Barve, *Free Radic. Biol. Med.*, 2009, **47**, 47–54.
138. S. J. Mitchell and S. N. Hilmer, *Therapeutic Advances in Drug Safety*, 2010, **1**, 65–77.
139. J. G. Stine and J. H. Lewis, *Expert Opin. Drug Metab. Toxicol.*, 2011, **7**, 875–890.
140. J. Polson and W. M. Lee, *Hepatology*, 2005, **41**, 1179–1197.
141. W. M. Lee, *Best Practice & Research. Clinical Gastroenterology*, 2012, **26**, 3–16.
142. R. J. Andrade, M. I. Lucena, M. C. Fernandez, G. Pelaez, K. Pachkoria, E. Garcia-Ruiz, B. Garcia-Munoz, R. Gonzalez-Grande, A. Pizarro, J. A. Duran, M. Jimenez, L. Rodrigo, M. Romero-Gomez, J. M. Navarro, R. Planas, J. Costa, A. Borras, A. Soler, J. Salmeron and R. Martin-Vivaldi, *Gastroenterology*, 2005, **129**, 512–521.

CHAPTER 17

Immune System Disorders

RODNEY R. DIETERT

Department of Microbiology and Immunology, College of Veterinary Medicine, Cornell University, North Tower Rd. Ithaca, NY 14853, USA
E-mail: rrd1@cornell.edu

17.1 Introduction

The immune system is composed of a variety of different cell types that contribute in a coordinated manner to provide: 1) host defense, 2) tissue surveillance and integrity, and 3) the homeostatic regulation of function of tissue and organs. Because immune cells are distributed during early development to virtually every tissue and organ of the body, the functional status of these resident immune cells can greatly influence the overall function of the tissue or organ, as well as the risk of subsequent pathology. Besides systemic immune dysfunction, immune dysfunction of specialized populations such as microglia in the brain, alveolar macrophages in the respiratory tract, and Kupffer cells in the liver can directly mediate organ pathologies and diseases.

Therefore, immune system disorders should not be thought of as diseases restricted to the primary and secondary lymphoid organs (*e.g.*, thymus, spleen). Instead, immune disorder-based diseases span every medical categorization and coding.[1] Of course this also means that immune disorders are usually underestimated since they are likely to be given a different medical label. Examples of this would be for diseases such as psoriasis, atherosclerosis, asthma, autoimmune thyroiditis, and inflammatory bowel disease, which are likely to be categorized as dermal, cardiovascular, respiratory, endocrine, and gastrointestinal diseases respectively. However, in reality—if one examines the basis

Issues in Toxicology No. 16
Aging and Vulnerability to Environmental Chemicals: Age-related Disorders and their Origins in Environmental Exposures
Edited by Bernard Weiss

Published by the Royal Society of Chemistry, www.rsc.org

of these diseases and not just the involved tissues where the pathology occurs—these are all immune dysfunction-based diseases featuring inflammatory misregulation.[2]

A recent topic of interest has been the various ways in which environmental factors such as pollutants can cause immune alterations that then lead to chronic diseases. Historically, the focus of immunotoxicology was on ensuring the integrity of the immune system to provide host defense, protecting against infectious agents.[3] Detection of detrimental effects of the environment on immune-mediated host defense was seen as the foremost priority during the era where HIV/AIDS-associated immunosuppression was emerging as a critical health threat. Obviously, reduction of immune function remains a concern. But more recently, this priority was overshadowed by the potential for environmental risk factors to cause other adverse immune outcomes that are far more directly connected to the risk of major chronic diseases: inappropriate immune enhancement, autoimmunity, and misregulated inflammation.[1]

As will be described in this chapter, health risks tied to environmentally-induced immune system disorders are not restricted to a handful of random diseases and conditions, such as loss of host defense, increased risk of infections, and leukemia. In stark contrast, the immune system disorders that result from early-life environmental insult predispose individuals not just to acute illnesses, but also to chronic diseases. They also increase the probability that individuals will carry the burden of multiple chronic diseases over a lifetime.[4] New patterns of elevated health risks for several interlinked chronic diseases and conditions can emerge from a single ill-timed environmental exposure.[5] Many of these immune-based chronic diseases will emerge later in life during the normal aging process. This chapter describes the cause–effect relationships between problematic environmental conditions, developmental immunotoxicity (DIT), immune dysfunction, inflammatory misregulation, and chronic diseases. It also discusses opportunities that could reduce the risk of prevalence of chronic diseases that emerge during the aging process.

17.2 Immune Cells as Environmental Sentries at the Portals of Entry

Components of the immune system are dispersed throughout the body and are particularly concentrated at the portals where initial environmental exposure occurs (airways, gastrointestinal system, skin, and reproductive-excretory systems). It is here that these resident immune cells play a role in sampling the environment for danger signals, including the introduction of potential pathogens. But it is also these same cells that are among the first to encounter potentially harmful environmental factors. By location alone, virtually any environmental exposure is likely to involve the exposure of at least some immune cell populations (*via* the airways, skin, and gut). The question then becomes not whether any immune cell populations were exposed to a toxicant, but rather when are exposures significant relative to risk of immune dysfunction, pathology, and disease? Isolated exposure of small populations of specialized cells such as brain microglia, alveolar macrophages, gut intraepithelial lymphocytes, or skin dendritic cells might be viewed as having quite limited consequences. But the relative sensitivity and functional implications of environmental damage to these immune cell residents in tissues is often either underestimated or uncertain. For example in the child, environmental factors interact with both the gut microbial population and mucosal immune cells to produce significant local immune alteration.[6–8] But this alteration can result in immune problems and elevated risk of diseases that extend beyond the gut to several other tissues and organs. In mice, investigators recently demonstrated that the status of the gut microbiome and changes in gastrointestinal immune cell populations affect the risk of neurologically-based experimental autoimmune encephalomyelitis.[9] This is an important concept: that the status of gastrointestinal immune cell populations appears to affect the risk of neurological chronic disease. The implications are that environmentally-induced alterations of local resident immune cell populations may elevate health risks involving other tissues and organs, or even systemically. But how or why might this happen? At least one possible explanation lies in the observation that the immune system appears to exist as a fractal network, despite its dispersal in tissues. With this in mind, local effects have the potential to lead to functional or pathological ramifications in non-local tissues.[1]

17.3 Early-Life Origins of Adult Immune-Based Diseases

17.3.1 Development Origins of Disease: The Barker Hypothesis

One of the challenges in identifying the risk of immune-based diseases from exposure to environmental factors such as toxicants is the issue of the time interval between problematic exposures and disease onset. The concept of a developmental basis of adult disease was advanced in prior decades and became known as the "Barker Hypothesis".[10–12] But while the original concept was framed primarily as related to undernutrition and risk of subsequent cardiovascular disease,[13] it is now clear that the connection between fetal environment and adult disease is far more extensive in scope and impact.[14–16] The range of environmental factors that can produce a fetal linkage with risk of adult disease goes well beyond undernutrition, and the adverse outcomes are not restricted to just cardiovascular disease.[17] The concept of developmental origins of chronic diseases has become a major issue in toxicology.[18–20]

17.3.2 Critical Windows of Immune Vulnerability

While early-life insult and developmentally programmed dysfunction can affect any physiological system, the immune system represents a particular concern as a target. In general, environmentally-induced immune alterations in the young are termed developmental immunotoxicity (DIT), as the categorization encompasses many different types of environmental factors or agents.[21] Immune maturation occurs in discrete steps during both prenatal and postnatal development.[22,23] These steps must occur with precision and precise developmental timing to produce a functioning, effectively regulated, and well-balanced immune system in the child.

The basic concept that during development there are critical windows of vulnerability for the immune system has existed for more than a decade.[24–28] The conceptual framework states that specific maturational events are precisely timed with specific windows of prenatal and/or neonatal development. Because the maturational events are both critical for integrity of the child's immune system and may be restricted to one or a few windows of development, their disruption can have not only devastating effects on subsequent immune function, but also environmentally-mediated effects that are likely distinct from those produced by similar exposures at other periods of development. Examples of critical windows for the immune system would be: 1) emergence of myelomonocytic cells and seeding of tissues and organs, 2) first appearance of microglia cells, 3) seeding and expanded distribution of microglia cells in the cerebral wall, 4) appearance and expansion of astrocyte populations, 5) seeding of thymus with thymocytes and selection against autoreactive T-cell clones, 6) emergence, seeding, and expansion of Treg populations as well as Th17 cells, 7) emergence and expansion of intraepithelial lymphocytes (IELs) contributing to the gastrointestine-associated lymphoid tissue (GALT), 8) alteration of macrophages and macrophage-related cells in response to collectins (surfactants), 9) maturation of dendritic cells to promote Th1 responses, and 10) maturation of innate immune cells in response to neonatal intestinal microbiota (information adapted from ref. 29).

While this conceptual framework for "critical windows" emerged for the immune system and had strong biological plausibility,[28] proof of concept was needed. Data supporting proof of concept for the existence and significance of critical developmental windows of immune vulnerability were obtained *via* examination of the effects of developmental exposure to the heavy metal lead.[30] When lead exposure was restricted to different narrow windows of early development, different immune alterations were observed in the offspring. Developmentally-restricted exposure to lead produced both quantitatively and qualitatively different adverse immune outcomes in the young. Because similar results were obtained comparing development windows using two different test species,[30] the "critical window" of lead exposure appeared to be paramount in determining what kind of immune alterations would be seen in the offspring. This and other studies indicated that developmental timing is of vital importance when it comes to both dose–response sensitivity and the spectrum of toxicant-induced immune alterations that will result.

Age-based comparisons among several chemicals and drugs led to the conclusion that children are more susceptible to immmuntoxicity than are adults.[31] This increased susceptibility can take several forms. Lower doses of chemicals and drugs are likely to produce adverse immune effects following exposure of the young, compared to adults. Additionally, immunotoxic exposures of the young are more likely to produce a broader spectrum of adverse effects than exposures of adults. The adverse effects of immunotoxicity in the young (*i.e.*, DIT) are more likely to persist than those in the adult. Immunotoxicity following exposure of the young is more likely to appear at a much later age following some second environmental exposure (or conditions, *e.g.*, stress). The early-life, seemingly innocuous, exposure developmental programming for dysfunction becomes apparent following a later, often adult, environmental exposure. A classic example of this is described where prenatal exposure of mice to disethylstilbesterol (DES) appears to permanently alter the cytokine programming of lymphocytes, which becomes physiologically evident after a second low-level adult exposure to DES.[32] It is important to recognize that: 1) some maturational steps are systemic, while others occur only in specific organs or tissues, and 2) even organ-specific maturational steps may affect immune status of other tissues later in life. An example of the latter is the ability of the environmental influences on the immune–gut microbiome interaction in the neonate to affect the risk of multiple manifestations of allergic diseases in the child.[33,34]

This concept of "critical windows" in the young becomes important in estimations of health risk in the absence of age-relevant data. For example, if only adult exposure data exist for the immune system, it is not possible to know whether environmental exposure might disrupt a key immune maturation event that is restricted to early development. This is not a matter of simple dose-sensitivity differences, but rather, it is an issue of whether critical targets are lacking in the adult test system. In effect, it nullifies the utility for the adult exposure test system for non-adults. For this reason, four immunotoxicologists recently called for required DIT testing of chemicals and drugs.[5]

17.3.3 The Scope of Adverse Outcomes Occurring with DIT

As mentioned briefly in the introduction, the historical focus of immunotoxicity testing had two primary goals: 1) detection of immunosuppression,[35] and 2) the identification chemicals that could serve as sensitizers.[36,37] Assays and biomarkers were designed accordingly and many were intended to serve as surrogates of host resistance challenges (again, where a loss of host defense was measured).[38] These were quite effective for their intended purposes, and it was found that a small collection of assays were capable of providing reliable indications of chemically-induced immunosuppression in animal models.[39]

However, the scope of the required detection of adverse immune outcomes, and particularly that associated with early developmental exposures, has changed dramatically. It is no longer risk of immunosuppression that is the preeminent concern. Given current disease prevalences, identification of the risk of allergic, autoimmune, and inflammatory diseases is a major priority in safety testing. This shift in safety testing focus was recently discussed in the content of immune-based diseases.[5] Because of the broader scope of potentially problematic immune alterations that can occur and the disease ramifications,

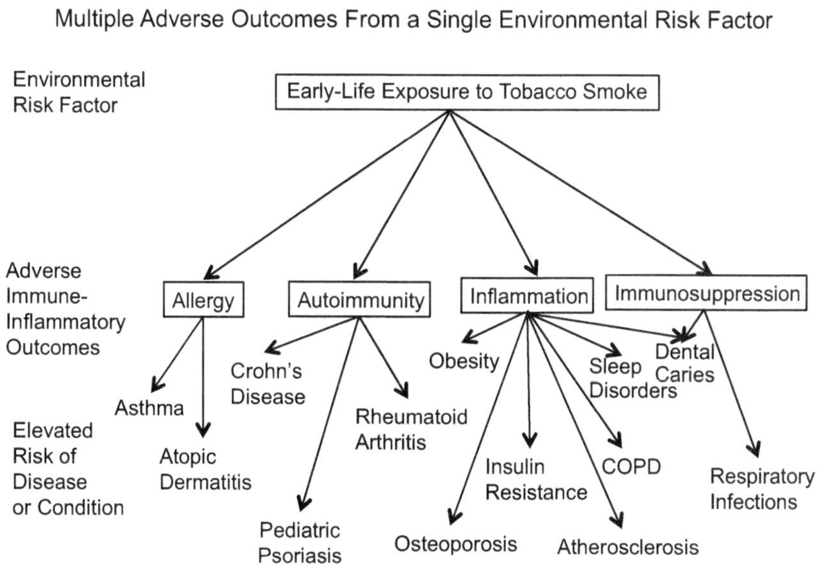

Figure 17.1 The figure illustrates the multiple immune dysfunctions and/or inflammatory-based health risks associated with early-life exposure to tobacco smoke. Immunosuppression (*i.e.*, reduced host resistance) is far from the only concern. In fact, improper immune enhancement, including elevated risk of allergic, autoimmune, and inflammatory diseases, is a significant chronic health concern.

new approaches are needed to ensure protection of the developing immune system.[1] To emphasize the range of immune dysfunction-based outcomes that can occur from a single toxicant source, Figure 17.1 illustrates the elevated immune-inflammatory disease risks reported to be linked with early-life exposure to tobacco smoke. The elevated risks of disease run the full gamut of adverse immune outcomes, ranging from elevated risk of infections and cancer to increased risk of allergic, autoimmune and inflammatory diseases. While tobacco smoke contains numerous immunotoxicants, it is still only one of many sources for environmental insult of the immune system. Among the diseases and conditions characterized by inflammatory misregulation and linked with early-life exposure to tobacco smoke are: asthma,[40] atherosclerosis,[41] atopic dermatitis,[42,43] Crohn's disease,[44] dental caries,[45] early-onset chronic obstructive pulmonary disease,[46] insulin resistance,[47] obesity,[48] osteoporosis,[49] pediatric psoriasis,[50] rheumatoid arthritis,[51] susceptibility to respiratory infections,[52] and sleep disorders.[53]

Environmental events that affect immune development and programming have significant ramifications in later life, and there is increasing appreciation of the potential impact of these exposures across all aspects of immune system function (*e.g.*, both adaptive and innate immunity). Maternal exposures have been reported to alter the course of innate immune development in the offspring such that the risk of immune imbalances[54] and inflammatory disease is increased.[55] Figure 17.2 provides examples of innate immune cell immunotoxicity by chemicals and drugs that result in inappropriate inflammation in tissues. It is precisely these types of adverse immune outcomes, particularly in children, that can establish a life course of inflammation-driven chronic diseases.

Feltes *et al.*[56] postulated that prenatal programming establishes the pathway to aging in adults, in which inflammation plays a major role. Microbes in the gastrointestinal tract and possibly the respiratory tract play a significant role in the early-life immune programming process.[57] This means that environmental conditions that affect the microbiome can exert a disproportionate influence on immune programming for risk of adult disease.[58] Other groups have shown that early neonatal exposure can have similar effects in which the developing immune system is programmed for later dysfunctional responses in the adult when the immune system is challenged.[59] Several research groups have attributed the rise in inflammatory-based diseases, including allergic and autoimmune diseases, to suboptimum early-life environmental effects on the prenatal and neonatal immune system.[60] Even inappropriately timed immune activation can have later life ramifications. For example, prenatal immune challenges can establish a cascade of metabolic and immune-inflammatory alterations that contribute to the risk of schizophrenia.[61,62]

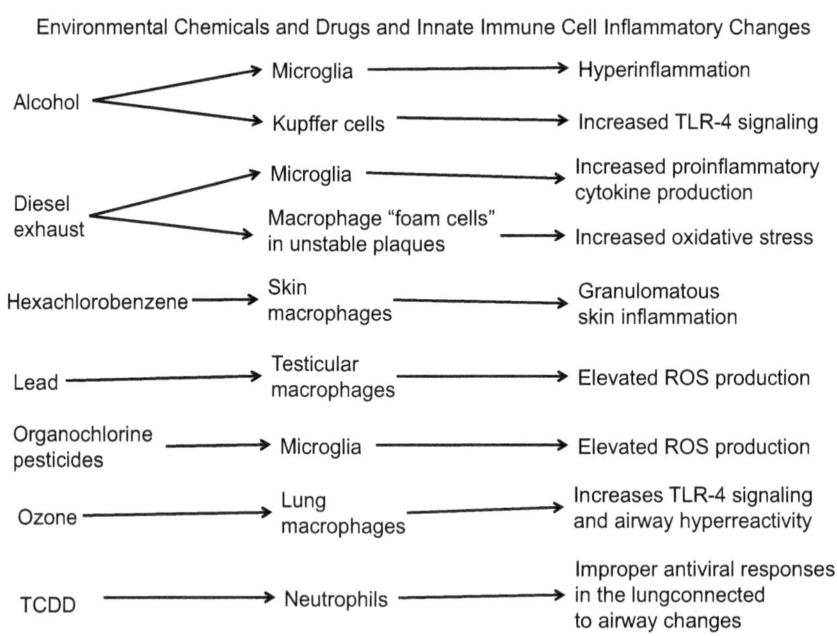

Figure 17.2 Environmental chemicals and drugs can produce immunotoxicity in resident innate immune cells in tissues, resulting in inappropriate inflammatory responses and subsequent pathology. (Information adapted from Dietert, 2009a).

Examples of specific chronic diseases and conditions that are connected to immune-inflammatory dysfunction, have environment determinants, and are thought to have earlier-in-life origins include: Alzheimer's disease,[63] asthma,[64] atherosclerosis,[65] atopic dermatitis,[42] autism,[4,66] autoimmune thyroiditis,[67] celiac disease,[68] chronic kidney disease,[69,70] chronic obstructive pulmonary disease,[71] depression,[72,73] endometriosis,[74] food allergies,[75,76] inflammatory bowel disease,[44,77] myalgic encephalomyelitis,[78] multiple sclerosis,[79] psoriasis,[80] rheumatoid arthritis,[81] schizophrenia,[61,62] sleep disorders,[53] systemic lupus erythematosus,[82] and type 1 diabetes.[83,84]

17.3.4 Sex-Specific Adverse Outcomes and Diseases Implications

One of the more recent findings concerning DIT and health risks is that males and females can differ in the specific adverse outcomes that may occur following an early-life immune insult. In fact, a majority of chemicals and drugs examined thus far exhibit strong sex-specificity for the nature of the immune alterations that are seen with DIT. It is useful to recognize that if the same exposure can induce differences in immune alterations between males and females, then it is likely to result in sex-specific chronic disease outcomes as well. For example, exposure of the young to the same dose of an immunotoxicant might produce an elevated risk of atherosclerosis in males and systemic lupus erythematosus (SLE) in females. Environmental epigenetic programming also appears to exhibit sexual dimorphism.[85] As a result it is important to consider the likelihood that early-life immunotoxic exposures will produce different outcomes in males *vs.* females and different elevated risks of specific immune-dysfunction-based diseases.

Examples of sex-specific adverse immune outcomes have been reported for the following: atrazine,[86] lead,[87] genistein,[88] mercury,[89] TCDD,[90] and nonylphenol.[91]

This also translates to differences among sexes for environmentally-influenced immune dysfunction-based diseases. For example, Caesarian (*vs.* vaginal) delivery has been reported to increase the risk for Crohn's disease in boys but not in girls.[92] In mice, a neonatal chlamydial respiratory infection was reported to differentially alter the immune gene expression pathways of males *vs.* females. An infection-driven Th2 helper bias was observed in adult females after the neonatal exposures, but did not occur in infected male mice.[93]

The existence of sex-specific differences in immunotoxicity in many ways parallels, and may partially explain, observed sex-specific difference in the prevalences of specific inflammatory diseases. For example, autoimmune diseases occur in both sexes, yet for the majority of autoimmune diseases, there is sexual dimorphism with a strong preponderance of females affected compared with males.[94,95] This is seen in diseases such as SLE, multiple sclerosis, Hashimoto's thyroiditis, Sjogren syndrome, and rheumatoid arthritis.[96–98] An environmental component has been suggested for a least part of the sex bias that has been observed in autoimmune diseases.[99] There are some possible clues as to the basis for this sex-determine difference. In general, the greater prevalence of the disease and the later that it emerges in life, the more likely it is to have a major bias in females.[95] Even in men and women with the same autoimmune disease, there can be marked differences in the presentation and characteristics of the disease.[100,101] In a Taiwanese population study, Weng et al.[98] reported that females were 10 times more likely to have SLE, while SLE-related mortality was 3 times greater in males than females. This difference in mortality is consistent with the report that male SLE patients tend to have increased severity of the disease compared with female patients.[102]

Other inflammatory-based diseases also show a strong gender bias. Myalgic encephalomyelitis (also termed chronic fatigue syndrome) is thought to be more prevalent in females than males,[103] as is Alzheimer's disease.[104] However, the latter may be affected, at least in part, by the longer lifespan of women.[105] In contrast, autism spectrum disorders[106] and Parkinson's disease are thought to be more prevalent in males than females.[107]

In many cases where the males and females have similar prevalences for an immune-inflammatory-based disease across a lifetime, there are major differences in the age of onset. For example, despite males and females having similar overall lifetime prevalences, males tend to be diagnosed with atopy and/or asthma at an earlier age than females.[108] The reverse of this age-of-diagnosis trend occurs with psoriasis. For this autoimmune-inflammatory disease, there is a greater prevalence in younger females than in younger males.[109]

17.4 Chronic Misregulated Inflammation Links Most Chronic Diseases

Chronic inflammation as a result of immune and inflammatory dysregulation is proving to be the thread that connects otherwise apparently disparate diseases that: 1) arise in different tissues, 2) are more prevalent in different genders and, 3) appear at different ages. In fact, immune dysfunction-based chronic inflammation is a probable cause of most chronic diseases today.[110–112] Prasad *et al.*[112] argued that these diseases are age-associated and that the solution to these leading causes of worldwide death and disability is a reduction in the inflammation-associated risk factors. If one begins to view diseases and conditions such as obesity, arthritis, osteoporosis, psoriasis, and frailty as merely different manifestations or adverse outcomes of a common underlying problem, misregulated inflammation, then health management over a lifetime would take a very different path from current practices. Comorbid patterns of chronic diseases become clear and more useful solutions and can be pursued once a target of underlying immune and inflammatory dysfunction is seen as the target for correction.

Once a child or young adult is diagnosed with an immune-based chronic disease, they automatically acquire elevated risks for several other chronic diseases.[3,5,113] Some of these additional diseases are likely to emerge later in life. The individual patterns may be identified based on the initially-diagnosed disease. For example, childhood asthma might be an entryway disease for an allergy pattern, type 1 diabetes initiates an autoimmune disease pattern, psoriasis initiates an inflammatory disease pattern, schizophrenia begins an immune activation pattern, and obesity starts a metabolic disease pattern. But in reality, these patterns have major overlaps and intersection points.[5] For example, depression and sleep disorders fall at the center of many inflammatory-based disease patterns because of the specific cytokine imbalances that are associated with the underlying immune dysfunction. Additionally, frailty is an end-stage inflammatory-based condition[114] that is comorbid for numerous other earlier-age-of onset diseases.[110,115]

Figure 17.3 illustrates the point that chronic diseases have many intersections and overlaps. Each childhood- or young adult- initiated disease pattern has both unique features as well a common ground in terms of predictable later-onset chronic diseases and conditions. Skin cancer is a predicted elevated later life risk of children and young adults with psoriasis. It is not a likely outcome for cohorts diagnosed with chronic kidney disease or type 1 diabetes. Yet, individuals with all of these conditions are at an elevated risk of inflammation-associated depression.

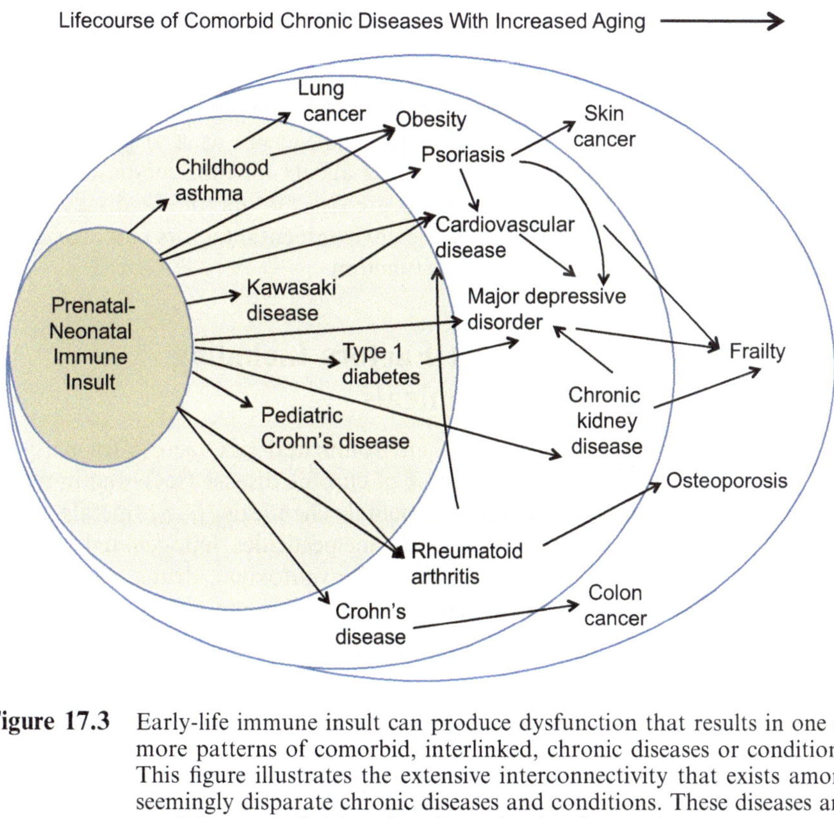

Figure 17.3 Early-life immune insult can produce dysfunction that results in one or more patterns of comorbid, interlinked, chronic diseases or conditions. This figure illustrates the extensive interconnectivity that exists among seemingly disparate chronic diseases and conditions. These diseases and conditions are all driven by misregulated inflammation.

Among the defects that appear common to many chronic diseases is the inability to resolve acute inflammation and, as a result, avoid inappropriate chronic inflammatory insults in the tissues.[116] Even low levels of chronic inflammation persisting over decades in tissues can result in loss of organ function, oxidative damage to cells increasing the risk of cancer in that tissue, and autoimmune reactions to components of the damaged tissue. Molecules that can correct this defect and permit acute inflammation to resolve appropriately offer significant promise as a more potential therapeutic of several chronic diseases.[117–119]

17.5 Environmental Triggers of Chronic Diseases

When immune dysfunction and a predisposition for misregulated inflammation is established in the young following environmental insult, there can still be a missing piece that is needed before the onset of many chronic diseases. That piece is a challenge for the immune system, which triggers the dysfunctional and inappropriate response in the tissues. In the case of childhood asthma, that is likely to be a combination of a propensity for IgE production against innocuous antigens, mobilization of eosinophils, and inappropriate inflammatory responses in the lung resulting in airway hyperreactivity and damage.[64] What has become clear is that many immune-based chronic diseases are diagnosed shortly after an infection. In the case of asthma, it is usually a respiratory infection. For gastrointestinal tract autoimmune conditions, it could well be a gastrointestinal infection that serves as a trigger. Dietert[3] discusses the role of infections as triggering agents for immune-based chronic disease. In this case, while the infections are risk factors for the diseases, they are not causative in the same way as the environmental factors (*e.g.*, toxicants) that cause the underlying immune dysfunction.

17.6 Environmental Risk Factors Including Environmental Chemicals

The literature contains a number of environmental risk factors for early-life immune programming and elevated risk of chronic disease (reviewed in ref. 1). Different categories include environmental chemicals (*e.g.*, metals, polychorinated biphenyls, dioxins, organochlorine pesticides, halogenated aromatic hydrocarbons, polyaromatic hydrocarbons, mycotoxins), drugs, diet, various stressors, infections, and birth delivery mode. Among drugs, examples of reported developmental immunotoxicants include alcohol,[120] antibiotics,[121] paracetamol,[122] dexamethasone,[123] and diethylstilbesterol.[124] Prenatal dietary factors include minerals,[125] vitamins,[126] fatty acids,[127] and phytoestrogens.[128]

In addition to external environmental risk factors such as chemicals and drugs, stress is major contributor to early-life programmed adverse immune outcomes.[129] This can come in the form of physical-psychological stress,[130,131] as well as stress from infectious challenges.[132] Additionally, the birth delivery mode (Caesarian *vs.* vaginal delivery) plays a major role in the immune status of the child. It is not yet clear which factors linked with delivery mode might mediate this immune effect (*e.g.*, use of prophylatic drugs, delivery stress, differences in microbial exposure).

Environmental chemicals represent a prominent category of developmental immunotoxicants, many of which produce multiple adverse immune outcomes following early-life exposure.[3] The chemicals are not toxic solely to the immune system. However, in some cases, the immune system represents one of the more sensitive targets for toxicity. Grandjean and colleagues reported that high intake of marine-based dietary PCBs by pregnant women in the Faroe Islands increased the risk of both allergic sensitization[133] and suppressed vaccine responses[133,134] in the offspring. Additionally, in mouse studies 2,3,7,8-tetrachlorodibenzodioxin (TCDD), a dioxin, appears to disrupt early immune development in several ways, resulting in inappropriate inflammatory responses,[135] a predisposition for some forms of autoimmunity,[136] and suppression of cell-mediated immunity.[137] Based on animal and human studies, developmental exposure to organochlorine pesticides can affect both adaptive immune responses,[138] as well as innate immune cell function such as inducing the elevated production of tumor necrosis factor-alpha (TNF-α), a pro-inflammatory cytokine.[139] Several studies in mice and humans suggest a role for trichloroethylene in causing immunosuppression[140] and in promoting auto-immunity, as reviewed by Cooper *et al.*[141] Also, from animal and humans studies, early-life exposure to Pb is able to elevate IgE levels,[142] particularly in children who are also exposed to cigarette smoke.[143] Early-life exposure to bisphenol A appears to promote a Th2 bias.[88,144] Perfluorinated compounds used in various industrial applications have also been reported to be immunotoxic in rodents and to promote inappropriate inflammation.[145]

17.7 Summary

Early-life immune insult, also known as developmental immunotoxicity (DIT), is a serious component of current health risks. Environmental risk factors for DIT, including environmental chemicals and drugs, can program the developing immune system toward dysfunction, including misregulation of inflammation. The inability to resolve acute inflammation and resulting ongoing chronic inflammation in tissues is a major health threat, and chronic inflammation is a common adverse outcome of DIT. It is also a unifying feature and likely requirement of a majority of chronic diseases and conditions. Males and females often respond differently to early-life environmental exposures that affect the immune system. Sex-based differences in DIT have been reported for a significant percentage of immunotoxic chemicals and drugs examined to date, and these can extend to the very nature of the immune alterations that are produced. The ramifications are that the specific health risks for males *vs.* females can be markedly different after DIT-inducing environmental exposures. For this reason, sex-based immunotoxicological evaluation and health risk reduction planning is needed.

Effective measures to prevent chronic diseases should include: 1) the detection of DIT that contributes to life-long inflammatory misregulation, and 2) the management of chronic diseases to correct underlying immune dysfunction and reduce the risk of additional comorbidities. A focus on early life should be a research and safety testing priority given the uniqueness of the critical developmental windows of immune vulnerability and the chronic disease burdens that are associated with disruption of immune maturation and early-life programming for immune dysfunction.

Acknowledgements

The author thanks Janice Dietert, Performance Plus Consulting, for her editorial assistance.

References

1. R. R. Dietert, *J. Immuntoxicol.*, 2011, **8**, 101.
2. R. R. Dietert and R. W. Luebke (eds), Immunotoxicity, *Immune Dysfunction, and Chronic Disease*, Springer, New York, 2012.
3. R. R. Dietert and J. T. Zelikoff, *Curr. Pediatr. Rev.*, 2009, **5**, 36.
4. R. R. Dietert, J. M. Dietert and J. C. DeWitt, *Emerging Health Threats Journal*, 2011, **4**, 7111.
5. R. R. Dietert, J. C. DeWitt, D. R. Germolec and J. T. Zelikoff, *Environ. Health. Perspect.*, 2010, **118**, 1091.
6. D. A. Peterson and R. A. Cardona, *Adv. Immunol.*, 2010, **107**, 71.
7. N. H. Salzman, *Curr. Opin. Microbiol.*, 2011, **14**, 95.
8. A. L. Kau, P. P. Aherrn, N. W. Griffin, A. L. Goodman and J. I. Gordon, *Nature*, 2011, **474**, 327.
9. Y. K. Lee, J. S. Menezes, Y. Umesaki and S. K. Mazmanian, *Proc. Natl. Acad. Sci. USA*, 2011, **108**, 4615.
10. D. J. Barker and C. Osmond, *Lancet*, 1986, **1**(8489), 1077.
11. D. J. Barker and C. N. Martyn, The maternal and fetal origins of cardiovascular disease, *J. Epidemiol. Community Health*, 1992, **46**, 8.
12. D. J. Barker, *J. Intern. Med.*, 2007, **261**, 412.
13. D. J. Barker, *Brit. Med. Bull.*, 1997, **53**, 96.
14. E. J. Tokar, W. Qu and M. P. Waalkes, Arsenic, stem cells, and the developmental basis of adult cancer, *Toxicol. Sci*, 2011, **120**(Suppl 1), S192.
15. D. I. Phillips and S. G. Matthews, *World J. Diabetes*, 2011, **2**, 211.
16. L. Harvey, T. H. Burne, J. J. McGrath and D. W. Eyles, *J. Steroid Biochem. Mol. Biol.*, 2010, **121**, 239.
17. S. Darney, B. Fowler, P. Grandjean, J. Heindel, D. Mattison and W. Slikker Jr., *Reprod. Toxicol.*, 2011, **31**, 271.
18. X. Zhang, J. H. Sliwowska and J. Weinberg, *Exp. Biol. Med. (Maywood)*, 2005, **230**, 376.
19. S. Bezek, E. Ujházy, M. Mach, J. Navarová and M. Dubovický, *Interdiscip. Toxicol*, 2008, **1**, 29.

20. M. Vahter, *Basic Clin. Pharmacol. Toxicol.*, 2008, **102**, 204.
21. M. I. Luster, R. R. Dietert, D. R. Germolec, R. W. Luebke, and S. L. Makris in *Encyclopedia of Children Health*, ed., J. O. Nriagu, Elsevier, Oxford, 2011, pp. 44–50; Developmental immuntoxicants, pp. 44–50. In [ed.], J. O. Nriagu, *Encyclopedia of Children Health.* ISBN: 978-0-444-52272-6.
22. K. S. Landreth, *Hum. Exp. Toxicol.*, 2002, **21**, 493.
23. M. P. Holsapple, L. J. West and K. S. Landreth, *Birth Defects Res. B Dev. Reprod. Toxicol.*, 2003, **68**, 321.
24. J. B. Barnett, *Environ. Toxicol. Pharmacol.*, 1997, **4**, 315.
25. T. E. Miller, K. A. Golemboski, R. S. Ha, T. Bunn, F. S. Sanders and R. R. Dietert, *Toxicol. Sci.*, 1998, **42**, 129.
26. S. E. Moore, *Proc. Nutr. Soc.*, 1998, **57**, 241.
27. S. D. Holladay and R. J. Smialowicz, *Environ. Health. Perspect.*, 2000, **108**(Suppl 3), 463.
28. R. R. Dietert, R. A. Etzel, D. Chen, M. Halonen, S. D. Holladay, A. M. Jarabek, K. Landreth, D. B. Peden, K. Pinkerton, R. J. Smialowicz and T. Zoetis, *Environ. Health. Perspect.*, 2000, **108**(Suppl 3), 483.
29. R. R. Dietert and J. M. Dietert, *J. Toxicol. Environ. Health B Crit. Rev.*, 2008, **11**, 660.
30. T. L. Bunn, P. J. Parsons, E. Kao and R. R. Dietert, *J. Toxicol. Environ. Health A*, 2001, **64**, 223.
31. R. W. Luebke, D. H. Chen, R. Dietert, Y. Yang, M. King, M. I. Luster and Immunotoxicology Workgroup, *J. Toxicol. Environ. Health B Crit. Rev.*, 2006, **9**, 1.
32. E. Karpuzoglu-Sahin, Y. Zhi-Jun, A. Lengi, N. Sriranganathan and S. Ansar Ahmed, Effects of long-term estrogen treatment on IFN-gamma, IL-2 and IL-4 gene expression and protein synthesis in spleen and thymus of normal C57BL/6 mice, *Cytokine*, 2001, **14**, 208.
33. N. P. Ly, A. Litonjua, D. R. Gold and J. C. Celedón, *J. Allergy Clin. Immunol.*, 2011, **127**, 1087.
34. R. M. McLoughlin and K. H. Mills, *J. Allergy Clin. Immunol.*, 2011, **127**, 1097.
35. M. I. Luster, C. Portier, D. G. Pait and D. R. Germolec, *Toxicology*, 1994, **92**, 229.
36. I. Kimber, G. F. Gerberick, H. Van Loveren and R. V. House, *Fundam. Appl. Toxicol.*, 1992, **19**, 479.
37. G. F. Gerberick, R. V. House, E. R. Fletcher and C. A. Ryan, *Fundam. Appl. Toxico.l*, 1992, **19**, 438.
38. M. I. Luster, C. Portier, D. G. Pait, G. J. Rosenthal, D. R. Germolec, E. Corsini, B. L. Blaylock, P. Pollock, Y. Kouchi, W. Craig, K. L. White, A. Munson and C. H. Comment, *Fundam. Appl. Toxicol.*, 1993, **21**, 71.
39. M. I. Luster, C. Portier, D. G. Pait, K. L. White, C. Jennings, A. E. Munsen and G. J. Rosenthal, *Fund. Appl. Toxicol.*, 1992, **18**, 200.
40. M. Kanoh, Y. Kaneita, M. Hara, S. Harada, Y. Gon, H. Kanamaru and T. Ohida, *Prev Med*, 2012, **54**, 94.

41. C. C. Geerts, M. L. Bots, D. E. Grobbee and C. S. Uiterwaal, *Arterioscler. Thromb. Vasc. Biol.*, 2008, **28**, 2296.
42. I. J. Wang, W. S. Hsieh, K. Y. Wu, Y. L. Guo, Y. H. Hwang, S. H. Jee and P. C. Chen, *Pediatr. Allergy Immunol.*, 2008, **19**, 580.
43. D. Hinz, M. Bauer, S. Röder, S. Olek, J. Huehn, U. Sack, M. Borte, J. C. Simon, I. Lehmann and G. Herberth for the LINA study group, *Allergy*, 2012, **67**, 380.
44. S. E. Roberts, C. J. Wotton, J. G. Williams, M. Griffith and M. J. Goldacre, *World J. Gastroenterol.*, 2011, **17**, 743.
45. K. Tanaka, Y. Miyake, M. Arakawa, S. Sasaki and Y. Ohya, *BMC Public Health*, 2010, **10**, 335.
46. M. G. Foreman, L. Zhang, J. Murphy, N. N. Hansel, B. Make, J. E. Hokanson, G. Washko, E. A. Regan, J. D. Crapo, E. K. Silverman, D. L. DeMeo and COPD Gene Investigators, *Am. J. Respir. Crit. Care Med.*, 2011, **184**, 414.
47. E. Thiering, I. Brüske, J. Kratzsch, J. Thiery, S. Sausenthaler, C. Meisinger, S. Koletzko, C. P. Bauer, B. Schaaf, A. von Berg, D. Berdel, I. Lehmann, O. Herbarth, U. Krämer, H. E. Wichmann, J. Heinrich and GINIplus and LISAplus Study Groups, *Int. J. Hyg. Environ. Health,*, 2011, **214**, 361.
48. E. Raum, J. Küpper-Nybelen, A. Lamerz, J. Hebebrand, B. Herpertz-Dahlmann and H. Brenner, *Obesity (Silver Spring)*, 2011, **19**, 2411.
49. M. K. Javaid and C. Cooper, *Best Pract. Res. Clin. Endocrinol. Metab*, 2002, **16**, 349.
50. M. G. Ozden, N. S. Tekin, M. A. Gürer, D. Akdemir, C. Doğramacı, S. Utaş, A. Akman, S. E. Evans, S. Bahadır, S. Oztürkcan, G. Ikizoğlu, N. Sendur, O. Köse, Y. Bek, S. Yaylı, T. Cantürk and A. Y. Turanl, *Pediatr. Dermatol.*, 2011, **28**, 306.
51. A. N. Colebatch and C. J. Edwards, *Clin. Exp. Immunol.*, 2011, **163**, 11.
52. L. L. Jones, A. Hashim, T. McKeever, D. G. Cook, J. Britton and J. Leonardi-Bee, *Respir. Res.*, 2011, **12**, 5.
53. K. Yolton, Y. Xu, J. Khoury, P. Succop, B. Lanphear, D. W. Beebe and J. Owens, Associations between secondhand smoke exposure and sleep patterns in children, *Pediatrics*, 2010, **125**, e261.
54. T. H. Nesterenko and H. Aly, *Am. J. Perinatol.*, 2009, **26**, 191.
55. N. A. Hodyl, M. J. Stark, A. Osei-Kumah and V. L. Clifton, *Expert. Rev. Clin. Immunol.*, 2011, **7**, 579.
56. B. C. Feltes, J. de Faria Poloni and D. Bonatto, *Biogerontology*, 2011, **12**, 293.
57. J. L. Kaplan, H. N. Shi and W. A. Walker, *Pediatr. Res.*, 2011, **69**, 465.
58. T. M. Marques, R. Wall, R. P. Ross, G. F. Fitzgerald, C. A. Ryan and C. Stanton, *Curr. Opin. Biotechnol.*, 2010, **21**, 149.
59. S. J. Spencer, M. A. Galic and Q. J. Pittman, *Am. J. Physiol. Endocrinol. Metab.*, 2011, **300**, E11.
60. J. G. Lisciandro and A. H. van den Biggelaar, *Clin. Exp. Allergy*, 2010, **40**, 1719.

61. U. Meyer, *Prog Neuropsychopharmacol Biol Psychiatr*, 2011, Nov 15, [Epub ahead of print] http://dx.doi.org/101016/j.pnpbp.2011.11.003.
62. G. Pacheco-López, S. Giovanoli, W. Langhans and U. Meyer, *Schizophr Bull*, 2011, Dec 19. [Epub ahead of print] PMID: 22186136.
63. D. E. Barnes and S. J. Lee, *Alzheimers Res. Ther.*, 2011, **3**, 33.
64. R. R. Dietert, *Reproduct. Toxicol.*, 2011b, **32**, 198.
65. W. Palinski, T. Yamashita, S. Freigang and C. Napoli, *Nutr. Rev.*, 2007, **65**, S182.
66. C. Onore C, M. Careaga and P. Ashwood, *Brain Behav. Immun.*, 2012, **26**, 383.
67. G. E. Krassas, K. Tziomalos, N. Pontikides, H. Lewy and Z. Laron, *Eur. J. Endocrinol.*, 2007, **156**, 631.
68. E. Decker, G. Engelmann, A. Findeisen, P. Gerner, M. Laass, D. Ney, C. Posovszky, L. Hoy and M. W. Hornef, *Pediatrics*, 2010, **125**, e1433.
69. V. M. Vehaskari, *Curr. Opin. Pediatr.*, 2010, **22**, 176.
70. A. Shankar, L. Sun, B. E. Klein, K. E. Lee, P. Muntner, F. J. Nieto, M. Y. Tsai, K. J. Cruickshanks, C. R. Schubert, P. C. Brazy, J. Coresh and R. Klein, *Kidney Int.*, 2011, **80**, 1231.
71. A. Bush, *COPD*, 2008, **5**, 53.
72. R. Dantzer, *Biol. Psychiatry*, 2012, **71**, 4.
73. D. K. Kinney and M. Tanaka, *J. Nerv. Ment. Dis.*, 2009, **197**, 561.
74. M. Umezawa, C. Sakata, N. Tanaka, M. Tabata, K. Takeda, T. Ihara and M. Sugamata, *J. Toxicol. Sci.*, 2011, **36**, 493.
75. P. Grandjean, L. K. Poulsen, C. Heilmann, U. Steuerwald and P. Weihe, *Environ. Health Perspect.*, 2010, **118**, 1429.
76. A. Mišak, *Proc. Nutr. Soc.*, 2011, **70**, 465.
77. H. Renz, P. Brandtzaeg and M. Hornef, *Nat. Rev. Immunol.*, 2012, **12**, 9.
78. C. Heim, U. M. Nater, E. Maloney, R. Boneva, J. F. Jones and W. C. Reeves, *Arch. Gen. Psychiatry*, 2009, **66**, 72.
79. D. A. Fernandes de Abreu, V. Landel and F. Féron, *J. Neurol. Sci.*, 2011, **311**, 64.
80. A. R. Setty, G. Curhan and H. K. Choi, *Am. J. Med.*, 2007, **120**, 953.
81. J. J. Jaakkola and M. Gissler, *J. Epidemiol.*, 2005, **34**, 664.
82. C. J. Edwards, H. Syddall, R. Goswami, P. Goswami, E. M. Dennison and C. Cooper, *Lupus*, 2006, **15**, 213.
83. M. A. D'Angeli, E. Merzon, L. F. Valbuena, D. Tirschwell, C. A. Paris and B. A., *Arch. Pediatr. Adolesc. Med.*, 2010, **164**, 732.
84. J. Virk, J. Li, M. Vestergaard, C. Obel, M. Lu and J. Olsen, *PLoS One*, 2010, **5**, e11523.
85. A. Gabory, L. Attig and C. Junien, *Mol. Cell. Endocrinol.*, 2009, **304**, 8.
86. A. A. Rooney, R. A. Matulka and R. W. Luebke RW, *Toxicol. Sci.*, 2003, **76**, 366.
87. T. L. Bunn, P. J. Parsons, E. Kao and R. R. Dietert, *Toxicol. Sci.*, 2001, **64**, 57.
88. H. Guo, T. Liu, Y. Uemura, S. Jiao, D. Wang, Z. Lin, Y. Narita, M. Suzuki, N. Hirosawa, Y. Ichihara, O. Ishihara, H. Kikuchi, Y. Sakamoto, S. Senju, Q. Zhang and F. Ling, *Cell Mol. Immunol.*, 2010, **7**, 227.

89. I. A. Silva, M. El Nabawi, D. Hoover and E. K. Silbergeld, *Dev. Comp. Immunol.*, 2005, **29**, 171.
90. B. C. Gehrs and R. J. Smialowicz, *Toxicology*, 1999, **134**, 79.
91. N. A. Karrow, T. L. Guo, K. B. Delclos, R. R. Newbold, C. Weis, D. R. Germolec, K. L. White Jr. and J. A. McCay JA., *Toxicology*, 2004, **196**, 237.
92. P. Malmborg, S. Bahmanyar, L. Grahnquist, H. Hildebrand and S. Montgomery, Cesarean section and the risk of pediatric Crohn's disease, *Inflamm. Bowel Dis.*, 2011, Apr 27. doi: 10.1002/ibd.21741.
93. O. Wynne, J. C. Horvat, A. Osei-Kumah, R. Smith, P. M. Hansbro, V. L. Clifton and D. M. Hodgson, *Stress*, 2011, **14**, 247.
94. P. A. McCombe, J. M. Greer and I. R. Mackay, *Curr. Mol. Med.*, 2009, **9**, 1058.
95. O. L. Quintero, M. J. Amador-Patarroyo, G. Montoya-Ortiz, A. Rojas-Villarraga and J. M. Anaya, *J. Autoimmun.*, 2012, **38**, 109.
96. R. Voskuhl., *Biology of Sex Differences*, 2011, **2**, 1.
97. J. Sellner, J. Kraus, A. Awad, R. Milo, B. Hemmer and O. Stüve, *Autoimmun. Rev.*, 2011, **10**, 495.
98. M. Y. Weng, Y. T. Huang, M. F. Liu and T. H. Lu, *J. Rheumatol.*, 2011, **38**, 706.
99. K. M. Pollard, *J. Autoimmun.*, 2012, **38**, J177.
100. U. Nussinovitch and Y. Shoenfeld Y., *Autoimmun Rev*, 2012, **11**, A377.
101. M. M. Schoonheim, H. E. Hulst, S. Landi, O. Ciccarelli, S. D. Roosendaal, E. J. Sanz-Arigita, H. Vrenken, C. H. Polman, C. J. Stam, F. Barkhof and J. J. Geurts, *Mult Scler*, 2012, **18**, 164.
102. K. L. Crosslin and K. L. Wiginton, *Gend. Med*, 2011, **8**, 365.
103. B. Evengård, A. Jacks, N. L. Pedersen and P. F. Sullivan, *Psychol. Med.*, 2005, **35**, 1317.
104. M. Musicco, *Funct. Neurol.*, 2009, **24**, 89.
105. L. E. Hebert, P. A. Scherr, J. J. McCann, L. A. Beckett and D. A. Evans, *Am. J. Epidemiol.*, 2001, **153**, 132.
106. Centers for Disease Control and Prevention, *MMWR Surveill. Summ.*, 2009, **58**, 1.
107. G. F. Wooten, L. J. Currie, V. E. Bovbjerg, J. K. Lee and J. Patrie, *J. Neurol. Neurosurg. Psychiatry*, 2004, **75**, 637.
108. A. J. Lowe, J. B. Carlin, C. M. Bennett, C. S. Hosking, M. J. Abramson, D. J. Hill and S. C. Dharmage, *J. Allergy Clin. Immunol.*, 2008, **121**, 1190.
109. J. M. Gelfand, R. Weinstein, S. B. Porter, A. L. Neimann, J. A. Berlin and D. J. Margolis, *Arch. Dermatol.*, 2005, **141**, 1537.
110. I. Manabe, *Circ. J.*, 2011, **75**, 2739.
111. R. R. Dietert, J. C. DeWitt and R. W. Luebke in *Immunotoxicity, Immune Dysfunction, and Chronic Disease*, eds. R. R. Dietert and R. W. Luebke, Springer, New York, 2012, pp. 419–440.
112. S. Prasad, B. Sung and B .B. Aggarwal, *Prev. Med.*, 2012, **54**, S29.
113. R. R. Dietert and J. T. Zelikoff, *World J. Pediatr.*, 2010, **6**, 111.
114. X. Yao, H. Li and S. X. Leng, *Clin. Geriatr. Med.*, 2011, **27**, 79–87.

115. S. S. Chang, C. O. Weiss, Q. F. Xue and L. P. Fried, *Arch. Gerontol. Geriatr.*, 2012, **54**, 9.
116. C. N. Serhan, *J. Thromb. Haemost.*, 2009, **7**(Suppl 1), 44.
117. G. Bannenberg and C. N. Serhan, *Biochim. Biophys. Acta.*, 2010, **1801**, 1260.
118. T. Ishida, M. Yoshida, M. Arita, Y. Nishitani, S. Nishiumi, A. Masuda, S. Mizuno, T. Takagawa, Y. Morita, H. Kutsumi, H. Inokuchi, C. N. Serhan, R. S. Blumberg and T. Azuma, *Inflamm. Bowel Dis.*, 2010, **16**, 87.
119. M. Spite and C. N. Serhan, *Circ. Res.*, 2010, **107**, 1170.
120. F. Sozo, L. O'Day, G. Maritz, K. Kenna, V. Stacy, N. Brew, D. Walker, A. Bocking, J. Brien and R. Harding, *Am. J. Physiol. Lung Cell. Mol. Physiol*, 2009, **296**, L510.
121. M. B. Azad and A. L. Kozyrskyj, *Clin. Dev. Immunol.*, 2012, **2012**, 9. Article ID 932072, doi: 10.1155/2012/9320720.
122. S. O. Shaheen, R. B. Newson, G. D. Smith and A. J. Henderson, *Int. J. Epidemiol.*, 2010, **39**, 790.
123. S. Roque, T. G. Oliveira, C. Nobrega, P. Barreira-Silva, C. Nunes-Alves, N. Sousa, J. A. Palha and M. Correia-Neves, *Front. Behav. Neurosci.*, 2011, **5**, 4.
124. N. Brown, M. Nagarkatti and P. S. Nagarkatti, *Toxicol. Appl. Pharmacol.*, 2006, **212**, 119.
125. M. T. Sharkar, M. Y. Jou, M. B. Hossain, B. Lönnerdal, C. B. Stephensen and R. Raqib, *J. Nutr.*, 2011, **141**, 1559.
126. A. A. Ginde, J. M. Mansbach and C. A. Camargo Jr., *Curr. Allergy Asthma Rep.*, 2009, **9**, 81.
127. L. S. Kremmyda, M. Vlachava, P. S. Noakes, N. D. Diaper, E. A. Miles and P. C. Calder, *Clin. Rev. Allergy Immunol.*, 2011, **41**, 36.
128. T. L. Guo, K. L. White Jr., R. D. Brown, K. B. Delclos, R. R. Newbold, C. Weis, D. R. Germolec and J. A. McCay, *Toxicol. Appl. Pharmacol.*, 2002, **181**, 219.
129. E. Merlot, D. Couret and W. Otten, *Brain. Behav. Immun.*, 2008, **22**, 42.
130. M. Von Korff, J. Alonso, J. Ormel, M. Angermeyer, R. Bruffaerts, C. Fleiz, G. de Girolamo, R. C. Kessler, V. Kovess-Masfety, J. Posada-Villa, K. M. Scott and H. Uda, *Pain*, 2009, **143**, 76–83.
131. N. M. Nielsen, A. V. Hansen, J. Simonsen and A. Hviid, *Am. J. Epidemiol.*, 2011, **173**, 990.
132. C. S. Algert, J. R. Bowen, S. L. Lain, H. D. Allen, J. M. Vivian-Taylor and C.L. Roberts, *Pediatr. Allergy Immunol.*, 2011, **22**, 836.
133. C. Heilmann, E. Budtz-Jørgensen, F. Nielsen, B. Heinzow, P. Weihe and P. Grandjean, *Environ. Health Perspect.*, 2010, **118**, 1434.
134. C. Heilmann, P. Grandjean, P. Weihe, F. Nielsen and E. Budtz-Jørgensen, *PLoS Med*, 2006, **3**, e311.
135. J. P. Hogaboam, A. J. Moore and B. P. Lawrence, *Toxicol. Sci.*, 2008, **102**, 160.
136. A. Mustafa, S. D. Holladay, S. Witonsky, D. P. Sponenberg, E. Karpuzoglu and R. M. Gogal Jr., *Toxicology*, 2011, **290**, 157.

137. B. C. Gehrs, M. M. Riddle, W. C. Williams and R. J. Smialowicz, *Toxicology*, 1997, **122**, 229.
138. K. L. White Jr., D. R. Germolec, C. D. Booker, D. M. Hernendez, J. A. McCay, K. B. Delclos, R. R. Newbold, C. Weis and T. L. Guo, *Toxicology*, 2005, **207**, 271.
139. M. F. Schaalan, S. M. Abdelraouf, W. A. Mohamed and F. S. Hassanein, *J Immunotoxicol.*, 2012, **9**, 15.
140. M. M. Peden-Adams, J. G. Eudaly, L. M. Heesemann, J. Smythe, J. Miller, G. S. Gilkeson and D. E. Keil, *J. Environ. Sci. Health. A Tox. Hazard Subst. Environ. Eng.*, 2006, **41**, 249.
141. G. S. Cooper, S. L. Makris, P. J. Nietert and J. Jinot, *Environ. Health Perspect.*, 2009, **117**, 696.
142. J. E. Snyder, N. M. Filipov, P. J. Parsons and D. A. Lawrence, *Toxicol. Sci.*, 2000, **57**, 87.
143. P. M. Lutz, E. A. Kelty, T. D. Brown, T. J. Wilson, G. Brock and R. E. Neal, *Toxicology*, 2012, **291**, 43.
144. H. Yan, M. Takamoto and K. Suganem, *Environ. Health Perspect.*, 2008, **116**, 514.
145. J. C. Dewitt, M. M. Peden-Adams, J. M. Keller and D. R. Germolec, *Toxicol. Pathol.*, 2012, **40**, 300.

CHAPTER 18

Aging and Vulnerability to Ambient Air Pollution

MORTON LIPPMANN

New York University School of Medicine, Nelson Institute of Environmental Medicine, 57 Old Forge Road, Tuxedo, NY, USA 10987
E-mail: morton.lippmann@nyumc.org

18.1 Background

We have had solid quantitative evidence of the role of age in the vulnerability to adverse effects of ambient air pollution since the publication of the Interim Report of the Committee on Air Pollution[1] on the December 1952 "killer fog" in London, England. As shown in Table 18.1, the number of deaths in Greater London in the four weeks following the killer fog episode was much higher than that of the four weeks that preceded it, with the relative risks (RRs) being highest for bronchitis (6.7), influenza (5.1), other respiratory (4.0), and pneumonia (3.5). It should also be noted that while the RRs were greatest for pulmonary endpoints, the numbers of excess deaths were greatest for heart disease. Table 18.2 shows the deaths for this period by age range, with the RR being about 2 for those older than 65. An RR of 2 was also seen for children between 1 month and 1 year of age. Lung capacity is growing very rapidly in the first year of life and is dropping markedly, especially for smokers, in the last decades, and greater RRs attributable to the added stress to health and survival for vulnerable individuals resulting from inhaling the dirty air could have been anticipated.

Issues in Toxicology No. 16
Aging and Vulnerability to Environmental Chemicals: Age-related Disorders and their Origins in Environmental Exposures
Edited by Bernard Weiss

Published by the Royal Society of Chemistry, www.rsc.org

Table 18.1 Greater London Deaths Divided According to Cause – Nov. and Dec. 1952.

Cause	*Av. Number of deaths in weeks ending 8th, 15th, 22nd, 29th Nov.*	*Number of deaths registered in week ending* 6th Dec.	13th Dec.	20th Dec.	27th Dec.	*For weeks ending 6th, 13th, 20th, 27th Dec.* Av. No. of deaths	RR
Pulmonary Tuberculosis	17	14	77	37	21	37.25	2.19
Lung Cancer	34	45	69	32	36	45.50	1.34
Heart Disease	226	273	707	389	272	410.25	1.82
High Blood Pressure	14	19	47	36	21	30.75	2.20
Other Circulatory	22	26	46	31	32	33.75	1.53
Influenza	2	2	24	9	6	10.25	5.13
Pneumonia	31	45	168	125	91	107.25	3.46
Bronchitis	51	76	704	396	184	340.00	6.67
Other Respiratory	6	9	52	21	13	23.75	3.96
Ill-defined Causes	20	25	79	35	37	36.50	1.83
All Other Causes	340	411	511	412	316	412.50	1.21
All causes	763	945	2,484	1,523	1,029	1,495	1.96

From: Comm. on Air Pollution: Interim Report, Cmd 9011, London. H.M. Stationery Office (Dec. 1953).

Table 18.2 Greater London Deaths Divided According to Age – Nov. and Dec. 1952.

Dec. Age	*Av. Number of deaths in weeks ending 8th, 15th, 22nd, 29th Nov.*	*Number of deaths registered in week ending* 6th Dec.	13th Dec.	20th Dec.	27th Dec.	*For weeks ending 6th, 13th, 20th, 27th* Av. No. of deaths	RR
Weeks:							
0–4	20	16	28	19	12	18.75	0.94
4–52	8	12	26	15	11	16.00	2.00
Years:							
1–4	7	6	7	13	7	8.25	1.18
5–14	4	4	6	6	2	4.50	1.18
15–24	7	9	7	14	7	9.25	1.32
25–34	11	16	28	17	11	18.00	1.64
35–44	26	36	64	29	34	40.75	1.57
45–54	70	80	204	96	83	115.75	1.65
55–64	133	157	448	251	167	255.75	1.92
65–74	211	254	717	444	258	418.25	1.98
75 and over	266	355	949	619	437	590.00	2.22
All ages	763	945	2,484	1,523	1,029	1,495.00	1.96

From: Comm. on Air Pollution: Interim Report, Cmd 9011, London, H.M. Stationery Office (Dec. 1953).

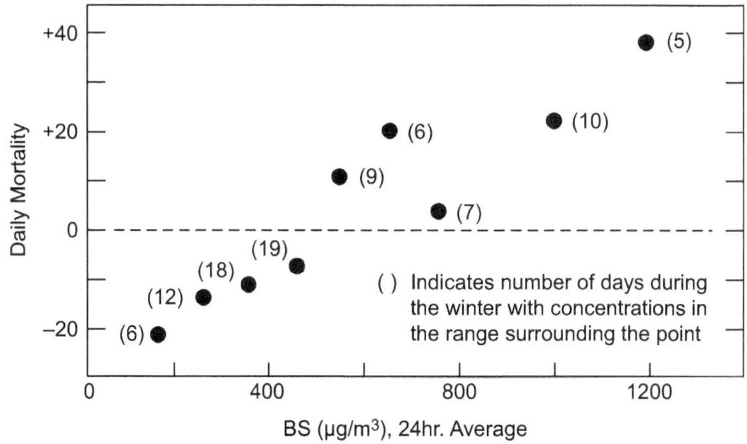

Figure 18.1 Martin and Bradley (1960) data for winter of 1958–1959 in London, as summarized by Ware *et al.* (1981), showing average deviations of daily mortality from 15-day moving average by concentration of black smoke.

The only air quality indices being measured in London in that era were Black Smoke (BS), as measured by light reflectance of the blackish particles collected on a filter, and the acidity in a water-filled bubbler flask that collected both water-soluble gases and particles. The BS readings were expressed in mg m^{-3}, based on gravimetric laboratory calibrations. The acidity was expressed as the concentration of sulfur dioxide (SO_2) in mg m^{-3}. The peak day BS concentrations exceeded the calibration range limit of ~2 mg m^{-3}, and the visual range was so limited that all surface traffic had to cease. At lower BS concentrations, the excess daily mortality in London for the winter of 1958–1959 varied in an almost linear fashion,[2] as illustrated in Figure 18.1.

Contemporary concentrations of particulate matter (PM) suspended in the outdoor air are based on gravimetric measurements on filter discs, and peak levels are typically about two orders of magnitude lower than those of the 1952 killer smog episode. However, as discussed later in this chapter, we still have statistically significant excesses of daily mortality associated with PM mass concentrations, and still have the greatest RRs for mortality in the elderly.

We have also seen substantial declines of long-term or cumulative exposures to ambient air PM in the UK and the US since the end of World War II, which has resulted in much lower rates of annual mortality and the burdens of chronic diseases. Table 18.3 illustrates the declines in chronic bronchitis and respiratory tract cancer mortality rates in 64 UK county boroughs as the UK Clean Air Act was implemented.[3] As shown later in this chapter, contemporary studies still show significant associations of annual mortality from lung cancer and from cardiac and respiratory causes with PM concentrations, albeit at much lower rates.

Table 18.3 Standardized annual mortality rate regression coefficients on smoke[a] for 64 UK county boroughs.

Sex	*Ages*	*Mortality in*	*Cancer of Trachea, Bronchus & Lung*	*Chronic Bronchitis*
Males	45–64	1969–1973	0.07	0.02
		1958–1964	0.53[b]	0.32[a]
		1948–1954	0.71[c]	0.48[c]
	65–74	1969–1973	0.15	−0.06
		1958–1964	0.68[c]	0.31
		1948–1954	0.87[c]	0.37[a]
Females	45–64	1969–1973	−0.02	−0.02
		1958–1964	−0.64[b]	0.33[a]
		1948–1954	0.49[a]	0.49[b]
	65–74	1969–1973	0.07	0.03
		1958–1964	0.25	0.40[a]
		1948–1954	0.61[b]	0.31

[a]Based on index of black smoke pollution 20 years before death (*Br. J. Prev. Soc. Med.*, 1959, **13**, 14–27).
[b]$p < 0.05$.
[c]$p < 0.01$.
[d]$p < 0.001$.
Source: Adapted from Ref. 3.

18.2 Introduction to Contemporary Ambient Air Pollution and its Health Effects

Ambient air pollution, *i.e.*, the gaseous pollutants, such as ozone (O_3), nitrogen dioxide (NO_2), SO_2, and carbon monoxide (CO), and PM suspended in the outdoor air, are well-established risk factors affecting public health in terms of excess mortality, morbidity, and function. The risks are highly variable among pollutants due to their differing physical and chemical properties. They are also highly variable within the members of populations due to: 1) substantial variations in pollutant concentrations in the outdoor air; 2) attenuation in concentration of the concentrations in indoor microenvironments where most people spend most of their time; 3) respiratory rates and air volumes inhaled; 4) fractional depositions within respiratory tract regions (upper respiratory tract, tracheobronchial airways, and gas exchange region) that depend on particle size distributions and solubility; 5) retention at deposition sites and/or translocation *via* surface transport or within blood to other organs; 6) chemical transformations within the airways, at deposition sites, along translocation pathways, and within other organ systems; and 7) factors affecting inter-individual vulnerability.

18.2.1 Vulnerability

Health-related responses to ambient air pollutants depend greatly on inter-individual differences within a population that determine whether they respond and the extent of their responses, *i.e.*, their vulnerability. The major factors affecting an individual's vulnerability to the adverse effects of inhaled ambient air pollutants include: 1) age; 2) genetic predispositions; 3) prior epigenetic changes resulting from earlier lifetime exposures to ambient air pollutants, indoor air pollutants, and other toxicants: 4) pre-existing diseases; 5) smoking history; 6) occupational exposures; 7) prenatal exposures; 8) nutritional deficiencies. This chapter is focused on age as a determinant of vulnerability, and the other factors enumerated above will be cited as they influence the effects of age.

18.2.2 Age

Health risks associated with ambient air pollution vary with age, with a tendency to decrease during childhood, and to increase with age in our last few decades. Parental exposures, and especially maternal exposures, to ambient air pollutants and cigarette smoke components and their metabolites affect fetuses *in utero* and early childhood development in ways that can predispose the fetus and young child to health risks later in life. In young children, the lungs are not yet fully developed and they therefore differ from those of adults in terms of the deposition and retention of inhaled pollutants. Also, infants and young children have much higher ratios of inhaled volumes to body size than adults, even when at rest, and still further increases when they are in motion with associated increases in their ventilation rates and volumes.

Lung volumes reach their peaks in our third decade, and ventilatory capacity begins an accelerating rate of decline in our fourth decade. The rate of decline is predictive of premature mortality, and is much greater in smokers and workers with emphysema than in healthy nonsmokers.

18.2.3 Ambient Air Pollutants

The literature on the effects of age on human responsiveness to exposures to ambient air pollutants is largely limited to pollutants that have been regulated because of widespread exposures and the extent of their public health impacts, *i.e.*, the criteria pollutants having National Ambient Air Quality Standards (NAAQS).[4] There are currently six criteria pollutants, which are expressed in terms of mass concentrations. In addition to PM, which covers all solid and liquid particles irrespective of chemical composition, there are NAAQS for photochemical oxidants, expressed as the concentrations of CO and O_3; nitrogen oxides, expressed as the concentration of NO_2; sulfur oxides, expressed as the concentration of SO_2; and lead (Pb) in terms of the metal and all of its compounds. Of these, there is extensive literature on variation in vulnerability by age only for PM, O_3, CO, and Pb. The gaseous pollutants are specific molecules. Pb and PM can be present in varying particle size distributions. PM includes a vast array of chemicals, ranging from mineral dusts, soot, pollens, and other biological particles emitted as primary particles, to a broad range of secondary PM composed of inorganic and organic chemicals that are condensed from vapors or formed in the ambient air by chemical reactions.

The current PM NAAQS are specified in terms of mass concentrations within two particle size ranges, those less than 10 μm in aerodynamic diameter (PM_{10}) and those below 2.5 μm in aerodynamic diameter ($PM_{2.5}$). PM_{10} excludes particles larger than 10 μm on the basis that they do not penetrate beyond the larynx to deposit in the lungs. The distinction at 2.5 μm is based on the differences in particle composition, with most of the larger particles being mechanically generated, irregular in shape, and alkaline, while the smaller particles are carbonaceous and/or acidic. Furthermore, most of the mass of PM_{10} particles deposit within the lung conductive airways within the thorax, while the smaller (fine) particles penetrate the conductive airways and deposit within the gas exchange region, where they have greater access to the bloodstream.[5]

18.2.4 Human Responses to Ambient Air Pollutants

The known population-based human responses to inhaled pollutants have been largely limited to the pulmonary, cardiovascular, and nervous systems, and described in terms of premature mortality, excess hospital and/or emergency room admissions, and loss of functional capacity. Short-term human responses of limited numbers of volunteer subjects undergoing controlled, short-term laboratory exposures have provided data on acute functional responses, symptoms, and biomarkers. In addition, there have been studies of short-term functional responses in field studies of volunteers engaged in normal recreational outdoor exercise. Long-term and cumulative exposures have been associated with lifespan shortening and the prevalence of chronic diseases and functional losses.

Pulmonary responses in humans have most often been associated with exposures to O_3, SO_2, and PM_{10}. Cardiovascular responses have most often been associated with exposures to PM_{10}, CO, and Pb. Nervous system responses have most often been associated with exposures to Pb. These and some other responses are described and discussed in greater detail for criteria air pollutants in the next section.

18.3 Health-Related Effects of Ambient Air Pollutants

18.3.1 Ozone

O_3 is an especially strong oxidant, but is relatively low in terms of aqueous solubility. Thus it is poorly taken up in passage through the upper respiratory tract or the mucus lining the larger tracheobronchial airways. Much of it penetrates to the gas exchange region of the lungs, where the mucus barrier is patchy or absent, and where it reacts with lung surfactant and with bronchiolar and alveolar epithelial cells.[6]

18.3.1.1 Short-Term Effects on Respiratory Function

Even at atmospheric concentrations that conform to the NAAQS, the reactions at the lung surfaces cause constriction of C-fibers within the lung airways in many people, resulting in small, but significant short-term reductions in the lung volumes and maximal flow rates of forced expiratory maneuvers, *i.e.*, forced vital capacity (FVC), forced expiratory flow rate in 1 second (FEV_1), and peak expiratory flow rate (PEFR). In controlled laboratory O_3 exposure studies in healthy children and young adults engaged in moderate exercise, such effects can readily be measured in most subjects, but with a very wide range of reproducible responsiveness in the individual subjects.[6] Figure 18.2 shows the extent of the decline in FEV_1 as a function of the O_3 concentration for healthy young adults after 6.6 hours of exposure while mildly exercising. Shorter exposures would cause smaller FEV_1 decrements, while more vigorous exercise would increase the decrements.[7] Field studies of healthy children at summer camps in wooded northeastern US sites, performed to determine whether there were similar O_3-associated pulmonary function decrements as those seen in the controlled laboratory studies, showed greater average decrements in the natural settings.[8]

Upon repetitive daily exposures, the maximal functional responses are seen on the first or second days, with lesser responses on successive days. However, after several weeks without further exposures, their initial responsiveness is restored.[6] Such functional adaptation is also seen on a seasonal basis in areas with prolonged high levels of O_3. Subjects are more responsive in the Spring than in the Summer, and they are minimally responsive in the Winter.

However, as illustrated in Figure 18.3, the acute responsiveness to O_3 seen in children and young adults diminishes with age. It is also noteworthy that

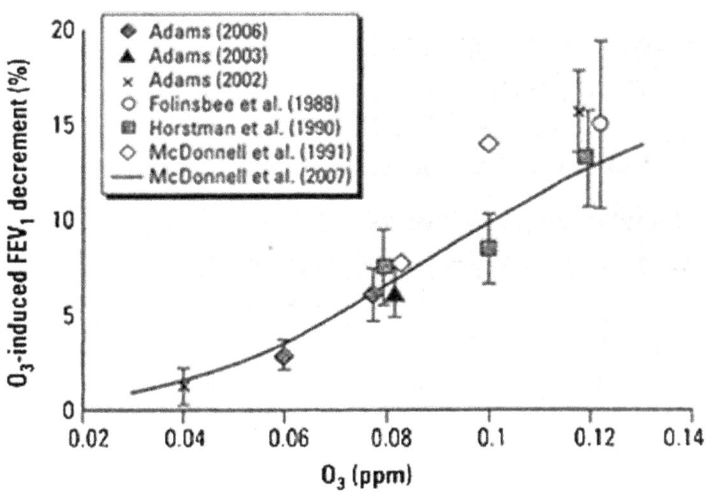

Figure 18.2 Comparison of mean O_3-induced FEV_1 decrements due to 6.6 h exposures with mild exercise in the various studies described (inset).

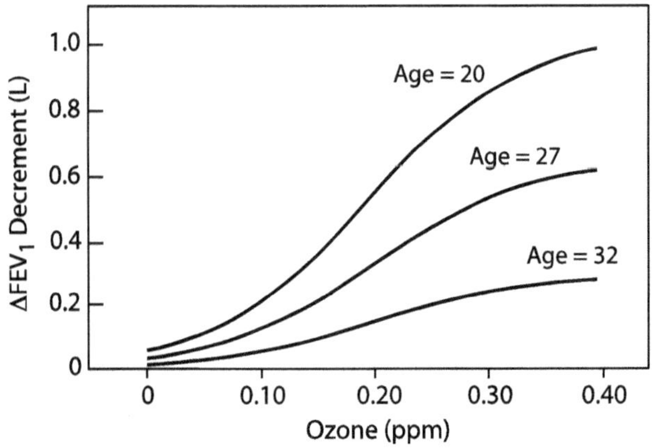

Figure 18.3 Predicted mean decrements in forced expiratory volume in L(ΔFEV_1) following 2 hour exposures to ozone while undergoing heavy intermittent exercise for three ages.
From: Ref. 9.

responsiveness is usually lower in people who smoke or have asthma than in healthy nonsmokers, which may possibly be due to the thicker mucus layers on their airways.[9]

In a field study of children with moderate to severe asthma at a summer camp in the Connecticut River Valley,[10] the associations between decrements in peak expiratory flow rates and ambient O_3 concentration were similar in magnitude to those reported by the same group of investigators for other, healthy, children.[8] However, the level of physical activity, and hence the O_3 uptake, of the asthmatic children was lower, and they needed, and were provided with, rescue medication by an on-site physician.

18.3.1.2 Other Short-Term Respiratory System Effects

Controlled exposure studies, sometimes conducted simultaneously with the respiratory function studies described previously, have shown responses in terms of respiratory symptoms, airway reactivity, pulmonary inflammation, pulmonary permeability, mucociliary particle clearance rates, and aerosol dispersion within the airways. However, the effects of age or aging on such functional responses were not studied for any of these effects.[6]

18.3.1.3 Epidemiological Studies

18.3.1.3.1 Long-Term Effects on Respiratory Function. Since O_3 was the only criteria pollutant that consistently produced short-term changes in respiratory function at current NAAQS levels, it was anticipated that it would also be associated with chronic functional losses. However, the Children's Health Study (CHS) of cohorts of 4th through 12th grade children in 12 Southern California communities found that lung development was not related to long-term average O_3 concentration, but was significantly associated with the long-term average concentrations of PM_{10}, $PM_{2.5}$, NO_2, and acidic vapors.[11]

18.3.1.3.2 Long-Term Effects on Hospital Admissions. As summarized by Thurston and Ito,[12] studies by Schwartz and colleagues reported increases associated with ambient O_3 concentrations for respiratory hospitalizations of Medicare patients in eleven US cities, as illustrated in Figure 18.4. This figure also shows comparable increases in European cities, with higher rates indicated for those over 65 years of age than for those under 65.

18.3.1.3.3 Short- and Long-Term Effects on Mortality. The National Mortality and Morbidity Air Pollution Study (NMMAPS) of 95 US communities reported statistically significant associations in seven of them and for the 95 as a whole. The lag effects for a 20 ppb increase in 24 h average O_3 are shown in Figure 18.5 for the 95-city data.[13]

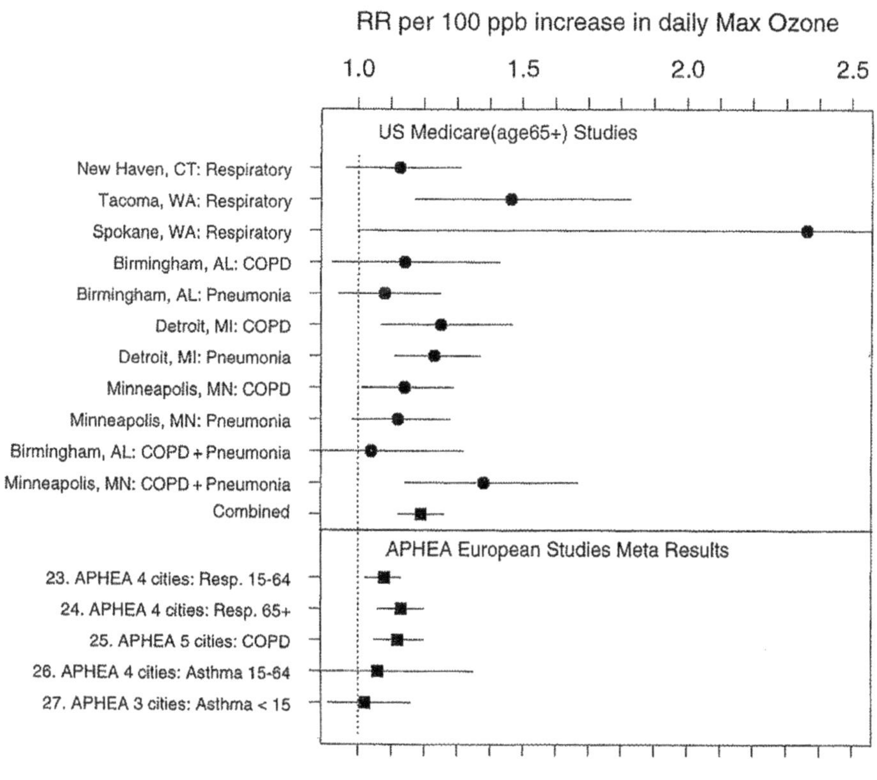

Figure 18.4 Reported relative risk of respiratory hospital admission associated with a 100 ppb increase in daily 1 h maximum O_3 (with 95% CI). From: Ref. 12.

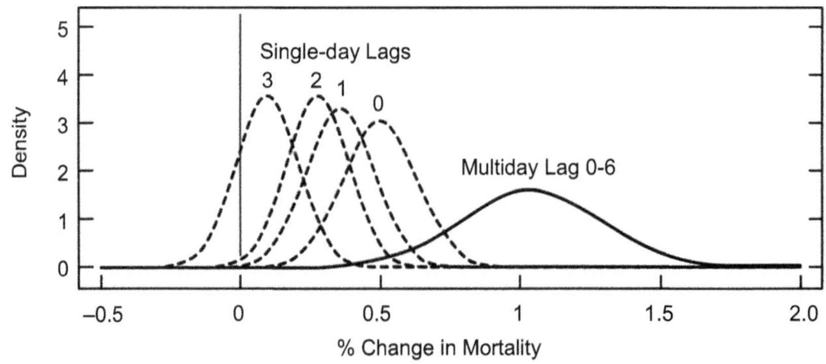

Figure 18.5 Comparison of single-day lags (0-,1-,2-, and 3-day) to a cumulative multi-day lag (1- to 6-day) for % changes in all cause mortality per 20 ppb increase in 24 h average O_3 in all age groups.
Source: From EPA O_3 Criteria Document, 2005.

While O_3 has an impact on short-term mortality, primarily in the warmer months, its long-term average concentration has not been shown to be associated with annual mortality.[14]

18.3.2 Particulate Matter

The major source of the PM in London in 1952, as described in Section 18.1, was the inefficient burning of soft coal for space heating within individual dwellings. It had high concentrations of acidic sulfates as well as a variety of hydrocarbons that were products of incomplete combustion. The UK Clean Air Act mandated the replacement of soft coal with coke, resulting in major reductions in the sulfur and hydrocarbon concentrations of the ambient air PM, as well as major reductions in air pollution-associated health impacts. Coke was subsequently replaced by natural gas from the North Sea deepwater wells, leading to further improvements in air quality. In the US, the switch to natural gas for urban space heating during the 2nd half of the 20th Century had similar beneficial effects, and the more recent switch of many coal-fired power plants to natural gas is further reducing the sulfur and hydrocarbon concentrations in our ambient air.

PM in contemporary ambient air has always been, and will continue to be, a complex mixture of solid and liquid particles of varying sizes, originating from a variety of sources of varying strengths. The chemical composition of the PM mixture has changed, as motor vehicles became a major source category, and is continuing to change as new engine technologies and better exhaust emission controls are substantially reducing tailpipe emissions. In every densely populated region there are sources of PM associated with traffic, including tailpipe emissions from diesel- and gasoline-powered engines, brake and tire wear, and dusts that are re-suspended from roadway surfaces by the vehicle motions. The proportions contributed by each source vary with the size of the fleet, types and sizes of the engines, traffic density, road surfaces, wind speeds, solar intensity, and moisture on the roadway and in the air.

There will also always be emissions from local and regional fossil fuel powered electric power plants, but the mixtures vary with fuel source. The eastern US is still heavily impacted by coal combustion effluents, but it and the western US have seen reduced emissions as natural gas has replaced coal as the fuel of choice. Major port cities in the US are impacted by the residual oil burned in power plants and by the effluents of bunker oil fuels consumed by international shipping. Mining, materials processing, and industrial emissions are highly variable across the US, as are the organic products of secondary aerosol formation such as PAHs, and inorganic products of secondary aerosol formation such as sulfuric acid. The more acidic atmosphere in the eastern US can also increase the solubility and bioavailability of trace toxic metals in the ambient air, while the greater solar radiation in the southwestern US may lead to greater atmospheric photochemical formation of PAH compounds.

18.3.2.1 Associations of $PM_{2.5}$ and its Components with Annual Mortality and Hospital Admissions

The significant associations of PM mass concentrations with premature mortality, combined with the high valuation of human life, drives the high benefit/cost ratio established for EPA's implementation of the US Clean Air Act. The Harvard Six-Cities study, a prospective cohort study of annual adult mortality rates in 6 eastern and midwestern US cities, showed that there were significant, almost linear relationships between mortality and various components of PM mass.[15,16] As shown in Figure 18.6, the association becomes stronger as one goes from total suspended PM mass to thoracic PM (PM_{10}), to fine PM ($PM_{2.5}$), and is approximately equally strong for the sulfate and nonsulfate components fraction of the $PM_{2.5}$. The $PM_{2.5}$ contains most of the sulfuric acid and toxic transition metals originating from the combustion of coal and of bunker and residual oils, as well as most of toxic PAH and other semi-volatile organic compounds in the ambient air, and has been more closely associated with cardiovascular mortality than the $PM_{10-2.5}$ mass. By contrast, the $PM_{10-2.5}$ mass has been more closely associated with respiratory mass than the $PM_{2.5}$ mass. Since both $PM_{2.5}$ and $PM_{10-2.5}$ are complex mixtures that vary in composition both spatially and temporally, it has been impractical to reproduce exposures for controlled chamber exposures and their short-term functional effects. Thus the information that we have on the health-related effects of $PM_{2.5}$ have come from observational studies of human populations in relation to $PM_{2.5}$ mass concentrations in most cases, with some more recent studies demonstrating associations with specific $PM_{2.5}$ constituents and/or source categories.

Ito *et al.*[17] performed an analysis of total daily mortality and hospital admissions for Medicare recipients (people over 65 years of age) that investigated the influences of $PM_{2.5}$ constituents. They used factor analysis of short-term fluctuations of $PM_{2.5}$ chemical constituents and gaseous pollutants in 64 individual US cities, and identified six major sources of ambient air

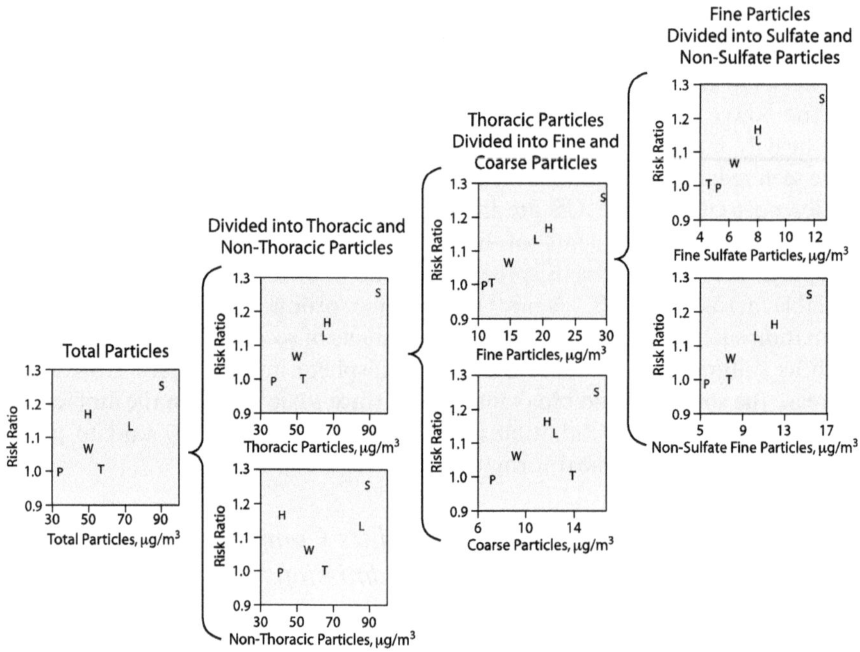

Figure 18.6 Relative Risks for annual mortality in six U.S cities (P = Portage, WI; W = Watertown, MA; T-Topeka, KS; H = Harriman, TN; L = Saint Louis, MO; and S = Steubenville, WV), expressed in terms of different indices of PM component concentrations.
From: Ref. 16.

pollution: traffic, soil, coal, salt, metals, and residual oil combustion in 64 individual US cities and identified traffic and soil factors in the majority of these cities. In time-series analysis, $PM_{2.5}$ chemical constituents and gaseous pollutants were often at least as strongly associated with the health outcomes as $PM_{2.5}$ mass concentrations. As shown on the right side of Figure 18.7, SO_4^{2-} and $PM_{2.5}$ mass were more closely associated with mortality in the second stage analysis, to identify the most influential constituents, than were the other measured constituents of the pollution mixture, while for cardiovascular hospital admissions on the left side of Figure 18.7, transition metals (Cu, Ni, V, and Fe) appeared to be more influential than $PM_{2.5}$ mass and SO_4^{2-}.

In another recent study of hospital admissions, using the same $PM_{2.5}$ speciation and Medicare data resources, Bell[18] performed a second stage analysis to identify influential constituents. Table 18.4 summarizes her findings on cardiovascular and respiratory hospital admissions, as well as PM_{10}-associated daily mortality rates from the NMMAPS study, which are associated with $PM_{2.5}$ constituents in the same communities. It can be seen that the only $PM_{2.5}$ constituents that were significantly associated with the hospital admissions (in both categories) were EC, Ni, and V. Ni was the only $PM_{2.5}$ constituents that was significantly associated with mortality.

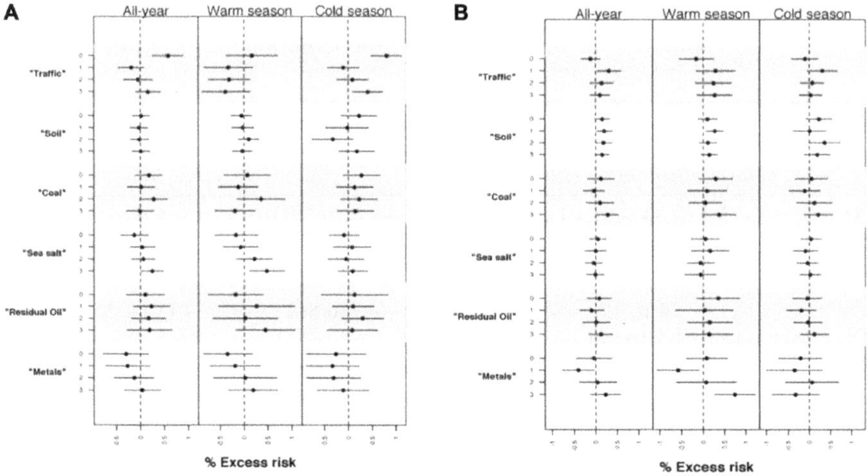

Estimated percent excess risk of CVD hospitalizations (left) and all-cause mortality (right) for factor scores computed from factor analysis in each city, per the median of inter-quartile-range of the pollutants across the cities at lag 0 through 3 days, combined across 64 cities

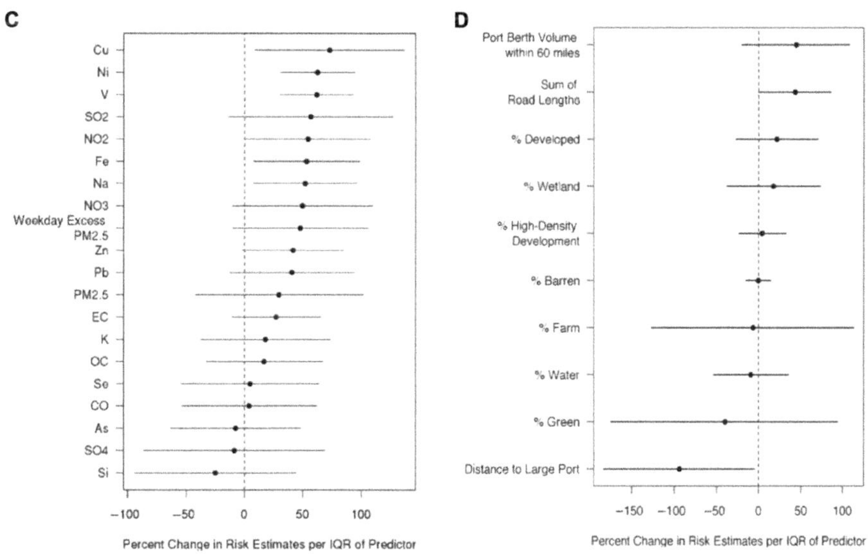

Percent change in lag 0 day $PM_{2.5}$ CVD hospitalizations (left) and all-cause mortality (right) risk estimates per inter-quartile-range of predictor variables in the second-stage meta-regression analysis: influence of city-average pollutants/chemical constituents

Figure 18.7 Risks of acute exposure to components of ambient air PM for cardiovascular hospitalizations (left) and all-cause mortality (right), in terms of PM sources (top), PM components (bottom left), and other factors(bottom right).
From: Ref. 17.

Table 18.4 Percentage Change in the Lag-0 PM Total Mass Health Effect Estimates per IQR Increase in the Component Fraction of $PM_{2.5}$ Total Mass (95% PI).[a,b,c,d]

	$PM_{2.5}$ and Cardiovascular Hospitalization n = 106	*$PM_{2.5}$ and Respiratory Hospitalization on n = 106*	*PM_{10} and Mortality n = 100*
Al	− 5.4 (− 14.9 to 4.1)	856 (− 122 to 293)	− 6.6 (− 15 to 1.5)
NH_4^+	− 1.9 (− 43 to 39)	− 687 (− 1500 to 129)	27 (− 11 to 66)
As	− 9.4 (− 38 to 19)	− 106 (− 706 to 495)	− 15 (− 56 to 26)
Ca	− 11 (− 34 to 12)	408 (− 45 to 861)	− 11 (− 26 to 3.0)
Cl	13 (− 1.1 to 26)	200 (− 75 to 475)	− 8.2 (− 26 to 10)
Cu	4.4 (− 20 to 29)	243 (− 277 to 762)	− 4.3 (− 30 to 21)
EC	**26 (4.4 to 47)**	**511 (81 to 941)**	− 9.9 (− 35 to 15)
Fe	− 7.2 (− 27 to 12)	− 125 (− 535 to 285)	1.1 (− 13 to 15)
Pb	2.6 (− 20 to 25)	− 76 (− 546 to 395)	− 8.9 (− 40 to 22)
Mg	− 18 (− 41 to 4.3)	87 (− 375 to 548)	− 7.2 (− 25 to 11)
Ni	**19 (9.9 to 28)**	**223 (37 to 410)**	**145 (4.0 to 25)**
NO_3^-	16 (− 11 to 42)	37 (− 514 to 588)	− 10 (− 48 to 28)
OCM	− 5.6 (− 38 to 27)	350 (− 289 to 989)	− 17 (− 50 to 16)
K	− 13 (− 35 to 8.0)	35 (− 424 to 495)	− 23 (− 50 to 4.3)
Si	− 11 (− 26 to 4.5)	186 (− 139 to 511)	− 10 (− 21 to 1.3)
Na^+	8.2 (− 12 to 28)	355 (− 55 to 766)	− 13 (− 39 to 13)
SO_4=	− 15 (− 38 to 8.9)	− 321 (− 810 to 167)	31 (− 2.7 to 64)
Ti	− 22 (− 44 to 0.3)	155 (− 315 to 624)	− 7.0 (− 26 to 12)
V	**28 (11 to 44)**	**392 (46 to 738)**	29 (− 0.5 to 58)
Zn	7.9 (− 8.0 to 24)	− 38 (− 384 to 308)	6.4 (− 14 to 27)

[a]The IQR increase In the fraction of $PM_{2.5}$ represented by each component is based on the IQR values displayed in Figure 7.
[b]Bell *et al.* 2009b.
[c]*n* = number of counties.
[d]**Bold** values are statistically significant.

18.3.2.2 Long-Term Effects of $PM_{2.5}$ on Chronic Disease Prevalence

The Chemical Speciation Network (CSN) PM component concentration data, when averaged over seasonal and annual averages, have been used to determine the associations of the component concentrations with annual mortality rates for members of the American Cancer Society (ACS II) cohort residing in CSN communities.[19] Figure 18.8 A shows the associations of annual mortality rates for individual measured $PM_{2.5}$ constituents, while Figure 18.8 B shows the associations for source-related $PM_{2.5}$ factors. It can be seen that the coal combustion source, and its most characteristic components (Se, As, and Br) are significantly, and more closely, associated with annual mortality rates than the others.

18.3.3 Carbon Monoxide

CO binds firmly to caboxyhemoglobin (COHb), reducing the capacity of COHb to carry inhaled oxygen to the bloodstream.

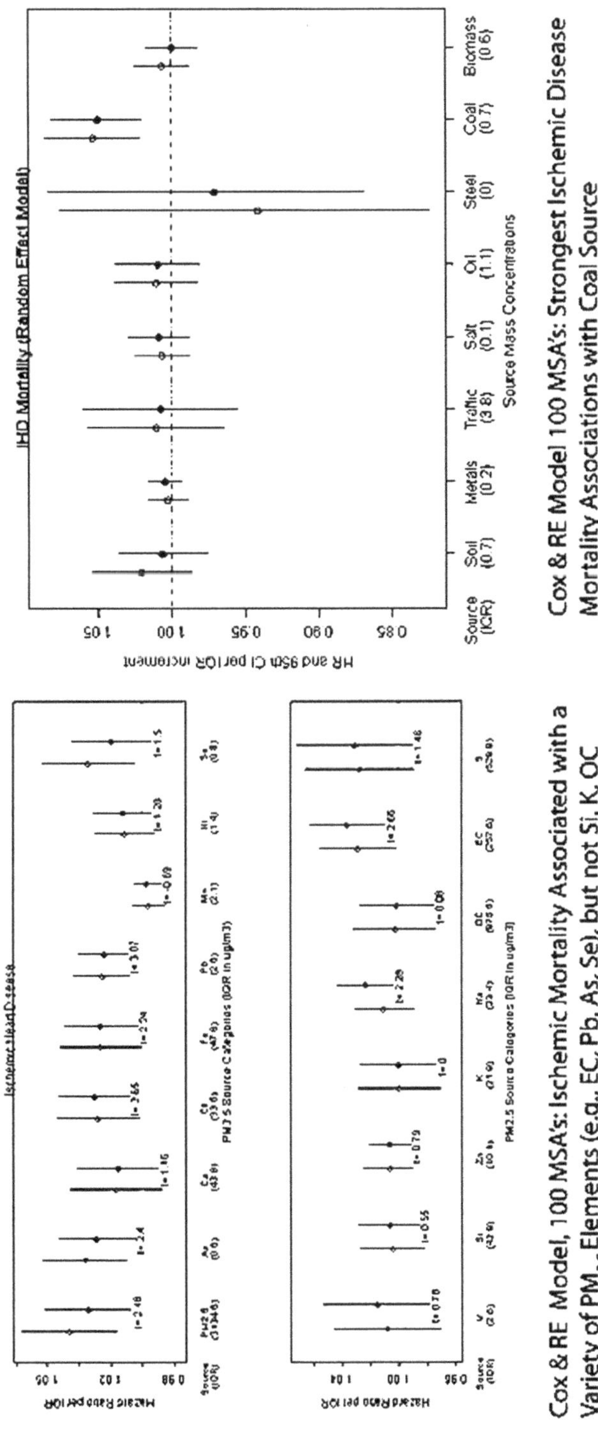

Figure 18.8 Influences of PM components (left) and sources (right) on annual ischemic disease mortality. From: Ref. 19.

18.3.3.1 Effects of CO on the Onset of Angina in Cardiovascular Patients

Each NAAQS is based on the need to protect the most vulnerable segment of the population. For CO, the people needing the greatest degree of protection are cardiovascular patients subject to recurring bouts of angina (mostly elderly people), and controlled clinical exposure studies of volunteers demonstrated that a shortening of the time to angina was observed at COHb concentrations of 2.9 to 4.5%.[20]

18.3.4 Lead

Pb was, until the 1970s, added to gasoline in the US as an antiknock agent in the form of tetraethyl and tetramethyl lead. When the fuel was consumed, most of the oxidized Pb was emitted into the roadway air as fine particles, and most of the Pb that accumulated within the exhaust piping was eventually discharged from the tailpipe as larger particles. Some of the lead-bearing particles in the ambient air were inhaled, while others were deposited on plant and ground surfaces and incorporated into foods consumed by humans or into fodder consumed by animals that were in turn consumed by humans. With the removal of organic Pb compounds from gasoline, air concentrations of Pb dropped precipitously, and blood levels of Pb (PbB) also fell precipitously, with an approximate 3 to 6 month lag.

When Pb concentrations were elevated, many studies of the NHANES populations showed strong associations of PbB and indices of health in children and adults.[21] The effects in children include decreased IQ, increased auditory thresholds, decreased postural stability, and an increase in behavioral problems. In adults, PbB elevations were associated with increased blood pressure.

18.3.5 Sulfur Dioxide

SO_2 exposures of volunteers in controlled laboratory studies have produced transient bronchoconstriction responses in people with asthma, when engaging in moderate to heavy exercise, at concentrations as low as 0.04 ppm. However, this response does not appear to be age-dependent.[22]

Epidemiological studies show associations of SO_2 with a variety of health effects at lower concentrations over longer averaging times, but it is highly likely that the effects are more related to other components of the ambient air pollution mixture than to SO_2.

18.3.6 Nitrogen Dioxide

NO_2 concentrations in ambient air have been significantly associated with a variety of health effects in human populations, but there have been no consistent studies linking NO_2 to health-related effects in controlled exposure studies in human volunteers at levels approaching typical or even maximal ambient concentrations. There is no evidence that these responses were age-dependent.[23]

As with SO_2, epidemiological studies show associations of NO_2 with a variety of health effects at lower concentrations, but it is highly likely that the effects are more closely related to other components of the ambient air pollution mixture than to NO_2.

References

1. Committee on Air Pollution, Interim Report, Cmd 9011. London, H.M. Stationery Office. 1953, p. 58.
2. J. H. Ware, L. A. Thibodeau, F. E. Speizer, S. Colome and B. G. Ferris Jr., *Environ. Health Perspect*, 1981, **41**, 255–276.
3. S. Chinn, C. Florey, V. Du, I. G. Baldwin and M. Gorgol, *J. Epid. Comm. Health*, 1981, **35**, 174–179.
4. M. Lippmann, Air in Air Pollutants and the Respiratory Tract, ed. W. M. Foster and D. L. Costa, Marcel Dekker, New York, 2nd edn, 2005, pp. 405–441.
5. M. Lippmann in Environmental Toxicants: Human Exposures and their Health Effects, ed. M. Lippmann, Wiley, Hoboken, 2009, pp. 317–365.
6. M. Lippmann in Environmental Toxicants: Human Exposures and their Health Effects, ed. M. Lippmann, Wiley, Hoboken, 2009, pp. 869–936.
7. W. F. McDonnell, D. H. Horstman, M. J. Hazucha, E. Seal, E. D. Haak, S. A. Salaam and D. E. House, *J. Appl. Physiol.*, 1983, **54**, 1345–1352.
8. D. M. Spektor, G. D. Thurston, J. Mao, D. He, C. Hayes and M. Lippmann, *Environ. Res.*, 1991, **55**, 107–122.
9. W. F. McDonnell, K. E. Muller, P. A. Bromberg and C. M. Shy, *Am. Rev. Respir. Dis.*, 1993, **147**, 818–825.
10. G. D. Thurston, M. Lippmann, M. B. Scott and J. M. Fine, *Am. Rev. Respir. Crit. Care Med*, 1997, **155**, 654–660.
11. W. J. Gauderman, E. Avol, F. Gillil, H. Vora, D. Thomas, K. Berhane, R. McConnell, N. Kunzli, F. Lurmann, E. Rappaport, H. Margolis, D. Bates and M. Peters, *N. Engl. J. Med.*, 2005, **351**, 1057–1067.
12. G. D. Thurston and K. Ito in Air Pollution and Health, ed. S. T. Holgate, J. M. Samet, H. S. Koren and R. L. Maynard, Academic Press, London, 1999, pp. 485–510.
13. M. L. Bell, F. Dominici and J. M. Samet, *Epidemiol*, 2005, **16**, 436–445.
14. C. A. Pope III, R. T. Burnett, M. J. Thun, E. E. Calle, D. Krewski, K. Ito and G. D. Thurston, *J. Am. Med. Assoc*, 2002, **287**, 1132–1147.
15. US EPA, Review of the National Ambient Air Quality Standards for Particulate Matter: OAQPS Staff Paper, 1996, EPA-452/R-96-013, Research Triangle Park, US Environmental Protection Agency.
16. D. W. Dockery, C. A. Pope III, X. Xu, J. D. Spengler, J. H. Ware, M. E. Fay, B. G. Ferris Jr. and F. E. Speizer, *N. Engl. J. Med.*, 1993, **329**, 1753–1759.

17. K. Ito in Characteristics of PM Associated with Health Effects, HEI Research Report No. 165, 2012. Health Effects Institute, Boston.
18. M. L. Bell, HEI Research Report No. 161, 2012, Health Effects Institute, Boston.
19. G. D. Thurston in Characteristics of PM Associated with Health Effects, HEI Research Report No. 165, 2012. Health Effects Institute, Boston.
20. M. T. Kleinman in Environmental Toxicants: Human Exposures and their Health Effects, ed. M. Lippmann, Wiley, Hoboken, 2009, pp. 499–528.
21. L. T. Grant in Environmental Toxicants: Human Exposures and their Health Effects, ed. M. Lippmann, Wiley, Hoboken, 2009, pp. 757–809.
22. M. Lippmann in Environmental Toxicants: Human Exposures and their Health Effects, ed. M. Lippmann, Wiley, Hoboken, 2009, pp. 957–1000.
23. R. B. Schlesinger in Environmental Toxicants: Human Exposures and their Health Effects, ed. M. Lippmann, Wiley, Hoboken, 2009, pp. 823–868.

Subject Index

References to figures are given in italic type. Reference to tables are given in bold type.